AACN Handbook of

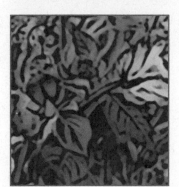

Critical
Care
Nursing

AACN Handbook of

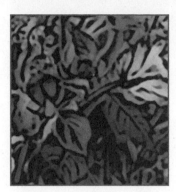

Critical Care Nursing

Marianne Chulay, RN, DNSc, FAAN
Consultant, Critical Care Nursing and Clinical Research, Chapel Hill, North Carolina
Director, Nursing Research and Practice
Moses Cone Health System
Greensboro, North Carolina

Cathie Guzzetta, RN, PhD, FAAN
Director, Holistic Nursing Consultants
Nursing Research Consultant
Parkland Memorial Hospital and Children's Medical Center
Dallas, Texas

Barbara Dossey, RN, MS, FAAN
Director, Holistic Nursing Consultants
Santa Fe, New Mexico
Co-Director, BodyMind Systems
Temple, Texas

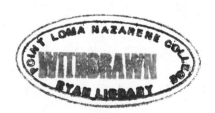

Appleton & Lange
Stamford, Connecticut

Notice: The authors and the publisher of this volume have taken care to
make certain that the doses of drugs and schedules of treatment are correct
and compatible with the standards generally accepted at the time of
publication. Nevertheless, as new information becomes available, changes in
treatment and in the use of drugs become necessary. The reader is advised to
carefully consult the instruction and information material included in the
package insert of each drug or therapeutic agent before administration.
This advice is especially important when using new or infrequently used drugs.
The authors and publisher disclaim all responsibility for any liability,
loss, injury, or damage incurred as a consequence, directly or indirectly,
or the use and application of any of the contents of the volume.

97 98 99 00 / 10 9 8 7 6 5 4 3 2 1

Prentice Hall International (UK) Limited, *London*
Prentice Hall of Australia Pty. Limited, *Sydney*
Prentice Hall Canada, Inc., *Toronto*
Prentice Hall of Hispanoamericana, S. A., *Mexico*
Prentice Hall of India Private Limited, *New Delhi*
Prentice Hall of Japan, Inc., *Tokyo*
Simon & Schuster Asia Pte. Ltd., *Singapore*
Editora Prentice Hall do Brasil, Ltda., *Rio de Janeiro*
Prentice Hall, *Upper Saddle River, New Jersey*

Library of Congress Cataloging-in-Publication Data
Chulay, Marianne.
    AACN handbook of critical care nursing / Marianne Chulay, Cathie
Guzzetta, Barbara Dossey.
        p.   cm.
    Includes index.
    ISBN 0-8385-3609-3 (pbk: :   alk. paper)
    1. Intensive care nursing—Handbooks, manuals, etc.   I. Guzzetta,
Cathie E.   II. Dossey, Barbara Montgomery.   III. Title.
    [DNLM: 1. Critical Care—methods—handbooks.   2. Nursing Care—
methods—handbooks.   3. Holistic Nursing—methods—handbooks.   WY
49 C559h 1996]
RT120.I5C48   1996
610.73'61—dc20
DNLM/DLC
for Library of Congress   96-13093
                                                                  CIP

Acquisitions Editor: David P. Carroll
Production: Andover Publishing Service
Designer: Janice Barsevich Bielawa
Original Illustrations by: Kerry Bassett, Raleigh, NC

PRINTED IN THE UNITED STATES OF AMERICA

ISBN: 0-8385-3609-3

9 780838 536094

90000

*To our critical care nursing colleagues around the world
who journey on the path of caring, healing, and excellence.*

■ Contents

■ Contributors

Michael H. Ackerman, DNS, RN, CCRN
Advanced Practice Nurse/Critical Care
Strong Memorial Hospital
Associate Professor of Clinical Nursing
School of Nursing
University of Rochester
Rochester, New York
*Chapter 3, Planning Care for Critically Ill Patients and
Families*
Chapter 14, Multisystem Problems

Thomas Ahrens, RN, DNSc
Clincial Nurse Specialist, MICU
Barnes Hospital
St. Louis, Missouri
Chapter 5, Hemodynamic Monitoring

Sandi O'Brien Brettler, RN, MSN, CCRN
Clinical Nurse Specialist, Neuroscience
Moses Cone Health System
Greensboro, North Carolina
Chapter 15, Neurologic System

Suzi Burns, RT, RN, MSN, LNP
Practitioner-Teacher, Critical Care
School of Nursing
University of Virginia Health Sciences Center
Charlottesville, Virginia
Chapter 23, Advanced Respiratory Concepts

Debra Byram, RN, MS
Clinical Nurse Specialist
Warren G. Magnuson Clinical Center
National Institutes of Health
Bethesda, Maryland
Chapter 2, Assessment of Critically Ill Patients and Families

Karen K. Carlson, RN, MN
Critical Care Clinical Nurse Specialist
The Carlson Consultant Group
Bellevue, Washington
and
Clinical Faculty
School of Nursing
University of Washington
Seattle, Washington
Chapter 18, Renal System

Marianne Chulay, RN, DNSc, FAAN
Consultant, Critical Care Nursing and Clinical Research
Chapel Hill, North Carolina
and
Director, Nursing Research and Practice
Moses Cone Health System
Greensboro, North Carolina
Chapter 1, Caring for Critically Ill Patients and Families
*Chapter 3, Planning Care for Critically Ill Patients and
Families*
Chapter 5, Hemodynamic Monitoring
Chapter 6, Airway and Ventilatory Management
Chapter 11, Safety Issues
Chapter 13, Respiratory System

Maria A. Connolly, RN, DNSc, CCRN
Associate Professor of Medical-Surgical Nursing
Niehoff School of Nursing
Loyola University of Chicago
Chicago, Illinois
*Chapter 3, Planning Care for Critically Ill Patients and
Families*
Chapter 6, Airway and Ventilatory Management
Chapter 13, Respiratory System

Barbara Dossey, RN, MS, FAAN
Director, Holistic Nursing Consultants
Santa Fe, New Mexico
Co-Director, BodyMind Systems
Temple, Texas
Chapter 1, Caring for Critically Ill Patients and Families
Chapter 8, Alternative Therapies
Chapter 28, Alternative Therapies Table
"What Heals" Inserts

Dorrie K. Fontaine, RN, DNSc, FAAN
Clinical Associate Professor
Coordinator, Acute Care Nurse Practitioner Program
School of Nursing
Georgetown University
Washington, DC
Chapter 3, Planning Care for Critically Ill Patients and Families
Chapter 20, Trauma

Bradi Bartrug Granger, RN, MSN
Clinical Nurse Specialist, Cardiology
Duke University Medical Center
Durham, North Carolina
Chapter 12, Cardiovascular System

Ann Smith Gregoire, RN, MSN, CRNP, CCRN
Clinical Nurse Specialist
Surgical Intensive Care Unit
Thomas Jefferson University Hospital
Philadelphia, Pennsylvania
Chapter 22, Advanced Cardiovascular Concepts

Cathie Guzzetta, RN, PhD, FAAN
Director, Holistic Nursing Consultants
Nursing Research Consultant
Parkland Memorial Hospital and Children's Medical Center
Dallas, Texas
Chapter 1, Caring for Critically Ill Patients and Families
Chapter, 3, Planning Care for Critically Ill Patients and Families
Chapter 8, Alternative Therapies
Chapter 28, Alternative Therapies Table
"What Heals" Inserts

Carol Jacobson, RN, MN, CCRN
Director, Quality Educational Services
Critical Care Consultant and Educator
Seattle, Washington
Chapter 21, Advanced ECG Concepts

Susan Johnson, RN, MSN
Unit Manager, Infectious Disease Unit
University of Syracuse Hospital System
Syracuse, New York
Chapter 11, Safety Issues

Deborah G. Klein, RN, MSN, CCRN, CS
Clinical Nurse Specialist
Trauma/Critical Care Nursing
MetroHealth Medical Center
Cleveland, Ohio
Chapter 24, Advanced Neurologic Concepts

Joanne Krumberger, RN, MSN, CCRN
Critical Care Clinical Nurse Specialist
Clement J. Zablocky Veterans Affairs Medical Center
Milwaukee, Wisconsin
Chapter 17, Gastrointestinal System
Chapter 19, Endocrine System

Debra J. Lynn-McHale, RN, MSN, CS, CCRN
Staff Development Coordinator
Thomas Jefferson University Hospital
Philadelphia, Pennsylvania
Chapter 22, Advanced Cardiovascular Concepts

Diane J. Mick, MSN, RN, CCRN
Doctoral Student
Research Assistant
School of Nursing
University of Rochester
Rochester, New York
Chapter 14, Multisystem Problems

Mary Beth Egloff Parr, MSN, RN, CCRN
Senior Clinical Nurse Specialist & Educator
Pulmonary and Special Services
Sharp Health Care
San Diego, California
Chapter 6, Airway and Ventilatory Management

Carol A. Rauen, RN, MS, CCRN
Nursing Coordinator and Clinical Nurse Specialist
Georgetown University Hospital
Washington, DC
Chapter 20, Trauma

Juanita Reigel, RN, MSN, CCRN, LNP
Practioner-Teacher, Cardiology
Ethics Consultant
School of Nursing
University of Virginia Health Sciences Center
Charlottesville, Virginia
Chapter 10, Ethical and Legal Considerations

Anita Sherer, RN, MSN
Clinical Pathway Coordinator
Moses Cone Health System
Greensboro, North Carolina
Chapter 3, Planning Care for Critically Ill Patients and Families

Sue Simmons-Alling, RN, MSN
Advanced Practice Psychiatric Nurse
Therapist
Spring Lake Heights, New Jersey
Chapter 2, Assessment of Critically Ill Patients and Families
Chapter 3, Planning Care for Critically Ill Patients and Families

Gerri Stegall, RN, BSN, CCRN
Research Coordinator
East Alabama Medical Center
Opelika, Alabama
Chapter 11, Safety Issues

Gregory M. Susla, PharmD, FCCM
Critical Care Pharmacist
Warren G. Magnuson Clinical Center
National Institutes of Health
Bethesda, Maryland
Chapter 9, Pharmacology
Chapter 26, Pharmacology Tables

Debbie Tribett, MS, RN, CS, LNP
Adult Nurse Practitioner
Infectious Diseases Physicians
Fairfax, Virginia
Chapter 16, Hematology and Immunology Systems

Lorie Rietman Wild, RN, MN
Clinical Nurse Specialist
University of Washington Medical Center
Seattle, Washington
Chapter 7, Pain Management

Susan L. Woods, PhD, RN
Professor of Nursing
Department of Biobehavioral Nursing and Health Systems
School of Nursing
University of Washington
Seattle, Washington
Chapter 4, Interpretation and Management of Basic Cardiac Rhythms
Chapter 32, Cardiac Rhthyms, ECG Characteristics and Treatment Guide

Marlene S. Yates, RN, BSN
Clinical Nurse Educator
Moses Cone Health System
Greensboro, North Carolina
Chapter 3, Planning Care for Critically Ill Patients and Families

■ Reviewers

We gratefully acknowledge the expertise, interest, and assistance of the following individuals who reviewed sections of this text:

Alexandria Berg, RN, MSN
Clinical Specialist, Transplantation
The Emory Clinic, Inc.
Atlanta, Georgia

Melissa Biel, RN, MSN
Director of Practice
American Association of Critical-Care Nurses
Aliso Viejo, California

Wanda Bride, RN, BSN
Nurse Manager, Coronary Care Unit
Duke University Medical Center
Durham, North Carolina

Cindy Carter-Cole, RN, MSN
Case Manager
Moses Cone Health System
Greensboro, North Carolina

Joanie Ching, RN, MN
Clinical Nurse Specialist—Pain Management
University of Washington Medical Center
Seattle, Washington

Trish Dalkin, RN, MSN
Thoracic-Cardiovascular Post-Operative Unit
University of Virginia Health Sciences Center
Charlottesville, Virginia

Ross W. Davis, MD, FCCM
Clinical Professor of Medicine
East Alabama Medical Center
Opelika, Alabama

Susan Flewelling Goran, RN, MSN, CCRN
Staff Education Specialist, SCU
Maine Medical Center
Portland, Maine

Diane E. Fritsch, MSN, RN, CCRN, CS
Clinical Nurse Specialist/Trauma Critical Care Nursing
MetroHealth Medical Center
Cleveland, Ohio

Randall Harris, RRT
Senior Respiratory Therapist
University of Virginia Health Sciences Center
Charlottesville, Virginia

Kim Hoffman, RN, MN
Assistant Nurse Manager - Critical Care
University of Washington Medical Center
Seattle, Washington

Carol Jacobson, RN, MN, CCRN
Director, Quality Educational Services
Critical Care Consultant and Educator
Seattle, Washington

Tammara L. Jenkins, MSN, RN, CCRN
Clinical Nurse Specialist/Pediatric Critical Care
Warren G. Magnuson Clinical Center
National Institutes of Health
Bethesda, Maryland

Anne McCreary Juhasz, PhD, CFLE
Professor Emeritus
Loyola University
Chicago, Illinois

Lynn Keegan, RN, PhD, FAAN
Associate Professor
University of Texas Health Science Center
San Antonio, Texas

Christine Kessler, RN, MNCS
Director Critical Care Consultants
Alexandria, Virginia

Timothy W. Lane, MD
Professor of Medicine
University of North Carolina at Chapel Hill
Chapel Hill, North Carolina

Pauline LeBlanc, RN
University of Virginia Health Sciences Center
Charlottesville, Virginia

Susan Liles, RN, MSN, CIC
Infection Control Practitioner
Moses Cone Health System
Greensboro, North Carolina

Sharon Mavroukakis, MS, RN
Clinical Nurse Educator, Critical Care
Warren G. Magnuson Clinical Center
National Institutes of Health
Bethesda, Maryland

Rebecca J. McKenzie, RN, MSN
Nurse Manager, CV Surgical Units
Duke University Medical Center
Durham, North Carolina

William S. Minor, Jr, BSN, RN, CCRN
Level III Staff Nurse
Moses Cone Health System
Greensboro, North Carolina

Barbara Mitchell, RN, MSN
Trauma Coordinator
Georgetown University Hospital
Washington, DC

Kate Muzzarelli, RN, RNC, BSN
Clinical Practice Specialist
American Association of Critical-Care Nurses
Aliso Viejo, California

Laura K. Newby, MD
Assistant Professor of Medicine
Cardiology Department
Duke University Medical Center
Durham, North Carolina

Frederick P. Ognibene, MD, FCCM
Senior Investigator/Critical Care Medicine Department
National Institutes of Health
Bethesda, Maryland

Donna Peter, RN, MSN(c)
Nurse Manager, Cardiology Telemetry Units
Duke University Medical Center
Durham, North Carolina

Lori M. Rhudy, RN, MSN, CRRN
Clinical Educator
Moses Cone Health System
Greensboro, North Carolina

Judy Salter, RN, MSN, CRRN, CNRN
Clinical Nurse Specialist
MetroHealth Medical Center, Center for Rehabilitation
Cleveland, Ohio

Rose B. Shaffer, RN, MSN, CCRN
Case Manager
Thomas Jefferson University Hospital
Philadelphia, Pennsylvania

Lori L. Taylor, RRT
Senior Respiratory Therapist, Medicine Service
University of Virginia Health Sciences Center
Charlottesville, Virginia

Martha Taylor, RN, MSN
Director of Heart Center Nursing
Duke University Medical Center
Durham, North Carolina

Barbara A. Todd, RN, MSN, CRNP
Director, Clinical Services Cardiac and Thoracic Surgery
Temple University Hospital
Philadelphia, Pennsylvania

Susan Allyn Turcke, MSN, RN, CEN
Staff Nurse
Hospital of the University of Pennsylvania
Philadelphia, Pennsylvania

Hobie Vaughn, BS
Clinical Research Associate
East Alabama Medical Center
Opelika, Alabama

Linda G. Waite, RN, MN, CCRN
Clinical Nurse Specialist/ICU
Fairview Southdale Hospital
Edina, Minnesota

Debra Wilmoth, RN, BSN, CCRN
Clinician III/MICU
University of Virginia Medical Center
Charlottesville, Virginia

Susan L. Woods, PhD, RN
Professor of Nursing
Department of Biobehavioral Nursing and Health Systems
School of Nursing
University of Washington
Seattle, Washington

Joseph P. Zbilut, RN, PhD, DNSc, C-ANP
Professor, Dept. of OR/Surgical Nursing
Rush University
Chicago, Illinois

■ Preface

Critical care nursing is a complex, challenging area of nursing practice, where clinical expertise is developed over time by integrating critical care knowledge, clinical skills, and caring practices. One of the difficulties when educating new practitioners entering critical care nursing is the dearth of textbooks that succinctly present essential information for the safe and competent care of critically ill patients and their families. Current textbooks deal with critical care content by combining basic and advanced concepts in each body system chapter, rather than by staging the introduction of more advanced concepts until after basic concepts have been mastered. In-depth discussion of the pathophysiology, while meaningful and important for advanced practitioners, overwhelms the novice practitioner with information that is not essential to providing safe and competent care.

Current texts also include too much information for entry level courses in critical care nursing or for use as a review tool for the critical care certification (CCRN) exam. Orientation programs in most hospitals are extremely short (2 to 6 weeks), and undergraduate programs that provide critical care content do so in electives of three credits or less or integrate the content into an advanced medical-surgical nursing course. Instructors in both settings are reluctant to suggest or require students to buy expensive books that include more information than they need at that time or that repeat material that appears in other student-owned textbooks (anatomy and physiology, nursing diagnosis, noncritical care assessment, major medical diagnoses). While clinicians may purchase these currently available books to prepare for certification exams, many would prefer a more concise textbook and reference source.

The *AACN Handbook of Critical Care Nursing* is designed to provide essential information on the care of adult critically ill patients and families, recognizing the learner's need to assimilate basic, foundational knowledge before attempting to master complex concepts of critical care nursing. Written by nationally acknowledged clinical experts in critical care nursing, this handbook sets a new standard for critical care nursing education.

The *AACN Handbook of Critical Care Nursing* represents a departure from the way in which most critical care books are written because it:

- Succinctly presents essential information for the safe and competent care of critically ill adult patients and their families, building on the clinician's significant medical-surgical nursing knowledge base, avoiding repetition of previously acquired information.
- Stages the introduction of advanced concepts in critical care nursing after basic concepts have been mastered.
- Presents practical approaches to patient and family teaching when time is short and acuity is high.
- Emphasizes what it means to practice holistic critical care nursing. It recognizes that bodily illness can no longer be treated exclusively with body-oriented therapies and that total healing can occur only when the emotional and spiritual, as well as the physical, needs of patients are addressed. This book emphasizes that even in the midst of critical illness, catastrophic disease, or death, meaning, wholeness, and healing can take place.
- Describes in detail how alternative therapies (for example, relaxation, imagery, music, touch) can be incorporated into critical care practice.

- Provides a one-hour audiotape as a "right brain" experiential approach to understanding and integrating alternative therapies at the bedside, such as relaxation, imagery, and music therapy, and presents auscultatory findings of cardiac and respiratory abnormalities.
- Provides clinicians with clinically relevant tools and guides to use as they care for critically ill patients and families.

Our book is intended for all clinicians, students, educators, and researchers who are interested in updating their critical care knowledge within a holistic or body-mind-spirit framework. Clinicians will find the book particularly useful because of the development of autonomous, alternative therapeutic nursing interventions and the emphasis on the scientific data to support both technologic and holistic modalities.

The *AACN Handbook of Critical Care Nursing* is divided into four sections:

- *Section I* presents essential information that new clinicians must understand to provide safe, competent nursing care to all critically ill patients, regardless of their underlying medical diagnoses. This section includes content on basic concepts of holistic critical care practice; assessment, diagnosis, planning, and interventions common to critically ill patients and families; interpretation and management of cardiac rhythms; hemodynamic monitoring; airway and ventilatory management; pharmacology and pain management; safety issues; and the incorporation of alternative therapies into critical care practice. Chapters in Section I present content in enough depth to insure competence for the new critical care clinician, while deferring more advanced content related to those concepts to a later section of the handbook (*Section III*).
- *Section II* of the *Handbook* covers pathologic conditions commonly encountered in medical and surgical critical care units, closely paralleling the blueprint for the CCRN exam. Chapters in this section are organized by body system (cardiovascular, respiratory, neurologic, hematology and immunology, gastrointestinal, renal, endocrine) and also include chapters on trauma and multisystem problems. Case studies assist clinicians in understanding the magnitude of the pathological problems and their impact on patients and families. Following the case study presentation, a brief description of the pathophysiology, etiology, clinical manifestations, diagnostic testing, and complications associated with the con-

dition are presented. The focus of each pathological presentation is the multidisciplinary management of key patient needs and problems.
- *Section III* of the *Handbook* presents advanced critical care concepts or pathologic conditions that are frequently not found in general medical-surgical critical care units. The format of this section is identical to *Section II*.
- *Section IV* contains reference information that clinicians will find helpful in the clinical area (normal laboratory and diagnostic values; algorithms for advanced cardiac life support; troubleshooting guides for hemodynamic monitoring and ventilator management; and summary tables of critical care drugs, alternative therapies, and cardiac rhtythms). Content is presented primarily in table format for quick reference.

Each chapter begins with *Knowledge Competencies* that can be used to guide informal or formal teaching and to gauge the learner's progress. These are followed by a section entitled *What Heals*, an exploration of what clinicians do to facilitate healing within their patients. These sections explore body-mind-spirit concepts and translate theoretical notions of holism and healing into understandable nursing actions that can make the critical difference in achieving optimal patient outcomes. These discussions include topics such as nourishing the human spirit, creative pain management, enhancing the placebo response, teaching correct biologic images, fostering intuition, using intentional touch, and integrating alternative therapies with patients. Case studies are presented in many of the chapters and can be read before proceeding with the chapter to obtain an overall picture of the clinical problem, as a review and summary after finishing the chapter, or as a teaching tool for clinical conferences. A *Critical Thinking* case study concludes many of the chapters to challenge the clinician to apply chapter information to a realistic clinical scenario.

Our Vision

We believe that the *AACN Handbook of Critical Care Nursing* provides the essence of what it means to practice holistic critical care nursing. To this end, the implications for nursing practice are limitless because caring-healing practices have always been an inherent part of nursing. The challenge then is for each of us to find our own path in this caring-healing journey.

Marianne Chulay
Cathie Guzzetta
Barbara Dossey

■ Foreword

Every so often one comes upon a resource that is usable, practical, and written in an understandable, yet highly professional manner. The *AACN Handbook of Critical Care Nursing* is such a resource. This handbook provides state-of-the-art information that novice critical care nurses can use in their care of patients and families all along the continuum and in any setting. Finally, here is a handbook which is easy to read and easy to refer to when time is of the essence!

The *AACN Handbook of Critical Care Nursing* is unique in many ways when compared to other critical care texts. The format used is easy to navigate, is nonthreatening, and truly serves as a guide to help the new critical care nurse to think and not just to act. I found the "Thinking Critically" case studies especially helpful in this way. They spark the reader to consider a variety of aspects of care and to approach critical illness in a thoughtful and logical manner. The diagrams, figures, and tables are not intimidating, as is so often the case. Rather, they serve as great companions to the written text. The reference tables are perfect for use in the clinical area and will be a valued support to critical care providers.

Critical care education is an essential part of the delivery of high quality and compassionate care. This handbook takes a unique and exciting approach to critical care education by blending traditional and nontraditional therapeutic provision of care. The reader is taught to view the patient holistically and to consider the implications of critical illness on all aspects of the patient's life, including the impact on family members and their response to it. Interdisciplin-

ary collaboration is emphasized throughout the handbook as the essential core of effective critical care delivery. The case studies and exemplars are as "real life" as they get, helping the reader to apply the principles described. The audiotape also serves as an excellent adjunct to the written text, and can be used to reinforce some of the key concepts.

Perhaps the most striking difference between the *AACN Handbook of Critical Care Nursing* and other critical care texts, and probably my favorite distinction, is that it was written primarily BY clinicians, FOR clinicians. Marianne, Cathie, and Barbara have brought together a group of expert authors who "walk the talk" of critical care and don't merely "talk the talk." These authors share cutting edge information on clinical assessment and therapeutic interventions and deliver their unique perspectives on critical care in a way which is readable and applicable to hands-on clinicians. These authors make a significant difference for patients and families every day, and you will feel their impact and care each time you pick up the *AACN Handbook of Critical Care Nursing*. Most of them have taught critical care principles and practices to bedside clinicians for decades and they are impeccably qualified to write these chapters and to share their wealth of knowledge and "real life" experiences with you.

I was not surprised by the caliber of this handbook for a variety of reasons. Probably the most telling reason to me is that the editors, Marianne Chulay, Cathie Guzzetta, and Barbara Dossey, are consummate professionals who have dedicated their careers to patients and families who require critical and holistic care. These nurses work every day to create a health care system that places the needs of patients and families as the top priority and that demands the provision of competent caring. They also work diligently to foster an environment in which all providers can contribute and can feel good about their work.

I am thrilled that, through this handbook, you will get to know some of the many talented and caring people I know, and that you will be able to use their expertise to make a difference in the care of patients and families where you live.

Melissa A. Fitzpatrick, RN, MSN
Immediate Past President, American Association of Critical-Care Nurses
Vice President, Adult Critical Care and Cardiac Services
Dartmouth-Hitchcock Medical Center
Lebanon, New Hampshire

■ *Acknowledgements*

We thank the following sources for permission to use excerpts from their audiotapes:

W.B. Saunders Company, Philadelphia (Tilkian AG, Conover MB. Understanding Heart Sounds and Murmurs, 3rd edition, 1993).

American College of Chest Physicians, Chicago (Cugell D, Weiss E. Introduction to Breath Sounds, 1969).

Sounds True Audio, Boulder, CO (Dossey BM, Keegan L, Guzzetta CE. The Art of Caring: Holistic Healing Using Relaxation, Imagery, Music Therapy, and Touch, 1996).

And, for all their love, understanding, and encouragement one more time, we thank our families—Jeff Chulay; Philip, Angela, and P.C. Guzzetta; and Larry Dossey—who are a part of our caring-healing journey.

AACN Handbook of

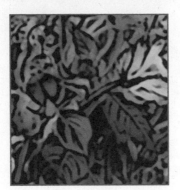

Critical Care Nursing

Key Concepts in Caring for the Critically Ill Patient and Family

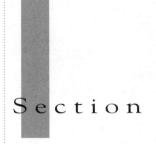

Section I

Caring for Critically Ill Patients and Families

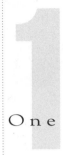

One

► Knowledge Competencies

1. Discuss the tenets of critical care nursing practice guided by the holistic model.

2. Explore the three components of relationship-centered care necessary to implement holistic critical care practice.

3. Examine ways that alternative therapies might be integrated into critical care practice.

4. Identify sources for updating critical care practice based on current research.

5. Describe the steps of a continuous quality improvement program for critically ill patients.

■ *What Heals: Clinical Expertise*

Patricia Benner's research has helped us to understand how expertise develops in nursing practice. It explains so clearly why the advanced beginner can never view the world of critical care nursing from the same perspective as the expert. It explains a hierarchy of thinking, judgment, behavior, and experience that clearly differentiates one level of practice from another.

Based on this research, Benner has described four levels of proficiency through which critical nurses pass: advanced beginner, competent, proficient, and expert. *Advanced beginner* nurses rely on learned procedures, classic textbook knowledge, and rules and regulations to guide nursing care of the immediate clinical situation. They are task oriented and place great emphasis on recording certain activities such as vital signs and medication flow rates. Their view of a particular clinical situation is often constricted. They tend to miss subtle cues to patient problems and are not able to grasp the importance of clinical changes because they have not worked with patients through various illness trajectories. They have trouble understanding the big picture because of a lack of experience and understanding.

As nurses progress to the level of *competence,* specific changes in thinking and behaving become evident. At this level, nurses frequently experience crisis when they find out that all their coworkers are not perfect. They begin to question their trust in the judgments and actions of others. Such questioning brings forth a new sense of responsibility and obligation to manage clinical problems. Competent nurses still rely on rules and principles, however, as the most important elements required to guide actions. At the level of *proficiency,* nurses are able to rely on long-range goals and can differentiate between significant and insignificant findings. They gain increased skill in understanding the relevance of rapidly changing clinical situations and are no longer task driven in their clinical practice.

Finally, *expert* nurses possess an intuitive grasp of each situation, enabling them to zero in on the problem and act in a timely fashion. At this level, their perception of the clinical world is vastly different from the prior three levels of proficiency. These nurses have sufficient confidence in their understanding of the clinical situation to consider advocating for what needs to be done. They know when a situation is urgent, they are comfortable with rapidly changing situations, and they know when to take action.

Benner's research makes a considerable contribution to nursing practice by putting into words what many of us have observed in practice. When you understand the rationale for why various nurses think and act differently in a clinical situation based on their level of proficiency, a higher level of tolerance and patience can emerge in the profession. Likewise, this understanding provides direction about how to help less experienced nurses progress to a higher level of practice.

For example, what is the best way to assist the advanced beginner to progress beyond the institution-driven rules and procedures to patient-driven needs and actions? Can we structure opportunities for them to observe an expert nurse who can show them that talking to the family or implementing methods to reduce pain may be more important than recording hemodynamic monitoring values on the flow sheet? How can we transform the clinical setting into a learning environment to capture these rich moments for teaching?

As nurses progress to the level of competence, they begin to question the judgments and actions of more experienced staff and become quick to criticize their errors and mistakes. How might we help these nurses work through such feelings? How might an expert nurse monitor and direct this criticism constructively? Is it possible for expert nurses to capture the opportunities that arise spontaneously in practice as teaching moments to demonstrate that the needs of the patient take precedence over and frequently overturn stringent rules and organizational goals?

As nurses progress to the level of proficiency, their clinical world increasingly becomes differenti-

ated. Subtle signs and symptoms automatically claim their attention. They are comfortable plotting a new course when expectations are overturned. How might these nurses be commissioned as role models for those with less experience to help them recognize significant patient cues and the need to direct their actions based on rapidly changing clinical situations?

And then there is the expert. We have all seen this person. He or she can walk into a patient's room, where the health care team has been struggling for hours to get things under control, and in less than a minute, can figure out what is going on with the patient and know instinctively when the situation is urgent and warrants immediate action. Experts see the big picture. They understand what the patient needs. Their practice is patient driven. These individuals are our ultimate teachers and mentors.

Where would you place yourself on this continuum of clinical practice (i.e., at the advanced beginner, competent, proficient, or expert level)? Although it would be wonderful to believe that each nurse will eventually mature from the beginner to the expert, for various reasons some of us get stuck at a particular level. Although experience, book learning, and clinical knowledge make a difference, all of us, no matter at what level, need a mentor. Two critical rules apply in the mentorship process. For the process to work, first, a mentor must desire to mentor and second, the person with less experience must desire to be mentored.

If you have not reached the expert level yet, then perhaps it is time that you find a nurse who is willing to mentor you. Tell this mentor where you are headed and what you would like to accomplish. Invite your mentor to challenge you and allow him or her to structure some of your goals. Ask your mentor to evaluate and help you augment your clinical thinking, judgment, and actions to foster your development and empower you to progress to a higher level of practice.

CEG & BMD

Adapted from: Guzzetta CE: Comments. Capsules and Comments in Critical Care Nursing. *1993; 2:55–56.*

INTRODUCTION

The ultimate goal in critical care is to meet the needs of the patient and family,[1] as those needs are defined by them. The health care system should be driven, or organized, around those needs, not by what works best for the hospital or clinicians. It is important that clinicians not lose sight of this goal, even when the patient's acuity or the intensity of the situation tends to overshadow patient and family needs.

Meeting critically ill patients' and family needs requires a high level of clinical expertise and functioning from all members of the health care team. Excellence in critical care practice requires more than a requisite amount of knowledge and technical skills in critical care. Clinical excellence involves the integration of a variety of important capabilities: up-to-date clinical knowledge and technical skills, a holistic approach, ethical decision making, compassion and understanding of the critical illness experience for the patient and family, strong leadership skills, collaboration with the multidisciplinary team, and a commitment to continuous quality improvement.

This chapter addresses several of these aspects of clinical excellence, emphasizing their importance to optimal patient care. Many of these aspects of clinical excellence are also presented throughout other chapters.

---

[1]Throughout this text, use of the term *family* refers broadly to family members, significant others, and whomever the patient identifies as important in his or her life (e.g., friends or pets).

HOLISTIC CRITICAL CARE PRACTICE

Embedded in the goal or vision of meeting patient and family needs is an inherent mandate that critical care practice be guided from a holistic framework, rather than from the traditional biomedical or allopathic model. Allopathy is the method of combating disease with techniques that produce effects different from those produced by the disease. At present, much of critical care practice operates from an allopathic model that separates an individual into biologic, psychologic, sociologic, and spiritual fragments. Within the allopathic model, *disease* is viewed from the biological dimensions of nonhealth, breakdown, or disability. The focus of this model is on curing disease—a focus which concentrates solely on the body side of the body-mind equation.

Many clinicians have long recognized the inadequacies of the allopathic model in caring for the whole patient and have embraced the more comprehensive holistic model to guide practice. A primary assertion of the holistic model is that illness impacts not just the body but also the psycho-social-spiritual dimensions of living human beings. The primary emphasis is on helping and healing individuals from a bio-psycho-social-spiritual perspective, even if there is no cure. The focus is on body-mind-spirit healing which combines the best of biotechnology with the best of caring, love, compassion, and creativity to expand human potential, seek wholeness in human existence, and find balance, harmony, meaning, and purpose in life. Table 1–1 provides a comparison of the allopathic and holistic models.

TABLE 1–1. ASSUMPTIONS OF ALLOPATHIC AND HOLISTIC MODELS OF CARE

Allopathic Model	Holistic Model
Treatment of symptoms	Search for patterns, causes
Specialized	Integrated; concerned with the whole patient
Emphasis on efficiency	Emphasis on human values
Professional should be emotionally neutral	Professional's caring is a component of healing
Pain and disease are wholly negative	Pain and disease may be valuable signals of internal conflicts
Primary intervention with drugs, surgery	Minimal intervention with appropriate technology, complemented with a range of noninvasive techniques (psychotechnologies, diet, exercise)
Body seen as a machine in good or bad repair	Body seen as a dynamic system, a complex energy field within fields (family, workplace, environment, culture, life history)
Disease or disability seen as an entity	Disease or disability seen as a process
Emphasis on eliminating symptoms and disease	Emphasis on achieving maximum body-mind health
Patient is dependent	Patient is autonomous
Professional is authority	Professional is therapeutic partner
Body and mind are separate; psychosomatic illnesses seen as mental; may refer (patient) to psychiatrist	Body-mind perspective; psychosomatic illness is the province of all health care professionals
Mind is secondary factor in organic illness	Mind is primary or coequal factor in all illness
Placebo effect is evidence of power of suggestion	Placebo effect is evidence of mind's role in disease and healing
Primary reliance on quantitative information (charts, tests, and dates)	Primary reliance on qualitative information, including patient reports and professional's intuition; quantitative data an adjunct
"Prevention" seen as largely environmental; vitamins, rest, exercise, immunization, not smoking	"Prevention" synonymous with wholeness in work, relationships, goals, body-mind-spirit

From Fergurson M: The aquarian conspiracy: Personal and social transformations in our time. Tarcher, 1987. With permission.

Within this holistic model, *health* is viewed not simply as the absence of disease but as an ideal state, an integrated balance, and an ability to maximize individuals' potential for functioning despite changes occurring within themselves and their relationships with their environment. Health is a process by which individuals maintain their sense of coherence—a sense that life is understandable, manageable, and meaningful. *Illness,* in contrast, is not the absence of health nor is it the same as disease. Illness focuses on an individual's unique lived experiences involved in searching for meaning and purpose surrounding symptoms and suffering as well as in discovering ways to live within the limitations of symptoms or disability. The human experience of these events, rather than the pathophysiologic state, is placed at the core of what it means to be healthy or sick. For example, when a person experiences chest pain and undergoes angioplasty, he or she is not the heart disease patient but rather a person with an illness related to cardiovascular disease. Following the angioplasty, this person must seriously evaluate his or her life and reflect on lifestyle and events leading up to this event. This reflective process helps the patient and family make treatment decisions and reorganize their life and family structure to make specific lifestyle changes which contribute to future health.

Although critical care has made enormous advances in confronting disease, critical care nurses must play a vital part in creating the necessary changes to reform the health care system from one that is driven by biotechnology to one that is driven by the body-mind-spirit needs of patients with critical illness.

Holism in Critical Care

Holistic nursing is recognized as the most complete way to conceptualize and practice professional nursing. The American Holistic Nurses' Association (AHNA) working description of holistic nursing is as follows:[2]

> Holistic nursing embraces all nursing practice which has healing the whole person as its goal. Holistic nursing recognizes that there are two views regarding holism: that holism involves studying and understanding the interrelationships of the bio-psycho-social-spiritual dimensions of the person, recognizing that the whole is greater than the sum of its parts; and that holism involves understanding the individual as an integrated whole interacting with and being acted upon by both internal and external environments. Holistic nursing accepts both views, believing that the goals of nursing can be achieved within either framework.

---

[2]Reproduced with permission from the American Holistic Nurses' Association (AHNA), 1994. For information on AHNA Standards of Holistic Nursing Practice, Holistic Ethics, Holistic Nursing, and Healing Touch Certificate Programs: AHNA, 4101 Lake Boone Trail, Suite #201, Raleigh, NC 27607; (919)787-5181; FAX (919)787-4916.

Holistic practice draws on nursing knowledge, theories, expertise, and intuition to guide nurses in becoming therapeutic partners with clients/patients in strengthening the clients'/patients' responses to facilitate the healing process and achieve wholeness.

Practicing holistic nursing requires nurses to integrate self-care in their own lives. Self-responsibility leads the nurse to a greater awareness of the interconnectedness of all individuals and their relationships to the human and global community, and permits nurses to use this awareness to facilitate healing.

Thus the concepts of holistic nursing are based on broad and eclectic academic principles. Holistic concepts incorporate a sensitive balance between art and science, analytic and intuitive skills, and the interconnectedness of body-mind-spirit. Holism is a way of viewing individuals in terms of patterns and processes that combine to form a whole, instead of seeing them as fragments, pieces, or parts.

Holistic critical care nursing involves much more than caring for only the patient's bodily illness. It involves assessing and identifying the patient's bio-psycho-social-spiritual problems, determining desired patient outcomes, and implementing and evaluating interventions to achieve these outcomes. Within this framework, patients' rights and choices are respected. Nurses actively engage patients in making mutual decisions regarding goals of care, treatment options, and outcome evaluation. Health education, illness prevention, and health promotion become core ingredients in assisting patients to take responsibility for their health and participate in self-care. Nurses advocate for patients based on the patients' cultural background, health beliefs, and values. Holistic critical care nurses are flexible and able to give up control of routines, procedures, and institutional policies (or a sense of "I know what is best for the patient") to provide relationship-centered care driven by the needs of the patient. Cultural diversity, cultural health care practices, and alternative therapies are integrated into nursing practice to treat the whole patient. An environment conducive to spiritual growth and assisting patients to search for meaning and purpose in life and during illness is fostered. Respect for privacy and confidentiality as well as ensuring environmental safety and emergency preparedness is maintained.

Standards of Holistic Critical Care Practice

The American Association of Critical-Care Nurses (AACN) has developed process and outcome standards for nursing care of the critically ill, and the American Holistic Nurses' Association has developed standards of holistic nursing. These standards define and establish the scope of holistic critical care nursing practice that has guided the development of this book.

The nursing process and outcome standards for critical care nursing and for holistic nursing provide the criteria by which to measure the quality of holistic critical care nursing rendered to patients. Because the process standards for holistic nursing have been developed based on the universal language of the nursing process, they easily may be combined with the more physiologically based process standards of critical care nursing to ensure the delivery of not only quality physiologic but also quality psycho-social-spiritual care to critically ill patients.

These standards provide model statements that direct the nurse in delivering care during each step of the nursing process. They also are used as the basis for evaluating the effectiveness and quality of the care. Because the standards of practice are written in general terms, it is usually necessary to use them with more specific standards of care tailored to the patient's illness and modified according to hospital policy, as well as to state nurse practice acts.

Relationship-Centered Care

In 1994 the PEW-Fetzer Task Force published its report[3] on relationship-centered care. Relationship-centered care provides a road map for delivering holistic critical care which addresses the interdependence of bio-psycho-social-spiritual dimensions in health and illness. It is based on the belief that relationships and interactions among people form the foundation for any therapeutic or healing activity.

There are three components to relationship-centered care: (1) the patient-practitioner relationship, (2) the community-practitioner relationship, and (3) the practitioner-practitioner relationship. These three components are central to delivering holistic critical care and provide concrete guidelines for putting into action a model of health care that integrates caring, healing, and holism.

Patient-Practitioner Relationship

The foundation of care given by any practitioner is the relationship between the practitioner and the patient. In the patient-practitioner relationship, the practitioner incorporates comprehensive biotechnological as well as psycho-social-spiritual care. Active collaboration with the patient and the patient's family in the decision-making process and in promoting health and preventing illness within the family is fostered. Part of this relationship involves understanding the patient's experience of health and illness and the meaning of this experience. Understanding the patient's experience involves appreciating the patient as a whole person, exploring the individual's life and illness stories, being able to imagine the life events of a patient, and discovering the role of the patient's family, culture, and community. To develop and maintain caring healing relationships with patients, practitioners need to be open and fully focused

[3]Pew-Fetzer Task Force on Advancing Psychosocial Health Education: *Health professions education and relationship-centered care.* San Francisco: Pew Health Professions Commission and the Fetzer Institute, 1994.

AT THE BEDSIDE

Nurse: "I met Jack the night before surgery when I did his preop teaching. He was this joking, funny guy. After surgery, he never woke up. He remained in a coma for 4 months and ended up with every complication in the book.

"His wife and kids were so disconnected from him at first—he wasn't the same person they had known all those years. I knew it would be important for them to reconnect with him because I feared he would never wake up. So we planned times when we'd sit by Jack's bed and talk about things that Jack was interested in.

"And I'd joke a lot with Jack when I was taking care of him. I knew the town he was from in New Jersey so I could say things like, 'Oh Jack, you should see the Giants. They are a mess this year!' You can imagine how much it freaked out the doctors and others when I did this!

"His wife, though, went from being afraid to enter the room to telling Jack all about the kids, who was dating whom, that sort of thing.

"It hurt a lot when Jack died, because it was the end of a 4-month relationship with someone I actually got to know a lot about. But when he died, it was peaceful for everyone. And the family had reconnected with their husband and their father.

"You know, it feels so good when you can do something like that for other people. It makes you feel so good about what you're doing in nursing."

with patients, actively listen and communicate effectively, establish respect for the patient's dignity and uniqueness, accept and compassionately respond to patients, and strive to reduce the power inequalities between practitioner and patient with regard to race, sex, education, occupation, and socioeconomic status. To work effectively within the patient-practitioner relationship, the practitioner must develop the knowledge, skills, and values summarized in Table 1–2.

Community-Practitioner Relationship

Forming a relationship with the patient also necessitates developing a relationship with the patient's community. Critically ill patients and their families simultaneously belong to many types of communities (e.g., immediate family, relatives, friends, coworkers, neighborhoods, religious and community organizations). Critical care practitioners must be sensitive to the various characteristics of the patient's communities and work to bring together the best of these communities as they interact with the critically ill patient. The harmful elements within the community that block the patient's healing must be identified and improved

TABLE 1–2. PATIENT-PRACTITIONER RELATIONSHIP

Area	Knowledge	Skills	Values
Self-awareness	Knowledge of self Understanding self as a resource to others	Reflect on self and work	Importance of self-awareness, self-care, self-growth
Patient experience of health and illness	Role of family, culture, community in development Multiple components of health Multiple threats and contributors to health as dimensions of one's reality	Recognize patient's life story and its meaning View health and illness as part of human development	Appreciation of the patient as a whole person Appreciation of the patient's life story and the meaning of the health-illness condition
Developing and maintaining caring relationships	Understanding of threats to the integrity of the relationship (e.g., power inequalities) Understanding of potential for conflict and abuse	Attend fully to the patient Accept and respond to distress in patient and self Respond to moral and ethical challenges Facilitate hope, trust, and faith	Respect for patient's dignity, uniqueness, and integrity (mind-body-spirit unity) Respect for self-determination Respect for person's own power and self-healing processes
Effective communication	Elements of effective communication	Listen Impart information Learn Facilitate the learning of others Promote and accept patient's emotions	Importance of being open and nonjudgmental

From Tresolini CP and the Pew-Fetzer Task Force: Health professions education and relationship-centered care. San Francisco: Pew Health Professions Commission and the Fetzer Institute, 1994. With permission.

to enhance the patient's health and well-being. Moreover, practitioners need to understand the various types of care offered by the community such as self-help groups, home care, and care given by community-based institutions such as schools, clinics, churches, homes for the aged, and halfway houses. The knowledge, skills, and values needed by practitioners to effectively participate in and work with various communities are summarized in Table 1–3.

Practitioner-Practitioner Relationship

Providing comprehensive holistic care for critically ill patients and their families cannot be accomplished in isolation. It involves the many contributions from diverse practitioners. The *quality* of the relationships formed among these practitioners plays an integral role in all therapeutic or healing activities. To develop effective practitioner-practitioner relationships, it is necessary to understand and respect one another's roles. Practitioners need to learn about the different roles of conventional and alternative practitioners and the therapeutic and healing modalities they use.

Collaborative practice relationships begin by affirming the shared mission, tasks, goals, and values of the health care team. These relationships require that practitioners listen openly, communicate effectively, learn cooperatively, and work together. Although collaboration among practitioners is the cornerstone to all effective practice, collaboration among practitioners in the critical care setting assumes an enormous level of importance. One has to only

visualize the degree of collaboration necessary among the many diverse practitioners to achieve successful outcomes and prevent complications in patients undergoing cardiac transplantation or those suffering from a traumatic spinal cord injury. During critical illness characterized by uncertainty, complexity, and unpredictability, the demand for information and coordinated efforts becomes more crucial to allow critical thinking, correct decision making, rapid responses, and optimal performance to occur. Perhaps most important, collaborative practice relationships have been shown to enhance desired patient outcomes. Knaus and colleagues have found, for example, that collaborative relationships among critical care practitioners significantly correlated with decreased mortality in critically ill adults.[4]

The effectiveness of collaborative practice, however, depends on the relationships developed among the multidisciplinary practitioners. Collaboration, simply stated, means working together on behalf of patients by sharing in problem solving, goal setting, and decision making within a trusting, collegial, and caring environment. It implies that practitioners work interdependently rather than autonomously with each assuming responsibility and accountability for patient care. The knowledge, skills, and values needed to form effective practitioner-practitioner relationships are summarized in Table 1–4. Thus develop-

---

[4]Knaus W, Draper E, Wagner D, et al: An evaluation of the outcomes from intensive care in major medical centers. *Annals of Internal Medicine.* 1986; 104:410–418.

TABLE 1–3. COMMUNITY-PRACTITIONER RELATIONSHIP

Area	Knowledge	Skills	Values
Meaning of community	Various models of community Myths and misperceptions about community Perspectives from the social sciences, humanities, and systems theory Dynamic change—demographic, political, industrial	Learn continuously Participate actively in community development and dialogue	Respect for the integrity of the community Respect for cultural diversity
Multiple contributors to health within the community	History of community, land use, migration, occupations, and their effect on health Physical, social, and occupational environments and their effects on health External and internal forces influencing community health	Critically assess the relationship of health care providers to community health Assess community and environmental health Assess implications of community policy affecting health	Affirmation of relevance of all determinants of health Affirmation of the value of health policy in community services Recognition of the presence of values that are destructive to health
Developing and maintaining community relationships	History of practitioner-community relationships Isolation of the health care community from the community at large	Communicate ideas Listen openly Empower others Learn Facilitate the learning of others Participate appropriately in community development and activism	Importance of being open-minded Honesty regarding the limits of health science Responsibility to contribute health expertise
Effective community-based care	Various types of care, both formal and informal Effects of institutional scale on care Positive effects of continuity of care	Collaborate with other individuals and organizations Work as member of a team or healing community Implement change strategies	Respect for community leadership Commitment to work for change

From Tresolini CP and the Pew-Fetzer Task Force: Health professions education and relationship-centered care. *San Francisco: Pew Health Professions Commission and the Fetzer Institute, 1994. With permission.*

TABLE 1–4. PRACTITIONER-PRACTITIONER RELATIONSHIP

Area	Knowledge	Skills	Values
Self-awareness	Knowledge of self	Reflect on self and needs Learn continuously	Importance of self-awareness
Traditions of knowledge in health professions	Healing approaches of various professions Healing approaches across cultures Historical power inequities across professions	Derive meaning from others' work Learn from experience within healing community	Affirmation and value of diversity
Building teams and communities	Perspectives on team building from the social sciences	Communicate effectively Listen openly Learn cooperatively	Affirmation of mission Affirmation of diversity
Working dynamics of teams, groups, and organizations	Perspectives on team dynamics from the social science	Share responsibility responsibly Collaborate with others Work cooperatively Resolve conflicts	Openness to others' ideas Humility Mutual trust, empathy, support Capacity for grace

From Tresolini CP and the Pew-Fetzer Task Force: Health professions education and relationship-centered care. *San Francisco: Pew Health Professions Commission and the Fetzer Institute, 1994. With permission.*

TABLE 1–5. VISION PARTNERS

V **Values Driven**—Partners are driven by values, not by environment, emotions, or circumstances. Do you "walk the talk" of the values you share with your partners?

I **Interdependence**—Interdependence involves the "we" of a partnership. We can do it. We can get there. We can create something greater together. Do you partner with a "we" or a "me" focus?

S **Shifting Paradigms**—"You can't change the fruit without changing the root." Our paradigms—the models or context in which we do our thinking—frame our attitudes and behaviors. Do you think from the inside out—starting with yourself and putting ethics ahead of personality and popularity? If not, you may need to change your thinking (shift your paradigm). If the fruit is our partnership and the root is how we think, some shifting may be necessary to genuinely achieve your partnership's goals. Are you "root bound"? Do you need to replant your ideas so you can grow better fruit?

I **Integrity**—Integrity is the value we place on ourselves. Personal integrity generates trust by keeping us from judging another before checking our perceptions with that person. Integrity stops us from talking behind another's back; from dishonest communication and behaviors; and from self-serving motivation. Are you honest in your communications? Do you participate in conversations about another person without bringing your concerns to that person directly? Do you voice your convictions even if they are unpopular?

O **Organizational Outcomes**—Focusing on organizational outcomes is a characteristic of organizational excellence. This holds true for partners, too. When partners focus on outcomes, they gain a shared purpose and direction for progress. Are you focused on outcomes and driven by the ones you share with your partner?

N **Negotiation**—In negotiating, partners focus on interests, not positions. A win-win situation is where one partner doesn't succeed at the other's expense. How are your negotiation skills?

P **Principle-Centered Leadership**—Principles drive every work, action, and priority of effective partners. Are you a principle-centered leader? Do your actions with your partners reflect your values and principles?

A **Accountability**—Each of us is accountable to our own effectiveness, for our own happiness, and for most of our circumstances. Are you accountable for your behaviors, words, and priorities in your partnerships?

R **Renewal**—With renewal, we can replace old patterns of self-defeating and noncollaborative behavior with new patterns of effectiveness, happiness, and trust. What was the most recent thing you did to renew yourself and your partnerships?

T **Trust**—Trust nurtures the self-esteem of each partner, enabling him or her to focus on issues rather than personalities and positions. Are you a trustworthy partner? Do you operate above the table at all times?

N **Novelty**—Partnerships are only as much fun and as invigorating as the partners make them. What novel approaches do you use to energize your partnerships?

E **Evolution**—Evolution happens as partners open up the gates for change. Sometimes this may feel like revolution, but it's really a gradual metamorphosis toward interdependence in the partnership. Where are your partnerships compared to where they began?

R **Respect**—Only in an environment of mutual respect, where each viewpoint is truly heard, will partners express their most important and truthful thoughts. Are you respectful in your interactions, even in the face of debate and disagreement? Do you listen well without interruption, seeking first to understand before being understood?

S **Synergy**—Synergy happens when the combined actions of people working together create a greater effect than each person can achieve alone. Synergistic partnerships value differences, respect them, and build on strengths to compensate for weakness. Do your partnerships focus on the contributions of each partner with the goal of creating a greater good for all?

From Miccolo M: Effective partnering. AACN News. *Aliso Viejo, CA: American Association of Critical-Care Nurses, 1993.*

ing collaborative practice relationships becomes the foundation for delivering holistic relationship-centered care. When such effective relationships are developed, we become vision partners with our colleagues. The qualities of vision partners are outlined in Table 1–5.

Alternative Therapies

In 1993, a landmark study was published by David M. Eisenberg, MD, and colleagues at Harvard Medical School and Beth Israel Hospital that caused conventional health care practitioners to take notice.[5] Dr. Eisenberg wanted to find out how many Americans used alternative (or unconventional or complementary) therapies. He described

unconventional or alternative therapies as those therapies not normally taught in medical schools and those not normally offered in hospital settings. The results of the study revealed that in 1990 about one third of all American adults used some form of alternative therapies (e.g., acupuncture, hypnosis, herbs, biofeedback, imagery, touch).

The findings also revealed that Americans made 425 million visits to practitioners of alternative medicine, which exceeded the total number of visits to primary care physicians in the United States. Moreover, expenditures for alternative care were $14 billion, most of which were out of pocket and not reimbursed by insurance plans.

About the same time that the Eisenberg study was published, the federal government recognized the existence of underground networks offering alternative therapies to patients with such illnesses as AIDS and cancer. The government also recognized that Americans were pursuing alternative methods of health care with unprecedented

[5]Eisenberg DM, et al: Unconventional medicine in the United States: Prevalence, costs, and patterns of use. *New England Journal of Medicine.* 1993; 328(4):246.

enthusiasm and felt, in this era of health care reform, that the time had come to determine whether any of these therapies were effective in treating illness and had the potential to reduce health care costs.

In 1992, as directed by Congress, the National Institutes of Health (NIH) created the Office of Alternative Medicine (OAM) to evaluate whether alternative therapies had the potential to change the clinical course and outcomes of an illness. The mission of the OAM is to support research investigations to determine which alternative therapies work, which ones do not, and which ones have the potential to do harm. The results of these studies will validate the efficacy of some alternative therapies and will lay to rest those that offer no promise. The ultimate mission of the OAM is to integrate validated alternative medical practices with current conventional medical practices to create a more humanistic health care system.

Alternative therapies targeted for evaluation include body-mind or biobehavioral interventions (biofeedback, relaxation, imagery, meditation, hypnosis, psychotherapy, prayer, therapeutic touch, distant or psychic healing, art, dance, and music), nutritional approaches, traditional and ethnomedicine, Native American approaches, traditional oriental medicine, structural and energetic therapies (acupressure, chiropractic, massage, reflexology, rolfing), pharmacologic and biologic treatments (antioxidizing agents, cell treatments, metabolic therapy, oxidizing agents such as ozone and hydrogen peroxide), and electromagnetic applications. Two Centers of Excellence for Alternative Medical Research Grants have been established by the OAM. The first is Bastyr University in Seattle, which is investigating alternative therapies in treating patients with HIV/AIDS, and the second is the Minneapolis Center for Addiction, which is evaluating alternative therapies in treating patients with substance abuse. Eight other Centers of Excellence have recently been established.

Alternative therapies must be considered as adjuncts or complements to conventional critical care biotechnology and pharmacology and not as replacements for them. A "both/and" instead of an "either/or" approach in interfacing alternative therapies with traditional medical and surgical therapies is necessary. Many of these alternative therapies flow from our holistic philosophy, can be used independently by the nurse, and have the potential to help individuals access their inner healing resources. The time has come to integrate effective alternative therapies in the critical care setting which have the potential to augment conventional medical therapies in meeting the body-mind-spirit needs of our patients to enhance desired patient outcomes. When body-mind-spirit needs are addressed, healing will enter into the health care arena. Nurses have the opportunity to play a major role in the future direction, investigation, and implementation of many of these therapies.

AT THE BEDSIDE

Nurse: "People aren't always willing to give up things or aren't always sure what to give up to facilitate or to meet patients' needs. For example, we've proven, through research, that using the bedside monitor to 'count' heart rate is more accurate than apical auscultation. So why are we so reluctant to give it up and use the monitor?

"And our studies show that a closed loop titrator controls blood pressure significantly better than traditional manual control of the drugs so that patients have less postoperative bleeding and fewer returns to the OR.

"Something is wrong in our system when we do things for tons of reasons except because it's what's best for patients and families."

RESEARCH-BASED PRACTICE

The primary method for determining the best way to care for critically ill patients is through the systematic objective study of clinical phenomena and interventions. The management of critically ill patients is continually being updated with the acquisition of new knowledge, primarily through clinical research. Updating clinical policies, procedures, and standards of care with this new knowledge should occur on at least a yearly basis through systematic review of these documents.

Sources of the most up-to-date research-based information on critical care topics include journals, procedure manuals, recent text books on critical care, or practice guidelines from expert consensus, federal, or professional groups (Table 1–6). Practice guidelines are a particularly good source of research-based recommendations for clinical practice. Review articles which summarize research on specific critical care topics are also another good source for identifying the current research-based recommendations for practice (Table 1–7).

The latest research studies should be used whenever decisions are made about clinical practice routines. This approach will balance the tendency to make clinical practice decisions based exclusively on historical practice, the "we always do it this way" mentality, with a sound scientific basis for best clinical practices. For example, cardiac output measurements may have been done with iced injectates. Reviewing the research on cardiac output injectates would provide clinicians with information on the efficacy of room temperature injectates in most clinical situations. This latter practice may well decrease clinician time and costs associated with cardiac output measurements.

TABLE 1–6. RESOURCES FOR CRITICAL CARE RESEARCH INFORMATION

Journals
AACN Clinical Issues: Advanced Practice in Acute and Critical Care
American Journal of Critical Care
Applied Nursing Research
Critical Care Nursing Clinics of North America
Critical Care Nursing Quarterly
Critical Care Quarterly
Critical Care Medicine
Heart and Lung
Alternative Therapies in Health and Medicine
Nursing Research

Abstracting Publications
Capsules and Comments in Critical Care Nursing
AACN Nursing Scan in Critical Care

Professional Societies/Nonprofit Groups/Federal Agencies
Agency for Health Care Policy and Research, Department of Health and
    Human Services, Rockville, MD
American Association of Critical-Care Nurses, Aliso Viejo, CA
Centers for Disease Control, Department of Health and Human Services,
    Atlanta, GA
ECRI, Plymouth Meeting, PA
National Institutes of Health Consensus Panels, Department of Health and
    Human Services, Bethesda, MD
Society of Critical Care Medicine, Anaheim, CA

In addition to integrating current research findings into practice, designing and supporting clinical research studies on critical care practice are also important. Research priorities developed by professional nursing organizations can be an excellent source of ideas for clinically relevant

TABLE 1–7. EXAMPLES OF RECENT LITERATURE REVIEWS ON CRITICAL CARE TOPICS

Bridges E, Woods S: Pulmonary artery pressure measurement: State of the
    art. *Heart and Lung.* 1993;22:99–111.
Copel L: Continuous Svo$_2$ monitoring: A research review. *Dimensions of
    Critical Care Nursing.* 1991;10(4):202–209.
Doering L: The effect of positioning on hemodynamics and gas exchange
    in the critically ill: A review. *American Journal of Critical Care.*
    1993;2(3):208–216.
Drew B: Bedside ECG monitoring: State of the art for the 1990's. *Heart
    and Lung.* 1990;20:610–623.
Hickey M: What are the needs of families of critically ill patients? A review
    of the literature since 1976. *Heart and Lung.* 1990;19:401–415.
Mancinelli-Van Atta J, Beck S: Preventing hypoxemia and hemodynamic
    compromise related to endotracheal suctioning. *American Journal of
    Critical Care.* 1992;1(3):62–79.
Rudy E, Baun M, Stone K, Turner B: The relationship between endotracheal
    suctioning and changes in intracranial pressure: A review of the litera-
    ture. *Heart and Lung.* 1986;15:488–493.
Simpson T, Wahl G, DeTraglia M, Speck E, Taylor D: The effects of eipdural
    versus parenteral opiod analgesics on postoperative pain and pulmonary
    function in adults who have undergone thoracic and abdominal surgery:
    A critique of research. *Heart and Lung.* 1992;21:125–140.
US Department of Health and Human Services: Acute pain management:
    Operative or medical procedures and trauma. Clinical practice guide-
    lines. Rockville, MD: Agency for Health Care Policy and Research, Public
    Health Service, US Department of Health and Human Services, 1992.

TABLE 1–8. SELECTED RESEARCH PRIORITIES FOR CRITICAL CARE NURSING

- Techniques to optimize pulmonary functioning and prevent pulmonary complications
- Weaning of mechanically ventilated patients.
- Effect of nursing activities/interventions on hemodynamic parameters.
- Techniques for real-time monitoring of tissue perfusion and oxygenation.
- Nutritional support modalities and patient outcomes.
- Interventions to prevent infection.
- Pain assessment and pain management techniques.
- Accuracy and precision of invasive and noninvasive monitoring devices.
- Effect of nursing activities, environmental stimuli, and human interactions on intracranial and cerebral perfusion pressure.
- Ethical issues related to initiation, maintenance, and withdrawal of life support technology.
- Collaboration and communication among health care professionals.

From Lindquist R, Barnsteiner J, Murdaugh C, Beecroft P: Critical care nursing research priorities. American Journal of Critical Care. 1992;1(1):15–20.

research projects. Some examples of research priorities published by the AACN are listed in Table 1–8.

CONTINUOUS QUALITY IMPROVEMENT

Continuous quality improvement (CQI) activities in critical care are one of several approaches used to identify and correct clinical practice problems and to focus the health care team on refinements in practice. CQI involves the ongoing monitoring of patient outcomes, processes of care delivery, and organizational structures by members of the health care team to assure an optimal level of patient care.

As in other areas of the hospital, CQI in critical care follows the 10-step process advocated by the Joint Commission on the Accreditation of Healthcare Organizations (JCAHO). Table 1–9 provides an example of a CQI program for a critical care unit primarily caring for medical patients. Although the CQI program for each critical care unit will vary depending on the types of patient care services provided, many of the indicators for monitoring are similar (Table 1–10).

The primary focus in CQI monitoring should be on patient and family outcomes, rather than the processes of care. Monitoring the process by which nursing or medical care is delivered is important when monitoring indicates a less than acceptable level on patient outcomes. For example, the incidence of artificial airway complications, such as oral or nasal skin breakdown or self-extubation rates, would be monitored first, rather than monitoring compliance with the unit's endotracheal (ET) tube taping procedure. Monitoring the process of taping ET tubes would only occur if the complication rate exceeded the thresholds for evaluation set by the practice committee.

The other emphasis in CQI activities in critical care units is the monitoring of quality control indicators related to safety of equipment in the critical care environment and

TABLE 1–9. TEN-STEP PROCESS TO CONTINUOUS QUALITY IMPROVEMENT ACTIVITIES

JCAHO 10-Step CQI Process	Medical ICU Example
Step 1: Assign responsibility	The unit clinical practice committee is responsible for all CQI activities.
Step 2: Identify scope of care	The MICU is a 12-bed unit caring primarily for adult critically ill patients: Critical pathway patients: sepsis, asthma, pneumonia, CHF, and arrhythmias High-volume, high-risk patients not on critical pathways: airway management, hemodynamic instability, ventilator dependency, neuromuscular blockade, immobility Low-volume, high-risk patients: IABP therapy, CAVH, pediatric patients
Step 3: Aspects of care	The following clinical outcomes measures are routinely monitored through multidisciplinary critical pathways: Pain Incidence of complications Functional ability Patient satisfaction Length of stay Cost In addition, aspects of care related to organizational structure and nursing standards are monitored through routine quality control activities: Safety and emergency preparedness Accuracy of bedside laboratory tests Environmental controls Assessing, diagnosing, planning, implementing, and evaluating standards for critical care nursing practice
Step 4: Indicators	Indicators are selected by the critical pathway teams or the unit practice committee based on identification of key patient care issues and quantified with objective measurement tools or instruments; for example: Airway management: self-extubation rate, oral/nasal skin integrity, nosocomial pneumonia rate IABP management: complication rates Pain: pain rating on visual analogue scale Patient satisfaction: responses on hospital survey Bedside laboratory test: analysis of quality control samples
Step 5: Threshold for evaluation (TFE)	Thresholds for evaluation are determined by the unit practice committee based on the mandated regulatory standards or associated risk to the patient; quality control TFEs are: Crash cart checks: 97% Refrigerator temperature: 97% Bedside laboratory tests: 97% Assessment and documentation standards: 90% Complications associated with artificial airways and IABP: 95% Patient satisfaction: 85%
Step 6: Collection of data	Critical pathway outcome data will be collected by unit clinicians at the point of care and collated by the outcomes management department.
Steps 7 and 8: Evaluation of care and development of action plans	The unit practice committee is responsible for evaluation of data from critical pathways, unit-specific indicators, and quality control indicators. Action plans will be developed for all indicators below TFE. Monthly CQI data analysis and corrective action plans will be communicated to unit nursing staff, the nurse manager, and appropriate personnel.
Step 9: Assess action and document	Ongoing monitoring will occur to determine the effectiveness of action plans.
Step 10: Communicate relevant information	Quarterly reporting of CQI activities will be submitted to the unit nurse manager, nursing staff, divisional practice committee, and other appropriate individuals within the organization. Multidisciplinary information will be submitted to critical pathway teams.

the accuracy of bedside laboratory tests (Table 1–9). These monitoring activities are anticipated to result in a high level of performance, often in the 95 to 97% range, but are routinely done on a frequent basis to insure optimal patient care. Many of the quality control indicators are monitored each shift or once a day, depending on the level of risk to the patient. For example, crash cart checks are routinely done each shift in critical care environments because arrests occur frequently in critically ill patients and represent a high-risk situation if the necessary equipment is not present and/or operating properly. It is not uncommon for critical care units to have a greater emphasis on quality control monitoring activities than other nonacute units in the hospital.

The optimal approach to CQI involves members of the multidisciplinary team in CQI activities. Achieving optimal patient outcomes requires the energies and efforts of every member of the health care team. It is rare that one discipline alone impacts the outcomes in critically ill patients. For example, optimal pain management involves nursing and

TABLE 1–10. EXAMPLES OF ASPECTS OF CARE COMMONLY MONITORED IN CRITICAL CARE CQI ACTIVITIES.

Patient Outcomes
Complications associated with the primary disease process and/or critical illness:
  Morbidity
  Mortality
  Infection
  Immobility
Readmission rates
Pain
Patient and family satisfaction
Length of stay
Cost

Processes of Patient Care Delivery
Standards of care for critically ill patients:
  Assessing diagnosing, planning, implementing, and evaluating of patient care
  Transportation
  Neuromuscular blockade
  Airway management and ventilatory support
  Advanced cardiac life support
Documentation

Quality Control Activities
Preparedness of emergency equipment (e.g., crash cart checks, O_2 and electrical back-up systems)
Laboratory and equipment quality control (e.g., arterial blood gas analyzer, glucometer, Hemacron)

medicine to insure appropriate medication orders, timely drug administration, coordination of painful interventions, and assessment of response to pain medication. Approaches by a single discipline to improve care delivery are not usually as effective as a multidisciplinary approach.

CQI activities can be easily incorporated into existing multidisciplinary programs, such as critical pathways or Care Maps, by including the monitoring of patient outcomes or processes of care into variance analysis mechanisms (See Chapter 3, Planning Care for Critically Ill Patients and Families). This approach increases the number of patients being monitored, with a dramatic decrease in time spent on CQI monitoring activities. This method also optimizes the opportunities to intervene quickly for individual patients when monitoring identifies a variance from the expected norms.

SELECTED BIBLIOGRAPHY

What Heals: Clinical Expertise

Benner P: *From novice to expert: Excellence and power in clinical nursing practice.* Menlo Park, CA: Addison-Wesley, 1984.

Benner P, Tanner C: Clinical judgment: How expert nurses use intuition. *American Journal of Nursing.* 1987;87:23.

Benner P, Tanner C, Chesla C: From beginner to expert: Gaining a differentiated clinical world in critical care nursing. *Advances in Nursing.* 1992;14:13–28.

Guzzetta C: Comments. *Capsules & Comments in Critical Care Nursing.* 1993;2:55–56.

Holistic Critical Care Practice

Achterberg J, Dossey B, Kolkmeier L: *Rituals of healing.* New York: Bantam, 1994.

Allred CA, Arford PH, Michel Y, Veitch JS, Dring R, Carter V: Case management: The relationship between structure and environment. *Nursing Economics.* 1995;13:32–41.

American Holistic Nurses' Association Working Description of Holistic Nursing. Raleigh, NC: American Holistic Nurses' Association, 1994.

Baggs J, Ryan S, Phelps C, Richeson JF, Johnson J: The association between interdisciplinary collaboration and patient outcomes in a medical intensive care unit. *Heart and Lung.* 1992;21(1):18–24.

Barnsteiner J, et al: Defining and implementing a standard for therapeutic relationships. *Journal of Holistic Nursing.* 1994;12:35–49.

Burkhardt M: Spirituality: An analysis of the concept. *Holistic Nursing Practice.* 1989;3:69–77.

Clark C, Heidenreich T: Spiritual care for the critically ill. *American Journal of Critical Care.* 1995;4:77.

Dossey B, Keegan L, Guzzetta CE. *The art of caring: Holistic healing using relaxation, imagery, music therapy, and touch.* Boulder, CO: Sounds True Audio, 1995 (audiotapes).

Dossey B, Keegan L, Guzzetta CE, Kolkmeier L: *Holistic nursing: A handbook for practice,* 2nd ed. Gaithersburg, MD: Aspen, 1995.

Dossey L: *Meaning and medicine.* New York: Bantam, 1991.

Dossey L: What does illness mean? *Alternative Therapies in Health and Medicine.* 1995;1:6–10.

Dracup K, Bryan-Brown W: Humane care in inhumane places. *American Journal of Critical Care.* 1995;4(1):1.

Evans JA: The role of the nurse manager in creating an environment for collaborative practice. *Holistic Nursing Practice.* 1994;8:22–31.

Flynn J: Shifting paradigms. *Nursing Leadership Forum.* 1995;1(1):12.

Gilje F: Being there: An analysis of the concept of presence. In Gaut D (ed.): *The presence of caring in nursing.* New York: National League for Nursing, 1992, pp. 53–67.

Gould LK, Ornish D, Scherwitz L, Brown S, Edens P, et al.: Changes in myocardial perfusion abnormalities by positron emission tomography after long-term, intense risk factor modification. *Journal of the American Medical Association.* 1995;274:894–901.

Grossman D, Taylor R: Cultural diversity on the unit. *American Journal of Nursing.* 1995;95(2):64.

Keegan L: *Nurse as healer.* New York: Delmar, 1994.

Knaus W, Draper E, Wagner D, et al.: An evaluation of the outcomes from intensive care in major medical centers. *Annals of Internal Medicine.* 1986;104:410–418.

McKivergin M: The essence of therapeutic presence. *Journal of Holistic Nursing.* 1994;12:65–81.

Meyer C: Visions of tomorrow's ICU. *American Journal of Nursing.* 1993;93(5):27.

Miccolo M: Effective partnering. *AACN News.* Aliso Viejo, CA: American Association of Critical-Care Nurses, 1993, p. 2.

Miller B, Haber J, Byrne M: The experience of caring in the acute care setting: Patient and nurse perspectives. In Gaut D (ed.): *The presence of caring in nursing.* New York: National League for Nursing, 1992, pp. 137–156.

Pew-Fetzer Task Force on Advancing Psychosocial Health Education: *Health professions education and relationship-centered care.* San Francisco: Pew Health Professions Commission and the Fetzer Institute, 1994.

Sanford S, Disch J. *Standards of nursing care of the critically ill.* Stamford CT: Appleton & Lange, 1989.

Shadick, KM: A practice model for cultural diversity. *American Nephrology Nurses' Association Annual Conference Proceedings.* Dallas, TX, 1994.

Watson J: *Nursing: Human science and human care.* New York: National League for Nursing, 1985, p. 16.

Watson J: Nursing caring-healing paradigm as exemplar for alternative therapies. *Alternative Therapies in Health and Medicine.* 1995;1:64–69.

Alternative Therapies

Eisenberg DM, et al: Unconventional medicine in the United States: Prevalence, costs, and patterns of use. *New England Journal of Medicine.* 1993;328(4):246.

OAM Report: *Alternative Therapies in Health and Medicine.* 1995;1(4):14–20.

Continuous Quality Improvement

Cassidy D, Friesen M: QA: Applying JCAHO's generic model. *Nursing Management.* 1990;21(6):22–27.

Larson E, Oram L: From process to outcome in infection control. *Journal of Nursing Quality Assurance.* 1989;4(1):18–26.

Lower M, Burton S: Measuring the impact of nursing interventions on patient outcomes—The challenges for the 1990's. *Journal of Nursing Quality Assurance.* 1989;4(1):27–34.

Marek K: Outcome measurement in nursing. *Journal of Nursing Quality Assurance.* 1989;4(1):1–9.

O'Leary D: CQI—A step beyond QA. *Joint Commission Perspectives.* 1990; March/April:2–3.

Rowe M, Jackson J: Multidisciplinary QA in a critical care unit. *Journal of Nursing Quality Assurance.* 1989;3(2):35–40.

Research-Based Practice

Boggs R, Wooldrige-King M: *AACN procedure manual for critical care,* 3rd ed. Philadelphia: WB Saunders, 1993.

Campbell G, Chulay M: Establishing a clinical nursing research program. In J Spicer, MA Robinson (eds.): *Environmental management in critical care nursing.* Baltimore: Williams & Wilkins, 1990, pp. 52–60.

Chulay M, White TM: Nursing research: Instituting changes in clinical practice. *Critical Care Nurse.* 1989;9:106–113.

Lindquist R, Barnsteiner J, Murdaugh C, Beecroft P: Critical care nursing research priorities. *American Journal of Critical Care.* 1992;1(1):15–20.

Notter L: *Essentials of nursing research.* New York: Springer Publishing, 1994.

Polit D: *Essentials of nursing research: Methods, appraisal, and utilization.* Philadelphia, JB Lippincott: 1993.

Sanford S, Disch J. *Standards of nursing care of the critically ill.* Stamford, CT: Appleton & Lange, 1989.

Tanner C: Evaluating research for use in practice: Guidelines for the clinician. *Heart and Lung.* 1987;16(4):424–431.

Waltz C: *Measurement in nursing research.* Philadelphia: FA Davis, 1991.

Assessment of Critically Ill Patients and Families

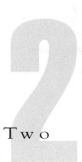

Two

▶ Knowledge Competencies

1. Discuss the importance of a consistent and systematic approach to assessment of critically ill patients and their families.
2. Identify the assessment priorities for different stages of a critical illness:
   • Prearrival assessment
   • Admission quick check
   • Comprehensive admission assessment
   • Ongoing assessment
3. Describe how the assessment is altered based on the patient's clinical status.

■ *What Heals: The Human Spirit*

Spiritual well-being is at the core of meaning and healing. When we address spiritual well-being, we assist patients in accessing their inner healing resources of hope, strength, faith, and connectedness to their world. Clark and Heidenreich[1] have identified three factors that are integral to the spiritual well-being of critically ill patients: care practitioners, family and friends, and religion and faith. Nursing interventions focusing on these three factors include establishing trusting relationships, providing in-depth spiritual assessment, conveying technical competence, and acting as a facilitator among patient, family, clergy, and other practitioners. Because of fluctuation in patients' health status and environmental factors, patients' perception of hope and well-being may change. Therefore, critical care nurses need to conduct ongoing spiritual assessments both on admission and intermittently

throughout the hospital stay. *Spiriting,* a more representative term for spirituality, has several defining characteristics: unfolding mystery, inner strengths, and harmonious interconnectedness. *Unfolding mystery* refers to one's experience about life's purpose and meaning, mystery, uncertainty, and struggles. *Inner strengths* refer to a sense of awareness, self, consciousness, inner resources, sacred source, unifying force, inner core, and transcendence. *Harmonious interconnectedness* includes connections and relationships, and harmony with self, other, higher power or God, and the environment (see Table 2–6 for assessment components).

An assessment of spirituality provides reflective questions for assessing, evaluating, and increasing awareness of spirituality in patients, families, and self (see Table 2–6 for key questions). These reflective questions can facilitate healing because they stimulate spontaneous, independent, meaningful initiatives to enhance the individuals's capacity for recovery and restoration.

---

[1]Clark C, Heidenreich T: Spiritual care for the critically ill. *American Journal of Critical Care.* 1995;4:77.

Spiritual assessment is not only critical for a holistic patient assessment but is also mandated by the Joint Commission on Accreditation of Healthcare Organizations (JCAHO) to support the Patient Bill of Rights and improve the quality of health care.* The Patient Bill of Rights states that "care of the patient must include consideration of the psychosocial, spiritual, and cultural variables that influence the perception of illness. The provision of patient care reflects consideration of the patient as an individual with personal values and belief systems that impact upon his/her attitude and response to the care that is provided by the organization."

CEG & BMD

*Patient Rights: Accreditation Manual for Hospitals (Suppl). Chicago: Joint Commission on Accreditation of Healthcare Organizations, 1992.

INTRODUCTION

The assessment of critically ill patients and their families is an essential competency for critical care practitioners. Information obtained from an assessment identifies the immediate and future needs of the patient and family so a plan of care can be initiated to address or resolve these needs.

Traditional approaches to patient assessment include a complete evaluation of the patient's history and a comprehensive physical examination of all body systems. This approach, while ideal, rarely is possible in critical care as clinicians struggle with life-threatening problems during admission and must balance the need to gather data while simultaneously prioritizing and providing care. Traditional approaches and techniques for assessment must be modified in critical care to balance the need for information, while considering the critical nature of the patient and family's situation.

This chapter outlines an assessment approach that recognizes the emergent and dynamic nature of a critical illness. This approach emphasizes the collection of assessment data in a phased, or staged, manner consistent with patient care priorities. The components of the assessment can be used as a generic template for assessing most critically ill patients and families. The assessment can then be individualized by adding more specific assessment requirements depending on the specific patient diagnosis. These specific components of the assessment are identified in subsequent chapters.

Crucial to developing competence in assessing critically ill patients and their families is a consistent and systematic approach to assessments. Without this approach, it would be easy to miss subtle signs or details that may identify a problem or indicate a patient's changing status. Assessments should focus first on the patient, then on the technology. The patient needs to be the focal point of the critical care practitioner's attention, with technology augmenting the information obtained from the direct assessment.

There are two standard approaches to assessing patients, the head-to-toe approach and the systems approach. Most critical care nurses use a combination of both, a systems approach applied in a "top-to-bottom" manner. The admission and ongoing assessment sections of this chapter are presented with this combined approach in mind.

ASSESSMENT FRAMEWORK

Assessing the critically ill patient and family begins from the moment the nurse is made aware of the pending admission of the patient and continues until transfer to a less acute setting. The assessment process can be viewed as four distinct stages: prearrival, admission quick check ("just the basics"), comprehensive admission, and ongoing assessment.

- *Prearrival assessment.* A prearrival assessment begins the moment information is received about the upcoming admission of the patient. This notification comes from the initial health care team contact. The contact may be paramedics in the field reporting to the Emergency Department (ED), a transfer from another facility or from other areas within the hospital such as the Emergency Room (ER), Operating Room (OR), or medical/surgical nursing unit. The prearrival assessment paints the initial picture of the patient and allows the critical care nurse to begin anticipating the patient's physiologic and psychologic needs.
- *Admission quick check.* An admission quick check assessment is obtained immediately upon arrival and

TABLE 2–1. *ABCDE* **ACRONYM**

*A*irway
*B*reathing
*C*irculation, *C*erebral perfusion, and *C*hief complaint
*D*rugs and *D*iagnostic tests
*E*quipment

---

is based on assessing the parameters represented by the *ABCDE* acronym (Table 2–1). The admission quick check assessment is a quick overview of airway patency and the adequacy of ventilation and perfusion, to ensure early intervention for any life-threatening situations. Energy is also focused on exploring the chief complaint and obtaining essential diagnostic tests to supplement physical assessment findings.

- *Comprehensive admission assessment.* A comprehensive admission assessment is performed as soon as possible, with the timing dictated by the degree of physiologic stability and emergent treatment needs of the patient. The comprehensive assessment is an in-depth assessment of the past medical history and social and relevant family history, and a complete physical examination of each body system.

- *Ongoing assessment.* After the baseline comprehensive assessment is completed, ongoing assessments, an abbreviated version of the comprehensive admission assessment, are performed at varying intervals. The assessment parameters outlined in this section are usually completed for all patients, in addition to other ongoing assessment requirements related to the patient's specific condition, treatments, and/or response to therapy.

PREARRIVAL ASSESSMENT: BEFORE THE ACTION BEGINS

A prearrival assessment begins when information is received about the pending arrival of the patient. The prearrival report, though abbreviated, provides key information about the chief complaint, diagnosis or reason for admission, pertinent history details, and physiologic stability of the patient (Table 2–2). It also contains the gender and age of the patient and information on the presence of invasive tubes and lines and pending or completed laboratory or diagnostic tests. This information assists the clinician to anticipate the patient's physiologic and emotional needs prior to admission and to ensure that the bedside environment is set up to provide all monitoring, supply, and equipment needs prior to the patient's arrival.

Many critical care units have a standard room setup, guided by the major diagnosis-related groups of patients each unit receives. The standard monitoring and equipment

AT THE BEDSIDE
▶ *Prearrival Assessment*

The charge nurse notifies Sue that she will be receiving a 26-year-old male from the Emergency Room who was involved in a serious car accident. He suffered a closed head injury and chest trauma with collapsed left lung. The patient was intubated and placed on a mechanical ventilator. IV access had been obtained, and a left chest tube had been inserted. After obtaining a CT of the head, the patient will be transferred to the ICU.

Sue goes to check the patient room prior to admission and begins to do a mental check of what will be needed. "OK, the patient is intubated so I'll connect the ambu bag to the oxygen source, check for suction catheters, and make sure the suction systems are working. The ventilator is ready to go. I have an extra suction gauge to connect to the chest tube system. I'll also turn on the ECG monitor and have the ECG electrodes ready to apply. The arterial line flush system and transducer are also ready to be connected. The IV infusion devices are set up. This patient has an altered level of consciousness, which means frequent neuro checks and potential insertion of an intracranial pressure catheter for monitoring. I have my pen light handy, but I better check to see if we have all the equipment to insert the ICP catheter in case the physician wants to perform the procedure here after the CT scan. I think I'm ready."

list for each unit varies; however, there are certain common requirements (Table 2–3). The standard room setup is modified for each admission to accommodate patient-specific needs (e.g., additional equipment, IV fluids, medications). Proper functioning of all bedside equipment should be verified prior to the patient's arrival.

It is also important to prepare the medical records forms, which usually consist of a manual flowsheet or computerized data entry system to record vital signs, intake and output, medication administration, and patient care activities. The prearrival report may suggest pending procedures, necessitating the organization of appropriate supplies at the bedside. Having the room prepared and all equipment available facilitates a rapid, smooth, and safe admission of the patient.

ADMISSION QUICK CHECK ASSESSMENT: THE FIRST FEW MINUTES

From the moment the patient arrives in the critical care unit (ICU) setting, his or her general appearance is immediately observed and assessment of *ABCDE*s is quickly performed (Table 2–2). The seriousness of the problem(s) is deter-

TABLE 2–2. SUMMARY OF PREARRIVAL AND ADMISSION QUICK CHECK ASSESSMENTS

Prearrival Assessment
- Abbreviated report on patient (age, sex, chief complaint, diagnosis, pertinent history, physiologic status, invasive devices, equipment and status of laboratory/diagnostic tests)
- Room setup complete, including verification of proper equipment functioning

Admission Quick Check Assessment
- General appearance (consciousness)
- *A*irway:
  Patency
  Position of artificial airway (if present)
- *B*reathing:
  Quantity and quality of respirations (rate, depth, pattern, symmetry, effort, use of accessory muscles)
  Breath sounds
  Presence of spontaneous breathing
- *C*irculation and *C*erebral Perfusion:
  ECG (rate, rhythm, and presence of ectopy)
  Blood pressure
  Peripheral pulses and capillary refill
  Presence of bleeding
  Level of consciousness, responsiveness
- *C*hief Complaint:
  Primary body system
  Associated symptoms
- *D*rugs and *D*iagnostic Tests:
  Drugs prior to admission (prescribed, over-the-counter, illegal)
  Current medications
  Review diagnostic test results
- *E*quipment:
  Patency of vascular and drainage systems
  Appropriate functioning and labeling of all equipment connected to patient
- Allergies

mined so that life-threatening emergent needs can be addressed first. Simultaneous with the *ABCDE* assessment, the patient's allergy status is determined, including the type of reaction that occurs and what, if any, treatment is used to alleviate the allergic response. The patient is connected to

TABLE 2–3. EQUIPMENT FOR STANDARD ROOM SETUP

- Bedside ECG and invasive pressure monitor with appropriate cables
- ECG electrodes
- Blood pressure cuff
- Suction gauges and canister setup
- Suction catheters
- Bag-valve mask device
- Oxygen flow meter, appropriate tubing, and appropriate oxygen delivery device
- IV poles
- Bedside supply cart that contains such things as alcohol swabs, nonsterile gloves, syringes, needles, and chux
- Admission kit that usually contains bath basin and general hygiene supplies
- Critical care documentation forms

the appropriate monitoring and support equipment, critical medications are administered, and essential laboratory tests are obtained.

There may be other health care professionals present to receive the patient and assist with admission tasks. The critical care nurse, however, is the primary leader of the receiving team. While assuming the primary responsibility for assessing the *ABCDE*s, the critical care nurse directs the team in completing delegated tasks. Without a leader of the receiving team, care can be fragmented and vital assessment clues overlooked.

The critical care nurse rapidly assesses the *ABCDE*s in the sequence outlined below. If any aspect of this preliminary assessment deviates from normal, interventions are begun immediately to address the problem before continuing with the assessment.

Airway and Breathing

Patency of the patient's airway is verified by having the patient speak and/or watching the patient's chest rise and fall. If the airway is compromised, verify that the head has been positioned properly to prevent the tongue from occluding the airway and insert an oral airway as needed. Inspect the upper airway for the presence of blood, vomitus, and foreign objects. If the patient already has an artificial airway, such as a cricothyrotomy, endotracheal (ET) tube, or tracheostomy, ensure that the airway is secured properly. Note the size marking on the ET tube that is closest to the teeth or nares to assist future comparisons for proper placement. Suctioning of the upper airway, either through the oral cavity or artificial airway, may be required to ensure that the airway is free from secretions. Note the amount, color, and consistency of secretions removed.

If the patient is breathing on his or her own, note the rate, depth, pattern, and symmetry of breathing, the effort it is taking to breathe, and the use of accessory muscles. Observe for nonverbal signs of respiratory distress such as restlessness, anxiety, or change in mental status. Auscultate the chest for presence of bilateral breath sounds, quality of breath sounds, and bilateral chest expansion. Optimally, both anterior and posterior breath sounds are auscultated, but during this admission quick check assessment, time generally dictates that just the anterior chest is assessed. If noninvasive oxygen saturation monitoring is available, observe and quickly analyze the values. If the patient is receiving assistive breaths from a bag-valve mask or mechanical ventilator, note the presence of spontaneous breaths and evaluate whether ventilation requires excessive pressure.

Circulation and Cerebral Perfusion

Assess circulation by quickly palpating a pulse and viewing the electrocardiogram (ECG) monitor for the heart rate, rhythm, and presence of ectopy. Obtain blood pressure and temperature quickly. Assess peripheral perfusion by evalu-

AT THE BEDSIDE
▶ *Admission Quick Check*

Assessment Parameter	Findings
Airway	Oral ET, airway clear of secretions.
Breathing	Clear breath sounds, bilateral chest expansion. No spontaneous breathing, ventilator settings at A/C 12/minute, V_T 900, FIO_2 .40. Pulse oximetry reading 99%.
Circulation	BP 130/75, MAP 93, NSR with HR 96. Peripheral pulses +3. Skin warm & dry.
Cerebral perfusion	Unresponsive except to pain.
Nervous system	Glasgow Coma Scale 7. Pupils round, midline, with brisk reaction. Right pupil 3 mm, left pupil 5 mm. Spontaneous movement left side, no movement noted on right. Babinski absent.
Respiratory system	Left chest tube to 20-cm suction, 50 ml bloody drainage past 2 hours. No air leak. No crepitus around insertion site.

ating the color and temperature of the skin and capillary refill. Inspect the body for any signs of blood loss and determine if active bleeding is occurring.

Evaluating cerebral perfusion in the admission quick check assessment is focused on determining the functional integrity of the brain as a whole, which is done by rapidly evaluating the gross level of consciousness (LOC). Evaluate whether the patient is alert and aware of his or her surroundings, whether it takes a verbal or painful stimulus to obtain a response, or whether the patient is unresponsive. Observing the response of the patient during movement from the stretcher to the ICU bed can supply additional information about the LOC. Note whether the patient's eyes are open and watching the events around him or her. For example, does the patient follow simple commands such as "Place your hands on your chest" or "Slide your hips over"? If the patient is unable to talk because of trauma or the presence of an artificial airway, note whether the patient's head nods appropriately to questions.

Chief Complaint

Optimally, the description of the chief complaint is obtained from the patient, but this may not be realistic. The patient may not speak English or may be unable to respond.

Data may need to be gathered from bystanders, family, and/or friends. In the absence of a history source, practitioners must depend exclusively on the physical findings and knowledge of pathophysiology to identify the potential causes of the admission.

Assessment of the chief complaint focuses on determining the body systems involved, and the extent of associated symptoms. Additional questions explore the time of onset and precipitating factors. Though the admission quick check phase is focused on obtaining a quick overview of the key life-sustaining systems, a more in-depth assessment of a particular system may need to be done at this time. For example, in the prearrival case study scenario presented earlier, completion of the *ABCDE*s is followed quickly by more extensive assessment of both the nervous and respiratory systems.

Drugs and Diagnostic Tests

Information about drugs and diagnostic tests is integrated into the priority of the admission quick check. If intravenous access is not already present, it should be immediately obtained and intake and output records started. Ascertain whether the patient has taken any drugs recently, including prescribed, over-the-counter, or illegal substances. If intravenous medications are presently being infused, check the drug(s) and verify the correct infusion of the desired dosage and rate.

Obtain critical diagnostic tests. Augment basic screening tests (Table 2–4) by additional tests appropriate to the underlying diagnosis and chief complaint. Review any available laboratory or diagnostic data for abnormalities or indications of potential problems requiring immediate intervention. The abnormal laboratory and diagnostic data for specific pathologic conditions will be covered in subsequent chapters.

Equipment

Quickly evaluate all vascular and drainage tubes for location and patency, and connect them to appropriate monitoring or suction devices. Note the amount, color, consistency, and odor of drainage secretions. Verify the appropriate functioning of all equipment attached to the patient and label as required.

The admission quick check assessment is accomplished in a matter of a few minutes. After completion of

TABLE 2–4. COMMON DIAGNOSTIC TESTS OBTAINED DURING ADMISSION QUICK CHECK ASSESSMENT

Serum electrolytes

Glucose

Complete blood count with platelets

Coagulation studies

Arterial blood gases

Chest x-ray

the *ABCDE*s assessment, the comprehensive admission assessment will begin. If at any phase during the admission quick check a component of the *ABCDE*s has not been stabilized and controlled, energy is focused first on resolving the abnormality before proceeding to the comprehensive admission assessment.

COMPREHENSIVE ADMISSION ASSESSMENT

Comprehensive admission assessments determine the physiologic and psychosocial baseline so that future changes can be compared to determine whether the status is improving or deteriorating. The comprehensive admission assessment also defines the patient's pre-event health status, determining problems or limitations that may impact patient status during this admission. The content presented in this section is a template to screen for abnormalities and determine the extent of injury to the patient. Any abnormal findings or changes from baseline warrant a more in-depth evaluation of the pertinent system.

The comprehensive admission assessment includes the patient's medical, social, and family history, and physical examination of each body system. The comprehensive admission assessment of the critically ill patient is similar to admission assessments for non-critically ill patients. This section will describe only those aspects of the assessment that are unique to critically ill patients, or require more extensive information than is obtained from a non-critical care patient. The entire assessment process is summarized in Tables 2–5 and 2–6.

Changing demographics of critical care units indicate that an increasing proportion of patients are elderly, requiring assessments to incorporate the effects of aging. Though assessment of the aging adult does not differ significantly from the younger adult, understanding how aging alters the physiologic and psychologic status of the patient is important. Key physiologic changes pertinent to the critically ill elderly adult are summarized in Table 2–7. Additional emphasis must also be placed on the past medical history as the aging adult frequently has multiple coexisting illnesses and is taking several prescriptive and over-the-counter medications. Social history must address issues related to home environment, support systems, nutritional habits, and self-care abilities. The interpretation of clinical findings in the elderly must also take into consideration the fact that the coexistence of several disease processes and the diminished reserves of most body systems often result in more rapid physiologic deterioration than in younger adults.

Past Medical History

Besides the primary event that brought the patient to the hospital, it is important to determine prior medical and surgical conditions, hospitalization, medications, and symp-

TABLE 2–5. SUMMARY OF COMPREHENSIVE ADMISSION ASSESSMENT REQUIREMENTS

Past Medical History
Medical conditions, surgical procedures
Psychiatric/emotional problems
Hospitalizations
Previous medications (prescription, over-the-counter, illicit drugs) and time of last medication dose
Allergies
Review of body systems (see Table 2–6)

Social History
Age, sex
Ethnic origin
Height, weight
Highest educational level completed
Occupation
Marital status
Primary family members/significant others
Religious affiliation
Durable power of attorney (DPA) or living will
Substance use (alcohol, drugs, caffeine, tobacco)

Family History
Cancer, heart disease, hypertension, diabetes, seizures, stroke, or ulcers

Psychosocial Assessment
Mental status
General communication
Coping styles
Perception of illness
Expectations of critical care unit
Current stresses
Family needs

Spirituality
Meaning and purpose
Inner strength
Inner connections

Physical Assessment
Nervous system
Cardiovascular system
Respiratory system
Renal system
Gastrointestinal system
Endocrine, hematologic and immune systems
Integumentary system

toms (Table 2–6). For every positive symptom response, additional questions should be asked to explore the characteristics of that symptom (Table 2–8).

Social History

Inquire about the use and abuse of caffeine, alcohol, tobacco, and other substances. As the use of these agents can have major implications for the critically ill patient, questions are aimed at determining the frequency, amount,

TABLE 2–6. SUGGESTED QUESTIONS FOR REVIEW OF PAST HISTORY CATEGORIZED BY BODY SYSTEM

Body System	History Questions
Nervous	• Have you ever had a seizure? • Have you ever fainted, blacked out, or had delirium tremens (DTs)? • Do you ever have numbness, tingling, or weakness in any part of your body? • Do you have any difficulty with your hearing, vision, or speech? • Has your daily activity level changed due to your present condition? • Do you require any assistive devices such as canes?
Cardiovascular	• Have you experienced any heart problems or disease such as heart attacks? • Do you have any problems with extreme fatigue? • Do you have an irregular heart rhythm? • Do you have high blood pressure? • Do you have a pacemaker or an implanted defibrillator?
Respiratory	• Do you ever experience shortness of breath? • Do you have any pain associated with breathing? • Do you have a persistent cough? Is it productive? • Have you had any exposure to environmental agents that might affect the lungs?
Renal	• Have you had any change in frequency of urination? • Do you have any burning, pain, discharge, or difficulty when you urinate? • Have you had blood in your urine?
Gastrointestinal	• Has there been any recent weight loss or gain? • Have you had any change in appetite? • Do you have any problems with nausea or vomiting? • How often do you have a bowel movement and has there been a change in the normal pattern? Do you have blood in your stools? • Do you have dentures?
Integumentary	• Do you have any problems with your skin?
Endocrine and Hematologic	• Do you have any problems with bleeding?
Immunologic	• Do you have problems with chronic infections?
Psychosocial	• Do you have any physical conditions which make communication difficult (hearing loss, visual disturbances, language barriers, etc.)? • Is it difficult for you to ask questions or let others know what you need? • How do you best learn? Do you need information repeated several times and/or require information in advance of teaching sessions? • What are the ways you cope with stress, crises, or pain? • Who are the important people in your "family" or network? Who do you want to make decisions with you, or for you? • Have you had any previous experiences with critical illness? • Have you ever been abused? • Do you have problems with attention, problem solving, or memory? • Have you ever experienced trouble with agitation, irritability, being confused, mood swings, or suicide attempts? • What is the impact of illness on the family? • What are the cultural practices, religious influences, and values that are important to the family? • What are family members' perceptions and expectations of the critical care staff and the setting? • What are the crisis or coping skills of family members? • What are the learning styles of family members?
Spiritual*	Meaning and purpose: • What gives your life meaning? • Do you have a sense of purpose in life? • Does your illness interfere with your life goals? • Why do you want to get well? • How hopeful are you about obtaining a better degree of health? • What is the most motivating or powerful thing in your life? Inner strengths: • What brings you joy and peace in your life? • What are your personal strengths? • What do you believe in? • Is faith important to you? • How has your illness influenced your faith? • Does faith play a role in regaining your health? Interconnections: • How do you feel about yourself right now? • What do you do to heal your spirit?

*Adapted from: Guzzetta C, Dossey B: Cardiovascular nursing: Holistic practice. St. Louis, MO: Mosby-Year Book, 1992, p. 9.

TABLE 2–7. PHYSIOLOGIC EFFECTS OF AGING

BODY SYSTEM	EFFECTS
Nervous	Diminished hearing and vision, short-term memory loss, altered motor coordination, decreased muscle tone and strength, slower response to verbal and motor stimuli, decreased ability to synthesize new information, increased sensitivity to altered temperature states, increased sensitivity to sedation (confusion or agitation), decreased alertness levels.
Cardiovascular	Increased effects of atherosclerosis of vessels and heart valves, decreased stroke volume with resulting decreased cardiac output, decreased myocardial compliance, increased workload of heart, diminished peripheral pulses.
Respiratory	Decreased compliance and elasticity, decreased vital capacity, increased residual volume, less effective cough, decreased response to hypercapnia.
Renal	Decreased glomerular filtration rate, increased risk of fluid and electrolyte imbalances.
Gastrointestinal	Increased presence of dentation problems, decreased intestinal mobility, decreased hepatic metabolism, increased risk of altered nutritional states.
Endocrine, Hematologic, and Immunologic	Increased incidence of diabetes, thyroid disorders, and anemia; decreased antibody response and cellular immunity.
Integumentary	Decreased skin turgor, increased capillary fragility and bruising, decreased elasticity.
Miscellaneous	Altered pharmacokinetics and pharmacodynamics, decreased range of motion of joints and extremities.
Psychosocial	Difficulty falling asleep and fragmented sleep patterns, increased incidence of depression and anxiety, cognitive impairment disorders, difficulty with change.

and duration of use. Honest information regarding alcohol and substance abuse, however, may not be always forthcoming. Family and/or friends might provide additional information that might assist in assessing these parameters.

Physical Assessment by Body System

The physical assessment section is presented in the sequence in which the combined system, head-to-toe approach is followed. Though content is presented as separate components, generally the history questions are integrated into the physical assessment. The physical assessment section uses the techniques of inspection, auscultation, and palpation. Though percussion is a common technique in physical examinations, it is infrequently used in critically ill patients.

Pain assessment is generally linked to each body system rather than considered as a separate system category.

TABLE 2–8. IDENTIFICATION OF SYMPTOM CHARACTERISTICS

Characteristic	Sample Questions
Onset	How and under what circumstances did it begin? Was the onset sudden or gradual? Did it progress?
Location	Where is it? Does it stay in the same place or does it radiate or move around?
Frequency	How often does it occur?
Quality	How intense is the discomfort? Is it dull, sharp, burning, throbbing, etc.?
Quantity	How long does it last?
Setting	What were you doing when it happened?
Associated findings	Are there other signs and symptoms that occur when this happens?
Aggravating and alleviating factors	What things make it worse? What things make it better?

For example, if the patient has chest pain, assessment and documentation of that pain is incorporated into the cardiovascular assessment. Rather than have general pain assessment questions repeated under each system assessment, they are presented here.

Pain and discomfort are clues that alert both the patient and the critical care nurse that something is wrong and needs attention. Pain assessment includes differentiating acute from chronic pain, determining related physiologic symptoms, and investigating the patient's perceptions and emotional reactions to the pain. Explore the qualities and characteristics of the pain by using the questions listed in Table 2–8. Pain is a very subjective assessment and critical care practitioners sometime struggle with applying their own values when attempting to evaluate the patient's pain. To resolve this dilemma, use the patient's own words and descriptions of the pain whenever possible and use a pain scale (Chapter 7, Pain Management) to objectively and consistently evaluate pain levels.

Nervous System

The nervous system is the "master computer" of all systems and is divided into the central and peripheral nervous systems. With the exception of the peripheral nervous system's cranial nerves, almost all attention in the critically ill patient is focused on evaluating the central nervous system (CNS). The physiologic and psychologic impact of critical illness, in addition to pharmacologic interventions, frequently alters CNS functioning.

The single most important indicator of cerebral functioning is the LOC. The LOC is assessed in the critically ill patient using the Glasgow Coma Scale (Chapter 15, Neurological System).

Assess pupils for size, shape, symmetry and reactivity to direct light. When interpreting the implication of altered pupil size, remember that certain medications such as atropine or morphine may affect pupil size. Baseline pupil assessment is important even in patients without a neurologic diagnosis since some individuals have unequal or unreactive pupils normally. If pupils are not checked as a baseline, a later check of pupils during an acute event could inappropriately attribute pupil abnormalities to a pathophysiologic event.

Level of consciousness and pupil assessments are followed by motor function assessment of the upper and lower extremities for symmetry and quality of strength. Traditional motor strength exercises include having the patient squeeze the nurse's hands and plantar flexing and dorsiflexing of the patient's feet. If the patient cannot follow commands, an estimate of strength and quality of movements can be inferred by observing activities such as pulling against restraints or thrashing around. Also note the size, shape, symmetry, and tone of muscles. If the patient has no voluntary movement or is unresponsive, check the gag, corneal, and Babinski reflexes.

If head trauma is involved or suspected, check for signs of fluid leakage around the nose or ears, differentiating between cerebral spinal fluid and blood (Chapter 15, Neurological System). Complete cranial nerve assessment is rarely warranted, with specific cranial nerve evaluation based on the injury or diagnosis. For example, extraocular movements are routinely assessed in patients with facial trauma. Sensory testing is a baseline standard for spinal cord injuries, extremity trauma, and epidural analgesia.

Laboratory data pertinent to the nervous system include serum and urine electrolytes and osmolarity and urinary specific gravity. Drug toxicology and alcohol levels may be evaluated to rule out potential sources of altered LOC. If the patient has an intracranial pressure monitoring device in place, note the type of device (e.g., ventriculostomy, epidural, subdural) and analyze the baseline pressure and waveform. Check all diagnostic values and monitoring system data to determine if immediate intervention is warranted.

Cardiovascular System

Cardiovascular system assessment factors are directed at evaluating central and peripheral perfusion. Revalidate your admission quick check assessment of the blood pressure, heart rate, and rhythm. Assess the ECG for ST segment changes and determine the PR, QRS, and QT intervals and the QT_c measurements. Note any abnormalities or indications of myocardial damage, electrical conduction problems, and/or electrolyte imbalances. Note the pulse pressure and any orthostatic changes. If treatment decisions will be based on the cuff pressure, blood pressure is taken in both arms. If a 10 to 15 mmHg difference exists, future blood pressures must be taken in the same arm. If a different arm is used inconsistently, changes in blood pressure might be inappropriately attributed to physiologic changes rather than anatomical differences.

TABLE 2–9. EDEMA RATING SCALE

Following the application and removal of firm digital pressure against the tissue, the edema is evaluated for one of the following responses:

- 0 No depression in tissue
- +1 Small depression in tissue, disappearing in less than 1 second
- +2 Depression in tissue disappears in less than 1 to 2 seconds
- +3 Depression in tissue disappears in less than 2 to 3 seconds
- +4 Depression in tissue disappears in 4 seconds or longer

Note the color and temperature of the skin, with particular emphasis on lips, mucous membranes, and distal extremities. Also evaluate nail color and capillary refill. Inspect for the presence of edema, particularly in the dependent parts of the body such as feet, ankles, and sacrum. If edema is present, rate the quality of edema by using a 0 to +4 scale (Table 2–9). Inspect the jugular veins for the presence or absence of distension.

Auscultate heart sounds for S_1 and S_2 quality, intensity, and pitch, and for the presence of extra heart sounds, murmurs, clicks, and/or rubs. Listen to one sound at a time, consistently progressing through the key anatomical landmarks of the heart each time. Note whether there are any changes with respiration or patient position.

While still at the chest, palpate for the apical impulse or point of maximum impulse (PMI), the only normal pulsation expected on the chest wall. The PMI's location, size, and character are important qualities to record. Note also the location, amplitude, duration, distribution, and timing in the cardiac cycle of abnormal pulsations such as heaves, lifts, and thrills. While palpating the chest, note any areas of tenderness.

Palpate the peripheral pulses for amplitude and quality, using the 0 to +4 scale (Table 2–10). Check all pulses simultaneously, except the carotid, comparing each pulse to its partner. If the pulse is difficult to palpate, an ultrasonic (Doppler) device should be used. To facilitate finding a weak pulse for subsequent assessments, mark the location of the pulse with an indelible pen.

Electrolyte levels, complete blood counts (CBCs), coagulation studies, and lipid profiles are common laboratory tests evaluated for abnormalities of the cardiovascular system. Cardiac enzyme levels are obtained for any complaint of chest pain or suspected chest trauma. Drug levels of commonly used cardiovascular medications, such as digoxin or Pronestyl, may be warranted for certain types of dysrhythmias. A 12-lead ECG is evaluated on all patients

TABLE 2–10. PERIPHERAL PULSE RATING SCALE

- 0 Absent pulse
- +1 Palpable but thready; easily obliterated with light pressure
- +2 Normal; cannot obliterate with light pressure
- +3 Full
- +4 Full and bounding

with complaints of chest pain, irregular rhythms, or suspected myocardial bruising from trauma (Chapter 21, Advanced ECG Concepts).

Note the type, size, and location of intravenous (IV) catheters, and verify the patency of the catheters. If continuous infusions of medications such as vasopressors or antidysrhythmics are being administered, ensure that they are being infused into an appropriately sized vessel and are compatible with any piggybacked IV solution.

Verify all monitoring system alarm parameters as active with appropriate limits set. Note the size and location of invasive monitoring lines such as arterial, central venous, and pulmonary artery (PA) catheters. For PA catheters, note the size of the introducer and the size (centimeters) marking where the catheter exits the introducer. Interpret hemodynamic pressure readings against normals and with respect to the patient's underlying pathophysiology. Assess waveforms to determine the quality of the waveform (e.g., dampened or hyperresonant) and whether the waveform appropriately matches the expected characteristics for the anatomic placement of the invasive catheter (Chapter 5, Hemodynamic Monitoring). For example, a right ventricular waveform for a central venous pressure line indicates a problem with the position of the central venous line that needs to be corrected. If the pulmonary artery catheter has continuous mixed venous saturation (Svo_2) capabilities and/or continuous cardiac output data, these numbers are also evaluated in conjunction with vital sign data and any pharmacologic and/or volume infusions.

Respiratory System

Oxygenation and ventilation are the focal basis of respiratory assessment parameters. Revalidate the rate and rhythm of respirations and the symmetry of chest wall movement. If the patient has a productive cough or secretions are suctioned from an artificial airway, note the color, consistency, and amount of secretions. Evaluate whether the trachea is midline or shifted. Inspect the thoracic cavity for shape, anterior-posterior diameter, and structural deformities (e.g., kyphosis or scoliosis). Palpate for equal chest excursion, presence of crepitus, and any areas of tenderness or fractures. If the patient is receiving supplemental oxygen, verify the mode of delivery and percentage of oxygen against physician orders.

Auscultate anterior and posterior bilateral breath sounds to determine the presence of air movement and the presence of adventitious sounds such as crackles or wheezes. Note the quality and depth of respirations, and the length and pitch of the inspiratory and expiratory phases.

Arterial blood gases (ABGs) are frequently used diagnostic tests to assess for both interpretation of oxygenation, ventilatory status, and acid/base balance. Hemoglobin and hematocrit values are interpreted for impact on oxygenation and fluid balance. If the patient's condition warrants, the

oxygen saturation values may be continuously monitored via connection to a noninvasive oxygen saturation monitor or Svo_2 pulmonary artery catheter monitoring device.

If the patient is intubated, note the size of the tube and record the centimeter marking at the teeth or nares to assist future comparisons for proper placement. If the patient is connected to a mechanical ventilator, verify the ventilatory mode, tidal volume, respiratory rate, positive end expiratory pressure, and percentage of oxygen against prescribed settings. Observe whether the patient has spontaneous breaths, noting both the rate and average tidal volume of each breath. Note the amount of pressure required to ventilate the patient for later comparisons to determine changes in pulmonary compliance. If available, continuous end tidal CO_2 is integrated into the respiratory picture and compared to the ABGs.

If chest tubes are present, assess the area around the insertion site for crepitus. Note the amount and color of drainage and whether an air leak is present. Verify whether the chest tube drainage system is under water seal or connected to suction.

Renal System

Urinary characteristics and electrolyte status are the major parameters used to evaluate the function of the kidneys. In conjunction with the cardiovascular system, the renal system's impact on the fluid volume status is also assessed.

Most critically ill patients have a Foley catheter in place to evaluate hourly urinary output. Note the amount and color of the urine and assess a sample for the abnormal presence of glucose, protein, and blood. Inspect the genitalia for inflammation, swelling, ulcers, and drainage. If suprapubic tubes or a ureterostomy are present, note the position and the amount and characteristics of the drainage. Observe whether any drainage is leaking around the drainage tube.

In addition to the urinalysis, serum electrolyte levels, blood urea nitrogen (BUN), creatinine, and urinary and serum osmolarity are common diagnostic tests used to evaluate the functioning of the kidneys.

Gastrointestinal System

The key factors when reviewing the gastrointestinal system are the nutritional and fluid status. Inspect the abdomen for overall symmetry, noting whether the contour is flat, round, protuberant, or distended. Note the presence of discoloration or striae. The nutritional status is evaluated by looking at the patient's weight and muscle tone, the condition of the oral mucosa, and laboratory values such as serum albumin and transferrin.

Auscultation of bowel sounds should be done in all four quadrants in a clockwise order, noting the frequency and presence or absence of sounds. Bowel sounds are usually rated as absent, hypoactive, normal, or hyperactive. Before noting absent bowel sounds, a quadrant should be listened to for at least 60 to 90 seconds. Characteristics and frequency of the sounds are noted. After listening for the presence of normal sounds, determine if any adventitious bowel sounds such as friction rubs, bruits, or hums are present.

Palpation of the abdomen is not consistently done, but light palpation helps determine areas of tenderness, pain, and guarding or rebound tenderness. Remember to auscultate before palpating because palpation may change the frequency and character of the patient's peristaltic sounds.

Assess any drainage tube for location and function, and for the characteristics of any drainage. Validate the proper placement of the nasogastric tube by using a catheter-tip syringe to instill about 20 to 30 ml of air while using a stethoscope to listen over the stomach for the swooshing sound of the air. Assess nasogastric secretions for pH and occult blood. Check every emesis and stool for occult blood. Evaluate ostomies for location, color of the stoma, and the type of drainage.

Endocrine, Hematologic and Immune Systems

The endocrine, hematologic, and immune systems often are overlooked when assessing critically ill patients. The assessment parameters used to evaluate these systems are included under other system assessments, but it is important to consciously consider these systems when reviewing these parameters. Assessing the endocrine, hematologic, and immune systems is based on a thorough understanding of the primary function of each of the hormones, blood cells, or immune components of each of the respective systems.

Assessing the specific functions of the endocrine system's hormones is challenging because much of the symptomatology related to the hyposecretion or hypersecretion of the hormones can be found with other systems' problems. The patient's history may help differentiate the source, but any abnormal assessment findings detected with regard to fluid balance, metabolic rate, altered LOC, color and temperature of the skin, electrolytes, glucose, and acid-base balance require the critical care nurse to consider the potential involvement of the endocrine system. For example, are the signs and symptoms of hypervolemia related to cardiac insufficiency or excessive amounts of antidiuretic hormone (ADH)? Tests for specific hormone levels may be required to rule out involvement of the endocrine system.

Assessment parameters specific to the hematologic system include laboratory evaluation of the red blood cells (RBCs) and coagulation studies. Diminished RBCs may affect the oxygen-carrying capacity of the blood as evidenced by pallor, cyanosis, light-headedness, tachypnea, and tachycardia. Insufficient clotting factors are evidenced by bruising, oozing of blood from puncture sites or mucous membranes, or overt bleeding.

The immune system's function of fighting infection is assessed by evaluating the white cell and differential counts from the CBC, and assessing puncture sites and mucous membranes for oozing drainage and/or inflamed, reddened areas. Spiking or persistent low-grade temperatures often are indicative of infections. It is important to keep in mind, however, that many critically ill patients have impaired immune systems and the normal response to infection, such as white pus around an insertion site, may not be evident.

Integumentary System

The skin is the first line of defense against infection so assessment parameters are focused on evaluating the intactness of the skin. Assessing the skin can be integrated while performing other system assessments. For example, while listening to breath sounds or bowel sounds, the condition of the thoracic cavity or abdominal skin can be observed, respectively.

Inspect the skin for overall integrity, color, temperature, and turgor. Note the presence of rashes, striae, discoloration, scars, or lesions. For any abrasions, lesions, or wounds, note the size, depth, and presence or absence of drainage.

Psychosocial Assessment

The rapid physiologic and psychologic changes associated with critical illnesses, coupled with pharmacologic and biologic treatments, can profoundly affect behavior. Patients are suffering illnesses that have psychologic responses which are predictable, and, if untreated, may threaten recovery or life. To avoid making assumptions about how a patient feels about his or her care, there is no substitute for asking the patient directly or asking a collateral informant, such as the family or significant other.

Mental Status

Components of mental status include mood, perception, attitude, thought, speech, orientation, memory, attention, judgment, insight, and capacity for abstraction. Assessment of these components is reflected through the patient's verbal responses to probing questions. Probes to assist you when assessing mental status are summarized in Table 2–11. As you ask the questions, observe for eye contact, pressured or muted speech, and rate of speech. Rate of speech is usually consistent with the patient's psychomotor status.

General Communication

Communication is the primary means by which a patient influences, or is influenced by, another person. Factors that affect communication include culture, developmental stage, physical condition, stress, perception, poor self-concept, neurocognitive deficits, emotional state, and language skills. The nature of a critical illness, coupled with pharmacologic and airway technologies, interferes with the patients' usual methods of communication. It is essential to determine preillness communication methods and styles to ensure optimal communication with the critically ill patient and family. The inability of many critically ill patients to verbally communicate necessitates that critical care practitioners become expert at assessing nonverbal clues to determine important

TABLE 2–11. TIPS FOR ASSESSING MENTAL STATUS

The following probes can be used to assess mental status:
- My name is _____.
- How do you like others to address you? Can you tell me what hospital you are in? (Orientation).
- Where's home? What did you last eat? (Orientation and memory)
- What is my name? (Short-term memory)
- Name five things that start with the letter D. (Attention)
- If your IV tube starts leaking, what would you do? (Abstraction)
- What do you understand is your trouble? (Insight and perception)
- What are your concerns? Do you think you have done some terrible thing to cause your illness? Have you had the feeling that people know what you are thinking? (Thought and speech)
- You sound as though you're not sure I can help you. (Attitude, guarded)
- I hear irritability in your talk. Would you agree? (Mood and observe for affect)

information from, and needs of, patients. Important assessment data is gained by observation of body gestures, facial expressions, eye movements, involuntary movements, and changes in physiologic parameters, particularly heart rate, blood pressure, and respiratory rate. Often, these nonverbal behaviors may be more reflective of the patients' actual feelings, particularly if they are denying symptoms and attempting to be the "good patient" by not complaining.

Communication is also the primary vehicle for teaching patients and families. Determining how they can learn best will be important for future teaching sessions, as well as for information supplied prior to beginning instruction. For some individuals, knowledge is control, while others may be overwhelmed with medical terminology or the sick role, or not value participation in their care, preferring to be passive or dependent. Assessment of factors that may impair learning (e.g., anxiety, delirium, cognitive processing limitations, fatigue, demoralization, past experiences, values, culture, mourning) should also be considered.

Coping Styles

Individuals vary in the manner in which they cope with stress. Assess with the family previous resources, coping skills, or defense mechanisms that strengthen their adaptation or problem-solving resolution. Examples might include alternative medicine practices such as biofeedback for pain, withdrawal or dissociation to manage a procedure, and silence to minimize rehashing of conflict. It is most important to understand the meaning assigned to the event by the patient/family and the purpose the coping defense serves. Does the coping resource fit with the event and meet the patient/family need?

Family Relations Needs

The concept of family is not simple today and extends beyond the nuclear family to any loving, supportive person regardless of social and legal boundaries. Identify the

important people in the patient's kinship/friendship network. Critical care practitioners need to be flexible around traditional legal boundaries of "next of kin" so that communication is extended to, and sought from, surrogate decision makers and whomever the patient designates.

The family is an extension of the patient and shares many of the same emotional needs and behaviors. Personal emotional concerns for the family include feelings of guilt, anger, changing role in the family, and anxiety about the future. Some family members will feel guilty because of something they did or failed to do, angry at the patient for being so ill, or guilty for wishing their loved one would die to end the suffering.

Each family system is unique and varies by culture, values, religion, previous experience with crisis, composition, structure, language, socioeconomic status, psychological integrity, role expectations, communication patterns, health beliefs, and ages. Areas of assessment include:

- Who is "family"?
- What is the impact of illness on the family?
- What are the cultural practices, religious influences, and values important to the family?
- What are their perceptions and expectations of the critical care staff and of the setting?
- What are their crisis or coping skills?
- What are current or past stressors?
- What are the communication patterns among the family?
- What social supports and networks are used?
- What are the learning styles of family members?

ONGOING ASSESSMENT

After the admission quick check and the comprehensive admission assessments are completed, all subsequent assessments are used to determine trends, evaluate response to therapy, and identify new potential problems and/or changes from the comprehensive baseline assessment. The frequency of ongoing assessments is driven by the stability of the patient; however, routine periodic assessments are the norm. For example, ongoing assessments can occur every few minutes for extremely unstable patients to every 2 to 4 hours for very stable patients. Assessments should be done when any of the following situations occur:

1. When caregivers change
2. Before and after any major procedural intervention, such as intubation or chest tube insertion
3. Before and after transport out of the critical care unit for diagnostic procedures or other events
4. Deterioration in physiologic or mental status

As with the admission quick check, the ongoing assessment section is offered as a generic template that can be used as a basis for all patients (Table 2–12). More

TABLE 2–12. ONGOING ASSESSMENT TEMPLATE

Body System	Assessment Parameters
Nervous	• LOC • Pupils • Motor strength of extremities
Cardiovascular	• Blood pressure • Heart rate and rhythm • Heart sounds • Capillary refill • Peripheral pulses • Patency of IVs • Verification of IV solutions and medications • Hemodynamic pressures and waveforms • Cardiac output data
Respiratory	• Respiratory rate and rhythm • Breath sounds • Color and amount of secretions • Noninvasive technology information (e.g., pulse oximetry, end-tidal CO_2) • Mechanical ventilatory parameters • Arterial and venous blood gases
Renal	• Intake and output • Color and amount of urinary output • BUN/creatinine values
Gastrointestinal	• Bowel sounds • Contour of abdomen • Position of drainage tubs • Color and amount of secretions • Bilirubin and albumin values
Endocrine, Hematologic, and Immunologic	• Fluid balance • Electrolyte and glucose values • CBC and coagulation values • Temperature • WBC with differential count
Integumentary	• Color and temperature of skin • Intactness of skin • Areas of redness
Pain/discomfort	• Assessed in each system
Psychosocial	• Mental status and behavioral responses • Reaction to critical illness experience (e.g., stress, anxiety, coping, mood) • Presence of cognitive impairments (dementia, delirium), depression, or demoralization • Family functioning and needs • Ability to communicate needs and participate in care • Sleep patterns

in-depth and system-specific assessment parameters are added based on the patient's diagnosis and pathophysiologic problems.

ASSESSMENT OF COMMON BEHAVIORAL ALTERATIONS DURING CRITICAL ILLNESS: ANXIETY AND COGNITIVE IMPAIRMENT

A variety of biobehavioral alterations, most of which occur after 1 to 2 days of a critical illness, are common in critically ill patients. Anxiety and cognitive impairments related

to, or as a response to, the underlying physiologic condition can be difficult to identify. Recognizing these abnormalities is important to decrease morbidity and mortality of the critical illness, since most cause an increase in physiologic demand. The following section summarizes the characteristics and assessment findings of some of the most common forms of anxiety and cognitive and mood impairments in the critically ill patient.

Anxiety and Stress

Protracted stress, as with chronic illness, affects the general adaptation syndrome in maladaptive ways. Areas to assess are:

- *Physical.* Sweating, headaches, dyspnea, hyperventilation, tachycardia, dry mouth, nausea, dizziness, anorexia, grinding teeth, choking sensation, increased urination, fatigue, and sleep disruption
- *Cognitive.* Difficulty with memory, poor concentration, fearful anticipation, and future preoccupation
- *Emotional.* Restlessness, irritability to rage, tension, worry, inability to relax, and depression
- *Behavioral.* Crying, avoidance, restlessness, strained facial expression, acting out, demanding, whining, and being more self-centered or manipulative
- *Social.* Withdrawn and disruptive

The level of anxiety that promotes pathologic consequences is the subjective identification of a perception or threat that is unrealistic or exaggerated, given the reality of the situation. The critical care setting may force isolation from social supports, dependency, loss of control, trust in unknown care providers, helplessness, and an inability to problem-solve or attend. Generalized anxiety will be characterized by excessive worry, or apprehensive expectation, motor tension, and autonomic hyperactivity. Cultural expression may be a factor in the exaggerated or diminished communication of anxiety. Intense sighing, yawning, and hyperventilation are cues of anxiety. Restlessness, distractibility, and unrealistic demands for attention are warning signs of escalating anxiety. Anxiety is both psychologically and physiologically exhausting. Being in a prolonged state of arousal is hard work and uses adaptive reserves needed for recovery.

Medications such as interferon, digitalis, corticosteroids, angiotensin-converting enzyme (ACE) inhibitors, and vasopressors can induce anxiety. Abrupt withdrawal from benzodiazepines, caffeine, nicotine, and narcotics, as well as akathisia from phenothiazines, may mimic anxiety. Additional etiologic variables associated with anxiety include pain, sleep loss, delirium, hypoxia, ventilator synchronization or weaning, fear of death, loss of control, high-technology equipment, and a dehumanizing setting. Admission to or repeated transfers to the critical care unit may also induce anxiety.

Denial, delusions, distortions, acting out, regression, dissociation, and repression are ways the self tries to minimize perceived danger or relieve anxiety. Perception is a person's reality. Defense mechanisms are adaptive if they assist the patient or family to cope. If the defense mechanism fails or becomes too rigid, then it is maladaptive.

Although individuals will cope with a critical illness in different ways, their preillness coping style, personality traits, or temperament will assist you in anticipating coping styles in the critical care setting. Persons who are stoic by personality or culture usually present as the "good" patient. Assess for behaviors of not wanting to "bother" the busy staff or not admitting pain because family or others are nearby. Review with the family the patient's preillness temperament and preillness presence of anger, lack of assertiveness, shyness, lack of meaning or commitment, feeling out of control, dependency, suspiciousness, or impatience; self-sacrificing, controlling, and superiority behaviors may be risk factors for mistrust, low self-esteem, anxiety, guilt, lack of intimacy, and hopelessness.

A challenge in the critical care setting is "manipulative" behavior. This behavior is common to all of us as we seek to get our needs met. We must understand that impulsivity, deception, low frustration tolerance, unreliability, superficial charm, splitting among the provider team, heavier use of pain medication, and general avoidance of rules or limits are modes of interacting and coping and attempts to feel safe. Lack of caring positive relationships, powerlessness, lack of self-trust, or avoidance of discomfort (anxiety) challenge personal growth and are antecedents of manipulation. If the nurse recognizes dislike or negative feelings toward a patient, that could be a cue of the discomfort the patient is experiencing.

Powerlessness is a variation of an anxious perception that the patient is helpless to control or change an outcome. Medical procedures are often repeated, painful, and intrusive, with the patient having little or no consent over their occurrence or intensity. The family shares this concept, as reflected by such frustrated phrases as "What can I do?, What do I know?, Can others help?" Blaming others or God, pessimism, never taking charge, fatalism, or giving up are other indicators of powerlessness.

Fear has an identifiable source and has an important role in self-development. Treatments, procedures, pain, and separation are common objects of fear. The dying process elicits specific fears, such as fear of the unknown, loneliness, loss of body, loss of self-control, suffering, pain, loss of identity, and loss of everyone loved by the patient. The family, as well as the patient, experiences the grieving process, which includes the phases of denial, shock, anger, bargaining, depression, and acceptance. Usually, no two individuals are experiencing the same emotional reactions of grief at the same time; thus assessment will vary with each unique individual. Additionally, the dying process involves the intrapsychic response and beliefs of the individual who is dying, the bodily changes that impact self-esteem, and the family roles and functioning. The care provider system may have its own philosophies that impact the dying process, such as self-deliverance versus maintenance of life support, visitation policies, or organ donation.

Cognitive Impairment

Common to most critical care settings are the "D" syndrome problems—dementia, delirium, depression, and demoralization.

Dementia

Dementia, or impairment in global cognitive function, memory, and personality, usually occurs without sensorium disturbance (level of alertness or consciousness). The syndrome develops slowly and is often overlooked or attributed to the normal aging process. Early symptoms of personality change, apathy, and labile emotions progress to recent memory impairment, loss of social skills, or the need for supervision with activities of daily living (ADL). Dementia in critical care units is found in patients who have a premorbid syndrome, such as HIV infection of the CNS. Dementia does not typically have its onset during the critical care stay, but is exacerbated by conditions common during a critical illness, such as trauma, increased anxiety or agitation (often associated with physical restraints), medication reactions, anorexia, and metabolic changes.

Delirium

The best predictor for delirium is prior delirium. The onset is rapid (over hours or days) and evidenced by disorientation, confusion, perceptual disturbance, psychomotor changes (restlessness), distractibility, and sleep-wake cycle disturbances. The syndrome fluctuates over a 24-hour period so assessment results may vary with each shift. Delirium is most common in postsurgical and elderly patients and is the most common cause of disruptive behavior. The mislabeled "ICU psychosis" is not a psychosis but a delirium. Risk factors that contribute to delirium include sensory underload (or deprivation) and overload.

Sensory underload includes isolation, confinement, lack of information, loss of 24-hour rhythm, and lack of perceptual stimulation. The patient may verbalize the symptoms as loss of time, boredom, restlessness, fear, or having psychotic or depressive symptoms. The patient may withdraw and minimize contact with staff to conceal his or her changing mental status. Staff often interpret this early phase of delirium as depression.

Sensory overload usually falls within the categories of (1) noises: monitors, mechanical ventilators, data printing machines, staff talking, visitors, televisions; (2) sights: procedures on other patients, families visiting, bodies covered for the morgue, uncovered patients, medical rounds, emergency admissions; (3) smells: cleaning chemicals, medications, body fluids and decay, food odors; and (4) constant interaction.

A disrupted sleep-wake cycle with patients drifting in and out of sleep renders them vulnerable to delusions or misperceptions (an IV pole looks like a person) and unable to distinguish reality from dreams. Cessation or rapid withdrawal of benzodiazepines or narcotics can also lead to delirium or severe anxiety. Patients who manifest delusions are often assumed to have a psychiatric illness, but with more refined assessment of the delusions, one finds an organic delusional syndrome which may remit as the medical condition improves. Persecutory delusions are the most common, and the syndrome includes lack of insight, poor concentration, flat affect, impaired sensorium, disorganized thoughts, and hallucinations (of smell, taste, or touch). In organic brain syndromes, the long-standing personality traits often become exaggerated. For example, a person with a history of abusive behavior becomes angry and aggressive while in isolation with diminished controls. Knowing the preillness temperament may assist in predicting the behavioral response.

Depression

Depression co-occurring with a medical illness affects the long-term recovery outcomes by lengthening the course of the illness and increasing morbidity and mortality. Risk factors that predispose for depression with medical disorders include social isolation, recent loss, pessimism, financial pressures, history of mood disorder, alcohol or substance abuse/withdrawal, previous suicide attempts, and pain. Depressive syndromes include somatic symptoms (weight loss, appetite change, sleep disturbance, fatigue), cognitive symptoms (fear, hopelessness, self-pity, negativity, poor concentration), and behavioral symptoms (depressed affect, apathy, pessimism, unreactive mood). If psychotic symptoms accompany the depression, the delusional content is commonly experienced as punishment for an unforgivable sin. Asking significant others or previous providers about a prior history of depression will minimize the time lag in obtaining a psychiatric evaluation or referral and maximize interventions. If you suspect a patient is suicidal or preoccupied with death, inquire about feelings of hopelessness, wanting to die, activation of advance directives when medical alternatives are positive, or refusal to participate in medical regimens. These probes will let the patient know you are listening, tuned into his or her feelings, care, and can tolerate despair that is symptomatic of the here and now. Asking about suicidal thoughts will not cause them to feel suicidal.

Depressive symptoms can also appear as pseudodementia, evidenced by faulty memory, complaints, irritabil-

ity, poor cognition, and little energy to perform tasks. Key features in assessment to distinguish pseudodementia from depression include short duration of symptoms, complaints of cognitive loss in detail, distress with loss, memory gaps for specific events, good attention, answering questions with "I don't know," loss of social skills, dominant mood change, and history of previous psychiatric disorder. Assessment criteria to contrast the syndromes of dementia, delirium, and depression are summarized in Table 2–13.

Demoralization

Lack of enthusiasm, diminished confidence, discouragement, or dispiritedness reflect the demoralization that often accompanies chronic illness or trauma. Social isolation and alienation, along with cognitive impairment or perceived distortions, provide the potential for the patient to experience an assault on the sense of self. How often have you heard a patient ask, "Who am I? Is it worth it? Why go on?" Often overlooked is the emotional impact of body image change or physical damage caused by illness or trauma and others' response. Today's culture places emphasis on physical appearance. The "emotional" scarring of a mastectomy can be more impairing than the loss of the breast. The loss of a body part can result in depression, isolation, low self-

TABLE 2–13. ASSESSMENT CRITERIA TO DIFFERENTIATE DEMENTIA, DELIRIUM, AND DEPRESSION

	Dementia	Delirium	Depression
Prodrome	Irritable, confused, forgetful	Restless, irritable	Withdrawn, guilty, sleep disturbance
Course	Slow onset over time	Rapid onset, waxes and wanes	Usually over time, may be recurrent episodes
Orientation	Not affected until late in course	Disoriented to place and time	Oriented
Perception	Usually intact	Illusions, delusions (smell, taste, touch)	Delusions (guilt, sin, worthlessness)
Communication	Slowed	Incoherent	Decreased rate and volume
Cognition	Altered, decreased ability to problem-solve	Disorganized, cannot comprehend	Slowed, negative ruminations
Memory	Not affected	Insomnia, daytime fatigue	Middle and terminal insomnia
Psychomotor	Mixed	Agitated, pulls tubing	Agitated, retardation
Mood	Depressed or labile	Labile or anxious	Depressed

esteem, insecurity, poor communication, conflict, avoidance of physical intimacy, and dependence. The patient will need help in making peace with his or her altered body. The patient in a critical care unit constantly confronts loss, change, and sometimes life and death.

AT THE BEDSIDE
■ *Thinking Critically*

A 37-year-old white male with non-Hodgkins lymphoma is admitted to the ICU for labored breathing and an elevated temperature 1 week after a stem-cell transplant. He complained of severe mouth pain and nightmares and was questioning if he wanted the "torture" to continue. He was given morphine sulphate 10 mg/h IV for 24 hours, then 4 mg/h IV for 24 hours, and finally 2 mg/h IV. He continued with irritability, was verbally abusive to family and staff, and had fragmented sleep. On the third day he became agitated and tried to pull out his IV. That evening he told the family that "they" had killed the man next to him and were trying to do the same to him. During report the next morning the nurses reported he was oriented, alert, and less difficult, tense, restless, and irritable, following lorazepam 1 mg IV every 6 hours for three doses. After assessing the patient at noon, the nurse noted that the patient couldn't follow instructions, was trying to get out of bed, didn't know where he was or who he was, and was muttering about the murders. What would you conclude from these data?

SELECTED BIBLIOGRAPHY

What Heals: Spirituality

Burkhardt M: Spirituality: An analysis of the concept. *Holistic Nursing Practice*. 1989;3:69–77.

Clark C, Heidenreich T: Spiritual care for the critically ill. *American Journal of Critical Care*. 1995;4:77.

Patient Rights: Accreditation Manual for Hospitals (Suppl). Chicago: Joint Commission on Accreditation of Healthcare Organizations, 1992.

Critical Care Assessment

Alpen MA, Halm MA: Family needs: An annotated bibliography. *Critical Care Nurse*. 1994;12(2):32–51.

Barry PD: *Psychosocial nursing assessment and intervention: Care of the physically ill person*, 2d ed. Philadelphia: JB Lippincott, 1989.

Bates B: *A guide to physical examination*, 6th ed. Philadelphia: JB Lippincott, 1995.

Bone RC: *Recognition, assessment, and treatment of anxiety in the critical care patient: Proceedings of a consensus conference.* Yardley, PA: The Medicine Group USA, Inc., 1994.

Bosker G, Schwartz G, Jones J, Sequeira M: *Geriatric emergency medicine.* St. Louis, MO: Mosby-Year Book, 1990.

Folstein M, Folstein S, McHugh P: Mini-mental state: A practical method for grading the cognitive state of patients for the clinician. *Journal of Psychiatric Research.* 1975;12:189–198.

Goleman D, Gurin J (eds): *Mind body medicine: How to use your mind for better health.* Yonkers, NY: Consumer Report Books, 1993.

Timiras P (ed.): *Physiologic basis of aging and geriatrics*, 2d ed. Ann Arbor, MI: CRC Press, 1994.

Wright J, Shelton B. (eds): *Desk reference for critical care nursing.* Boston: Jones & Bartlett, 1993.

Planning Care for Critically Ill Patients and Families

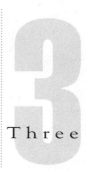

Three

► **Knowledge Competencies**

1. Discuss the importance of a multidisciplinary plan of care for optimizing clinical outcomes.
2. Describe common interventions in the care of critically ill patients with:
   • Altered nutritional status
   • Altered communication
   • Educational needs
   • Sleep pattern disturbances
   • Near-death experiences
3. Discuss interventions to maintain psychosocial integrity and minimize anxiety for the critically ill patient and family members.

■ *What Heals: Family Presence During Resuscitation*

Family presence during resuscitation is an emotionally charged topic among health care providers. In most hospitals, family members are prohibited from being present during resuscitation. But why do we deny access to the family? What are the problems involved? What might be the possible benefits to families as well as patients if they were allowed to be present? Consider the following case study:*

> *Nurse:* "I answered a code page for the cardiac ICU and asked how I could help. One of the nurses asked me to take care of the family. The patient's wife told me she was a nurse and that she just had to be with her husband. I went back to the code and talked with the cardiologist and the rest of the team. My head knew we'd never done this before. But my heart kept asking, 'Why not?'
> "On the way to the code, I explained what was going on to the patient's wife so she would know what to expect. With my arm

around her shoulder as an offering of support, I brought her to his side. She took his hand and talked to him the whole time, while everyone else did what they were supposed to.
> "When it became obvious that we weren't going to save him, his wife already knew that everything possible had been done. She thanked us profusely for allowing her to be with him as he died. But she didn't need to say a word. The look in her eyes and the touch of her hand said it all."

A family presence movement appears to be developing slowly across the country. In 1993, for example, the General Assembly of the Emergency Nurses Association (ENA) approved a resolution endorsing family presence during invasive procedures and/or resuscitation. In response to this endorsement, the ENA has published an 84-page manual on developing and implementing a family presence program. The manual includes a review of the literature and guidelines for setting up and evaluating the program, as well as a section (which includes slides) on educating health care providers about the program.

From: Chulay M: Presidential address. 1993 AACN National Teaching Institute and Critical Care Exposition, New Orleans, May 1993.

The family presence movement also can be verified by the appearance of articles being published on the topic (see reference list). Several of these articles describe how family presence had been successfully started or positively accepted at hospitals in Vermont, Maryland, Nevada, Wisconsin, Oregon, California, and England. The pioneers in this area, based at Foote Memorial Hospital in Michigan, have been offering the option of family presence in their hospital for several years. They point out, however, that family presence during resuscitation is not appropriate for everyone (currently only about 40% of families participate in family presence at Foote Memorial Hospital).

When implementing a family presence program, it has been recommended that families of patients undergoing CPR first be assessed by a support person (chaplain or nurse) to determine whether their presence would be appropriate. If appropriate, families can be offered the option. If they decline, their decision is supported. If they want to participate, the support person needs to explain the patient's status and brief the family about what they will see and hear in the resuscitation environment, including the appearance of the patient and equipment, as well as the procedures being performed. Families need to understand that it is expected that they will not disturb or disrupt the resuscitation.

Following the briefing, the support person then escorts the family into the room, clearing a space at the head of the bed if possible, encouraging the family to talk to and touch the patient, and explaining that even though the patient is unconscious, he or she still may be able to hear. The support person stays with the family to explain procedures, answer questions, and provide emotional support. Following the visitation, the support person escorts the family back to the waiting room and stays with them to address any questions and concerns and to continue emotional support.

Getting started with a family presence program is not an easy task. It probably does not begin with any formal program and standardized policies. It likely begins with one nurse advocating for one family during an exemplary situation in which bringing a family member in during a code is indisputably the right thing to do. It probably is launched by a nurse who is empowered to read the situation correctly, confident in arguing the case, and skillful in convincing others to overturn conventional protocol to make it happen to preserve the wholeness, dignity, and integrity of the family unit from birth to death.

CEG & BMD

INTRODUCTION

The achievement of optimal clinical outcomes in the critically ill patient requires a coordinated approach to care delivery by multidisciplinary team members. Experts in nutrition, respiratory therapy, critical care nursing and medicine, psychiatry and social work, as well as other disciplines, must work collaboratively to effectively, and efficiently, provide optimal care.

The use of multidisciplinary plans of care, also referred to as critical or clinical pathways or Care Maps, is a useful approach to facilitate the coordination of a patient's care by the multidisciplinary team and optimize clinical outcomes. These multidisciplinary plans of care are being used increasingly to replace individual, discipline-specific plans of care. Each clinical condition presented in this text will discuss the management of patient needs or problems with an integrated, multidisciplinary approach.

The following section will provide an overview of critical pathways, their benefits, and the processes used in their development.

In addition, this chapter discusses common patient management approaches to needs or problems during critical illnesses which are not diagnosis-specific, but common to a majority of critically ill patients, such as sleep deprivation, inadequate nutrition, or patient/family education. Additional discussion of these needs or problems is also presented in other chapters if management is different or critical to disease management.

MULTIDISCIPLINARY PLAN OF CARE/CRITICAL PATHWAYS

A critical pathway is a set of expectations for the major components of care a patient should receive during his or her hospitalization to manage a specific medical or surgical problem. The critical pathway expands the concept of a medical or nursing care plan and provides a multidisciplinary, comprehensive blueprint for patient care. The result is a diagnosis-specific plan of care that focuses the entire multidisciplinary care team on patient outcomes.

The critical pathway outlines what tests, medications, care, and treatments are needed to discharge the patient in a timely manner with all patient outcomes met (Figure 3–1). Other titles used to describe this concept are clinical pathways, care maps, or multidisciplinary care plans. Although the titles and formats differ somewhat for each of these plans, their purposes are similar.

Critical pathways have a variety of benefits to both patients and the hospital system:

- Improved patient outcomes
- Increased quality and continuity of care
- Improved communication and collaboration
- Identification of hospital system problems
- Coordination of necessary services and reduced duplication
- Prioritization of activities
- Reduced length of stay (LOS) and health care costs

Critical Pathway Development

Critical pathways are developed by a multidisciplinary team of individuals who closely interact with a specific patient population. Diagnoses appropriate for critical pathways are selected for high-volume, high-risk, or problem-prone patient populations. The process of path development typically includes five stages: groundwork, team selection, team meetings, approval, and education/implementation.

The groundwork phase involves a review of past performance data (e.g., LOS, cost, complications) with a comparison to other institutions' performance and current literature on standards/guidelines of care for the selected diagnosis. The institution's current practice is outlined based on retrospective chart reviews. Team member selection is a critical phase of critical pathway development. The inclusion of representatives from each discipline involved in primary patient care management activities for that diagnostic group in the critical pathway team optimizes collaboration, coordination, and commitment to the pathway process. Representatives of disciplines commonly involved in pathway development include physicians, nurses, respiratory therapists, physical therapists, social workers, and dieticians.

During the next phase, team meetings are held to formulate the multidisciplinary plan of care that will be used to care for patients in the institution. The format for the critical pathway typically includes the following categories:

- Discharge outcomes
- Progression outcomes (e.g., pain control, activity level, absence of complications)
- Assessment and evaluation
- Consultations
- Tests
- Medications
- Diet
- Activity
- Elimination
- Education
- Discharge planning

The suggested activities within each of these categories are divided into daily activities or grouped into phases of the hospitalization (e.g., preoperative, intraoperative, and postoperative phases).

Critical pathways usually require approval from relevant multidisciplinary committees and physician groups. All staff members who will use the path will require education as to the specifics of the path.

Documentation

Critical pathways are used by a wide range of disciplines; the users include nurses, physicians, respiratory therapists, social workers, pharmacists, physical therapists, occupational therapists, speech therapists, and dieticians. As individuals assess and implement various aspects of the critical pathway, documentation occurs directly on the pathway.

Each item on the pathway is evaluated as met, unmet, or not applicable. The appropriate column is then initialed by the caregiver. Items on the critical pathway that are not completed typically are termed *variances*. Variances are deviations from the expected activities planned on the critical pathway. Events planned on the critical pathway that occur early are termed *positive variances. Negative variances* are those planned events which are not accomplished on time. Negative variances typically include items not completed due to the patient's condition, hospital system problems, or lack of orders.

Monthly or quarterly summaries of the critical pathways outcomes assist the pathway team to evaluate the overall plan of care and to target areas for improvement activities. Trending pathway data provides an objective method for evaluating patient outcomes for specific groups of patients.

Quality Improvement Activities

Critical pathways offer an excellent tool for the continuous monitoring of patient outcomes and processes of care for quality improvement (QI) activities. QI data are collected concurrently while the pathway is being completed. Patient outcomes such as pain, complications, education, or functional mobility can be documented individually on a single patient and later compiled to measure overall outcomes across a patient population. Specific variance information can also be analyzed to measure processes that affect

Clinical Pathway: Elective Angioplasty, Stent, Atherectomy or Rotablator

PROCEDURE M.D. _____

Expected LOS: 2.0 Days   A.M. Admit: Y ☐ N ☐   Page 1 of 2

	PRE-PROCEDURE	Met	Unmet	N/A	PROCEDURE DAY	Met	Unmet	N/A
Progression Outcomes	Knowledge of procedure/pre & post care				Puncture site = Level I on Groin Assessment Scale Pain controlled or absent			
	Labs within acceptable limits and on chart				Distal pulses equal to baseline			
Assessments Evaluations	VS per unit protocol				*Assess groin, pulses, and VS per orders			
	Pedal pulse present				Groin Assessment Scale: Level I ___ Level II ___ Level III ___			
Consults	Consider Cardiac Rehab page 688, 8:30-4:30 p.m.				Physician explains procedure results			
	Procedure consent							
Tests	*EKG done				*EKG post-procedure CPK/ISO enzymes x1 8-12 hours post-procedure			
Treatments	Prep/Shave R & L groin				Analgesics if needed *ACT and remove sheath:_____ am/pm Pulled by:			
Medications	ECASA				*Discontinue heparin			
	IV Fluids as ordered							
Diet	FM 4gm Na diet — no caffeine				Liquids for 2h post- procedure			
	*NPO after midnight except meds or clear liquid breakfast then NPO				If liquids tolerated, resume diet; assist with feeding			
Activity	OOB ad lib				Bedrest and turn with assist, keep affected leg straight and restrained. *OOB to chair 6h after sheath out, then walk in room.			
Elimination					Discontinue Foley by 2400			
Education	Angina symptoms/call nurse				*Instruct to call RN if S/S angina *Instructions for groin protection and activity progression			
	Procedure book or fact sheet/video							
	Family waiting area location				*Risk factor assessment			
Discharge Planning	Consider Patient & Family Svcs referral							
Nursing Reviewed by	0700-1500 1500-2300 2300-0700				0700-1500 1500-2300 2300-0700			
Multidisciplinary Review								

Revised June 1, 1995 **PTCA-Elective**   Contact for Variances: CNS — (#152)   * Items for QI Monitoring

Figure 3-1. Critical pathway (critical pathway/multidisciplinary plan of care) for elective percutaneous transluminal coronary angioplasty (PTCA) patients. (*With permission from Moses Cone Health System, Greensboro, NC.*)

Clinical Pathway: Elective PTCA/Stent/DCA/Rotablator
Expected LOS: 2.0 Days   **Page 2 of 2**

	POST-PROCEDURE DAY 1	Met	Unmet	N/A	Extra Day	Met	Unmet	N/A
Progression Outcomes	DISCHARGE DATE:_____ DISCHARGED FROM: ☐ EAU, ☐ TCU, OTHER:_____				Describe Key Activities:			
Assessments Evaluations	VS stable with activity, pain free, and peripheral pulses equal to baseline. Groin Assessment = Level I (If unmet, rate & explain: II_____ III_____)				Groin Assessment Scale: Level I____ Level II ____ Level III ____			
Consults	Cardiac Rehab if ordered Dietition if complications affecting nutritional status							
Tests	EKG AM done							
Treatments	Discontinue saline lock or IV							
Medications	*Discontinue IV NTG by 0800 if infusing. *Discontinue heparin if infusing. Time:_____							
Diet	As ordered							
Activity	*Walk in hall up to 10 min							
Elimination								
Education	CAD Diet Packet Stent booklet if indicated **Review Instructions:** • Groin care • Medications • Activity/exercise booklet • Angina management/SL NTG • Resources for Risk Factor Modification • MD follow-up plan Discharge Instruction Sheet given							
Discharge Planning	Discharged							
Nursing Reviewed by	0700-1500 1500-2300 2300-0700				0700-1500 1500-2300 2300-0700			
Multidisciplinary Review								

Revised June 1, 1995 **PTCA-Elective**   Contact for Variances: CNS — (#152)   * **Items for QI Monitoring**

**The contents of this Clinical Path represent general guidelines for care for this diagnosis. The plan of care required may be altered or revised to meet the specific needs of each individual patient.

GROIN ASSESSMENT SCALE
(Score daily beginning procedure day)
Level I (mild):   •bruising/ecchymosis
                         •minimal bleeding/oozing
                         •palpable hematoma < 3cm

Level II (moderate):   •bleeding not affecting hemodynamic parameters
                         •pseudoaneurysm
                         •palpable hematoma > 3cm

Figure 3–1. (*Continued*)

patient outcomes. The multidisciplinary team reviews the outcome and variance data and develops action plans. These action plans lead to changes in practice which ultimately create improvements in quality and reductions in LOS and costs.

NUTRITIONAL SUPPORT

Critically ill patients have nutritional needs that are much different than healthy individuals. Generally, the demands of critical illness require higher amounts of calories and protein than that consumed by healthy individuals. In addition, the nature of critical illnesses often interferes with normal nutritional intake. This requires critical care clinicians to include nutrition in their daily assessment of the patient and to intervene aggressively to provide nutritional support when normal nutritional intake is disrupted.

The preferred route for providing nutrition to critically ill patients is orally. However, for a variety of reasons, the majority of critically ill patients cannot consume enough calories orally to meet daily nutritional needs. Some form of artificial nutrition is required to fill this caloric gap.

There are two choices to consider when making a decision as to the best method to feed patients artificially: enteral and parenteral nutrition.

Enteral Nutrition

Enteral nutrition is the preferred route of artificial nutrition when the patient is unable to take nutrition orally. The major advantages of enteral feeding over other approaches include the following:

- Least expensive
- Fewest complications associated with feeding, particularly infection-related
- Most natural method of feeding
- Neutralizes gastric acid

Complications of enteral feeding include gastrointestinal (e.g., diarrhea, nausea, vomiting), metabolic (e.g., fluid and electrolyte imbalance), and obstruction of the enteral tube (Table 3–1).

There are several choices to consider when deciding on the method of enteral feeding. In the critically ill patient, unless a gastrostomy or jejunostomy is present, the choice is usually confined to placement of a gastric (into the stomach) or transpyloric (past the stomach into the small bowel) tube for feeding. If the stomach is emptying properly, a gastric tube is the method of choice since access is most easily achieved with this method. However, if the stomach is not emptying properly, or if the patient is at risk for aspiration, a transpyloric tube should be selected. Different methods of enteral access and their indications, advantages, and disadvantages are summarized in Table 3–2.

Method of Enteral Administration

There is some debate as to which method of feeding, bolus or continuous, is best for critically ill patients. Each patient will be different, and what works best for one patient may not work well for another. In general, the continuous method of feeding is the most commonly used during a critical illness. The advantages of continuous feeding include ease of administration, possible better toleration for small continuous volumes than larger intermittent volumes, ability to feed into the small bowel, and decreased practitioner time to manage the feedings. The disadvantages include the dissimilarity to normal nutritional patterns, bloating, and potential increased risk of aspiration with gastric feedings. The choice of method for feeding always should be based on the individual patient's clinical situation and tolerance of feeding. If one method does not work, another should be attempted.

Types of Enteral Feedings

There are numerous types of feedings on the market today, making selection of the best type confusing (Table 3–3). The following list briefly summarizes the different classifications of feeding types:

- *Polymeric:* These formulas require digestion, and nutrients are provided in complete form. Formulas have from 1 to 2 kcal/ml, with 1.5 to 2.0 kcal formulas considered calorie dense. Typically, these formulas provide about 40 g/L of protein. Many of these formulas also come with the addition of fiber.
- *Elemental:* Nutrients in these formulas are in elemental form, requiring little or no digestion. These formulas also come with the addition of fiber. Similar amounts of kilocalories and proteins are provided as in polymeric formulas.
- *High-Protein:* These formulas contain higher amounts of protein than the standard 40 kcal/L. Typically these formulas contain approximately 60 g/L of protein and are available in both polymeric and elemental forms.
- *Peptide-Based Formulas:* These are similar to elemental formulas except that the proteins are peptides (shorter chains of amino acids).
- *Specialized or Disease-Specific Formulas:* A variety of products are available that are specific for different clinical conditions, such as hepatic, renal, or pulmonary failure, or for trauma patients.

Most critically ill patients can be fed polymeric formulas, and with appropriate monitoring, will have successful outcomes. More and more, practitioners are recognizing the need to use fiber-containing formulas. Fiber is useful in both controlling diarrhea and in reducing constipation. On certain occasions, elemental, peptide-based, and specialty formulas may be indicated. However, great caution should be used with these formulas because they are not without risks, and also are expensive.

TABLE 3–1. COMPLICATIONS OF ENTERAL FEEDING

Complications	Cause	Therapeutic Interventions
GI Complications		
Diarrhea	Low-residue formula	Select fiber formula
	Rapid formula administration	Initiate feeding at low rate
		Temporarily reduce rate
	Bolus feeding using syringe force	Reduce rate of administration; select alternative method
	Hypoalbuminemia	Use elemental or peptide-based formula or total parenteral nutrition until absorptive capacity of gut is restored
	Microbial contamination	Use good handling and administration technique
	Disuse atrophy	Use enteral nutrition whenever possible
	Rapid GI transit time	Select fiber formula; slow transit time
	Prolonged antibiotic treatment or other drug therapy	Review medical profile and eliminate causative agent if possible; question benefit of lactobacillus
	Nutrient malabsorption	Select formula that restricts offending nutrients
Cramping, gas, abdominal distention	Rapid, intermittent administration of refrigerated formula	Administer formula by continuous method and at room temperature
	Bolus feeding using syringe force	Reduce rate of administration; select alternative method
Nausea and vomiting	Rapid formula administration, gastric distention	Initiate feedings at low rate and gradually advance to desired rate of administration; temporarily reduce rate
		Consider postpyloric feeding tube
Constipation	Inadequate fluid intake	Supplement fluids
	Insufficient bulk	Fiber
	Inactivity	Get out of bed
Metabolic Complications		
Dehydration	Inadequate fluid intake or excessive losses	Supplement fluid intake; monitor I&O
Overhydration	Rapid refeeding, excessive fluid intake	Reduce rate of administration, especially in patients with severe malnutrition or major organ failure; monitor I&O
Hyperglycemia	Inadequate insulin production for the amount of formula given	Initiate feedings at low rate; monitor glucose; use oral hyperglycemia agents or insulin if necessary; select low-carbohydrate diet
	Stress	
	Inadequate fluid intake or excessive losses	Assess fluid and electrolyte status; supplement with appropriate fluid; monitor I&O
Hypernatremia	Inadequate intake, fluid overload, SIADH, excessive GI fluid losses	Assess fluid and electrolyte status; if necessary restrict fluids; use diuretics; replace with fluids of similar composition
Hyponatremia	Delayed gastric emptying, gastroparesis	Postpyloric feeding; select isotonic or low-fat formula; check residuals; reduce infusion rate; use concentrated formulas
Aspiration pneumonia	Gastrointestinal reflux, diminished gag reflex	Use small-bore feeding tubes to minimize compromise of LES HOB > 45°
		Initially and regularly check tube placement
Mechanical Complications		
Feeding tube plugging	Administering crushed medications	Administer as many medications in sorbitol-free elixir form as possible
		If crushing medications, make sure medications are finely crushed and tube is adequately flushed before and after delivery
		Use laser-bore tube for medication administration
	Administering sorbitol-based elixirs	Use sorbitol-free elixirs when available
		Adequately flush feeding tube
	Infrequent flushing of tube	Flush tube every 3–4 hours with warm water
		Flush tube before and after use with warm water
		If tube plugs, attempt to flush gently with warm water

Parenteral Nutrition

There are occasions when the critically ill patient cannot be fed enterally (e.g., major upper gastrointestinal surgery, high output fistula, or bowel obstruction) and the patient must be fed parenterally. Parenteral nutrition is typically administered in the critically ill patient via a subclavian or jugular catheter (single-lumen or multilumen). On rare occasions, parenteral nutrition is administered through a peripheral intravenous line.

The advantages of parenteral nutrition include patient tolerance, ease of administration, and the ability to feed patients during acute resuscitation periods when enteral nutrition could not be continued. The disadvantages of parenteral nutrition include cost, increased risk of infection, and the invasive nature of the feeding route.

TABLE 3–2. ENTERAL ACCESS DEVICES

Enteral Access	Tube Size, Length	Manufacturer, Product Name	Indications	Advantages	Disadvantages
Nasogastric Small-bore feeding tube	8–12 Fr 17–36 inches	Sherwood-Medical Kangaroo Ross Flexiflo	Functional stomach Upper gastrointestinal tract obstruction Dysphagia to solids Not at risk for aspiration	Placed at the bedside; low morbidity; easily inserted	Patient discomfort; potential for aspiration
Nasoenteric Nasoduodenal	18–14 Fr 36–45 inches	Corpak Silk Biosearch Entron Ross Flexiflo	Gastric atony Risk of aspiration	May decrease the risk of aspiration of tube feeding; continued use of the gastrointestinal tract	Patient discomfort; more difficult placement; easily malpositioned
Nasojejunal Combination tubes	18 Fr gastric port 9 Fr jejunal feeding port	Sandoz	High risk for pulmonary aspiration of gastric contents Functional small bowel	May decrease the risk of aspiration of tube feeding Continued use of the gastrointestinal tract	Increased cost for tube and skilled professional to place the tube; easily malpositioned
Gastrostomy Surgical	14–30 Fr	de Pezzer Malecot Foley	Unable to endoscopically place PEG† gastrointestinal surgery	Easily removed Traction removal; body image; placement without general anesthesia	Difficult removal; general anesthesia; invasive procedure Tube migration; easily obstructed; local stoma site complications
Percutaneous	14–22 Fr	Bard Sandoz Nuport Ross Flexiflo Inverta-PEG	Long-term tube feeding		Invasive procedure
Replacement tubes	14–22 Fr*	Ross Easy-Feed Sandoz Flow-Thru	Original gastrostomy in need of changing Long-term tube feeding in nonambulatory patients	External bumper to prevent tube migration; more durable plastic for longer tube life	
Low-profile gastrostomy device	18–22 Fr 24 Fr 28 Fr	Ross Stomate Bard Button Sandoz Gastro-port Corpak MIC MIC-KEY Surgitek One-Step	Long-term tube feeding; ambulatory patients; disoriented patients who pull at the gastrostomy tube	Increased mobility; decreased cost of over-time due to device longevity; decreased nursing time as compared with replacement tube change	Requires skilled professional for placement; increased trauma to patient as compared with replacement tube; increased cost as compared with gastrostomy tube change; requires second procedure after gastrostomy tube placement
Jejunostomy Temporary	11 gauge (5 Fr) Needle catheter Jejunostomy kit 14 Fr	Sandoz Vivonex MIC Jejunostomy Tube	Short-term enteral nutrition usually ≤ 2 weeks	Device placed at the time of initial gastrostomy, no need for second procedure Continued use of the gastrointestinal tract Silicone plastic	With weight gain, device may impact in abdominal wall Surgical placement; easily obstructed; costly elemental feeding products
Permanent	14–18 Fr Whistle tip	Bard	Long-term jejunal feeding catheter	Use of gastrointestinal tract; easily replaced when fistula tract formed; larger bore; location is proximal jejunum, therefore does not require elemental products	Requires continuous or slow intermittent tube feeding administration due to location
Combination tubes Gastric decompression	16–30 Fr gastric port; 9 Fr jejunal feeding port	MIC Gastro-enteric tube	Long-term feeding; dysfunctional stomach	Can decompress a dysfunctional stomach and prevent regurgitation of gastric contents while feeding the small intestine	Requires skilled professional to place the tube; expensive process; jejunal feeding
	18 Fr gastric 9 Fr jejunal 20 Fr gastric 9 Fr jejunal	Ross Sandoz	Functional small bowel		
	18 Fr	Moss	Short-term postoperative care	Use of gastrointestinal tract; plastic less durable	Placed during surgery

*Internal balloon size can vary from 5–30 ml.
†PEG, percutaneous endoscopic gastrostomy.
From Shuster MH, Mancino JM: Ensuring successful home tube feeding in the geriatric population. Geriatric Nursing. 1994;15:67–82. Adapted with permission.

TABLE 3–3. CATEGORIES OF ENTERAL FEEDING PRODUCTS AND EXAMPLES OF EACH

Polymeric
Nonfiber
Osmolyte (Ross)
Isocal (Mead Johnson)
IsoSource (Sandoz)
Calories Dense
Magnacal (Sherwood)
Twocal HN (Ross)
Fiber
Jevity (Ross)
Ultracal (Mead Johnson)

Elemental
Vivonex TEN (Sandoz)
Vivonex Plus (Sandoz)
L-emental (Nutrition Medical)

High–Protein
Promote/Promote with fiber (Ross)
Replete/Replete with fiber (Clintec)
IsoSource VHN (Sandoz)

Peptide-Based Formulas
Peptamen (Clintec)
Vital HN (Ross)
Accupep (Sherwood)

Specialty Formulas
Hepatic-aid (liver disease/McGaw)
Nephro (renal disease/Ross)
Pulmocare (pulmonary disease/Ross)
Impact (immune-enhancing/Sandoz)

PATIENT AND FAMILY EDUCATION

Patient and family education in the critical care environment is essential to providing the patient and family with information regarding diagnosis, prognosis, treatments, and procedures. In addition, education provides patients and family members a mechanism by which fears and concerns can be minimized and confronted so that they can become active members in the decisions made about care.

Providing patient and family education in critical care is challenging; multiple barriers (e.g., environmental factors, patient stability, patient/family anxiety) must be overcome, or adapted, in order to provide this essential intervention. The importance of education, coupled with the barriers common in critical care, necessitates that education be a continuous ongoing process engaged in by all members of the team.

Education in the critical care setting is most often done informally, rather than in traditional formal settings (e.g., classrooms). Education of the patient and family is often subtle, occurring with each interaction between the patient, family, and members of the health care team.

Assessment of Learning Readiness

Assessment of the patient's and family's learning needs should focus primarily on learning readiness. *Learning readiness* is a term that refers to that magic moment in time when the learner is able to comprehend and synthesize the shared information. Without learning readiness, teaching may not be useful. Questions to assess learning readiness are listed in Table 3–4.

Strategies to Address Patient and Family Education

Prior to teaching, the information gathered in the assessment is prioritized and organized into a format which is meaningful to the learner (Table 3–5). Next, the outcome of the teaching is established along with appropriate content, and then a decision should be made about how to share the information. The next step is to teach the patient, family, and/or significant others (Table 3–6). While this phase often appears to be the easiest, it's actually the most difficult. It is crucial during the communication of the content, regardless of the type of communication vehicle used (video, pamphlet, discussion), to listen carefully to the needs expressed by the learner and to provide clear and precise responses to those needs.

TABLE 3–4. ASSESSMENT OF LEARNING READINESS

Generic Principles

- Do the patient and the family have questions about the diagnosis, prognosis, treatments, or procedures?
- What do the patient and the family desire to learn about?
- What is the knowledge level of the individuals being taught? What do they already know about the issues that will be taught?
- What is their current situation (condition and environment) and have they had any prior experience in a similar situation?
- How does their current belief/value system influence their illness?
- Does the patient or the family have any communication barriers (e.g., language, illiteracy, culture, listening/comprehension deficits)?

Special Considerations in Critical Care

- Does the patient's condition allow you to assess this information from them (e.g., physiological/psychological stability)?
- Is the patient's support system/family/significant other available or ready to receive this information?
- What environmental factors (including time) present as barriers in the critical care unit?
- Are there other members of the health care team who may possess vital assessment information?

TABLE 3–5. PRINCIPLES FOR TEACHING PLANS

Generic Principles

- Establish the outcome of the teaching.
- Determine what content needs to be taught, given the assessment.
- Identify what support systems are in place to support your educational efforts (e.g., unit leadership, education department, standardized teaching plans, teaching materials such as pamphlets, brochures, videos).
- Familiarize yourself with the content and teaching materials.
- Contact resources to clarify and provide consistency in information and to also provide additional educational support and follow-up.
- Determine the most appropriate teaching strategy (video, written materials, discussion) and to whom (patient or family) it should be directed.

Special Considerations in Critical Care

- Plan the teaching strategy *carefully*. Patients and families in the critical care environment are stressed and an overload of information adds to their stress. When planning education, consider content and amount based on the assessment of the patient, nature and severity of the patient's illness, availability of significant others, and existing environmental barriers.

TABLE 3–6. PRINCIPLES FOR EDUCATIONAL SESSIONS

Generic Principles

- Consider the time needed to convey both the information and support system availability.
- Consider the situation the patient is currently experiencing. Postponement may need to be considered.
- Be aware of the amount of content and the patient's and the family's ability to process the information.
- Be sensitive in the delivery of the information. Make sure it is conveyed at a level that the patient and the family can understand.
- Refer to, and involve, resources as appropriate.
- Convey accurate and precise information. Make sure this information is consistent with previous information given to the patient.
- Listen carefully and solicit feedback during the session to guide the discussion and clarify any potential misinterpretations.

Special Considerations in Critical Care

- Keep the time frame and content brief. Education must be episodic due to the nature of the patient's condition and the environment.
- Provide repetition of the information. Stress and the critical care environment can alter comprehension; for this reason repetition is necessary.
- Avoid details unless the patient or family specifically requests them. Often, details can cloud the information given. Details can come later in the hospitalization, if necessary.

TABLE 3–7. PRINCIPLES FOR OUTCOME MONITORING

Generic Principles

- Measure the outcome. Was the outcome met? Was the outcome unmet?
- Communicate the outcome verbally and in a written format to other members of the health care team.
- Provide necessary follow-up and reinforcement of the teaching.
- Make referrals that may have been identified in or as a result of patient and family education.
- Evaluate the teaching process for barriers or problems, and then address those areas and be aware of these for future interactions.

Special Considerations in Critical Care

- Recognize that repetition of information is the rule, not the exception. Be prepared to repeat information previously given, many times if necessary.

Outcome Measurement of Patient and Family Education

Following educational interventions, it is essential to determine if the educational outcomes were achieved (Table 3–7). If the outcome was achieved, wonderful. If the outcome was not achieved, do not be discouraged. Patients and families experience a great deal of stress while in the critical care environment and reinforcement is *often* necessary.

NEAR-DEATH EXPERIENCES

A near-death experience (NDE) is a fascinating and unusual phenomenon encountered by some patients who have successfully survived a cardiopulmonary arrest. The NDE is comprised of perceptions and events experienced by patients during the clinical death phase of a cardiac arrest. In relating their experiences to others, survivors have described several features that characterize the perceptions and events of the NDE. The experiences seem to cluster around three common domains: affective, cognitive, and transcendental. During the clinical death phase, patients have described such affective feelings as being comfortable, pain free, relaxed, calm, and peaceful. Some also may be aware that they have died. The cognitive features include accelerated thoughts and time awareness (or a distortion of time) as well as a sudden understanding of life. Many patients report a panoramic memory or a sudden review of their entire past during the NDE.

The transcendental experiences involve visual images and out-of-body experiences. During the out-of-body experiences, called autoscopic observation, patients experience a separation of the body and mind, in which the mind positions itself in a corner of the room to observe the resuscitative efforts. In support of this phenomenon, some patients have been able to describe accurately such technicalities as the placement of equipment and personnel and the details of resuscitative procedures that could only be known if one was actually standing at the bedside observing the situation. Patients have described their inability to communicate with the health care team during the resuscitation as a distressing component of their NDE.

Some patients who experience a separation of body and mind describe their mind leaving the room and traveling through a long dark tunnel with loud noises or music associated with the journey. At the end of the tunnel, they frequently describe an unbelievably bright light, a beautiful meadow, or a heavenly world. Upon entering the light, some patients report encounters with persons, figures, guides, deceased relatives, or religious figures. Many also describe coming to a river or a mountain symbolizing a dividing line between life and death or a border of no return. Patients may know that crossing that line would mean they would remain forever. Many decide for themselves that they need to return although sometimes friends, relatives, or religious figures decide for them that they must go back.

AT THE BEDSIDE
▶ *Near-Death Experience*

Approximately 10 Minutes Into the Operation

"Her pressure's crashing!" What is it? What's the matter? At first there was a feeling of sweeping motion. It felt like my mind—the thinking and feeling part of me—quickly moved out of my body. I could see my body lying there on the table, but the real "me" hovered near my head.

It was clear that there was an emergency. The scene was frantic. People I didn't recognize were scurrying in and out of the room. I searched for my surgeon. I knew he was there, but he wasn't standing where I thought he should have been. Initially, I joined in the frenzy. I wanted to help. I am a nurse. I wanted to tell the doctors what was happening. Frantically, I tried to approach them. I tried to speak, but nothing came out. I reached to touch them, but a barrier kept me from getting close. Then I realized that no one could see or hear me. At that moment, an extraordinary calmness came over me. I moved toward a corner of the ceiling close to a "light."

I had an euphoric feeling of peace. It was as though warmth and acceptance were being communicated to me through the light. There was absolutely no fear. I felt safe and secure. There was a sense of timelessness—as though there was no time. I wanted to linger with the thoughts and feelings I was experiencing.

I heard someone say, "I don't think she's going to make it," but the words didn't concern me. I had no thought that I was dying, or that I was going to die. I felt very much alive. I heard my surgeon say, "She's hemorrhaging. We've got to open her up!"

I don't know how long my mind remained separated or when it rejoined my body. I remember feeling intense pain when the surgeon made the incision for the exploratory laparotomy. I remember using mental imagery to help myself deal with the pain. Inhale, exhale, relax; inhale, exhale, relax; . . . When I tired of the breathing exercise, I imagined myself in a very healthy state, jogging at the lake. One, two, three, four, five, . . . For the past 10 years, counting had been the technique I had used to keep a steady jogging cadence. I knew when I reached 500 I had jogged about a mile.

What are they doing now? Are they doing chest compressions? I've got to tell them I can feel this. Move your head, Carolyn, move your head.

"She feels that! I'm going to put her under again."

The Next Morning

I woke up. My chest was sore. My husband was at my side. I was in the intensive care unit. I remembered. "Jerry! I almost died. I could see. I was watching. I separated from my body. I was on the table, but I was watching. They did CPR." I began to drift off. I went back to the jogging trail. One-hundred-and-one, one hundred-and-two, . . .

Weeks Later

A few weeks after the surgery, I became very depressed. The reality of my close encounter with death set in. I now had new scars that were not there before. I felt somehow "different" because of this experience. There seemed to be too much to deal with at once. I spent time reflecting on how we get caught up in unimportant things and miss the beauty of life. There was a need to reset priorities and eliminate the trivia. I found myself concentrating on my family, friendships, and the development of my mind. I felt an intense commitment to my work. I had changed.

Adapted from: Guzzetta CE. Near-death experience. In: Dossey BM, Guzzetta CE, Kenner CV: *Critical care nursing: Body-mind-spirit.* Philadelphia: JB Lippincott, 1992, pp. 963–968. Copyright 1982 by Carolyn D. Henson, RN, MA. Reprinted by permission.

Although most NDEs are not described as negative experiences, a small percentage of patients have reported one of three types of distressing NDEs:

- An experience similar to a peaceful NDE but one that is interpreted by the patient as terrifying
- An experience that characterizes nonexistence or an eternal void characterized by despair and emptiness
- An experience with hellish imagery characterized by frightening events, strange creatures, sights of hell, flames, or burning, and feelings of loneliness, doom, terror, and helplessness[1]

At the completion of a successful resuscitation, patients may find their mind rapidly traveling back through the tunnel to be united with the body. They may see the body, know that pain is expected, and reenter the body. This reunion can be associated with not only physical discomfort but also with emotional pain and distress because frequently the mind desires to remain in the light or the place of peace and comfort.

Clinical Consequences of NDE

Patients who have had NDEs are profoundly affected by the experience. They report transcendental events and feelings of harmony, a sense of cosmic unity, and being at one with the universe. Patients may relate a sense of "all knowing"—understanding what truth is, what love is, and what life is all about. Many report a reordering of their lives following an NDE, in which personal values, attitudes, and beliefs are changed, resulting in a devaluation of material belongings and career success and an increased emphasis on altruistic and spiritual concerns. Patients describe feelings of invulnerability, a special sense of purpose and meaning in life, a greater concern for others, and a heightened belief in God and in an afterlife.

Factors Influencing NDE

Near-death experiences have been documented throughout history from such diverse near-death episodes as childbirth and sudden life-threatening events in which individuals encounter intense physical or emotional danger (e.g., trauma, surgery, combat, and drowning, and with mountaineers who have survived a lethal fall) to situations confronting the bedridden and terminally ill. It has been found that up to 48% of persons, from the young to the elderly, who have come close to death have experienced an NDE.

The principal features of NDEs also have been documented across various religious and cultural groups. These features (e.g., the affective, cognitive, and transcendental characteristics) are generally universal regardless of the country, religion, or culture. The symbolic imagery reported from the experience may differ, however, depending on the concepts of the afterlife and the cultural setting of the individual. There are many reports, for example, of religious divine beings visualized (e.g., God, angels, Hindu deities), but they are always named according to the individual's religious beliefs (e.g., no Hindu has reported seeing Jesus and no Christian has seen a Hindu deity). It appears that although the individual's images may be bound by cultural symbolism and beliefs, the NDE is essentially the same around the world and throughout time.

Causal Theories

There have been many theories developed to explain the near-death phenomenon. These include spiritual, organic, and psychologic theories, and some include combined models that incorporate components of each. Spiritual theories are developed on the assumption that the NDE phenomenon represents reports of individuals who have died and then returned. Thus, such theories assert that the NDE provides empirical evidence of the existence of an afterlife. Critics of such theories argue that a cardiac arrest does not really represent the death of an individual because death is characterized by a fixed and permanent state. Rather, the cardiac arrest represents the dying process, which is limited by time, and thus individuals who experience NDEs have entered the early phase of dying that can be reversed by successful cardiopulmonary resuscitation.

Organic theories focus on physical causes of NDEs. One theory asserts that the cerebral anoxia occurring during the dying process is responsible for the hallucinations and illusions of the NDE. Others believe that the panoramic memory and attitudinal changes that follow the NDE are an adaptive neurologic response to severe anxiety resulting from temporal lobe excitation. Another similar theory postulates that NDEs are the result of a stress-induced limbic lobe syndrome. Under extreme stress, the central nervous system secretes peptides that affect behavior, thereby accounting for the hallucinatory events associated with the NDE.

Psychologic theories explain NDEs as an emotional coping mechanism for dealing with dying. The person experiencing the NDE replaces the undesirable reality of death and substitutes pleasing apparitions. The peaceful feeling associated with the experience may be a stunning of psychologic responses rather than actual tranquility. The dissociative out-of-body experiences associated with NDEs allow the patient to watch the event as a disinterested third party. This depersonalization provides an adaptive mental response to devastating bodily danger, thereby protecting the individual from the trauma of the event.

None of the proposed theories accounts for all the characteristics and occurrences of NDEs, and there is little data to sustain any one of them although abundant theoretical hypotheses remain to be tested in the future.

---

[1]Greyson B, Bush NE: Distressing near-death experiences. *Psychiatry.* 1992;55:95–110.

Patient Problems and Principles of Management

The management of the patient who has had a NDE focuses on three phases of care: during the resuscitation, following the resuscitation, and following stabilization.

During the Resuscitation: Support the Patient

During the resuscitation, all health team members must remember (and perhaps be reminded) that clinically dead patients may have the ability to hear, see, and vividly describe the events surrounding the resuscitative efforts.

1. Avoid threatening or frightening language during the resuscitation.
2. Position someone at the head of the bed during the resuscitation to preserve a sense of reality orientation. Reassure, explain, and touch the patient as if he or she were alert and awake.
3. Offer the option of family visitation for those family members who wish to be present during the resuscitation. If a family wishes to be present, they should be briefed by a support person (e.g., a nurse or chaplain) on the patient's appearance, equipment, and procedures being performed. Instruct the family that it is expected that they will not interfere or disturb the resuscitation. Escort the family to the patient's room and position them at the head of the bed, if possible. Show the family how to touch and talk to the patient. Stay with the family to explain procedures, answer questions, and provide emotional support. Following the visitation, escort the family back to the waiting room and stay with them to address their questions and concerns and provide support.

AT THE BEDSIDE

Nurse: "A very powerful experience about communicating with a patient happened when I was new to critical care. We were doing CPR and a colleague of mine was at the head of the bed. I kept wondering, 'Why isn't she doing anything except talking to the patient? Why isn't she getting drugs?' She kept telling the patient what was going on, and to hang in there. I was being the good worker bee, running around, getting things done.

"After the code, one of the physicians made fun of her talking to the patient. But this nurse was someone who saw that maintaining contact with the person was just as important as everything else we were doing.

"By the way, the patient was successfully resuscitated and recalled everything that nurse told him. And he said so, over and over again—how important that was for him."

Following the Resuscitation: Monitor and Support the Patient

When the patient resumes consciousness following a successful resuscitation:

1. Stay with and support the patient while assessing levels of anxiety, restlessness, and orientation. Carefully observe for signs of an NDE occurrence such as changes in the patient's thinking, memory, personality, mood, attitudes, and beliefs. Patients may be angry, withdrawn, depressed, silent, or suddenly calm.
2. Slowly reorient the patient to time, place, person, and situation.

Following Stabilization: Facilitate Adaptive Coping

1. After the patient has stabilized, assess the patient's need to discuss the events of the preresuscitation, intraresuscitation, and postresuscitation periods.
2. Establish a pattern of active listening.
3. Provide the patient with behavioral, cognitive, and emotional support.
4. Honestly discuss the situation and events that occurred during the resuscitation. Patients frequently will request repeated explanations as a means of "reliving" the events in order to find meaning and understand what has happened. Often, patients will ask for more detailed information as time elapses.
5. Identify whether the patient has had an NDE. Although not all patients have NDEs during a cardiopulmonary arrest, discuss the possibility of NDEs associated with a cardiac arrest, thereby opening the door for discussion. Patients who have had such an experience may be reluctant to discuss the event because of the fear of ridicule or of being labeled as "crazy."
6. Relate that others also have had an NDE during a cardiac arrest. This explanation often is reassuring to patients who are afraid to discuss their own experience. Some patients already may be familiar with such experiences because near-death stories are being discussed with increasing frequency in popular magazines and on television shows, thereby expanding public awareness of this phenomenon.
7. Encourage patients to openly discuss their NDE, when they are ready to do so. Allow them to discuss the events at their own pace without pressure to provide the details surrounding the clinical death period. Most literature on the subject suggests that individuals have great difficulty finding the words to describe their NDEs.
8. Use techniques of relaxation, guided imagery, and music therapy to assist patients to tell their story

better, reflect on the experience, explore their feelings and attitudes, and focus on how the experience has impacted their lives (See Chapter 8, Alternative Therapies in Critical Care, and Chapter 28, Alternative Therapies Table).

9. Assist patients in explaining the NDE to their family if they so desire. Some patients are reluctant to discuss their NDE with their family and may request that a member of the health team be present to help explain the NDE to lend validity to their story.

10. Educate the family about NDEs to assist them in understanding and accepting the experience and to facilitate family discussion and support.

11. Provide the patient and family with written information on NDEs if they so desire (Table 3–8). Refer them to one of several books written on the topic (e.g., Moody's book *Life after Life*) or to the research and teaching organization, the International Association of Near-Death Studies (IANDS).[2] The organization has support groups called Friends of IANDS and publishes a journal called *Anabiosis*.

12. Evaluate the patient's ability to cope psychophysiologically with the events of the cardiac arrest and NDE to determine the effects of nursing interventions on desired patient coping outcomes.

13. Assess the patient for evidence of serious behavioral, emotional, or personality problems following the event. Refer any patient for long-term counseling if he or she demonstrates such problems.

COMMUNICATION WITH TEMPORARILY NONVOCAL PATIENTS

The ability to speak allows each of us to express our needs, wants, and desires. It allows us the opportunity to understand and be understood. In critical care, effective communication underlies all aspects of care. It affects self-esteem and is intertwined with quality of life. Those patients who cannot communicate have difficulty maintaining control over their lives and environment or participating in meaningful interchanges and activities.

Imagine how difficult it must be for patients in crisis to be unable to tell clinicians that they are in pain, are thirsty, or need to use the bedpan? Mechanically ventilated patients, common in critical care settings, experience this very situation. They are unable to speak due to a cuffed endotracheal (ET) or tracheostomy tube. Many times these patients have been near death and would give anything to

---

[2]International Association of Near-Death Studies (IANDS), Dept N88, PO Box 24665, Philadelphia, PA 19111.

TABLE 3–8. PATIENT RESOURCE LIST FOR NDES

Atwater PMH: *Coming back to life: The after effects of the near-death experience.* New York: Ballentine, 1988.

Cutner N, Hirshberg C, Hollister A, et al: Visions of life after death: The ultimate mystery. *Life.* March 1992:64–73.

The door to the secret city (story of a child's NDE). Kids Want Answers, Too, PO Box 297, Virginia Beach, VA 23458.

Eadie BJ: *Embraced by the light.* New York: Bantam, 1992.

Greyson B, Flynn C: *The near-death experience: Problems, prospects, perspectives.* Springfield, IL: CC Thomas, 1984.

International Association of Near-Death Studies (IANDS), Dept. N88, PO Box 24665, Philadelphia, PA 19111.

Lundahl CR: *A collection of near-death research readings.* Chicago: Nelson-Hall, 1982.

The magnificent journey: A window on life after death (video on near-death experience). Starpath Productions, PO Box 160, Fayetteville, AR 72702.

Moody RA: *Life after life.* New York: Bantam, 1975.

Moody RA: *Reflections on life after life.* New York: Bantam, 1977.

Morse M: *Closer to the light.* New York: Ivy, 1990.

Ring J: *Life after death: A scientific investigation of the near-death experiences.* New York: Coward, McCann, 1980.

Ring K: *Heading towards omega: In search of the meaning of the near-death experience.* New York: Morrow, 1984.

Zaleski C: *Otherworld journeys: Accounts of near-death experiences in medieval and modern times.* New York: Oxford, 1987.

---

be able to talk to their loved ones and express their feelings. The inability to speak is frustrating for the patients, family, and all members of the health care team.

Impaired communication results in patients experiencing anxiety and fear, emotions that can have a deleterious effect on their physical and psychological condition. Interviewing patients after removal of ET tubes reveals how isolated and alone they feel because of their inability to speak. Patients describe how terrified they become when the ventilator connecting tubing "pops off" the end of the ET tube, especially when the call light is nowhere within reach. Something as trivial as an itch in the middle of the back can be extremely difficult to communicate, and yet it is an uncomfortable, irritating situation for the patient.

Common Communication Problems

Patients' perceptions of communication difficulties related to mechanical ventilation include:

- Inability to communicate
- Insufficient explanations
- Inadequate understanding
- Fears and dangers of not being able to speak
- Difficulty with communication methods

Except for the problem of inability to vocalize, all of these problems could be resolved easily by clinicians. For instance, insufficient explanations and inadequate understanding can be remedied by frequent repetition of all plans and procedures. This is necessary because critically ill patients are often physically unstable and weak, receiving analgesics, sedatives, and/or anesthetic agents; sleep deprived; and/or stressed. These situations lead to decreased attention span and cognitive abilities, especially memory.

Patients often describe difficulties with communication methods used during mechanical ventilation. Many of these difficulties could be avoided if clinicians assessed the patient's communication abilities initially. Is the patient alert and oriented? Can the patient answer simple yes or no questions? Does the patient speak English? Can the patient use at least one hand to gesture? Does the patient have sufficient strength and dexterity to hold a pen and write? Are the patient's hearing and vision adequate? Additional assessment guidelines, tools, and algorithms for appropriate alternative communication interventions can be found in Chapter 6, Airway and Ventilatory Management.

Basic Needs

Communicating basic needs to critical care practitioners is usually difficult for temporarily nonvocal patients. Most adults are accustomed to attending to their own basic needs. During a critical illness, however, not only are they unable to physically perform certain activities, they cannot even communicate those needs effectively. Basic needs include such activities as bathing, brushing teeth, combing hair, urinating and defecating, eating, drinking, and sleeping. Other examples of important basic needs which are common to critically ill patients are related to body warmth, positioning, pain, breathing difficulties, comfort, and fear.

Critically ill patients often communicate needs which require immediate intervention by gesturing to the bedside clinician. For example, intubated patients will indicate that they need suctioning by curving an index finger (to resemble a suction catheter), raising a hand toward the endotracheal tube, and moving their hand back and forth; difficulty breathing will be indicated by pointing to the nose, mouth, or chest.

One important aspect of communicating by gesturing is for the clinician to "mirror" the gesture back to the patient, at the same time verbalizing the message or idea conveyed by the patient's gesture. This mirroring will ensure accuracy in interpretation and will assist the nurse and patient to form a repertoire of gestures to be used successfully in future conversations. When observing a patient's gestures, stand back from the bed and watch his or her arms and hands. Most gestures are easily understood, especially the one most frequently used by patients, the head nod indicating yes or no. Asking simple yes or no questions is helpful and facilitates communication, as long as clinicians avoid barraging the patient with questions. Before trying to guess the needs of temporarily nonvocal patients, give them the opportunity to use gestures to communicate their needs.

Teaching Communication Methods

The critical care environment presents many teaching/learning challenges. Patients and families are under a con-

siderable amount of stress, so the nurse must be a very creative teacher and offer communication techniques that are simple, effective, and easy to learn. The desire to communicate with loved ones makes the family very willing to learn new communication methods. Often it is the family members who make up large-lettered communication boards or purchase an erasable slate for the patient to use.

All patients should be informed prior to intubation that they will be unable to speak. A flipchart illustrating an ET or tracheostomy tube, with labeling in simple words, could be shown to patients awaiting elective intubation (e.g., prior to surgery). In addition, both the patient and family should be instructed in the use of appropriate, nonverbal communication techniques before intubation (e.g., gestures, alphabet boards, flash cards, paper and pencil). Another important point to emphasize with patients is that being unable to speak is usually temporary, just while the breathing tube is in place.

Implementation of Communication Strategies

Members of the critical care team should identify the common communication needs and characteristics of their patient population. For instance, similarities exist in surgical trauma units where patients typically are younger and were in relatively good health until the time of their accident or injury. Communication methods may include a set of 20 basic needs gestures that all the staff can perform, along with pen and paper on a clipboard and alphabet boards.

If the patient does not speak English, a picture board is sometimes useful along with well-understood gestures. Language flash cards that contain common ICU words or phrases in foreign languages, such as Italian or Spanish, can be made or purchased.

Once the most successful communication methods have been identified for a particular patient, they should be written into the plan of care. Continuity among critical care professionals in their approach to communication with nonvocal patients will improve the quality of care and increase patient satisfaction.

For more detailed information on communicating with temporarily nonvocal patients, see Chapter 6, Airway and Ventilatory Management.

SLEEP PATTERN DISTURBANCE

All critically ill patients experience altered sleep patterns. Sleep is a problem for patients because of the pain and anxiety of a critical illness within an environment that is busy with the life-saving activity of health care providers. Table 3–9 identifies the many reasons for patients to experience sleep deprivation. The priority of sleep in the hierarchy of patient needs is often perceived to be low by clinicians. This contradicts patients' own statements about the critical

TABLE 3–9. CAUSES OF SLEEP DEPRIVATION IN CRITICAL CARE

Patient Factors
Severity of underlying illness
Medications
    REM-suppressant drugs (narcotics, barbiturates, antidepressants)
    NREM (stages 3 and 4)-suppressant drugs
Pain
Fever
Loss of control (restraints, pharmacologic paralysis)
Fear, anxiety, psychological stress

Physician/Nursing Factors
Diagnostic testing
Nursing interventions
Invasive procedures

Environmental Factors
Lighting
Noise
    Mechanical devices, including ventilators and alarms
    Background noise
    Nursing or respiratory care
    Conversations between hospital staff
Noxious odors

From Schwab RJ: Disturbances of sleep in the intensive care unit. Critical Care Clinics. 1994;10:686.

care experience. Patients complain about lack of sleep as a major stressor along with the discomfort of unrelieved pain. The vicious cycle of undertreated pain, anxiety, and sleeplessness continues unless clinicians intervene to break the cycle with simple, but powerful, interventions individualized to each patient.

Noise, lights, and frequent patient interruptions are the hallmark of many critical care settings and the staff "tune it out" after they have worked in the setting for even a short while. However, patients do not leave after a shift and the sickest, most vulnerable patients may stay in the critical care unit for a week or longer. The symptoms of sleep deprivation can arise whenever an individual's normal amount of sleep is not achieved. In days to weeks of chronic sleep deprivation and the resulting fatigue, healthy adults experience notable psychologic changes such as confusion and irritability. Physiologic changes include depressed immune and respiratory systems and a decreased pain threshold. Healthy individuals are hardy and quickly make up lost sleep time when given the optimum opportunity to do so. Whether this is true with the fragile critically ill patient is unknown. It is believed that sleep has mysterious healing powers.

Enhancing patients' sleep potential in the critical care setting involves a knowledge of how the environment affects the patient and where to target interventions to best promote sleep and rest.

A nighttime sleep protocol where patients are closely monitored but untouched from 1 AM to 5 AM is an excellent example of eliminating the hourly disturbances to the critically ill. Encouraging blocks of time for sleep and careful

assessment of the quantity and quality of sleep are important to patient well-being. The middle-of-the-night bath should not be a standard of care for any patient. Table 3–10 details basic recommendations for sleep assessment, protecting or shielding the patient from the environment, and modifying the internal and external environments of the patient. When these activities are incorporated into standard practice routines, critically ill patients receive optimal opportunity to achieve sleep.

PSYCHOSOCIAL IMPACT OF CRITICAL ILLNESS

Basic Tenets

Keys to maintaining psychological integrity during a critical illness include keeping stressors at a minimum; encouraging family participation in care; promoting a proper sleep-wake cycle; encouraging communication, questions, and honest and positive feedback; empowering the patient to participate in decisions as appropriate; providing patient and family education about unit expectations and rules, procedures, medications, and the patient's physical condition; ensuring pain relief and comfort; and providing continuity of care providers. It's also important to have the patient's usual sensory and physical aids available, such as glasses, hearing aids, and dentures. Encourage the family to bring something familiar or personal from home, such as a family or pet picture.

Communication Needs

Promotion of psychological integrity occurs primarily through verbal communication. From the beginning, call the patient by his or her preferred name and introduce yourself. This shows respect and begins a trusting relationship. Actively listening to what the patient is saying or asking is preferable to talking *to* the patient. Facilitate listening by phrases such as, "Tell me more about . . . ." Keep eye contact with the patient and do not engage in other tasks while listening. Respond nonjudgmentally, and then clarify with phrases such as, "I hear you saying . . .," "Do I understand you to say . . .?", or "I wonder if you understand my point?"

Communication with the patient and family should be open and honest. Clinicians should keep promises (be careful about what you promise), describe expectations, not contract for secrets, elicit preferences, apologize for inconveniences and mistakes, and maintain confidentiality. Concise, simplistic explanations without medical jargon or alphabet shorthand (e.g., PEEP, IABP) will facilitate understanding. Contact interpreters, as appropriate, when language barriers exist.

Evaluate your communication by asking the patient and family for their understanding of the message you sent and its content and intent. When conflict occurs, find a private place for discussion. Avoid taking the confrontation personally. Ask yourself what is the issue and what needs to occur to resolve the issue or problem. If too much emotion is present, agree to address the issue at a later time, if possible.

For patients and families who are unable to discuss their stress, encourage them to write about it for 20 minutes or so. When you are unclear about a message, use reflective open-ended statements to ascertain the correct message. Referrals for consultation resources to offer more formal counseling, such as alcoholism rehabilitation, or complementary interventions should also be pursued.

Family Relations Interventions

Prior to surgery or the first visit to the critical care environment, the patient and family need a variety of information: where the patient will be; what they will see, hear, and smell; what losses to expect; and anticipatory guidance information. This information can be targeted to specific situations, such as a patient who is unable to see or is paralyzed and how the family can compensate for these losses.

Timing is important. If the patient is newly admitted, explain to the family who you are, what your role is, and that you need to be with the patient, but that you will return later to talk with them. Select a place where privacy and open communication can occur. Encourage the family to cry together, share loss, uncover unspoken fears, speak the unspeakable, and banish secrets. Involve children so they feel important and respected as family members. Find activities they can do to help, such as picking up toys in the waiting room or drawing a card for their loved one. Clarify what they see and hear. Mobilize resources and include them in patient care and problem solving, as appropriate. Some critical care units invite family members to medical rounds for the discussion of their loved one. Encourage the family to admit when they are overwhelmed, take breaks, go to meals, rest, sleep, take care of themselves, and not to abandon members at home. It is helpful to establish a communication tree so that one family member is designated to be called if there are changes in the patient's condition. Establish a time for that person to call the unit for updates. Reassure them you are there to help or refer them to other system supports.

Unit expectations and rules can be conveyed in a pamphlet for the family to refer to over time. Content that is helpful includes: orientation about the philosophy of care; routines as shifts change and during rounds; the varied roles of personnel who work with patients; and comfort information such as food services, bathrooms, waiting areas, chapel services, transportation, and lodging. Of primary importance to the family will be the unit visiting policies. Specifics to address are: the number of visitors allowed at one time, age restrictions, times if not flexible or open, and how to gain access to the unit.

For the family, the critical care setting symbolizes a variety of hopes, fears, and beliefs which range from magical cure to final sentence. A family-focused approach can promote coping and cohesion among family members and minimize the isolation and anxiety for patients. Anticipating family needs, focusing on the present, fostering open communication, and providing information are vital to promoting psychological integrity for families. By using the event of hospitalization as a point of access, critical care clinicians assume a major role in primary prevention and assisting families to cope positively with crisis and grow from the experience.

Delirium

Delirium is evidenced by disorientation, confusion, perceptual disturbance, psychomotor changes (restlessness), distractibility, and sleep-wake cycle disturbances. Delirium is

TABLE 3–10. STRATEGIES TO ENHANCE SLEEP IN THE CRITICALLY ILL PATIENT

Patient Assessment	Shielding the Patient	Modification of the Environment
Obtain and use sleep history to plan care	Increase nurses' awareness to sounds and lights in the critical care setting	Provide pain relief
Assess quality and quantity of sleep by observation and asking the patient	Prevent excessive noise, lights, and staff conversation near patients	Include backrubs in the nightly routine of "putting the patient to bed"
Document sleep-wake times	Evaluate the need for nursing care interruptions when a patient is resting or sleeping	Use relaxation techniques, imagery, or music therapy
Monitor for signs of sleep deprivation—unexpected confusion, fatigue	Block sleep times for naps and at night (1 AM to 5 AM) when possible	Administer a hypnotic with the least side effects and evaluate patient response
	Promote comfortable position for sleep and evaluate bed position	Maximize patient privacy
	Explain all environmental sounds to decrease anxiety	Post sign "Patient Sleeping"
		Provide large clocks and natural lighting
		Encourage family to stay with patient if valuable for patient healing and family well-being

(With permission from Fontaine D. Sleep disturbances in the critically ill patient. Critical Care Nursing Currents. 1987:5(4):22, Ross Products Division, Abbott Laboratories, Columbus, Ohio.)

most common in postsurgical and elderly patients and is the most common cause of disruptive behavior in the critically ill. Often mislabeled "ICU psychosis," delirium is not a psychosis. Sensory overload is a common risk factor that contributes to delirium in the critically ill.

Medication for managing delirious behavior is best reserved for those cases in which behavioral interventions have failed. Sedatives/hypnotics and anxiolytics may have precipitated the delirium and can exacerbate the sleep-wake cycle disturbances, causing more confusion. The agitated patient may require low-dose neuroleptics or short-acting benzodiazepines. Restraints are discouraged as they tend to increase agitation.

External stimulation should be minimized and a quiet, restful well-lighted room maintained during the day. Consistency in care providers is also important. Repeating orientation cues will minimize fear and confusion; for example, "Good morning Bill, my name is Sue. It's Monday morning in April and you are in the hospital. I'm a nurse and will stay here with you." Background noise from TVs and radios often increases anxiety as the patient has trouble processing the noise and content. Explain all procedures and tests concretely. Introduce one idea at a time, slowly, and have the patient repeat the information. Repeat and reinforce as often as needed.

If the patient demonstrates a paranoid element in his or her delirium, avoid confrontation and remain at a safe distance. Accept bizarre statements calmly, with a nod, but without agreement. Explain to the family that the behaviors are symptoms that will most likely resolve with time, resumption of normal sleep patterns, and medication. Delirious patients usually remember the events, thoughts, conversations, and provider responses that occur during delirium. The recovered patients may be embarrassed and feel guilty if they were combative during their illness.

Depression

Depression occurring with a medical illness affects the long-term recovery outcomes by lengthening the course of the illness and increasing morbidity and mortality. Risk factors that predispose for depression with medical disorders include social isolation, recent loss, pessimism, financial pressures, history of mood disorder, alcohol or substance abuse/withdrawal, previous suicide attempts, and pain. Depressive syndromes include somatic symptoms (weight loss, appetite change, sleep disturbance, fatigue), cognitive symptoms (fear, hopelessness, self-pity, negativity, poor concentration), and behavioral symptoms (depressed affect, apathy, pessimism, unreactive mood).

Educating the patient and family about the temporary nature of most depressions during critical illness will assist in providing reassurance that the patient is not crazy or stigmatized as having mental illness. Severe depressive symptoms will often respond to pharmacologic intervention, so a

psychiatric consult may be warranted. If you suspect a person is depressed, ask directly. Allow the patient to initiate conversation. Personal disclosure by staff may be burdensome, and offering opinions negates an opportunity for the patient to work through his or her feelings. However, if negative distortions about illness and treatment are communicated, it is appropriate to correct, clarify, and reassure with realistic information to promote a more hopeful outcome. Consistency in care providers will promote trust in an ongoing relationship and will enhance recovery.

A patient who has attempted suicide or is suicidal can be frightening to hospital staff. Staff are often uncertain of what to say when the patient says, "I want to kill myself . . . my life no longer has meaning." One approach is to reflect back what you hear or observed, for example, "You sound discouraged." Do not avoid asking if the person is feeling suicidal; there is little you can say that would be "wrong." Many times the communication of feeling suicidal is a cover for wanting to discuss fear, pain, or loneliness. A psychiatric referral is recommended for further evaluation and intervention.

Anxiety

Medical disorders can cause anxiety and panic–like symptoms which are distressing to the patient and family and may exacerbate the medical condition. Treatment of the underlying medical condition may decrease the concomitant anxiety. Both pharmacologic and nonpharmacologic interventions can be helpful in managing anxiety during critical illness. Pharmacologic agents for anxiety are discussed in Chapter 9, Critical Care Pharmacology. Goals of pharmacologic therapy are to titrate the drug dose so the patient can remain cognizant and interactive with staff, family, and environment; complement pain control; and assist in promoting sleep.

There are a variety of nonpharmacologic interventions to decrease or control anxiety (see also Chapter 8, Alternative Therapies in Critical Care):

- *Breathing Techniques.* Breathing techniques target somatic symptoms and include deep and slow abdominal breathing patterns. It is important to demonstrate and do the breathing with patients, as their heightened anxiety decreases their attention span. Practicing this technique may also decrease anxiety and promote synchrony for patients whom you anticipate may need ventilator support.
- *Sleep.* Restoration of the sleep-rest-wake cycle by planning care to permit 90 minutes of uninterrupted sleep (allows for rapid-eye-movement/restorative sleep) especially during the latter half of the night.
- *Muscle Relaxation.* Reduce psychomotor tension with muscle relaxation. Again, the patient will most likely be unable to cue himself or herself, so this is an excellent opportunity for the family to participate

as the cuing partner. Cuing might be, "The mattress under your head, elbow, heel, and back feels heavy against your body, press harder, and then try to drift away from the mattress as you relax." Commercial relaxation tapes are available but are not as useful as the cuing by a familiar voice.

- *Creation of a Calming Environment.* Presenting a calm, nonjudgmental attitude, acceptance, consistency, and confidence assists the patient to regain control. Assist other members of the health care team to mirror these behaviors, as well. Family members often benefit from support groups or educational presentations where they learn from others and realize they are not the only ones experiencing stress and anxiety. A referral for brief, focused psychotherapy may be an adjunct to pharmacologic therapy.

- *Imagery.* Interventions targeting cognition, such as imagery techniques, will depend upon the patient's capacity for attention, memory, and processing. Visualization imagery involves recalling a pleasurable, relaxing situation. For example, a hot bath, lying on a warm beach, listening to waves, or hearing birds sing. Guided imagery and hypnosis are additional therapies, but require some competency to be effective; thus a referral is suggested. Patients who practice meditation as an alternative for stress control should be encouraged to continue, but the environment may need modification to optimize the effects.

- *Preparatory Information.* Providing the patient and family with preparatory information is extremely helpful in controlling anxiety. Allowing the patient and family to control some aspects of the illness process, even if only minor aspects of care, can be anxiolytic.

- *Distraction Techniques.* Distraction techniques can also interrupt the "fear begets fear" cycle. Methods for distracting can be listening to familiar music or humorous tapes, watching videos, counting backward from 200 by 2 in a rapid manner, or singing (if previously enjoyed).

- *Use of Previous Coping Methods.* Identify how the patient and family have dealt with stress and anxiety in the past and suggest that approach if feasible. Supporting previous coping techniques, such as crying or being angry, may well be adaptive.

Supporting Patients and Family During the Dying Process

Caring for the dying patient and his or her family can be a most rewarding challenge. The use of advance directives provides an avenue for discussing values and beliefs associated with dying and living. Hopefully, discussions prior to a traumatic event or critical care admission have occurred

so the patient is empowered to institute stopping or continuing life support measures and has designated a surrogate decision maker. If advanced directives are in place, then advocating for those wishes and promoting comfort are primary responsibilities of clinicians. If previous discussions have not taken place, as with an unexpected traumatic accident, then requesting system resources to assist the family while you attend to the patient's critical needs is appropriate. Providing for clergy to assist with spiritual needs and rituals also can help the family to cope with the crisis.

It is important to have an awareness of your own philosophical feelings about death when caring for dying persons. Be genuine in your care, touch, and presence, and do not feel compelled to talk. Take your cue from the patient. Crying or laughing with the patient and family is an acknowledgment of humanness, an existential relationship, and a rare gift in a unique encounter. Following the death of a patient, it can be healing to have a group that includes everyone involved with the patient, including the family, review what went positively and what could have been improved. Attending the funeral service can also promote the grieving process.

SELECTED BIBLIOGRAPHY

What Heals: Family Presence During Resuscitation

Brown JR: Legally it makes good sense [commentary]. *Nursing 89*. March 1989:46.

Chalk S: More on family presence during resuscitation [letter]. *Journal of Emergency Nursing*. April 1994:97.

Doyle CJ, Post H, Burney RE, Maino J, Keefe M, Rhee KJ: Family participation during resuscitation: An option. *Annals of Emergency Medicine*. 1987; 16:107–109.

Eichhorn DJ, Meyers TA, Guzzetta CE: Letting the family say good-bye during CPR. *American Journal of Nursing*. 1995; 95:6.

Eichhorn DJ, Meyers TA, Guzzetta CE: Family presence during resuscitation: It is time to open the door. *Capsules & Comments in Critical Care Nursing*. 1995;3:8–13.

Eichhorn DJ, Meyers TA, Mitchell G, Guzzetta CE. Opening the doors: Family presence during resuscitation. *Journal of Cardiovascular Nursing*. 1996; 10:1–13

Emergency Nurses Association: Family presence at the bedside during invasive procedures and/or resuscitation. General Assembly 1993; Resolution 93:02.

Emergency Nurses Association Department of Nursing Resources: Presenting the option for family presence. ENA resources, publications, educational programs, professional resources 1995 pamphlet. Park Ridge, IL: ENA.

Espersen S: ED's code [commentary]. *Nursing 85*. June 1985:80.

Fina DK: A chance to say goodbye. *American Journal of Nursing*. May 1994:42–45.

Hanson C, Strawser D: Family presence during cardiopulmonary resuscitation: Foote hospital emergency department's nine-year perspective. *Journal of Emergency Nursing*. 1992;18:104–106.

Kuek L: The least we can do [letter]. *Journal of Emergency Nursing.* 1992;18:302.

Letting families in during a code. *AACN News.* September 1994:3.

Martin J: Rethinking traditional thoughts [letter]. *Journal of Emergency Nursing.* 1991;17:67–68.

Osuagwu C: ED codes: Keep the family out [letter]. *Journal of Emergency Nursing.* 1991;17:363–364.

Osuagwu C: Family presence during a code: More research is needed on patients' feelings. *Journal of Emergency Nursing.* 1995;21:196.

Post H: Letting the family in during a code. *Nursing 89.* March 1989:43–46.

Redheffer GM: A trauma nurses's opinion [commentary]. *Nursing 89.* March 1989:45.

Reese V: Her husband was dying and she wanted to watch the code. *Nursing 94.* April 1994:32S–32V.

Reynolds D (ed.): Death as a shared experience: Families in the resuscitation room. *ED Management.* December 1992:177–181.

Strawser D (personal communication), Foote Memorial Hospital, Jackson, MI, July 1994.

Swanson RW: Psychological issues in CPR. *Annals of Emergency Medicine.* 1993;22:84–87.

Ullman K: Hospital allows families in ER. *Medical World News.* June 13, 1988:29.

Villaire M: Beth Henneman's ICU passion is all in the family. *Critical Care Nurse.* October 1994:94.

Williams M: More on family presence during resuscitation [letter]. *Journal of Emergency Nursing.* 1993;19:477–478.

Yanks KK: More on family presence during resuscitation [letter]. *Journal of Emergency Nursing.* 1993;19:477–478.

Critical Pathways

Bueno M, Hwang R: Understanding variances in hospital stay. *Nursing Management.* 1993;24(11):51–57.

Hronek C: Implementing collaborative care. *Main Dimensions—Midwest Alliance in Nursing.* 1993;4(7):1–4.

Lunsdon K, Lord J: Architects of care. *Hospitals and Health Networks.* March 20, 1994:20–21.

Lunsdon K, Magland M: Mapping care. *Hospitals and Health Networks.* October 20, 1993:34–40.

Southwick K: Two approaches to better outcomes at lower cost. *Strategies for Healthcare Excellence.* 1994;7(3):1–8.

Nutrition

Ackerman MH (guest ed.): Nutrition. *AACN Clinical Issues in Critical Care Nursing.* 1994;1(5).

Ackerman MH, Ciechoski MJ, Marx LM: Current trends in enteral feeding. *Gastroenterology Nursing.* April 1992:233–236.

Ackermam MH, Evans NJ, Ecklund MM: Systemic inflammatory response syndrome, sepsis, and nutritional support. *Critical Care Nursing Clinics of North America.* 1994;6(2):321–340.

Zaloga G, Ackerman MH: A review of disease-specific formulas. *AACN Clinical Issues in Critical Care Nursing.* 1994;5(4):421–435.

Patient and Family Education

Bille DA: Patient and family teaching in critical care. In Dossey BM, Guzzetta CE, Kenner CV: *Critical care nursing: Body-mind-spirit* (3rd ed.). Philadelphia: JB Lippincott, 1992.

Joint Commission on Accreditation of Healthcare Organizations. *1995 Comprehensive accreditation manual for hospitals.* Joint Commission on Accreditation of Healthcare Organizations: Oakbook Terrace, IL, 1994, pp. 189–206.

Oka RA, Burke LE, Froelicher ES: Emotional responses and inpatient education. In Woods SL, Sivarajan Froelicher ES, Halpenny CJ, Motzer SU: *Cardiac nursing* (3rd ed.). Philadelphia: JB Lippincott, 1995.

Panchal JA, Kmetz LL: The puzzle of educating the client with a cardiovascular disorder: Making all the pieces fit. *Journal of Home Health Care Practice.* 1991;4(1):1–12.

Redman BK: *The process of patient education* (5th ed.). St. Louis, MO: CV Mosby, 1984.

Smith CE: *Patient education: Nurses in partnership with other health professionals.* New York: Grune & Stratton, 1987.

Spicer MR: *How to design and use a patient teaching module.* Atlanta, GA: Prichett & Hull, 1991.

Near-Death Experiences

Appleby L: Near death experience. *British Medical Journal.* 1989;298:977.

Association of the Scientific Study of Near-Death Phenomena: *Statement of purpose.* Peoria, IL: The Association for the Scientific Study of Near-Death Phenomena, 1979.

Clark K: Clinical interventions with near-death experiences. In Greyson B, Flynn CP : *The near-death experience: Problems, prospects, perspectives.* Springfield, IL: CC Thomas, 1984.

Corcoran DK: Helping patients who've had near-death experiences. *Nursing 88.* November 1988:34.

Gallup G, Proctor W: *Adventures in immortality: A look beyond the threshold of death.* New York: McGraw-Hill, 1982.

Greyson B, Bush NE: Distressing near-death experiences. *Psychiatry.* 1992;55:95–110.

Guzzetta CE: Near-death experience. In: Dossey BM, Guzzetta CE, Kenner CV: *Critical care nursing: Body-mind-spirit.* Philadelphia: JB Lippincott, 1992, pp. 963–968.

Guzzetta CE: The person with a near-death experience. In: Guzzetta CE, Dossey BM: *Cardiovascular nursing: Holistic practice.* St. Louis, MO: Mosby-Year Book, 1992, pp. 757–763.

Guzzetta CE: Near-death experiences: What if we could do more? *Capsules & Comments in Critical Care Nursing.* 1993;1:5–9.

Letting families in during a code. *AACN News.* September 1994:3.

Moody RA: *Life after life.* New York: Bantam, 1975.

Oakes AR: Near-death events and critical care nursing. *Topics in Clinical Nursing.* 1981;3:61.

Olson M: Near-death experiences and the elderly. *Holistic Nursing Practice.* 1992;7:16.

Ramaswami S: Omega as alpha: Implications of near-death experiences. In: Sheikh AA, Sheikh KS (ed.): *Death imagery: Confronting death can bring us to the threshold of life.* Milwaukee, WI: American Imagery Institute, 1991.

Reader AL: The internal mystery plays: The role and physiology of the visual system in contemplative practices. *ReVision.* 1994;17:3–13.

Ring J: *Life after death: A scientific investigation of the near-death experiences.* New York: Coward, McCann, 1980.

Ring J. Editorial. *Anabiosis.* 1981;2:21.

Roberts G, Owen H: The near-death experience. *British Journal of Psychiatry.* 1988;153:607.

Villaire M: Beth Henneman's ICU passion is all in the family. *Critical Care Nurse*. October 1994:94.

Sleep Deprivation

Edwards GB, Schuring LM: Sleep protocol: A research-based practice change. *Critical Care Nurse,* 1993;13:84–88.

Fontaine DK: Sleep in the critically ill patient. In Kinney M, Dunbar S, Packa D (eds.): *AACN's Clinical Reference for Critical Care Nursing.* St Louis, MO: Mosby-Year Book, 1993, pp. 351–364.

Richards KC: Sleep promotion in the critical care unit. *AACN Clinical Issues.* 1994;5:152–158.

Communication

Buckwalter K, Cusack D, Sidles E, Wadle K, Beaver M: Increasing communication ability in aphasic/dysarthric patients. *Western Journal of Nursing Research.* 1989;11(6):736–747.

Connolly M. Nonvocal treatments for short and long-term ventilator patients. In Mason M: Speech pathology for tracheotomized and ventilator dependent patients. Newport Beach, CA: Voicing, Inc.,1993.

Connolly M, Shekleton M: Communicating with ventilator dependent patients. *Dimensions of Critical Care Nursing.* 1991;10(2): 115–122.

Lawless C. Helping patients with endotracheal and tracheostomy tubes communicate. *American Journal of Nursing.* 1975;75: 2151–2158.

Riegel B, et al: Reviews and summaries of research related to AACN 1980 research priorities: Clinical topics. *American Journal of Critical Care.* 1993;2(5):413–425.

Psychosocial Support

Alpen MA, Halm MA: Family needs: An annotated bibliography. *Critical Care Nurse.* 1994;12(2):32–51.

Barry PD: *Psychosocial nursing assessment and intervention: Care of the physically ill person,* 2nd ed. Philadelphia: JB Lippincott, 1989.

Bone RC: *Recognition, assessment, and treatment of anxiety in the critical care patient: Proceedings of a consensus conference.* Yardley, PA: The Medicine Group USA, Inc., 1994.

Goleman D, Gurin J (eds.): *Mind body medicine: How to use your mind for better health.* Yonkers, NY: Consumer Reports Books, 1993.

Interpretation and Management of Basic Cardiac Rhythms

4

► Knowledge Competencies

1. Correctly identify key elements of electrocardiogram (ECG) waveforms, complexes, and intervals:
   • P wave
   • QRS complex
   • T wave
   • ST segment
   • PR interval
   • QT interval
   • RR interval
   • Rate (atrial and ventricular)

2. Compare and contrast the etiology, ECG characteristics, and management of common cardiac rhythms originating in the:
   • Sinus node
   • Atria
   • Atrioventricular junction
   • Ventricle

3. Describe the indications for, and use of, temporary pacemakers, defibrillation, and cardioversion for the treatment of serious cardiac arrhythmias.

■ What Heals: The Mind and Arrhythmias

Although the impact of emotional stress on the development of ventricular arrhythmias is well documented, often this topic is neglected as a part of an introduction to cardiac rhythms. Yet the data are hard to ignore. Wellens and coworkers, for example, documented the recurrent onset of ventricular fibrillation in a young girl whenever she was awakened by an alarm clock. The initial episode of fibrillation occurred after she was awakened by a thunderclap. In another report, an elderly woman, hospitalized for severe trauma following a motor vehicle accident, developed ventricular fibrillation and died immediately after being told that her husband had been killed during the accident. The authors (Grant and Weston) hypothesized that the emotional trauma of learning of her husband's death had lowered her threshold for ventricular fibrillation, causing ventricular ectopic activity, malignant arrhythmias, and ultimately sudden cardiac death. Likewise, Reich and colleagues found that 26 of 117 patients, referred to a major medical center for management of ventricular arrhythmias, had experienced emotional disturbances during the 24 hours before onset. The primary emotion identified was anger, but other common emotions such as depression and grief also were observed. Although those at highest risk for emotionally induced ventricular arrhythmias are patients with underlying cardiac disease, lethal ventricular arrhythmia also can be triggered by emotions in patients who have no structural cardiac disease (Hackett and colleagues).

Lown and associates described the case of a 39-year-old man who experienced two episodes of ventricular fibrillation. The initial episode occurred when he was roughhousing with his sexually mature daughters. This event was interrupted by a neighbor ringing the doorbell, at which time the man looked up, said "I'm sorry," developed ventricular fibrillation, and had a cardiac arrest. Following successful resuscitation, he underwent coronary angiography without any findings of structural heart disease. He was defensive and covertly hostile and denied being depressed or angry. Although outwardly calm and controlled, during psychiatric interviews he would develop ventricular premature beats. A second cardiac arrest occurred during sleep. When his arrhythmia could not be controlled with a variety of medications, he was taught to meditate and was successfully able to suppress his arrhythmias. Only through the combined used of medication and meditation could his arrhythmia be controlled.

Although it has been documented that a single emotional event can trigger ventricular arrhythmias, more frequently it has been reported that patients experience feelings of hopelessness, emotional vulnerability, grief, and depression (Green and coworkers) for several weeks prior to the major stressful event that culminates in a *giving-up–given-up* response (Engel). Thus, it is critical to assess patients for reports of recent stressful life events (i.e., loss of a loved one, loss of a job, severe disappointments) and newly identified anxiety-producing situations,

and to evaluate them for new signs and symptoms of fatigue and depression. Patients can be taught to record stressors during the day to become aware of which incidents trigger emotional responses. They can be instructed to avoid stressful settings, people, and situations whenever possible. They can be taught ways to change their perception of emotionally stressful situations and exert conscious control over their emotional responses (i.e., "Is this worth dying for?"). They also can be guided to learn a variety of strategies to reduce the impact of their emotional responses (i.e., deep breathing, muscle relaxation, biofeedback, imagery, music therapy).

Cases such as these suggest that the traditional way of regarding the heart as a mere object that can invariably be treated with mere surgical or pharmacologic approaches of therapy is incomplete. No matter how much we wish to objectify our approaches to cardiac disorders, research reports such as these remind us, perhaps uncomfortably, that disorders of the cardiac rate and rhythm are not always as objective as we might like them to be.

CEG & BMD

Adapted from: Dossey BM, Guzzetta CE: Stress and ventricular fibrillation. In Guzzetta CE, Dossey BM: Cardiovascular nursing: Holistic practice. St. Louis, MO: Mosby Year Book, 1992, p. 160.

INTRODUCTION

Continuous monitoring of cardiac rhythm in the critically ill patient is an important aspect of cardiovascular assessment. Frequent analysis of ECG rate and rhythm provides for early identification and treatment of alternations in cardiac rhythm, as well as abnormal conditions in other body systems. This chapter presents a review of basic cardiac electrophysiology and information essential to the identification and treatment of common cardiac arrhythmias. Advanced cardiac arrhythmias, as well as 12-lead ECG interpretation, are described in Chapter 21, Advanced ECG Concepts.

BASIC ELECTROPHYSIOLOGY

The sinus node is the normal pacemaker of the heart because it has the highest rate of the normal pacemaker

sites. The sinus node normally fires at a regular rate of 60 to 100 beats/minute. The impulse spreads from the sinus node through the atria and to the atrioventricular (AV) node, where it encounters a slight delay before it travels through the bundle of His, right and left bundle branches, and Purkinje fibers into the ventricles. The spread of this wave of depolarization through the heart gives rise to the classical surface ECG, which can be monitored continuously at the bedside.

The ECG is a graphic record of the electrical activity of the heart. Impulse formation and conduction throughout the heart produce weak electrical currents through the entire body. The difference in potential between a positive and a negative area within the body can be measured on the body surface by a galvanometer, an instrument consisting of a wire between the poles of an electromagnet. As current passes through the wire, the instrument is controlled by the magnetic field. The ECG machine contains a galvanometer

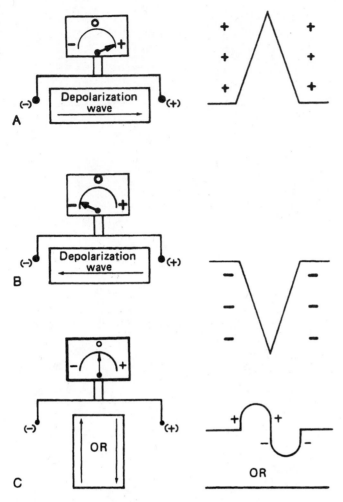

Figure 4–1. (A) Depolarization wave coursing toward a positive electrode results in a positive or upright deflection of the stylus. (B) Depolarization wave coursing away from a positive electrode results in a negative or downward deflection of the stylus. (C) Depolarization wave coursing in a direction that is perpendicular to the positive electrode results in a biphasic or isoelectric inscription. *(From: Gilmore SB, Woods SL: Electrocardiography and vectorcardiography. In Woods SL, et al (eds.): Cardiac nursing, 3rd ed. Philadelphia: JB Lippincott, 1995, p. 291.)*

that detects changes in surface potential, amplifies the signal, and records these body surface potential changes over time on calibrated moving paper.

By convention, if a positive electrode is placed on the side facing the advancing wave of depolarization, a positive deflection will be produced (Figure 4–1A). If the poles of the galvanometer are reversed, however, a negative deflection will be produced. The magnitude, or height, of the deflection represents the thickness of the muscle involved. If a positive electrode is placed on the side from which the wave of depolarization is receding, a negative deflection will result (Figure 4–1B). If an electrode is placed at right angles (perpendicular) to the wave of depolarization, a biphasic deflection or no deflection (isoelectric) will occur (Figure 4–1C).

ECG WAVEFORMS, COMPLEXES, AND INTERVALS

The ECG waves, complexes, and intervals are illustrated in Figure 4–2.

P Wave

The P wave represents atrial muscle depolarization. It is normally 2.5 mm or less in height and 0.11 second or less in duration. The voltage of positive deflections is measured from the upper portion of the baseline to the peak of the wave. The atrial repolarization (atrial T wave) is wide and of low amplitude and therefore is not seen or is buried in the QRS complex.

QRS Complex

The QRS complex (beginning of the Q wave to the end of the S wave) represents ventricular muscle depolarization. The first negative deflection is the Q wave, which is less than 0.03 second in duration and less than 25% of the R-wave amplitude; the first positive deflection is the R wave; and the S wave is the first negative deflection after the R wave. The voltage of negative deflections is measured from the lower portion of the baseline to the nadir of the wave. Figure 4–3 shows examples of various QRS complex configurations. When a wave is less than 5 mm vertically, small letters (q, r, s) are used; when a wave is 5 mm or more vertically, capital letters (Q, R, S) are used. When a complex is all negative, it is called a QS complex. Not all QRS complexes have all three waveforms. The QRS complex is measured from the beginning of the Q wave, or if no Q wave is present, from the beginning of R wave, to the end of the S wave. The QRS complex is normally 0.04 to 0.10 second in duration. The QRS complex in the chest leads (V_1 to V_6) can be 0.01 to 0.02 second longer than in the limb leads.

T and U Waves

The T and U waves represent ventricular muscle repolarization. They follow the QRS complex and are usually of the same deflection as the QRS complex. If a U wave is seen, it will follow the T wave. The presence of a U wave may indicate an electrolyte abnormality. It is thought to be the result of the slow repolarization of the intraventricular (Purkinje) conduction system.

ST Segment

The ST segment, which represents early repolarization of the ventricles, is from the end of the S wave (J point) to the beginning of the T wave.

PR Interval

The PR interval is measured from the beginning of the P wave to the beginning of the Q wave, or if no Q wave is present, to the beginning of the R wave, and represents the time required for the impulse to travel through the atria

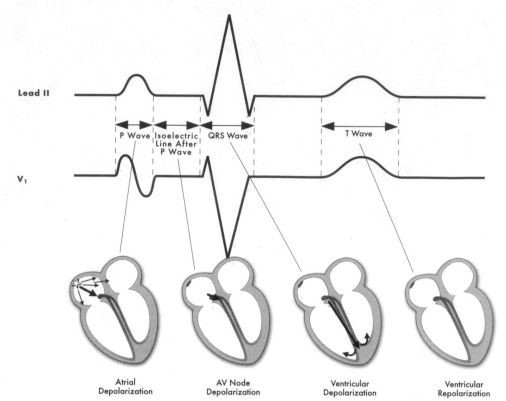

Figure 4–2. Electrocardiographic waves, complexes, and intervals in leads II and V$_1$.

Atrial Depolarization   AV Node Depolarization   Ventricular Depolarization   Ventricular Repolarization

and conduction system to the Purkinje fibers. In adults with normal heart rates, the PR interval usually ranges from 0.12 to 0.20 second in duration. The PR segment is isoelectric and is measured from the end of the P wave to the beginning of the QRS complex.

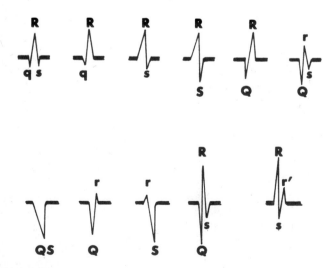

Figure 4–3. Examples of various QRS complexes and proper labeling of component waveforms. *(From: Gilmore SB, Woods SL: Electrocardiography and vectorcardiography. In Woods SL, et al (eds.): Cardiac nursing, 3rd ed. Philadelphia: JB Lippincott, 1995, p. 293.)*

QT Interval

The QT interval, which represents electrical systole, is measured from the beginning of the Q wave to the end of the T wave. If no Q wave is present, the beginning of the R wave is used for the QRS measurement. The QT interval varies with heart rate and must be corrected to a heart rate of 60/minute (QT$_c$) following measurement. This correction is done by use of a nomogram (Figure 4–4). The QT interval is usually less than half the RR interval (measured from the beginning of one R wave to the beginning of the next R wave) and usually is 0.32 to 0.40 second in duration if the heart rate is 65 to 95/minute. The QT$_c$ should not exceed 0.42 second in men or 0.43 second in women. The J point is the point where the QRS complex ends and the ST segment begins.

Cardiac Monitoring

Cardiac monitoring provides continuous observation of the patient's heart rate and rhythm, as well as ST-segment placement. Patients can be monitored using a three-lead or five-lead hardwire cable which attaches the patient to the cardiac monitor. Advantages of selected leads for monitoring are summarized in Table 4–1.

The electrodes are placed on the chest according to the leads selected for monitoring. A detailed description of electrode placement for all 12 leads of the ECG is presented

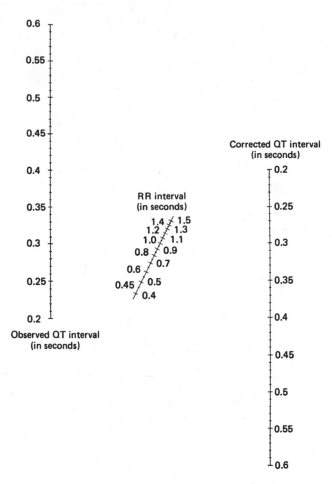

Figure 4–4. Nomogram for rate correction of QT interval. Measure the observed QT interval and the RR interval. Mark these values in the respective columns on the chart (left and middle). Place a ruler across these two points. The point at which the extension of this line crosses the third column is read as the corrected QT interval (QT$_c$). This nomogram is based on the following equation: QT$_c$ is equal to the observed QT interval divided by the square root of the RR interval. *(From: Kissen M, et al: A nomogram for rate correction of the QT interval in the electrocardiogram. American Heart Journal. 1948;35:991.)*

TABLE 4–1. ADVANTAGES OF COMMON ECG MONITORING LEADS

Lead	Advantages
Preferred Monitoring Leads	
MCL$_1$ and MCL$_6$	Allow distinction between left ventricular and right ventricular ectopy and between left ventricular and right ventricular artificial pacing
	Allow distinction between right and left bundle branch block
	Allow distinction between aberration and ectopy
	Assist in diagnoses that require well-formed P waves
	Apex of the heart is not covered by an electrode and is clear for auscultation and defibrillation without electrode interference
Other Monitoring Leads	
M$_3$	Allows identification of retrograde P waves
II	Assists in the diagnosis of hemiblock

(From: Osguthorpe SG, Woods SL: Myocardial ischemia and infarction. In Woods SL, et al (eds.): Cardiac nursing, 3rd ed. Philadelphia: JB Lippincott, 1995, p 479.)

in Chapter 21, Advanced ECG Concepts. This chapter describes the most commonly used monitoring leads and the corresponding electrode placement for continuous cardiac monitoring.

With a three-lead system, Lead MCL$_1$, Lead MCL$_6$, or Lead M$_3$ is commonly used (Figure 4–5A). Lead II may also be used in some cases. For MCL$_1$, MCL$_6$, or M$_3$, the positive electrode is placed in the V$_1$ position, the V$_6$ position, or the left upper abdomen, respectively, and the negative electrode is placed on the left posterior shoulder. The ground electrode is positioned on the right posterior shoulder. If you place the left arm electrode in the V$_1$ position, the right arm electrode on the left outer shoulder, and the left leg electrode in the V$_6$ position, you will get MCL$_1$ with the dial selector on Lead I and MCL$_6$ with the dial selector on Lead II. For Lead II, using a three-lead system,

the positive electrode is placed on the left upper abdomen and the negative electrode is placed on the right upper chest.

With a five-lead system, V$_1$, V$_6$, or Lead III is commonly used. With a five-lead system, the right arm electrode is placed on the right outer shoulder, the left arm electrode is placed on the left outer shoulder, the right leg electrode is placed on the lower right abdomen or hip, the left leg electrode is placed on the lower left abdomen or hip, and the chest electrode is placed in the V$_1$ or V$_6$ position (Figure 4–5B). With the electrodes in these positions, all 12 leads can be obtained. The chest electrode would need to be moved to the six chest lead positions to obtain the six V leads.

The electrode sites on the skin should be clean, dry, and relatively flat. Hair should be shaved, if present, and the skin cleansed with alcohol to remove any oils. Mildly abrading the skin with a gauze or abrading pad supplied on electrode packaging will improve transmission of the ECG signal. The pregelled electrodes are then applied to the chest. The alarm limits for heart rate are set (30% above and below patient's heart rate), the audio switch in the patient's room is turned off, and the alarm system is activated. Sources of artifacts, or distortions of the ECG signal, are shown in Figure 4–6. Electrodes should be changed often enough to prevent skin breakdown and provide artifact-free tracings. Placement of electrodes on the posterior shoulder, rather than on the anterior chest in the subclavicular area, will avoid skin breakdown in an area which is often used for percutaneous catheter insertion.

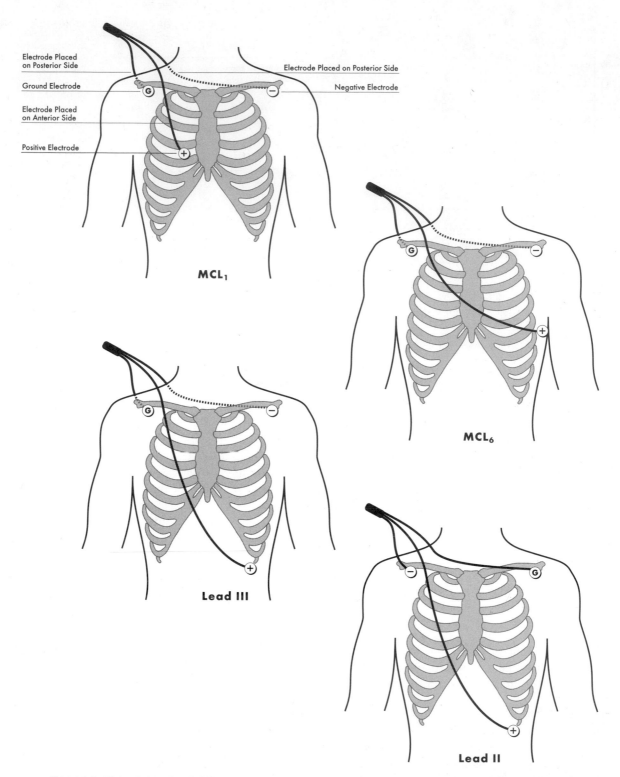

Figure 4–5. (A) Lead placement for constant cardiac monitoring using a three-wire system. Electrode placement for Lead MCL$_1$: ground electrode on the posterior right shoulder, negative electrode on the posterior left shoulder, and positive electrode in the V$_1$ position (fourth intercostal space, right of the sternum). Electrode placement for Lead MCL$_6$: ground electrode on the posterior right shoulder, negative electrode on the posterior left shoulder, and positive electrode in the V$_6$ position (horizontal from V$_4$ in the midaxillary line). To obtain M$_3$, the positive electrode is placed on the upper left abdomen (dashed line). Electrode placement for Lead II: ground electrode on the left shoulder, negative electrode on right shoulder, and positive electrode on the left lower rib cage.

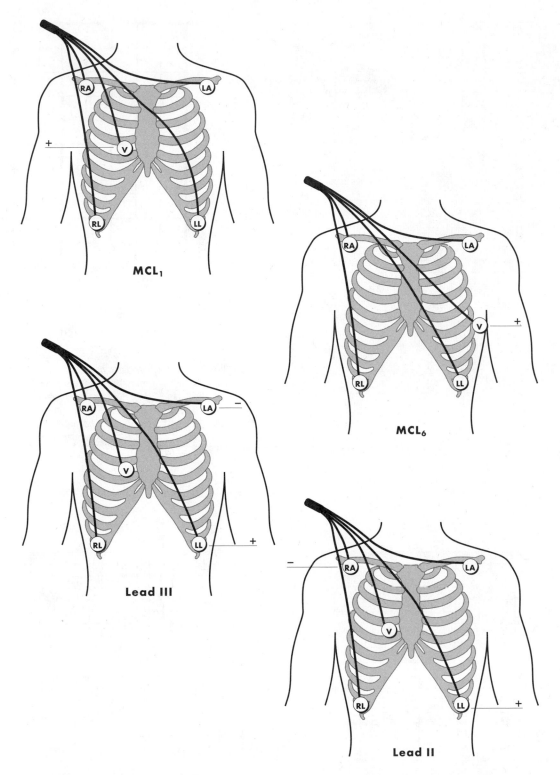

Figure 4–5 continued. (B) Lead placement for constant cardiac monitoring using a five-wire system. Electrodes are placed on the right and left shoulders, right and left lower chest areas, and in the V_1 or V_6 position. Selection of leads is made on the bedside monitor control panel.

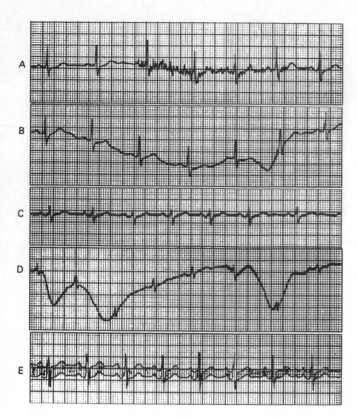

Figure 4–6. Sources of artifacts in ECG-monitored tracings. (A) Involuntary movement. (B) Voluntary movement. (C) Poor skin preparation. (D) Dried-out electrode. (E) Bad grounding. *(From: Graphic Controls, Medi-Trace R Products Division, Buffalo, NY, 1988.)*

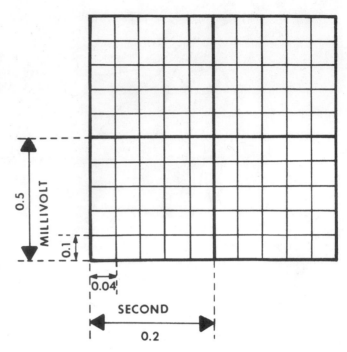

Figure 4–7. Time and voltage lines on ECG paper, at standard voltage and speed (one small box = 1 mm). Vertical measurements: 1 mm = 0.1 mV; 5 mm = 0.5 mV; 10 mm = 1 mV. Horizontal measurements: 1 mm = 0.04 second; 5 mm = 0.20 second; 25 mm = 1 second; 1500 mm = 60 seconds. *(From: Gilmore SB, Woods SL: Electrocardiography and vectorcardiography. In Woods SL, et al (eds.): Cardiac nursing, 3rd ed. Philadelphia: JB Lippincott, 1995, p. 291.)*

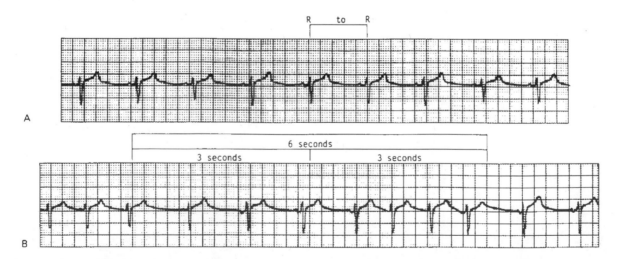

Figure 4–8. (A) Heart rate determination for a regular rhythm using little boxes between two R waves. One RR interval is marked at the top of the ECG paper. There are 25 little boxes between these two R waves. There are 1500 little boxes in a 60-second strip. By dividing 1500 by 25, one calculates a heart rate of 60 beats/minute. Heart rate can also be determined for a regular rhythm counting large boxes between R waves. There are five large boxes between R waves. There are 300 large boxes in a 60-second strip. By dividing 300 by 5, one calculates a heart rate of 60 beats/minute. (B) Heart rate determination for a regular or irregular rhythm using the number of RR intervals in a 6-second strip and multiplying by 10. There are seven RR intervals in this example. Multiplying by 10 gives a heart rate of 70/minute. *(From: Gilmore SB, Woods SL: Electrocardiography and vectorcardiography. In Woods SL, et al (eds.): Cardiac nursing, 3rd ed. Philadelphia: JB Lippincott, 1995, p. 295.)*

Determination of Heart Rate

ECG paper generally moves at a speed of 25 mm/second. Each small box horizontally is equal to 0.04 second. One large box (five small boxes) horizontally equals 0.20 second (5 × 0.04 second); one large box (five small boxes) vertically is equal to 5 mm (Figure 4–7).

Heart rate can be obtained from the ECG strip by several methods. The first, and most accurate if the rhythm is regular, is to count the number of small boxes (one small box = 0.04 second) between two R waves, and then divide that number into 1500. There are 1500 0.04-second interval boxes in a 1-minute strip (Figure 4–8A). Another method is to count the number of large boxes (one large box = 0.20 second) between two R waves, and then divide that number into 300 or use a standardized table (Table 4–2).

The third method for computing heart rate, especially useful when the rhythm is irregular, is to count the number of RR intervals in 6 seconds and multiply that number by 10. The ECG paper is usually marked at 3-second intervals (15 large boxes horizontally) by a vertical line at the top of the paper (Figure 4–8B). The RR intervals are counted, not the QRS complexes, to avoid overestimating the heart rate.

Any of these three methods can also be used to calculate the atrial rate by using P waves instead of R waves.

DETERMINATION OF CARDIAC RHYTHM

Correct determination of the cardiac rhythm requires a systematic evaluation of the ECG. The following steps should be used to determine the cardiac rhythm:

1. Calculate the atrial (P wave) rate.
2. Calculate the ventricular (QRS complex) rate.
3. Determine the regularity and shape of the P waves.
4. Determine the regularity, shape, and width of the QRS complexes.
5. Measure the PR interval.
6. Interpret the arrhythmia as described below.

COMMON ARRHYTHMIAS

An arrhythmia is any cardiac rhythm that is not normal sinus rhythm. An arrhythmia may result from altered impulse formation or altered impulse conduction. Arrhythmias are named by the place where they originate and by their rate. Arrhythmias are grouped as follows:

1. Rhythms originating in the sinus node
2. Rhythms originating in the atria
3. Rhythms originating in the junction
4. Rhythms originating in the ventricle
5. Atrioventricular blocks

TABLE 4–2. HEART RATE DETERMINATION USING THE ELECTROCARDIOGRAM LARGE BOXES

Number of Large Boxes Between R Waves	Heart Rate (Beats/Minute)
1	300
2	150
3	100
4	75
5	60
6	50
7	40
8	38
9	33
10	30

The etiology, ECG characteristics, and treatment of the basic cardiac arrhythmias are presented here and summarized in Chapter 32. (The following content is adapted with permission from Jacobson C: Cardiac arrhythmias and conduction disturbances. In Woods SL, et al (eds.): *Cardiac nursing,* 3rd ed. Philadelphia: JB Lippincott, 1995, pp. 324–337.

Rhythms Originating in the Sinus Node

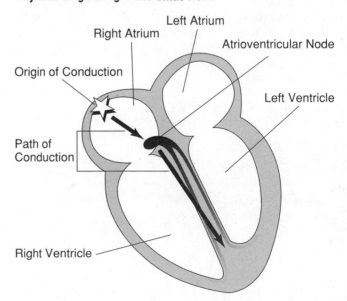

Normal Sinus Rhythm[1]

ECG Characteristics:

- *Rate:* 60 to 100 beats/minute
- *Rhythm:* Regular
- *P waves:* Precede every QRS complex; consistent in shape
- *PR interval:* 0.12 to 0.20 second
- *QRS complex:* 0.04 to 0.10 second
- *Example of normal sinus rhythm:*

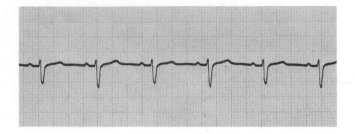

Sinus Bradycardia

All aspects of sinus bradycardia are the same as normal sinus rhythm except the rate is slower. It can be a normal finding in athletes and during sleep. Sinus bradycardia may be a response to vagal stimulation, such as carotid sinus massage, ocular pressure, or vomiting. Sinus bradycardia can be caused by inferior myocardial infarction, myxedema, obstructive jaundice, uremia, increased intracranial pressure, glaucoma, anorexia nervosa, and sick sinus syndrome. Sinus bradycardia can be a response to several medications, including digitalis, beta blockers, and some calcium channel blockers.

ECG Characteristics:

- *Rate:* Less than 60 beats/minute
- *Rhythm:* Regular
- *P waves:* Precede every QRS; consistent in shape
- *PR interval:* Usually normal (0.12 to 0.20 second)
- *QRS complex:* Usually normal (0.04 to 0.10 second)
- *Conduction:* Normal through atria, AV node, bundle branches, and ventricles
- *Example of sinus bradycardia:*

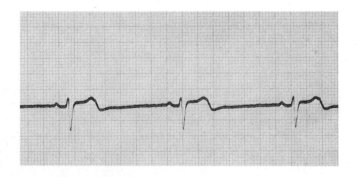

Except where indicated, all examples of arrhythmias in this section are from Dracup K: *Meltzer's intensive coronary care.* Stamford, CT: Appleton & Lange, 1995, pp. 131–252.

Treatment

Treatment of sinus bradycardia is not required unless the patient is symptomatic. If the arrhythmia is accompanied by hypotension, confusion, diaphoresis, chest pain, or other signs of hemodynamic compromise or by ventricular ectopy, atropine, 0.5 to 1.0 mg IV, is the treatment of choice. Attempts should be made to decrease vagal stimulation. If the arrhythmia is due to medications, they should be held until their need has been reevaluated.

Sinus Tachycardia

Sinus tachycardia is a sinus rhythm at a rate greater than 100 beats/minute. Sinus tachycardia is a normal response to exercise and emotion. Sinus tachycardia that persists at rest usually indicates some underlying problem, such as fever, acute blood loss, shock, pain, anxiety, heart failure, hypermetabolic states, or anemia. Sinus tachycardia is a normal physiologic response to a decrease in cardiac output, since cardiac output is the product of heart rate and stroke volume. Sinus tachycardia can be caused by the following medications: atropine, isoproterenol, epinephrine, dopamine, dobutamine, norepinephrine, nitroprusside, and caffeine.

ECG Characteristics:

- *Rate:* Greater than 100 beats/minute
- *Rhythm:* Regular
- *P waves:* Precede every QRS; consistent in shape; may be buried in the preceding T wave
- *PR interval:* Usually normal; may be difficult to measure if P waves are buried in T waves
- *QRS complex:* Usually normal
- *Conduction:* Normal through atria, AV node, bundle branches, and ventricles
- *Example of sinus tachycardia:*

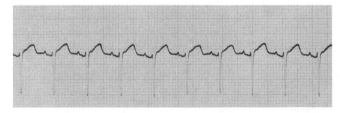

Treatment

Treatment of sinus tachycardia is directed at the underlying cause. This arrhythmia is a physiologic response to a decrease in cardiac output, and it should never be ignored, especially in the cardiac patient. Because the ventricles fill with blood and the coronary arteries perfuse during diastole, persistent tachycardia can cause decreased stroke volume, decreased cardiac output, and decreased coronary perfusion secondary to the decreased diastolic time that occurs with rapid heart rates. Carotid sinus pressure may slow the heart rate temporarily and thereby help in ruling out other arrhythmias.

Sinus Arrhythmia

Sinus arrhythmia occurs when the sinus node discharges irregularly. It occurs frequently as a normal phenomenon and is commonly associated with the phases of respiration. During inspiration, the sinus node fires faster; during expiration, it slows. Digitalis toxicity may also cause this arrhythmia. Sinus arrhythmia looks like normal sinus rhythm except for the sinus irregularity.

ECG Characteristics:

- *Rate:* 60 to 100 beats/minute
- *Rhythm:* Irregular; phasic increase and decrease in rate, which may or may not be related to respiration
- *P waves:* Precede every QRS; consistent in shape
- *PR interval:* Usually normal
- *QRS complex:* Usually normal
- *Conduction:* Normal through atria, AV node, bundle branches, and ventricles
- *Example of sinus arrhythmia:*

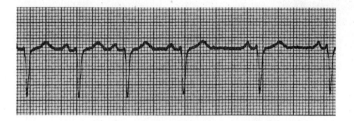

Treatment

Treatment of sinus arrhythmia usually is not necessary. If the arrhythmia is thought to be due to digitalis toxicity, then digitalis should be held. Atropine will increase the rate and eliminate the irregularity.

Sinus Arrest

Sinus arrest occurs when sinus node firing is depressed and impulses are not formed when expected. The result is an absent P wave at the expected time. The QRS complex is also missing, unless there is escape of a junctional or ventricular impulse (see below for description). If only one sinus impulse fails to form, this is usually called a *sinus pause*. If more than one sinus impulse in a row fails to form, this is termed a *sinus arrest*. Because the sinus node is not forming impulses regularly as expected, the PP interval in sinus arrest is not an exact multiple of the sinus cycle. Causes of sinus arrest include vagal stimulation, carotid sinus sensitivity, and myocardial infarction interrupting the blood supply to the sinus node. Drugs such as digitalis, beta blockers, and calcium channel blockers can also cause sinus arrest.

ECG Characteristics:

- *Rate:* Usually within normal range, but may be in the bradycardia range
- *Rhythm:* Irregular due to absence of sinus node discharge

- *P waves:* Present when sinus node is firing and absent during periods of sinus arrest, when present, they precede every QRS complex and are consistent in shape
- *PR interval:* Usually normal when P waves are present
- *QRS complex:* Usually normal when sinus node is functioning and absent during periods of sinus arrest, unless escape beats occur
- *Conduction:* Normal through atria, AV node, bundle branches, and ventricles when sinus node is firing; when the sinus node fails to form impulses, there is no conduction through the atria
- *Example of sinus arrest:*

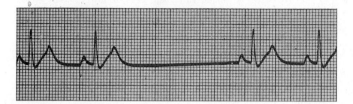

Treatment

Treatment of sinus arrest is aimed at the underlying cause. Drugs that are thought to be responsible should be discontinued and vagal stimulation should be minimized. If periods of sinus arrest are frequent and cause hemodynamic compromise, atropine 0.5 to 1.0 mg IV may increase the rate. Pacemaker therapy may be necessary if other forms of management fail to increase the rate to acceptable levels.

Arrhythmias Originating in the Atria

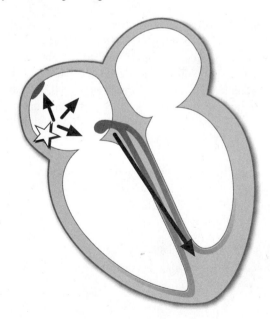

Premature Atrial Complexes

A premature atrial complex (PAC) occurs when an irritable focus in the atria fires before the next sinus node impulse is due to fire. PACs can be caused by caffeine, alcohol, nicotine, congestive heart failure, pulmonary disease, interruption of atrial blood supply by myocardial ischemia or infarction, anxiety, and hypermetabolic states. PACs can also occur in normal hearts.

ECG Characteristics:

- *Rate:* Usually within normal range
- *Rhythm:* Usually regular except when PACs occur, resulting in early beats. PACs usually have a noncompensatory pause (interval between the complex preceding and that following the PAC is less than two normal RR intervals) because premature depolarization of the atria by the PAC usually causes premature depolarization of the sinus node as well, thus causing the sinus node to "reset" itself
- *P waves:* Precede every QRS. The configuration of the premature P wave differs from that of the sinus P waves because the premature impulse originates in a different part of the atria, with atrial depolarization occurring in a different pattern. Very early P waves may be buried in the preceding T wave, altering the space of that T wave
- *PR interval:* May be normal or long depending on the prematurity of the beat; very early PACs may find the AV junction still partially refractory and unable to conduct at a normal rate, resulting in a prolonged PR interval
- *QRS complex:* May be normal, aberrant (wide), or absent, depending on the prematurity of the beat. If the ventricles have repolarized completely they will be able to conduct the early impulse normally, resulting in a normal QRS. If the PAC occurs during the relative refractory period of the bundle branches or ventricles, the impulse will conduct aberrantly and the QRS will be wide. If the PAC occurs very early during the complete refractory period of the bundle branches or ventricles, the impulse will not conduct to the ventricles and the QRS will be absent
- *Conduction:* PACs travel through the atria differently from sinus impulses because they originate from a different spot; conduction through the AV node, bundle branches, and ventricles is usually normal unless the PAC is very early
- *Example of PACs:*

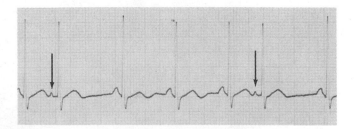

PAC conducted normally in the ventricle

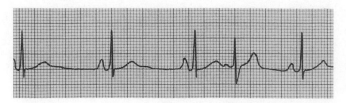

PAC conducted aberrantly in the ventricle

Treatment

Treatment of PACs usually is not necessary since they do not cause hemodynamic compromise. Frequent PACs may precede more serious arrhythmias such as atrial fibrillation. Treatment is directed at the cause. Drugs such as quinidine, disopyramide, or procainamide can be used to suppress atrial activity if necessary.

Wandering Atrial Pacemaker

Wandering atrial pacemaker (WAP) refers to rhythms that exhibit varying P-wave morphology as the site of impulse formation "wanders" from the sinus node to the atria to the AV junction. WAP can be due to increased vagal tone slowing the sinus pacemaker or to irritability of the atrial or junctional tissues, causing them to compete with the sinus node for control.

ECG Characteristics:

- *Rate:* 60 to 100 beats/minute; if the rate is faster than 100 beats/minute, it is called *multifocal atrial tachycardia* (MAT)
- *Rhythm:* May be slightly irregular
- *P waves:* Varying shapes (upright, flat, inverted, notched) as impulses originate in different parts of the atria or junction; at least three different P-wave shapes should be seen
- *PR interval:* May vary depending on proximity of the pacemaker to the AV node
- *QRS complex:* Usually normal
- *Conduction:* Conduction through the atria varies as they are depolarized from different spots; conduction through the bundle branches and ventricles is usually normal
- *Example of WAP:*

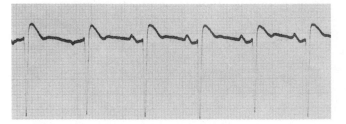

Treatment

Treatment of WAP usually is not necessary. If slow heart rates lead to symptoms, atropine can be given. If the heart rate is over 100 beats/minute (MAT), treatment of MAT is directed toward eliminating the cause and slowing the ventricular rate. Drugs such as quinidine to decrease atrial ectopy or verapamil or propranolol to slow the ventricular rate may be necessary.

Atrial Tachycardia

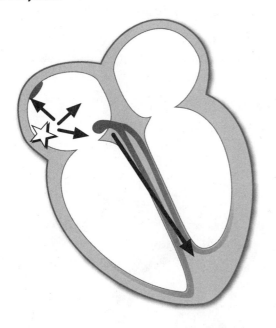

Atrial tachycardia is a rapid atrial rhythm occurring at a rate of 150 to 250 beats/minute. When the arrhythmia abruptly starts and terminates, it is called *paroxysmal atrial tachycardia* (PAT). Rapid atrial rate can be caused by emotions, caffeine, tobacco, alcohol, fatigue, or sympathomimetic drugs. Whenever the atrial rate is rapid, the AV node begins to block some of the impulses attempting to travel through it in order to protect the ventricles from excessively rapid rates. In normal healthy hearts the AV node can usually conduct each atrial impulse up to rates of about 180 to 200 beats/minute. In patients with cardiac disease or who have taken too much digitalis, the AV node may not be able to conduct each impulse and atrial tachycardia with block occurs.

ECG Characteristics:

- *Rate:* Atrial rate is 150 to 250 beats/minute
- *Rhythm:* Regular unless there is variable block at the AV node
- *P waves:* Differ in shape from sinus P waves because they are ectopic. Precede each QRS complex but may be hidden in preceding T wave. When block is present, more than one P wave will appear before each QRS complex.
- *PR interval:* May be shorter than normal but often difficult to measure because of hidden P waves
- *QRS complex:* Usually normal but may be wide if aberrant conduction is present

- *Conduction:* Usually normal through the AV node and into the ventricles. In atrial tachycardia with block some atrial impulses do not conduct into the ventricles. Aberrant ventricular conduction may occur if atrial impulses are conducted into the ventricles while the ventricles are still partially refractory.
- *Example of atrial tachycardia:*

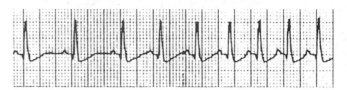

Treatment

Treatment of atrial tachycardia is directed toward eliminating the cause and decreasing the ventricular rate. Sedation may terminate the rhythm or slow the rate. Vagal stimulation, either through carotid sinus massage or Valsalva's maneuver, may slow the rate or convert the rhythm to sinus rhythm. Vasopressors reflexly stimulate the carotid sinus and may be effective in terminating the arrhythmia. Digitalis will slow the ventricular rate by increasing the block at the AV node, but it can also be the cause of atrial tachycardia with block and should be discontinued if that is the case. Propranolol, verapamil, and diltiazem increase block at the AV node and may either slow the ventricular rate or terminate the tachycardia. Quinidine may be used to prevent further recurrence of atrial tachycardia. If the patient is symptomatic, cardioversion may be necessary.

Atrial Flutter

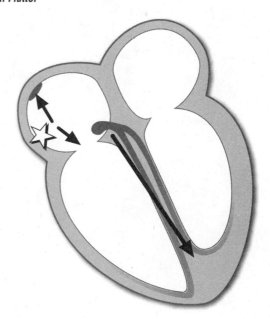

In atrial flutter, the atria fire at a rate of 250 to 350 times/minute, most commonly at 300. At such rapid atrial rates, the AV node will usually block at least half of the impulses in order to protect the ventricles from excessive rates. Causes of atrial flutter include rheumatic heart disease, atherosclerotic heart disease, thyrotoxicosis, heart failure, and myocardial ischemia or infarction. Because the ventricular rate in atrial flutter can be quite fast, symptoms associated with decreased cardiac output can occur. Mural thrombi may form in the atria due to the fact that there is no strong atrial contraction, and blood stasis occurs, leading to a risk of systemic or pulmonary emboli.

ECG Characteristics:

- *Rate:* Atrial rate varies between 250 to 350 beats/minute, most commonly 300; ventricular rate varies depending on the amount of block at the AV node, most commonly 150 beats/minute and rarely 300 beats/minute
- *Rhythm:* Atrial rhythm is regular; ventricular rhythm may be regular or irregular due to varying AV block
- *P waves:* F waves (flutter waves) are seen, characterized by a very regular, "sawtooth" pattern; one F wave is usually hidden in the QRS complex, and when 2:1 conduction occurs, F waves may not be readily apparent
- *FR interval (flutter wave to the beginning of the QRS complex):* May be consistent or may vary
- *QRS complex:* Usually normal; aberration can occur
- *Conduction:* Usually normal through the AV node and ventricles
- *Examples of atrial flutter:*

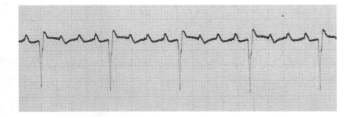

Atrial flutter with 4:1 conduction.

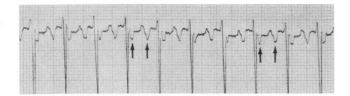

Atrial flutter with 2:1 conduction.

Treatment

Treatment of atrial flutter depends on the hemodynamic consequences of the arrhythmia. Excessively rapid ventricular rates need to be controlled immediately if cardiac out-

put is markedly compromised. Cardioversion may be necessary as an immediate treatment. Verapamil, diltiazem, and beta blockers can be used to slow the ventricular rate. Quinidine and procainamide may convert flutter to sinus rhythm, but should never be given without prior treatment to ensure adequate AV block. The danger of giving quinidine alone lies in the fact that quinidine slows the atrial rate. As the atrial rate slows from 300 to 220 beats/minute, for example, it is possible for the AV node to conduct each impulse rather than block impulses, thus leading to even faster ventricular rates.

Atrial Fibrillation

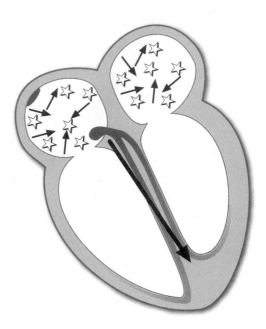

Atrial fibrillation is an extremely rapid and disorganized pattern of depolarization in the atria. Atrial fibrillation commonly occurs in the presence of atherosclerotic or rheumatic heart disease, heart failure, pulmonary disease, myocardial infarction, and congenital heart disease and following cardiac surgery. If the ventricular response to atrial fibrillation is very rapid, cardiac output can be reduced secondary to decreased diastolic filling time in the ventricles. Since the atria are quivering rather than contracting, atrial kick is lost, which can also reduce cardiac output. Another possible complication is mural thrombus formation in the atria due to stasis of blood as the atria quiver.

ECG Characteristics:

- *Rate:* Atrial rate is 400 to 600 beats/minute or faster. Ventricular rate varies depending on the amount of block at the AV node. In new atrial fibrillation, the ventricular response is usually quite rapid, 160 to 200 beats/minute; in treated atrial fibrillation, the ventricular rate is controlled in the normal range of 60 to 100 beats/minute.

- *Rhythm:* Irregular; one of the distinguishing features of atrial fibrillation is the marked irregularity of the ventricular response
- *P waves:* Not present; atrial activity is chaotic with no formed atrial impulses visible; irregular F waves are often seen, and vary in size from coarse to very fine
- *PR interval:* Not measurable since there are no P waves
- *QRS complex:* Usually normal; aberration is common
- *Conduction:* Conduction within the atria is disorganized and follows a very irregular pattern. Most of the atrial impulses are blocked within the AV junction. Those impulses that are conducted through the AV junction are usually conducted normally through the ventricles. If an atrial impulse reaches the bundle branch system during its refractory period, aberrant intraventricular conduction can occur.
- *Examples of atrial fibrillation:*

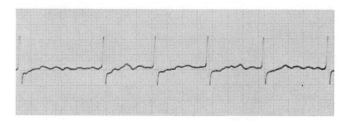

Atrial fibrillation with a controlled ventricular response.

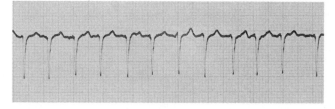

Atrial fibrillation with an uncontrolled ventricular response.

Treatment

Treatment of atrial fibrillation is directed toward eliminating the cause, decreasing atrial irritability, and decreasing the ventricular rate. Digitalis, verapamil, diltiazem, and propranolol are commonly used to reduce ventricular rate by increasing block at the AV node. Quinidine and procainamide are used to decrease atrial irritability and may convert the arrhythmia to sinus rhythm. Flecainide and amiodarone may also be used to control atrial fibrillation. If the patient is hemodynamically unstable due to very rapid ventricular rates, cardioversion may be necessary.

Arrhythmias Originating in the Atrioventricular Junction

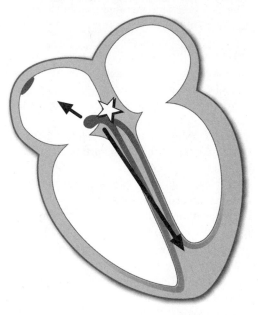

Introduction

Cells surrounding the AV node in the AV junction are capable of initiating impulses and controlling the heart rhythm. Junctional beats and junctional rhythms can appear in any of three ways on the ECG depending on the location of the junctional pacemaker and the speed of conduction of the impulse into the atria and ventricles:

- When a junctional focus fires, the wave of depolarization spreads backward (retrograde) into the atria as well as forward (antegrade) into the ventricles. If the impulse arrives in the atria before it arrives in the ventricles, the ECG will show a P wave (usually inverted because the atria are depolarizing from bottom to top) followed immediately by a QRS complex as the impulse reaches the ventricles. In this case the PR interval will be very short, usually 0.10 second or less.
- If the junctional impulse reaches both the atria and the ventricles at the same time, only a QRS will be seen on the ECG because the ventricles are much larger than the atria and only ventricular depolarization will be seen, even though the atria are also depolarizing.
- If the junctional impulse reaches the ventricles before it reaches the atria, the QRS will precede the P wave on the ECG. Again, the P wave will usually be inverted because of retrograde atrial depolarization, and the RP interval (distance from the beginning of the QRS to the beginning of the following P wave) will be short.

Premature Junctional Complexes

Premature junctional complexes (PJCs) are due to an irritable focus in the AV junction. Irritability can be due to coronary heart disease or myocardial infarction disrupting blood flow to the AV junction, nicotine, caffeine, emotions, or drugs such as digitalis.

ECG Characteristics:

- *Rate:* 60 to 100 beats/minute or whatever the rate of the basic rhythm
- *Rhythm:* Regular except for occurrence of premature beats
- *P waves:* May occur before, during, or after the QRS complex of the premature beat and are usually inverted
- *PR interval:* Short, usually 0.10 second or less when P waves precede the QRS
- *QRS complex:* Usually normal but may be aberrant if the PJC occurs very early and conducts into the ventricles during the refractory period of a bundle branch
- *Conduction:* Retrograde through the atria; usually normal through the ventricles
- *Example of a PJC:*

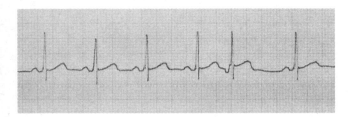

Treatment

Treatment is usually not necessary for PJCs. Frequent PJCs may precede junctional tachycardia. Antiarrhythmic therapy with quinidine or procainamide may be prescribed.

Junctional Rhythm, Accelerated Junctional Rhythm, and Junctional Tachycardia

Junctional rhythms can occur if the sinus node rate falls below the rate of the AV junctional pacemakers or when atrial conduction through the AV junction has been disrupted. Junctional rhythms commonly occur from digitalis toxicity or following inferior myocardial infarction due to disruption of blood supply to the sinus node and the AV junction. These rhythms are classified according to their rate: junctional rhythm usually occurs at a rate of 40 to 60 beats/minute, accelerated junctional rhythm occurs at a rate of 60 to 100 beats/minute, and junctional tachycardia occurs at rates of 100 to 250 beats/minute.

ECG Characteristics:

- *Rate:* Junctional rhythm, 40 to 60 beats/minute; accelerated junctional rhythm, 60 to 100 beats/minute; junctional tachycardia, 100 to 250 beats/minute

- *Rhythm:* Regular
- *P waves:* May precede or follow QRS
- *PR interval:* Short, 0.10 second or less
- *QRS complex:* Usually normal
- *Conduction:* Retrograde through the atria; normal through the ventricles
- *Examples of junctional rhythm, accelerated junctional rhythm, and junctional tachycardia:*

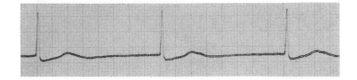

Junctional rhythm.

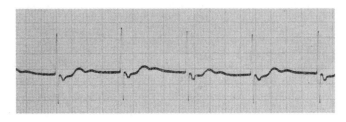

Accelerated junctional rhythm.

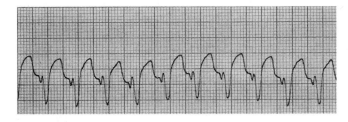

Junctional tachycardia.

Treatment

Treatment of junctional rhythm rarely is required unless the rate is too slow or too fast to maintain adequate cardiac output. If the rate is slow, atropine is given to increase the sinus rate and override the junctional focus or to increase the rate of firing of the junctional pacemaker. If the rate is fast, drugs such as verapamil, propranolol, quinidine, or digitalis may be effective in slowing the rate or terminating the arrhythmia. Cardioversion may be necessary if the rate is so rapid that cardiac output is severely limited. Since digitalis toxicity is a common cause of junctional rhythms, the drug should be held.

Arrhythmias Originating in the Ventricles

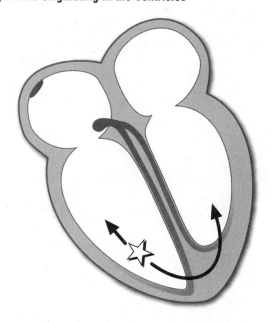

Ventricular arrhythmias originate in the ventricular muscle or Purkinje system. These arrhythmias are considered to be more dangerous than other arrhythmias because of their potential to severely decrease cardiac output and lead to death.

Premature Ventricular Complexes

Premature ventricular complexes (PVCs) are due to irritable foci in the ventricles and can be caused by hypoxia, myocardial ischemia, hypokalemia, acidosis, exercise, increased levels of circulating catecholamines, digitalis toxicity, and other causes. PVCs themselves are not harmful but may indicate increasing ventricular irritability, which may lead to more serious ventricular arrhythmias. The importance of PVCs depends on the clinical setting in which they occur. Many people have chronic PVCs that do not need to be treated. In the setting of an acute myocardial infarction or myocardial ischemia, whenever the heart is electrically unstable at the cellular level, PVCs can be precursors of more dangerous ventricular arrhythmias. PVCs are considered serious under the following circumstances:

1. Frequency of more than 6/minute
2. When they are multiformed (arising from more than one foci in the ventricle)
3. When they occur in pairs or triplets
4. When they fall on the T wave of the preceding beat (R on T)

ECG Characteristics:

- *Rate:* 60 to 100 beats/minute or the rate of the basic rhythm
- *Rhythm:* Irregular because of the early beats

- *P waves:* Not related to the PVCs. Sinus rhythm is usually not interrupted by the premature beats, so sinus P waves can often be seen occurring regularly throughout the rhythm. P waves may occasionally follow PVCs due to retrograde conduction from the ventricle backward through the atria; these P waves will be inverted
- *PR interval:* Not present before most PVCs; if a P wave happens, by coincidence, to precede a PVC, the PR interval is short
- *QRS complex:* Wide and bizarre; greater than 0.10 second in duration; may vary in morphology (size, shape) if they originate from more than one focus in the ventricles
- *Conduction:* Impulses originating in the ventricles conduct through the ventricles from muscle cell to muscle cell rather than through Purkinje fibers, resulting in wide QRS complexes. Some PVCs may conduct retrograde into the atria, resulting in inverted P waves following the PVC. When the sinus rhythm is undisturbed by PVCs, the atria depolarize normally
- *Example of a PVC:*

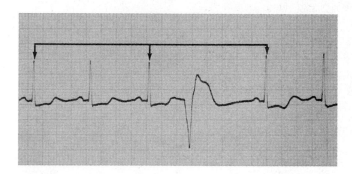

Treatment

Treatment of PVCs is directed toward the elimination of the cause. Drug treatment includes administration of an antiarrhythmic drug, usually lidocaine, intravenously. Procainamide or bretylium can also be used intravenously for acute control of PVCs. Drugs such as disopyramide, quinidine, propranolol, amiodarone, tocainide, mexiletine, and sotalol may be used for a long-term control of PVCs.

Ventricular Rhythm and Accelerated Ventricular Rhythm

Ventricular rhythm occurs when an ectopic focus in the ventricle fires at a rate under 50 beats/minute. This rhythm occurs as an escape rhythm when the sinus node and junctional tissue fail to fire or fail to conduct their impulses to the ventricle. Accelerated ventricular rhythm occurs when an ectopic focus in the ventricles fires at a rate of 50 to 100 beats/minute. The causes of this accelerated ventricular rhythm are similar to those of ventricular tachycardia (VT), but accelerated ventricular rhythm commonly occurs in the presence of inferior myocardial infarction when the rate of the sinus node slows below the rate of the latent ventricular pacemaker. Accelerated ventricular rhythm is a common arrhythmia after thrombolytic therapy, when reperfusion of the damaged myocardium occurs.

ECG Characteristics:

- *Rate:* Less than 50 beats/minute for ventricular rhythm and 50 to 100 beats/minute for accelerated ventricular rhythm
- *Rhythm:* Usually regular
- *P waves:* May be seen but at a slower rate than the ventricular focus, with dissociation from the QRS
- *PR interval:* Not measured
- *QRS complex:* Wide and bizarre
- *Conduction:* If sinus rhythm is the basic rhythm, atrial conduction is normal; impulses originating in the ventricles conduct via muscle cell-to-cell conduction, resulting in the wide QRS complex
- *Examples of ventricular rhythm and accelerated ventricular rhythm:*

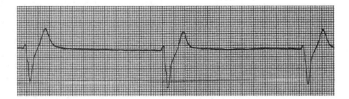

Escape ventricular rhythm.

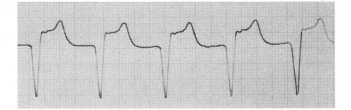

Accelerated ventricular rhythm.

Treatment

Treatment of accelerated ventricular rhythm depends on how it is tolerated by the patient. This arrhythmia is not harmful by itself because the ventricular rate is within normal limits and usually adequate to maintain cardiac output. If the patient is symptomatic due to the loss of atrial kick, suppressive therapy can be used, similar to that used to treat VT. It is important to know if there is an underlying rhythm at a reasonable rate when suppressive therapy is used, since abolishing the ventricular rhythm may leave an even less desirable heart rate. Often, accelerated ventricular rhythm is transient and benign and does not require treatment. If the ventricular rhythm is an escape rhythm, then treatment is

directed toward increasing the rate of the escape rhythm or pacing the heart temporarily.

Ventricular Tachycardia

Ventricular tachycardia is a rapid ventricular rhythm. The causes of VT are the same as the causes of PVCs, but VT is considerably more dangerous than PVCs because of its effect of decreasing cardiac output and tendency to degenerate into ventricular fibrillation.

ECG Characteristics:

- *Rate:* Ventricular rate is faster than 100 beats/minute.
- *Rhythm:* Usually regular but may be slightly irregular
- *P waves:* Dissociated from QRS complexes. If sinus rhythm is the underlying basic rhythm, they are regular. P waves may be seen but will not be related to QRS complexes. P waves are often buried within QRS complexes
- *PR interval:* Not measurable because of dissociation of P waves from QRS complexes
- *QRS complex:* Wide and bizarre; greater than 0.10 second in duration
- *Conduction:* Impulse originates in one ventricle and spreads via muscle cell-to-cell conduction through both ventricles; there may be retrograde conduction through the atria, but more often the sinus node continues to fire regularly and depolarize the atria normally
- *Example of ventricular tachycardia:*

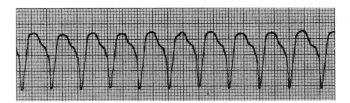

Treatment

Treatment of VT depends on how well the rhythm is tolerated by the patient. VT can be an emergency if there is no pulse or if cardiac output is severely decreased, due either to a very rapid rate or to the loss of atrial kick. The preferred immediate treatment for severely symptomatic VT is cardioversion, but defibrillation can be performed if there is not time to synchronize the shock. In pulseless VT, CPR must be initiated until defibrillation can be performed. If the patient is not severely symptomatic, lidocaine is the drug of choice for acute treatment of VT. Procainamide, bretylium, or magnesium sulfate can also be used for acute treatment. Maintenance therapy may be prescribed with the same drugs used for PVCs.

Ventricular Fibrillation

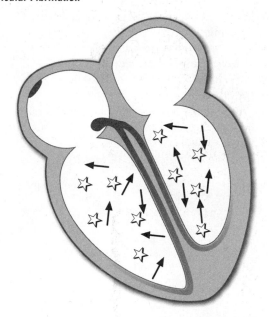

Ventricular fibrillation (VF) is rapid, ineffective quivering of the ventricles and is fatal without immediate treatment. Electrical activity originates in the ventricles and spreads in a chaotic, irregular pattern throughout both ventricles. There is no cardiac output or palpable pulse with VF.

ECG Characteristics:

- *Rate:* Rapid, uncoordinated, ineffective
- *Rhythm:* Chaotic, irregular
- *P waves:* None seen
- *PR interval:* None
- *QRS complex:* No formed QRS complexes seen; rapid, irregular undulations without any specific pattern
- *Conduction:* Multiple ectopic foci firing simultaneously in ventricles and depolarizing them irregularly and without any organized pattern; ventricles are not contracting
- *Example of VF:*

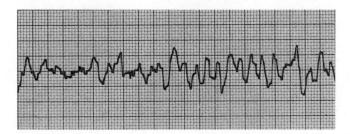

Treatment

Treatment of VF requires immediate defibrillation. Synchronized cardioversion is not possible since there are no formed QRS complexes on which to synchronize the machine. CPR must be performed until a defibrillator is available, and then defibrillation at 200 joules is recommended. If no pulse is obtained and VF continues, an immediate second shock at 300 joules is recommended followed by a pulse check and a third shock at 360 joules, if necessary. If VF does not convert after three shocks, CPR needs to be continued and drug therapy initiated. Lidocaine, procainamide, magnesium, and bretylium are commonly used in an effort to convert VF. Epinephrine may be given to help convert a fine fibrillation to a coarser fibrillation, since fine VF is often refractory to defibrillation. Once the rhythm has converted, maintenance therapy with intravenous antiarrhythmics is continued.

Ventricular Asystole

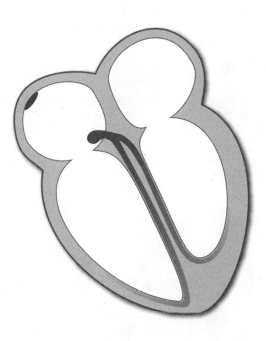

Ventricular asystole is the absence of any ventricular rhythm: no QRS complex, no pulse, and no cardiac output. Ventricular asystole is always fatal unless treated immediately.

ECG Characteristics:

- *Rate:* None
- *Rhythm:* None
- *P waves:* May be present if the sinus node is functioning
- *PR interval:* None
- *QRS complex:* None
- *Conduction:* Atrial conduction may be normal if the sinus node is functioning; there is no conduction into the ventricles

- *Example of ventricular asystole:*

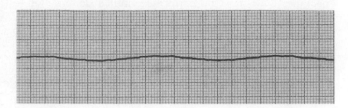

(From: Jones KM, Ochs GM: Interpretation of the electrocardiogram: A review for health professionals, *2nd ed. Stamford, CT: Appleton & Lange, 1990, p. 114.*)

Treatment

Treatment includes immediate CPR. Epinephrine is usually given intravenously in an effort to stimulate a rhythm. Atropine may also be given. A transcutaneous or transvenous pacemaker is often necessary.

Atrioventricular Blocks

The term *atrioventricular block* is used to describe arrhythmias in which there is delayed or failed conduction of supraventricular impulses into the ventricles. AV blocks have been classified according to location of the block and severity of the conduction abnormality.

First-degree Atrioventricular Block

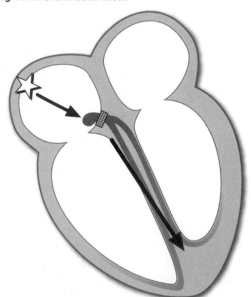

First-degree AV block (located at the AV node in this example) is defined as prolonged AV conduction time of supraventricular impulses into the ventricles. This delay usually occurs within the AV node; all impulses are conducted into the ventricles, but with delayed conduction times. First-degree AV block can be due to coronary heart disease, rheumatic heart disease, or administration of digitalis, beta blockers, or calcium channel blockers.

ECG Characteristics:

- *Rate:* Can occur at any sinus rate, usually 60 to 100 beats/minute
- *Rhythm:* Regular
- *P waves:* Normal; precede every QRS
- *PR interval:* Prolonged above 0.20 second
- *QRS complex:* Usually normal
- *Conduction:* Normal through the atria, delayed through the AV node, and normal through the ventricles
- *Example of first-degree AV block:*

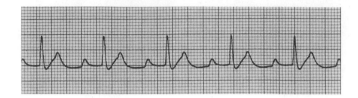

Treatment

Treatment of first-degree AV block is usually not required, but block should be observed for progression to more severe block.

Second-degree AV Block

Second-degree AV block occurs when selected atrial impulses fail to be conducted into the ventricles. Second-degree AV block can be divided into two distinct categories: type I block, occurring in the AV node, and type II block, usually occurring below the AV node in the bundle branch system.

Type I Second-degree AV Block

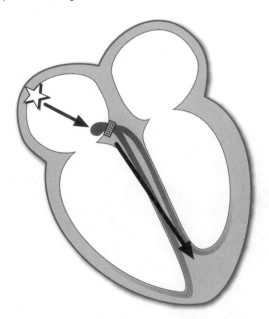

Type I second-degree AV block, often referred to as Wenckebach block, is a progressive increase in conduction times of consecutive atrial impulses into the ventricles until one impulse fails to conduct, or is "dropped." The PR intervals gradually lengthen until one P wave fails to conduct and is not followed by a QRS complex, resulting in a pause, after which the cycle repeats itself. This type of block is commonly associated with inferior myocardial infarction, coronary heart disease, aortic valve disease, mitral valve prolapse, atrial septal defects, and administration of digitalis, beta blockers, or calcium channel blockers.

ECG Characteristics:

- *Rate:* Can occur at any sinus or atrial rate
- *Rhythm:* Irregular; overall appearance of the rhythm demonstrates "group beating"
- *P waves:* Normal; some P waves are not conducted to the ventricles, but only one at a time fails to conduct to the ventricle
- *PR interval:* Gradually lengthens in consecutive beats; the PR interval preceding the pause is longer than that following the pause
- *QRS complex:* Usually normal unless there is associated bundle branch block
- *Conduction:* Normal through the atria; progressively delayed through the AV node until an impulse fails to conduct. Ventricular conduction is normal. Conduction ratios can vary, with ratios as low as 2:1 (every other P wave is blocked) up to high ratios such as 15:14 (every 15th P wave is blocked)
- *Example of second-degree AV block type I:*

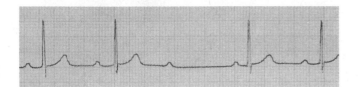

Treatment

Treatment of type I second-degree AV block depends on the conduction ratio, the resulting ventricular rate, and the patient's tolerance for the rhythm. If ventricular rates are slow enough to decrease cardiac output, the treatment is atropine to increase the sinus rate and speed conduction through the AV node. At higher conduction ratios where the ventricular rate is within a normal range, no treatment is necessary. If the block is due to digitalis or beta blockers, those drugs should be held. This type of block is usually temporary and benign, and seldom requires pacing, although temporary pacing may be needed when the ventricular rate is slow.

Type II Second-degree AV Block

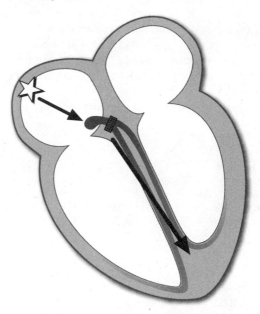

Type II second-degree AV block is sudden failure of conduction of an atrial impulse to the ventricles without progressive increases in conduction time of consecutive P waves. Type II block occurs below the AV node and is usually associated with bundle branch block; therefore, the dropped beats are usually a manifestation of bilateral bundle branch block. This form of block appears on the ECG much the same as type I block except that there is no progressive increase in PR intervals before the blocked beats. Type II block is less common than type I block, but is a more serious form of block. It occurs in rheumatic heart disease, coronary heart disease, primary disease of the conduction system, and in the presence of acute anterior myocardial infarction. Type II block is more dangerous than type I because of a higher incidence of associated symptoms and progression to complete AV block. When it occurs in the presence of anterior wall myocardial infarction, it is usually associated with a high mortality rate due to the extent of muscle damage necessary to produce this degree of block below the AV node.

ECG Characteristics:

- *Rate:* Can occur at any basic rate
- *Rhythm:* Irregular due to blocked beats
- *P waves:* Usually regular and precede each QRS; periodically a P wave is not followed by a QRS complex
- *PR interval:* Constant before conducted beats; the PR interval preceding the pause is the same as that following the pause
- *QRS complex:* Usually wide due to associated bundle branch block

- *Conduction:* Normal through the atria and through the AV node but intermittently blocked in the bundle branch system and fails to reach the ventricles. Conduction through the ventricles is abnormally slow due to associated bundle branch block. Conduction ratios can vary from 2:1 to only occasional blocked beats
- *Example of second-degree AV block type II:*

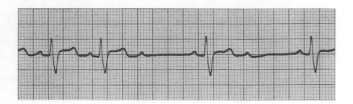

Treatment

Treatment usually includes pacemaker therapy, since this type of block is often permanent and progresses to complete AV block. Transcutaneous pacing can be used for treatment of symptomatic patients until transvenous pacing is initiated. CPR may be necessary if the ventricular rate is slow and cardiac output is greatly reduced.

High-grade AV Block

High-grade (or advanced) AV block is present when two or more consecutive atrial impulses are blocked when the atrial rate is reasonable (less than 135/minute) and conduction fails because of the block itself and not because of interference from an escape pacemaker. High-grade AV block may be type I, occurring in the AV node, or type II, occurring below the AV node. The significance of high-grade block depends on the conduction ratio and the resulting ventricular rate. Since ventricular rates tend to be slow, this arrhythmia is frequently symptomatic and requires treatment.

ECG Characteristics:

- *Rate:* Atrial rate less than 135 beats/minute
- *Rhythm:* Regular or irregular, depending on conduction pattern
- *P waves:* Normal; present before every conducted QRS, but several P waves may not be followed by QRS complexes
- *PR interval:* Constant before conducted beats; may be normal or prolonged
- *QRS complex:* Usually normal in type I block and wide in type II block
- *Conduction:* Normal through the atria. Two or more consecutive atrial impulses fail to conduct to the ventricles. Ventricular conduction is normal in type I block and abnormally slow in type II block
- *Example of high-grade AV block:*

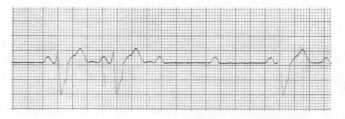

(From: Jones KM, Ochs GM: Interpretation of the electrocardiogram: A review for health professionals, 2nd ed. Stamford, CT: Appleton & Lange, 1990, p. 90.)

Treatment

Treatment of high-grade block is necessary if the patient is symptomatic. Atropine can be given and is generally more effective in type I block. A transcutaneous pacemaker may be required until transvenous pacing can be initiated, and permanent pacing is usually necessary in type II high-grade block.

Third-Degree AV Block (Complete Block)

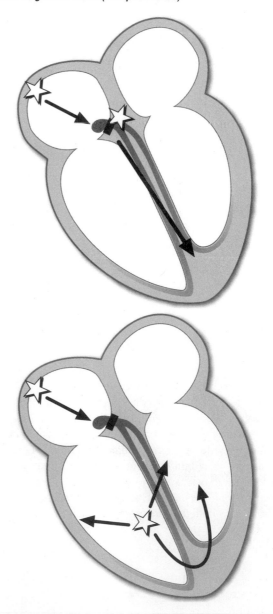

Third-degree AV block is complete failure of conduction of all atrial impulses to the ventricles. In third-degree AV block there is complete AV dissociation; the atria are usually under the control of the sinus node and the ventricles are controlled by either a junctional or ventricular pacemaker. The ventricular rate must be less than 45 beats/minute; a faster rate could indicate an accelerated junctional or ventricular rhythm that is interfering with conduction from the atria into the ventricles. Causes of complete AV block include coronary heart disease, myocardial infarction, Lev's disease, Lenègre's disease, cardiac surgery, congenital heart disease, and digitalis toxicity. Third-degree AV block can occur without significant symptoms if it occurs gradually and the heart has time to compensate for the slow ventricular rate. If it occurs suddenly in the presence of acute myocardial infarction, its significance depends on the resulting ventricular rate and the patient's tolerance.

ECG Characteristics:

- *Rate:* Atrial rate is usually normal; ventricular rate is less than 45 beats/minute
- *Rhythm:* Regular
- *P waves:* Normal but dissociated from QRS complexes
- *PR interval:* No consistent PR intervals because there is no relationship between P waves and QRS complexes
- *QRS complex:* Normal if ventricles controlled by a junctional pacemaker; wide if controlled by a ventricular pacemaker
- *Conduction:* Normal through the atria. All impulses are blocked at the AV node or in the bundle branches, so there is no conduction to the ventricles. Conduction through the ventricles is normal if a junctional escape rhythm occurs, and abnormally slow if a ventricular escape rhythm occurs
- *Examples of third-degree AV block:*

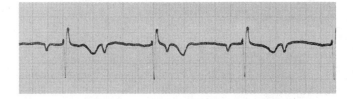

Third-degree AV block with a junctional rhythm.

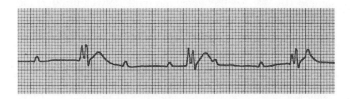

Third-degree AV block with a ventricular rhythm.

Treatment

Treatment of complete heart block with symptoms of decreased cardiac output includes transcutaneous pacing until transvenous pacing can be initiated. Atropine can be given but is not usually effective in restoring conduction. CPR should be performed until a pacemaker can be inserted if cardiac output is severely decreased.

TEMPORARY PACING

Indications

If the heart fails to generate or conduct impulses to the ventricle, the myocardium can be electrically stimulated using a cardiac pacemaker. A cardiac pacemaker has two components: a pulse generator and a pacing electrode or catheter. Temporary cardiac pacing is indicated in any situation in which bradycardia results in symptoms of decreased cerebral tissue perfusion or hemodynamic compromise. Signs and symptoms of hemodynamic instability are hypotension, change in mental status, angina, or pulmonary edema. Temporary pacing is also used to suppress rapid ectopic rhythms by briefly pacing the heart at a faster rate than the existing rate. Following pacing termination, return to a normal rhythm may occur if the rapid ectopic focus has been suppressed, allowing the sinus node to resume as the pacemaker. This type of pacing is termed *overdrive pacing* to distinguish it from pacing for bradycardic conditions.

Temporary cardiac pacing is accomplished by transvenous, epicardial, or transcutaneous methods. If continued cardiac pacing is required, insertion of permanent pacemakers is done under elective conditions. The following section presents an overview of temporary pacing principles. A more detailed explanation of pacemaker functions is covered in Chapter 21, Advanced ECG Concepts.

Transvenous Pacing

Transvenous pacing involves the placement of a pacing wire (electrode, catheter) into the right ventricle, with the tip of the catheter touching the ventricular wall (Figure 4–9A). The stiff pacing catheter is transvenously inserted and advanced into the heart until the tip of the catheter is positioned in the right ventricle. The other end of the pacing catheter is then connected to a pulse generator which delivers electrical impulses down the catheter to the ventricular tissue as required. In a properly functioning pacemaker system, the electrical stimulus from the pacemaker will then spread through ventricular tissue, depolarizing the ventricle. The term for this transference of an electrical impulse from the pacemaker catheter to the heart is *capture,* producing an ECG pattern which is typically very different from intrinsic electrical conduction in the heart (Figure 4–10).

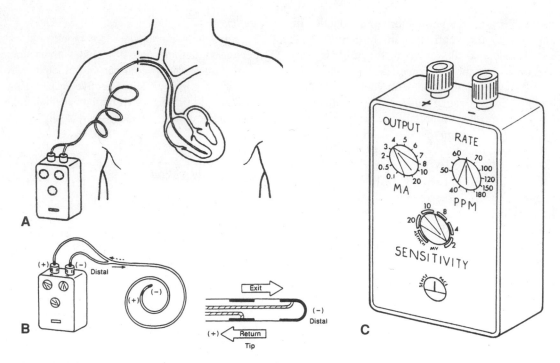

Figure 4–9. Temporary single-chamber ventricular pacemaker. (A) Transvenous pacemaker catheter in the apex of the right ventricle. (B) Bipolar catheter system. The impulse exits from the negative terminal of the pulse generator which is connected to the distal electrode. Intrinsic electrical activity is transmitted through the other catheter pole (positive sign) to the pulse generator. (C) Single-chamber pulse generator. *(From: Crawford M, et al: Common sense approach to coronary care, 6th ed. St. Louis, MO: Mosby-Year Book, 1995, pp. 453, 456, 460.)*

Pacing Catheter

The transvenous pacing catheter can be a thin flexible wire, with or without a balloon on the tip, or a larger and stiffer catheter. One of the most common types of catheters has a metal tip, labeled as the negative pole, and another metal area a few millimeters from the tip, labeled the positive pole (Figure 4–9B). This *bipolar* catheter has two separate wires within the catheter which connect to the metal areas on the catheter end and exit the catheter for connection to specific terminals on the pacing generator. The terminals on the pulse generator are labeled positive (+) and negative (−). The pacing-wire connections are labeled proximal and distal. The distal end of the pacing catheter is connected to the negative terminal of the pulse generator and the proximal end is connected to the positive terminal. The electrical impulse generated by the pacemaker is delivered from the negative terminal and is transmitted to the heart through the distal tip of the pacing catheter. Intrinsic electrical activity in the heart is sensed at the tip of the pacing catheter and transmitted to the pulse generator sensing circuit. This dual capability allows the pulse generator to "pace" the heart by sending electrical impulses down one wire and to "monitor" the ventricle for the presence of intrinsic electrical activity.

Proper functioning of these bipolar systems requires that the metal areas at the catheter end be in contact with cardiac tissue, rather than floating within the ventricular chamber. Anteroposterior and lateral chest x-ray films will confirm proper placement of the pacing catheter within the heart. The catheter is usually secured with a suture following insertion to prevent inadvertent movement.

Pulse Generator

The pulse generator can be programmed to deliver electrical impulses through the pacing catheter at varying rates, amplitudes (strengths), and modes by adjusting one of several dials on the generator front (Figure 4–9C). The strength or amplitude of the electrical stimulus is set on the output dial, with low numbers indicating small amounts of electrical output. The unit of measure of the electrical output is the milliampere (mA). The initial output setting for ventricular pacing is usually about 5 mA, with the final setting determined by stimulation threshold testing (see Chapter 21, Advanced ECG Concepts).

The rate of the electrical impulse generation is set on the rate knob. This designates the number of pulses per minute (PPM) that the generator will deliver through the pacing catheter. Although dependent on the clinical condition of the patient, typically settings are in the 60 to 80/minute range.

The third major component of the pulse generator is the sensitivity dial. These settings determine how the pacemaker generator will respond to the presence of intrinsic electrical activity. Setting the sensitivity at 20 or higher causes the

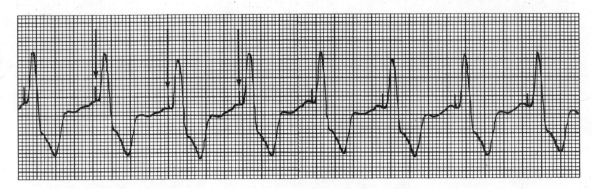

Figure 4–10. ECG of a fixed-rate ventricular pacemaker rhythm with 100% ventricular capture. *(From: Dracup K:* Meltzer's *intensive coronary care.* 5th ed. Stamford, CT: Appleton & Lange, 1995.)

generator to be insensitive to intrinsic electrical activity, delivering electrical impulses at the rate and amplitude set, regardless of the presence of intrinsic electrical activity. This approach to pacing is called *fixed mode,* or *asynchronous,* pacing. By turning the sensitivity control clockwise toward 0, the pacemaker sensitivity is increased to intrinsic electrical activity and pacing only occurs if the intrinsic rate is below the rate set on the pacemaker generator. This approach to pacing is called *demand-mode* pacing.

The last component of a simple pulse generator is the pacing/sensing indicator. This needle or light indicates whenever the generator is pacing the heart or is sensing the intrinsic electrical activity of the heart.

ECG Characteristics of Paced Rhythms

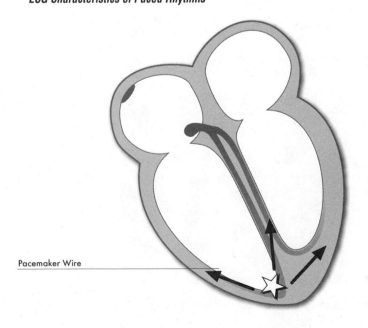

Pacemaker Wire

A paced ventricular beat begins with a pacing spike followed by a wide QRS complex and a wide T wave, oriented in the opposite direction of the QRS complex (Figure 4–10). This ECG strip shows all QRS complexes to be preceded by a pacemaker spike and is referred to as 100% ventricular capture. Note that the pacing spike is small, indicating that a bipolar pacing catheter is in place. Large pacing spikes indicate that a unipolar pacing catheter is in situ.

Figure 4–11 is the ECG of a ventricular pacemaker that is functioning correctly. The pacemaker generates an impulse when it senses that the heart rate has decreased below a set level. Therefore, the pacemaker senses the intrinsic cardiac rhythm of the patient and only generates an impulse when the rate falls below the predetermined level.

Refer to Chapter 21, Advanced ECG Concepts, for details of ECG characteristics for temporary ventricular pacemakers.

Transcutaneous Pacemakers

The emergent nature of many bradycardic rhythms requires immediate temporary pacing. Since transvenous catheter placement is difficult to accomplish quickly, a method for rapid easy pacing is necessary until implementation of more invasive approaches. Transcutaneous pacing is the preferred method for rapid, easy initiation of cardiac pacing in emergent conditions.

Transcutaneous pacing includes many of the same principles delineated for transvenous pacing. The primary difference is the transmission of the electrical impulse through the skin and chest wall, rather than directly to the myocardium through the transvenous pacing catheter. This type of pacing is accomplished by transmitting electrical impulses from a pulse generator through two electrode pads placed on the anterior and posterior chest walls (Figure 4–12). The pulse generator operates similarly to the trans-

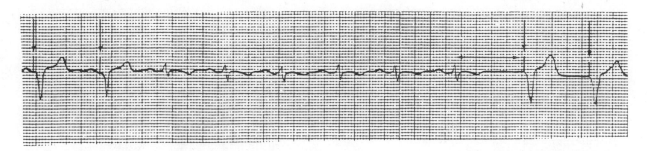

Figure 4–11. ECG of a demand pacemaker rhythm with appropriate sensing of inherent QRS complexes and appropriate pacing and ventricular capture when no inherent QRS complexes are present. *(From: Dracup K: Meltzer's intensive coronary care, 5th ed. Stamford, CT: Appleton & Lange, 1995.)*

venous unit; however, the electrical impulse's amplitude (mA) is set at a higher level for transcutaneous transmission to result in ventricular capture. Transcutaneous pacing spikes are usually very large, often distorting the QRS complex. The presence of a pulse with every pacing spike confirms ventricular capture.

The high-level transcutaneous electrical transmission to achieve ventricular capture results in inadvertent contraction of other muscles and discomfort for the patient, typically requiring sedation and analgesia. Despite sedation, many patients find the sensation associated with transcutaneous pacing to be very distressing.

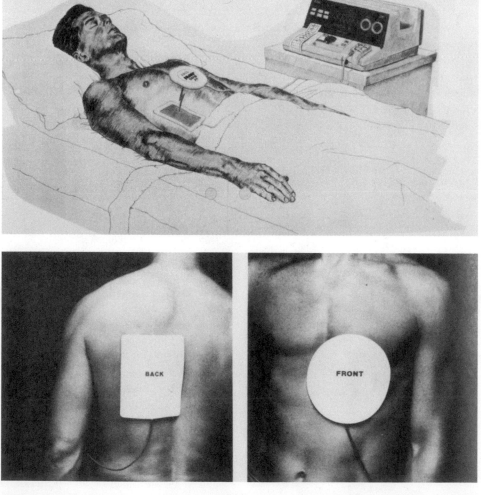

Figure 4–12. Transcutaneous pacemaker with electrode pads connected to the anterior and posterior chest walls. *(From: Zoll Medical Corporation, Burlington, MA.)*

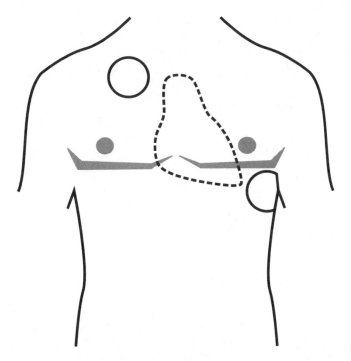

Figure 4–13. Anterior chest wall placement of paddles for cardioversion and defibrillation. *(From: Cummins RO (ed.): Textbook of advanced cardiac life support. Dallas, TX: American Heart Association, 1994, p. 4–4.)*

DEFIBRILLATION AND CARDIOVERSION

Defibrillation

Defibrillation is the therapeutic use of an electrical shock to temporarily depolarize an irregularly beating heart. Defibrillation is used immediately for ventricular fibrillation or ventricular tachycardia without a peripheral pulse. Defibrillation completely depolarizes all myocardial cells and ter-

minates the chaotic electrical activity, allowing the sinus node to regain control of the heart rhythm. If the myocardium is anoxic or acidotic, then it may not be possible to terminate the ventricular rhythm. The defibrillator paddles are placed appropriately on the chest (see below) and the defibrillator is discharged at 200 joules; if necessary, this is followed by a repeat shock at 200 to 300 joules. If the first two shocks fail to defibrillate, a third shock of 360 joules should be delivered immediately. Transthoracic impedance declines with repeated shocks. Thus, higher current flows will occur with subsequent shock, even at the same energy level.

When the defibrillator is in the synchronized mode, it may not fire on a disorganized rhythm because there are no predominant waves it recognizes. Thus the synchronizer switch must be turned off. In defibrillation, the electrode paddles are applied to the anterior chest before the defibrillator is discharged. The standard electrode position for the closed-chest procedure is as follows: one paddle just to the right of the upper sternum below the right clavicle and the other paddle just to the left of the cardiac apex (Figure 4–13). In order to reduce skin resistance to current flow and to prevent skin burns, defibrillator pads (adhesive pads with electrode gel) or electrode paste are used. Care should be taken to prevent contact between the two areas of conductive material because electrical bridging may occur. Self-adhesive defibrillator pads can also be used instead of the rigid metal paddles. In order to ensure good skin contact during defibrillation using hand-held paddles, 20 to 25 pounds of pressure should be exerted on each paddle. Do not let anyone touch the patient or the patient's bed when the defibrillator is fired. The electric shock is delivered by depressing both discharge buttons simultaneously. After defibrillation, the cardiac monitor and pulse are checked for signs of restored rhythm (Figure 4–14A).

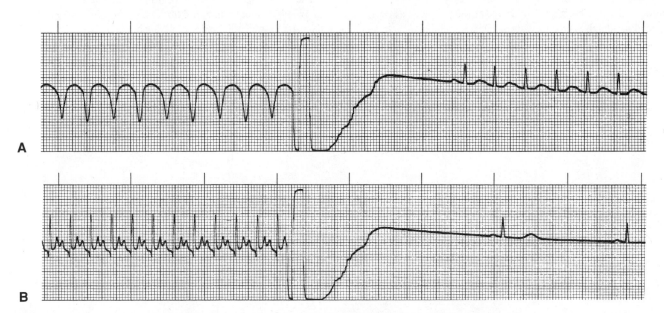

Figure 4–14. *ECG rhythms before and after: (A) Defibrillation. (B) Cardioversion.*

Cardioversion

Cardioversion, synchronized electrical countershock, is used to terminate arrhythmias that have QRS complexes and is usually an elective procedure. If the patient is alert and oriented, informed consent is obtained. The patient is given intravenous medication to promote short-acting anesthesia. The amount of voltage used varies from 50 to 200 joules. Digoxin is usually withheld for 48 hours prior to cardioversion to prevent arrhythmias after the procedure. The defibrillator is synchronized so that an electrical impulse is discharged during ventricular depolarization (QRS complex), thus avoiding the vulnerable period (T wave). The discharge buttons should be held until the synchronizer fires the defibrillator. If ventricular fibrillation occurs after cardioversion, the synchronizer is turned off, the defibrillator is recharged immediately, and defibrillation is repeated. Indications of successful response are conversion to sinus rhythm, strong peripheral pulses, and adequate blood pressure (Figure 4–14B). Airway patency should be maintained and the patient's state of consciousness assessed. Vital signs should be obtained at least every 15 minutes for 1 hour, every 30 minutes for 2 hours, and then every 4 hours following the procedure.

SELECTED BIBLIOGRAPHY

What Heals: The Mind and Arrhythmias

Engel G: A life setting conducive to illness: The giving-up-given-in complex. *Annals of Internal Medicine.* 1968;69:293.

Grant T, Yeston G: Cardiac arrest secondary to emotional stress. *Critical Care Medicine.* 1991;19:292.

Green WA, Goldstein S, Moss AJ: Psychosocial aspects of sudden death: A preliminary report. *Archives of Internal Medicine.* 1972;129:725.

Hackett RP, Rosenbaum JFM, Resar GE: Emotion, psychiatric disorders, and the heart. In Braunwald E (ed.): *Heart disease,* 3rd ed. Philadelphia: WB Saunders, 1988.

Lown B, Temte JV, Teich P, et al: Basis for recurring ventricular fibrillation in the absence of coronary artery disease and its management. *New England Journal of Medicine.* 1976; 294:623.

Reich P, et al: Acute psychological disturbances preceding life-threatening ventricular arrhythmias. *Journal of the American Medical Association.* 1981;246:233.

Wellens HJJ, Vermeulen A, Durrer D: Ventricular fibrillation upon arousal from sleep by auditory stimuli. *Circulation.* 1972;46:661.

ECG

Cummins RO: *Textbook of advanced cardiac life support.* Dallas, TX: American Heart Association, 1994.

Dracup K: *Meltzer's intensive coronary care,* 5th ed. Stamford, CT: Appleton & Lange, 1995.

Gilmore SB, Woods SL: Electrocardiography and vectorcardiography. In Woods SL, et al (eds.): *Cardiac nursing,* 3rd ed. Philadelphia: JB Lippincott, 1995, pp 241–295.

Goldschlager N, Goldman MJ: *Principles of clinical electrocardiography.* Stamford, CT: Appleton & Lange, 1989.

Jacobson C: Cardiac arrhythmias and conduction abnormalities. In Patrick M, et al (eds.): *Medical surgical nursing: Pathophysiological concepts.* Philadelphia: JB Lippincott, 1991, pp. 648–693.

Jacobson C: Arrhythmias and conduction disturbances. In Woods SL, et al (eds.): *Cardiac nursing,* 3rd ed. Philadelphia: JB Lippincott, 1995, pp. 324–337.

Jones KM, Ochs GM: *Interpretation of the electrocardiogram: A review for health professionals,* 2nd ed. Stamford, CT: Appleton & Lange, 1990.

Marriott HJL, Conover MB: *Advanced Concepts in Arrhythmias.* St. Louis, MO: CV Mosby, 1989.

Marriott HJL, Fogg E: Constant monitoring for cardiac dysrhythmias and block. *Modern Concepts of Cardiovascular Disease.* 1970;39(6):103–108.

Osguthorpe SG, Woods SL: Myocardial ischemia and infarction. In Woods SL, et al (eds.): *Cardiac nursing,* 3rd ed. Philadelphia: JB Lippincott, 1995, pp. 478–479.

Five

Hemodynamic Monitoring

> ## ▶ Knowledge Competencies
>
> 1. Identify the characteristics of normal and abnormal waveforms and normal pressures for the following hemodynamic monitoring parameters:
>   - Central venous pressure
>   - Pulmonary artery pressure
>   - Arterial blood pressure
>   - Cardiac output
> 2. Describe the basic elements of hemodynamic pressure monitoring equipment and methods used to ensure accurate pressure measurements.
>
> 3. Discuss the indications, contraindications, and general management principles for the following common hemodynamic monitoring parameters:
>   - Central venous pressure
>   - Pulmonary artery pressure
>   - Arterial blood pressure
>   - Cardiac output
> 4. Compare and contrast the clinical implications of, and management approaches to, abnormal hemodynamic values.

■ *What Heals: Creating a Healing Room*

What would be necessary for you to experience healing and energy at work rather than becoming physically and emotionally drained? What is it that you need to facilitate healing in yourself and your patients?

The following questions focus on creating a Healing Room. As you read the questions, consider the possibilities. If you can imagine the possibilities, it can be done.

- Is it possible for a room near the unit to be emptied and converted into a Healing Room to nourish the staff?
- Can you imagine signing up each day to go to the Healing Room on or near the unit for 15 or 20 minutes to nourish your body-mind-spirit with relaxation and rest?
- Is it possible for you to imagine that you have the support of your colleagues and administra-

tors to go to the Healing Room to nourish and heal yourself because they value and honor this time?

Can you imagine the Healing Room with comfortable pillows on a carpeted floor, restful pictures on the wall, and an audiocassette library with a wide range of music, relaxation, and imagery tapes, headphones, and tape recorders? There might also be a sign on the door that reads, "This Healing Room is for your relaxation and rest. Please enjoy." (For details on establishing an audiocassette library, refer to Chapter 8, Alternative Therapies.)

CEG & BMD

Adapted from: Dossey BM, Keegan L, Guzzetta CE, Kolkmeier L: Holistic nursing: Handbook for practice, 2nd ed. Gaithersburg, MD: Aspen, 1995, p. 70.

INTRODUCTION

Hemodynamic monitoring allows the clinician to have access to information which is normally not available from assessment of the cardiovascular system. Parameters such as cardiac output (CO) and intracardiac pressures can be directly measured and monitored through a special indwelling catheter connected to pressure monitoring equipment. The availability of these measurements can significantly contribute to management of the critically ill patient. While noninvasive assessment techniques such as physical examination, history taking, and laboratory analysis are helpful and necessary, they do not provide the specific parameters available from hemodynamic monitoring.

The bedside clinician is responsible for the accurate measurement and interpretation of hemodynamic data, as well as for the safe use of these devices in patient care.

BASIC COMPONENTS OF HEMODYNAMIC MONITORING SYSTEMS

Understanding hemodynamic monitoring starts with knowing the key components of monitoring systems. General components of a hemodynamic monitoring system include an indwelling catheter connected to a pressure transducer and flush system and a bedside monitor. All components which come in contact with the vascular system must be

sterile, with meticulous attention paid to maintaining a closed sterile system during use.

1. *Pulmonary artery (PA) catheter.* The PA catheter is a multilumen catheter inserted into the pulmonary artery (Figure 5–1). Each lumen or "port" has specific functions (Table 5–1). The PA catheter typically is inserted through an introducer sheath (large-diameter, short catheter with a diaphragm) placed in a major vein. Major veins used for PA catheter insertion include the internal jugular, subclavian, femoral, and less commonly, the brachial vein.

2. *Arterial catheter.* The arterial catheter, or "A-line," has only one lumen, which is used for measuring arterial pressures and for drawing arterial blood samples (Figure 5–2). Arterial catheters are inserted in any major artery, with the most common sites being the radial and femoral arteries.

3. *Pressure tubing.* The pressure tubing is a key part of any hemodynamic monitoring system (Figure 5–2). It is designed to be a stiff (noncompliant) tubing to ensure accurate transfer of intravascular pressures to the transducer. The pressure tubing connects the intravascular catheter to the transducer. Many pressure tubings have stopcocks in-line to facilitate blood sampling and zeroing the transducer (see below). Normally, the pressure tubing is kept as short as possible, with a minimal number of

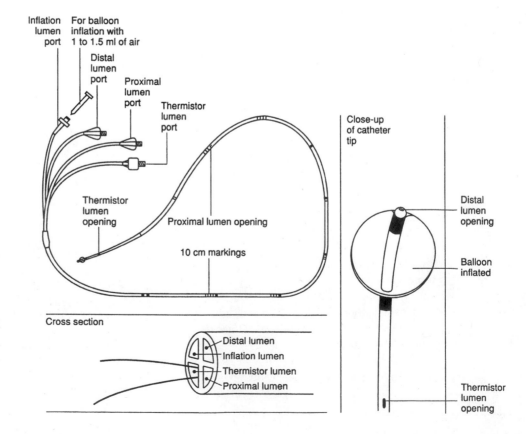

Figure 5–1. Flow directed pulmonary artery catheter (Swan-Ganz). *(From: Visalli F, Evans P: The Swan-Ganz catheter: A program for teaching safe, effective use.* Nursing 81, *1981;11:1.)*

TABLE 5–1. PULMONARY ARTERY (PA) PORT FUNCTIONS

Type of Port	Functions
Distal tip port	Measures pressure at the tip of the catheter in the PA. With proper inflation of the balloon, measures the pulmonary capillary wedge pressure (PCWP). Used to sample SvO_2 levels and for other blood sampling needs.
Proximal lumen port	Measures pressure 30 cm from the distal tip, usually in the right atrium (RA). Central venous pressure (CVP) and RA pressure (RAP) are synonymous terms. Injection site for cardiac output (CO) determinations. Used to draw blood samples for laboratory tests requiring venous blood. If coagulation studies are drawn, completely remove heparin from line prior to obtaining sample. Used for IV fluids and drug administration, if necessary.
Balloon inflation port	Inflated periodically with <1.5 ml of air to obtain PCWP tracing.
Ventricular port (on selected models of PA catheters)	Measures right ventricle (RV) pressure. Used for insertion of a temporary pacemaker electrode into the RV.
Ventricular infusion port (on selected models of PA catheters)	An additional lumen for IV fluid or drug administration. Located close to the proximal lumen exit area. May be used for CO determinations or CVP measurements, if necessary.
Cardiac output port (thermistor lumen)	Measures blood temperature near the distal tip when connected to the cardiac output computer. May be used to monitor body (core) temperature continuously.

stopcocks, to increase the accuracy of pressure measurements.

4. *Pressure transducer.* The pressure transducer is a small electronic sensor which has the ability to convert a mechanical pressure (vascular pressure) into an electrical signal (Figure 5–2). This electrical signal can then be displayed on the pressure amplifier.

5. *Pressure amplifier.* The pressure amplifier, or "bedside monitor," augments the signal from the transducer and displays the converted vascular pressure as an electrical signal (Figure 5–2). This signal is used to display a continuous waveform on the oscilloscope of the monitor and to provide a numerical display of pressure measurement (Figure 5–3). Most bedside monitors also have a graphic recorder to print out the pressure waveform.

6. *Pressure bag and flush device.* In addition to being attached to the pressure amplifier, the transducer is connected to an IV solution which is placed in a *pressure bag* (Figure 5–4). The IV solution is normally 500 to 1000 ml of normal saline (NS),

although 5% dextrose in water (D_5W) can be used. The IV solution is placed under 300 mm Hg of pressure to provide a slow, continuous infusion of fluid through the vascular catheter.

The IV solution is placed under pressure for another reason. Included in most pressure systems is a *flush device* (Figure 5–4). The flush device regulates fluid flow through the pressure tubing at a slow, continuous rate to prevent occlusion of the vascular catheter. Normally, the flush device restricts fluid flow to approximately 2 to 4 ml/hour. If the flush device is activated, normally by squeezing or pulling the flush device, a rapid flow of fluid will enter the pressure tubing. Flush devices are activated for two reasons: to rapidly clear the tubing of air or blood and to check the accuracy of the tubing/catheter system (square wave test). Measuring the fluid in the IV solution should be done on every shift to measure how much fluid has infused from the pressure bag. Depending on hospital procedures, heparin may be added to the IV solution to aid in keeping the system patent. If this is done, generally about 1 unit of 1:1000 heparin is added for every cubic centimeter (cc) of the IV solution.

7. *Alarms.* Bedside monitors have alarms for each of the hemodynamic pressures being monitored. Normally, every parameter that is being monitored has high and low alarms which can be set to detect variations from the current value. Alarm limits are generally set to detect significant decreases or increases in pressures or rates, typically ± 10% of the current values.

Ensuring System Accuracy

The information obtained from hemodynamic monitoring technology must be verified for accuracy by the bedside clinician. The following guidelines will produce consistently accurate readings.

Zeroing the Transducer

A fundamental principle in obtaining hemodynamic values is to zero the transducer amplifier system. Zeroing is the act of electronically compensating for any offset (distortion) in the transducer. This is normally done by exposing the transducer to air and pushing an automatic zero button on the bedside monitor. This step should be performed at least once before obtaining the first hemodynamic reading after catheter insertion. Since it is an electronic function, it normally has to be performed only once when the transducer and amplifier are first attached to the in-situ catheter.

Leveling the Transducer to the Catheter Tip

Leveling is the process of aligning the tip of the vascular catheter horizontal to a zero reference position, usually a

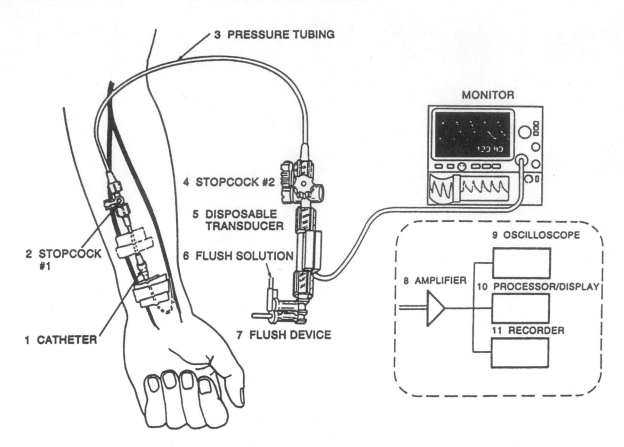

Figure 5–2. Components of a hemodynamic monitoring system. *(From: Gardner R, Hollingsworth K: Electrocardiography and pressure monitoring: How to obtain optimal results. In Shoemaker WC, Ayers S, Grenvik A, Holbrook P (eds): Textbook of critical care, 3rd ed. Philadelphia: WB Saunders, 1995, p. 272.)*

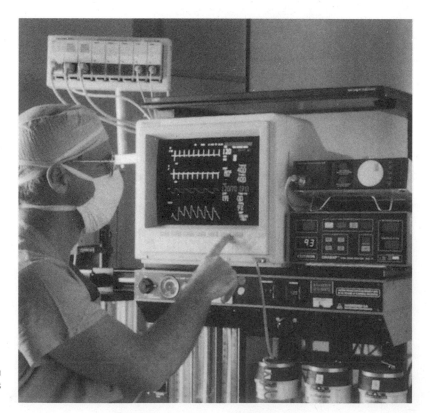

Figure 5–3. Bedside monitor (pressure amplifier) used in hemodynamic monitoring. *(From: Robinson JE: Advances for medicine. Andover, MA: Hewlett-Packard, 1992, cover.)*

stopcock in the pressure tubing close to the transducer (Figure 5–5). The location of the catheter tip varies with each type of catheter (Table 5–2). However, it is important to accurately estimate the tip of the catheter in order to ensure accurate readings from that catheter.

There are two basic methods for leveling. When the transducer and stopcocks are mounted on a pole close to the bed, the pole height is adjusted to have the stopcock opening horizontal to the external reference location of the catheter tip (Figure 5–5). To ensure horizontal positioning, a carpenter's level is usually necessary. Each time the bed height or patient position is altered, this leveling procedure must be repeated.

The other method for leveling places the transducer and stopcock at the correct location on the chest wall or arm (Figure 5–6). Taping or strapping the transducer to the appropriate location on the body eliminates the need for repeating the leveling procedure when bed heights are changed. As long as the transducer/stopcock position remains horizontal to the external reference location, no releveling need occur.

Leveling must be performed when obtaining the first set of hemodynamic information and any time the transducer is no longer horizontal to the external reference loca-tion. When obtaining the first set of readings, zeroing and leveling are frequently performed simultaneously. After this initial combined effort, zeroing does not need to be per-formed when leveling is done.

Calibration of the Transducer/Amplifier System

If the transducer/amplifier system is suspected of being inaccurate, calibration can be performed. Calibration is less important today since all disposable transducers are precal-ibrated by the manufacturer. If calibration needs to be checked prior to use, or if a reading is in doubt, a simple static pressure check can be done before the transducer is attached to the patient. Detailed descriptions of how to per-form static pressure checks can be found in most hemody-namic monitoring texts.

Ensuring Accurate Waveform Transmission

For hemodynamic monitoring to provide accurate informa-tion, the vascular pressure must be transmitted back to the transducer unaltered and then converted accurately into an electrical signal. In order for this waveform to be transmit-ted unaltered, no obstructions or distortions to the signal should be present along the transmission route. Distortion

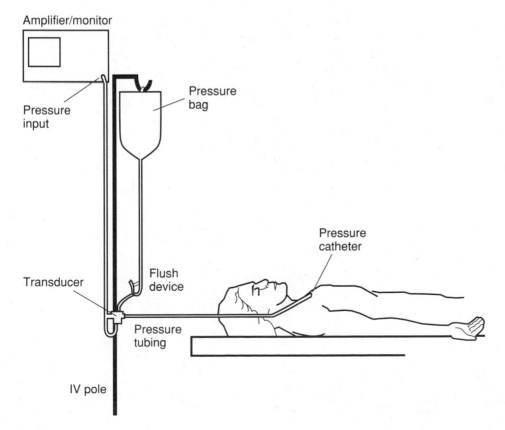

Figure 5–4. Pressure bag and flush device connected to a pressure trans-ducer and monitoring system. *(From: Ahrens TS, Taylor L:* Hemodynamic wave-form analysis. *Philadelphia: WB Saun-ders, 1992, p. 210.)*

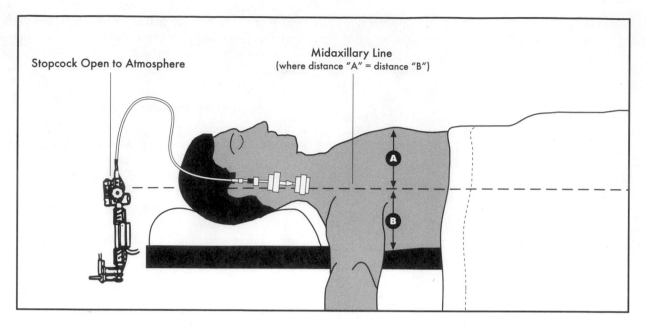

Figure 5–5. Typical leveling of pulmonary artery catheter with stopcock attached to the transducer for mounting on a pole. The stopcock close to the transducer is opened to atmospheric pressure (air) horizontal to the 4th intercostal space (ICS) at the midaxillary line.

of the waveform leads to inaccurate pressure interpretations. A variety of factors can cause distortions to the waveform, including catheter obstructions (e.g., clots, catheter bending, blood or air in tubing), excessive tubing or connectors, and transducer damage. Verification of an accurate transmission of the waveform to the transducer is checked by the bedside clinician by performing a square wave test.

Performing a Square Wave Test

The square wave test is performed on all hemodynamic pressure systems before assuming that the waveforms and pressures obtained are accurate. The square wave test is performed by recording the pressure waveform while fast-flushing the catheter (Figure 5–7). The fast-flush valve should be pulled or squeezed, depending on the model, for at least 1 second and then rapidly released. The tracing should show a rapid rise in the waveform to the top of the graph paper, with a square pattern. Release of the flush device should show a rapid decrease in pressure below the baseline of the pressure waveform (undershoot), followed immediately by a small increase above the baseline (over-

shoot) prior to resumption of the normal pressure waveform. Square wave tests with these characteristics are called *optimally damped tests* and represent an accurate waveform transmission. The square wave test is the best method available to the clinician to check the accuracy of hemodynamic monitoring equipment. For example, if an arterial line is to be examined for accuracy, a square wave test should be done. Do not compare the arterial line pressure with an indirect blood pressure reading with a sphygmomanometer, since the indirect method is always less accurate than the direct method (arterial line pressure). If the square wave test indicates optimal damping, then the arterial line pressure is accurate.

Two problems can exist with waveform transmissions, and are referred to as overdamping and underdamping (Table 5–3).

TABLE 5–2. IDENTIFICATION OF LEVELING LOCATION FOR DIFFERENT VASCULAR CATHETERS

Vascular Catheter	Leveling Location
Pulmonary artery catheter (PAP, PCWP, CVP)	Midaxillary line, 4th ICS
Radial Artery (BP)	1 cm below insertion site
Femoral Artery (BP)	1 inch below insertion site
Intraaortic Balloon Pump	Midaxillary line, 4th ICS

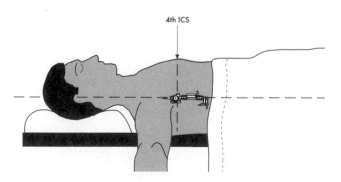

Figure 5–6. Leveling a transducer for mounting on the chest wall at the 4th ICS at the midaxillary line.

TABLE 5–3. ASSESSING DAMPING CONCEPTS FROM SQUARE WAVE TEST

Square Wave Test	Clinical Effect	Corrective Action
Optimally damped 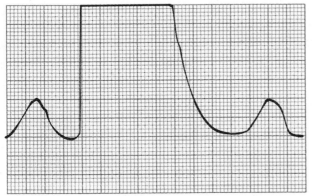	Produces accurate waveform and pressure.	None required.
Overdamped 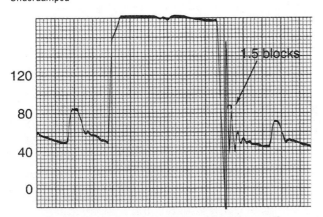	Produces a falsely low systolic and high diastolic value.	Check the system for air, blood, loose connections or kinks in the tubing or catheter.
Underdamped	Produces a falsely high systolic and low diastolic value.	Remove unnecessary tubing and stopcocks. Add a damping device.

Figure 5–7. Characteristics of an optimally damped square wave test. *(From: Ahrens TS:* Hemodynamic waveform analysis. *Philadelphia: WB Saunders, 1992, p. 347.)*

Figure 5–8. Overdamped square wave test. *(From: Ahrens TS:* Hemodynamic waveform analysis. *Philadelphia: WB Saunders, 1992, p. 216.)*

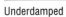

Figure 5–9. *Underdamped square wave test. (From Ahrens TS:* Hermodynamic waveform analysis. *Philadelphia: WB Saunders, 1992, p. 220.)*

Overdamped Square Wave Test

If something absorbs the pressure wave (like air or blood in the tubing, stopcocks, or connections), it is said to be overdamped. Overdamping decreases systolic pressures and increases diastolic pressures. An overdamped square wave test reflects the obstruction in waveform transmission. Characteristics of overdamping include a loss of the undershoot and overshoot waves after release of the flush valve and a slurring of the downstroke (Figure 5–8).

Underdamped Square Wave Test

If something accentuates the pressure wave (like excessive tubing), it is said to be underdamped. Underdamping increases systolic pressures and decreases diastolic pressures (Figure 5–9). An underdamped square wave test reflects the amplification of pressure waves and includes large undershoot and overshoot waves after the release of the flush valve.

Table 5–4 summarizes the methods of assessing and ensuring the accuracy of hemodynamic monitoring systems.

Care of the Tubing/Catheter System

The tubing/catheter system is a disposable, sterile setup and should remain closed to the atmosphere as much as possible. Nosocomial infections related to the tubing/catheter system are usually due to the entry of organisms through stopcocks. Stopcocks are opened for blood sampling and zeroing the transducer only when necessary. Closed, needleless systems should be used whenever feasible to decrease the risks to the patient and clinician.

Tubing changes, including flush device, transducer and flush solution, should occur every 4 days. The frequency of catheter device changes, while controversial, should occur whenever the catheter is suspected as a source of an IV infection or every 3 to 4 days.

Some clinicians believe it is safe to leave intravascular catheters in place until some sign of inflammation or infection develops. This approach may be safe, but it assumes more risk of developing catheter-related infection than the routine 4 to 5 day change guideline. Considering that the development of a single catheter-related infection can substantially increase the length of stay, it may be worthwhile to routinely change intravascular catheters. However, there is still a widespread variation in the practice of changing intravascular catheters at this time.

INSERTION AND REMOVAL OF CATHETERS FOR HEMODYNAMIC MONITORING

Pulmonary Artery Catheters

Pulmonary artery catheters are frequently inserted to assess cardiac and respiratory function, as well as to guide fluid and vasoactive drug administration in the critically ill patient.

Insertion

PA catheters can be inserted into most large-diameter veins, with the internal jugular vein as the most common insertion site. Typically, the PA catheter is placed into a percutaneously inserted introducer sheath with a sterile sleeve to maintain the sterility of the PA catheter after insertion (Figure 5–10). As the catheter is advanced into the right atrium,

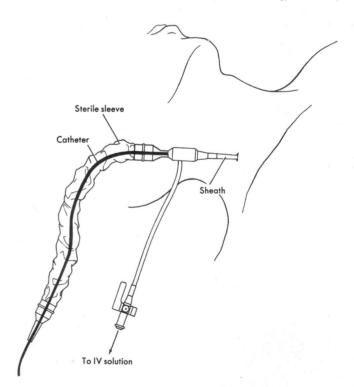

Figure 5–10. PA catheter inserted through an introducer sheath in the right internal jugular vein. The sterile sleeve of the introducer allows advancement of the PA catheter after insertion, if necessary. The side port of the sheath is connected to an IV to reduce clotting around the sheath and permit fluid administration. *(From: Daily E, Schroeder J: Techniques in bedside hemodynamic monitoring, 3rd ed. St. Louis, MO: CV Mosby, 1985, p. 93.)*

TABLE 5–4. SUMMARY OF METHODS FOR ASSESSING AND ENSURING ACCURACY OF HEMODYNAMIC MONITORING SYSTEMS*

Method	When Performed
Zero transducer	Should only be performed once. If the transducer zeros properly, a waveform should be visible on the monitor.
Level the transducer	Leveling should be done prior to each pressure reading and with any substantive change in pressures.
Square wave test	Should be performed prior to every reading and after blood has been withdrawn from the catheter.
Calibration	Calibration should be performed once prior to using the transducer.

*If a transducer has been zeroed, leveled, and calibrated and has an optimally damped square wave test, the monitor display is accurate.

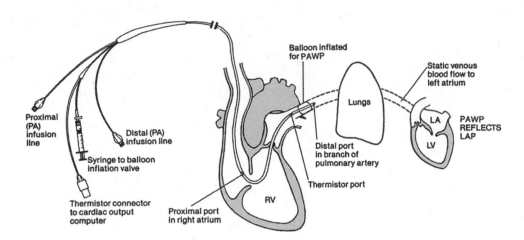

Figure 5–11. PA catheter inserted into the pulmonary artery.

the balloon at the tip of the catheter is inflated with 1 to 1.5 ml of air. Inflation of the balloon during insertion allows blood flow through the heart to direct, or pull, the catheter up into the pulmonary artery (Figure 5–11). Following placement of the catheter properly in the pulmonary artery, the balloon is deflated.

Pressure at the tip of the PA catheter is monitored continuously as the catheter is advanced through the right heart and into the pulmonary artery. Changes in pressure and waveform configurations allow clinicians to identify the location of the PA catheter as it is directed into the right atrium, through the tricuspid valve into the right ventricle, through the pulmonic valve, and into the pulmonary artery (Table 5–5). Normal pressures for each of the chambers are summarized in Tables 5–5 and 5–6. Occasionally, bedside fluoroscopy also is needed to assist with proper insertion of the catheter.

Following insertion, the PA pressure waveform is monitored continuously to identify inadvertent migration of the catheter tip into a small branch of the PA, obstructing blood flow to distal lung tissue or backward into the right ventricle. A chest x-ray is obtained after insertion to verify proper location and presence of pneumothorax, kinking of the catheter, or other complications.

Removal

Removing the PA catheter is a clinical decision based on the perception that the data from the catheter are no longer critical to the assessment process. This decision can be made anywhere from a few hours to several days after insertion. The removal of the pulmonary artery catheter is normally performed by a physician, although in some institutions nurses may perform this task.

Following the discontinuance of IV fluids, all stopcocks to the patient are turned off to avoid air entry into the venous system during catheter removal. The balloon of the catheter is deflated and the patient is placed in a supine position with the head of the bed flat. While the catheter is being gently withdrawn, the patient is instructed to exhale or hold his or her breath during removal to further decrease

the chance of air embolus. Resistance during catheter withdrawal could indicate catheter knotting and/or entrapment in a valve leaflet or chordae tendineae. A chest x-ray can confirm any problem and special removal procedures need to be performed to avoid cardiac structure damage.

Complications

Complications associated with PA catheters include those associated with insertion, maintenance, and removal of the device (Table 5–7). During insertion, the most common complication is ventricular ectopy (premature ventricular contractions, ventricular tachycardia or fibrillation) from catheter irritation of the ventricular wall. Similar to complications associated with central venous catheters, pneumothorax or air emboli also can occur during insertion or removal of a PA catheter. Infection also can occur with PA catheters. A rare but serious complication is damage to the tricuspid or pulmonic valves. Pulmonary hemorrhage or infarct may also occur during inadvertent migration of the PA catheter into small-diameter branches of the PA or from balloon rupture. Prevention and treatment strategies are summarized in Table 5–7 for each of these complications.

Arterial Catheters

Blood pressure (BP) measurement with the indirect method (sphygmomanometer) is not as accurate as direct BP measurement, particularly during conditions of abnormal blood flow (high- or low-cardiac-output states), systemic vascular resistance, or body temperature. The common occurrence of these conditions in critically ill patients necessitates insertion of an arterial catheter to directly measure BP.

Insertion

Arterial catheters are short (<4 inches) catheters which can be inserted into radial, brachial, axillary, femoral, or pedal arteries. The most common site is the radial artery. Arterial catheters can be placed by cutdown or with percutaneous insertion techniques, the latter being the most common insertion method.

TABLE 5–5. PRESSURE WAVEFORMS OBSERVED DURING PULMONARY ARTERY (PA) CATHETER INSERTION

Location	Pressure Waveform	Normal Pressures
Right atrium		0 to 6 mm Hg
Right ventricle		Systolic, 20 to 30 mm Hg Diastolic, 0 to 5 mm Hg
Pulmonary artery		Systolic, 20 to 30 mm Hg Diastolic, 10 to 15 mm Hg
Pulmonary capillary wedge		8 to 12 mm Hg

With permission from: Boggs R, Wooldridge-King M: AACN procedure manual, *3rd ed. Philadelphia: WB Saunders, 1993, pp. 308, 324, 326, 334.*

TABLE 5–6. NORMAL HEMODYNAMIC AND BLOOD FLOW PARAMETERS

Parameter	Normal	Calculations for Derived Values
Cardiac index (CI)	2.5–4 L/min/m^2	$\dfrac{CO}{BSA*}$
Cardiac output (CO)	4–8 L/min	
Stroke index (SI)	25–45 ml/m^2	$\dfrac{SV}{BSA}$
Stroke volume (SV)	50–100 ml	
Blood pressure		
Systolic (SBP)	90–140 mm Hg	$MAP = \dfrac{(2 \times DBP) + SBP}{3}$
Diastolic (DBP)	60–90 mm Hg	
Mean (MAP)	70–100 mm Hg	
Left ventricular ejection fraction (LVEF)	60–80%	
Pulmonary artery		
Systolic (PAS)	20–30 mm Hg	$PAM = \dfrac{(2 \times PAD) + PAS}{3}$
Diastolic (PAD)	10–15 mm Hg	
Mean (PAM)	10–20 mm Hg	
PCWP†	8–12 mm Hg	
CVP	2–6 mm Hg	
Left ventricular stroke work index (LVSWI)	35–85 g-m/m^2	(MAP – PCWP)(LVSI)(.0144)
Right ventricular stroke work index (RVSWI)	8.5–12 g-m/m^2	(PAM – CVP)(RVSI)(.0144)
Systemic vascular resistance (SVR)	900–1300 dynes/sec/cm^5	$\dfrac{MAP - CVP}{CO}$ (80)
Pulmonary vascular resistance (SVR)	40–220 dynes/sec/cm^5	$\dfrac{PAM - PCWP}{CO}$ (80)

*Body surface area.
† Pulmonary capillary wedge pressure.

General insertion steps for percutaneous insertion are similar to an intravenous catheter insertion. Prior to insertion of a radial artery catheter, however, an Allen test is performed to verify the adequacy of circulation to the hand in the event of radial artery thrombosis. The Allen test is performed by completely obstructing blood flow to the hand by compressing the radial and ulnar arteries for a minute or two. Release of the ulnar artery only will result in rapid return of color to the hand if good collateral blood supply exists.

During insertion, care should be exercised not to damage the arterial vessel by excessive probing or movement of the needle. Bleeding into the tissues can occur quite easily if the vessel is damaged, causing obstruction to distal blood flow and nerve pressure. Following artery cannulation, the catheter is connected to the pressure transducer and a high-pressure infusion system to prevent blood from backing up into the tubing and fluid container (Figure 5–2).

Removal

Arterial monitoring is discontinued when the patient has a stable blood pressure and tissue oxygenation status or when frequent arterial blood samples are no longer indicated. Removal of arterial catheters is commonly performed by nurses, using procedures similar to IV catheter removal.

The presence of the catheter in a high-pressure system, though, requires greater attention to achieving hemostasis with arterial catheters. Following catheter removal, holding firm pressure over the site for at least 5 minutes and until hemostasis occurs is important for preventing arterial bleeding. For patients with any coagulation disturbances, the time for site holding may be much longer than 5 to 10 minutes. Pressure dressings, rather than manual pressure, at the site are not recommended as a means to achieve hemostasis. Once hemostasis is achieved, a pressure dressing at the site can be used but is probably not needed in most cases.

Frequent assessment of the site after catheter removal is recommended to identify rebleeding and/or thrombosis of the artery. Checking the extremity for the presence of pulses, circulation, and bleeding is necessary for a few hours after catheter removal.

Complications

A variety of complications are associated with arterial catheters (Table 5–8). The most serious are related to bleeding from the arterial catheter. Loose connections in the arterial system can lead to rapid and massive loss of blood. The morbidity and mortality associated with these complications require stringent safeguards (Luer-lock connections, mini-

TABLE 5–7. PROBLEMS ENCOUNTERED WITH PULMONARY ARTERY (PA) CATHETERS*

Problem	Cause	Prevention	Treatment
Phlebitis or local infection at insertion site	Mechanical irritation or contamination.	Prepare skin properly before insertion. Use sterile technique during insertion and dressing change. Insert smoothly and rapidly. Use Teflon-coated introducer. Attach silver-impregnated cuff to introducer. Change dressings, stopcocks, and connecting tubing every 24 to 48 hours. Remove catheter or change insertion site every 4 days.	Remove catheter. Apply warm compresses. Give pain medication as necessary.
Ventricular irritability	Looping of excess catheter in right ventricle. Migration of catheter from PA to RV. Irritation of the endocardium during catheter passage.	Suture catheter at insertion site; check chest film. Position catheter tip in main right or left PA. Keep balloon inflated during advancement; advance gently.	Reposition catheter; remove loop. Inflate balloon to encourage catheter flotation out to PA. Advance rapidly out to PA.
Apparent wedging of catheter with balloon deflated	Forward migration of catheter tip caused by blood flow, excessive loop in RV, or inadequate suturing of catheter at insertion site.	Check catheter tip by fluoroscopy; position in main right or left PA. Check catheter position on x-ray film if fluoroscopy is not used. Suture catheter in place at insertion site.	Aspirate blood from catheter; if catheter is wedged, sample will be arterialized and obtained with difficulty. If wedged, slowly pull back catheter until PA waveform appears. If not wedged, gently aspirate and flush catheter with saline; catheter tip can partially clot, causing damping that resembles damped PAW waveform.
Pulmonary hemorrhage or infarction, or both	Distal migration of catheter tip. Continuous or prolonged wedging of catheter. Overinflation of balloon while catheter is wedged. Failure of balloon to deflate.	Check chest film immediately after insertion and 12 to 24 hours later; remove any catheter loop in RA or RV. Leave balloon deflated. Suture catheter at skin to prevent inadvertent advancement. Position catheter in main right or left PA. Pull catheter back to pulmonary artery if it spontaneously wedges. Do not flush catheter when in wedge position. Inflate balloon slowly with only enough air to obtain a PAW waveform. Do not inflate 7-Fr catheter with more than 1 to 1.5 ml of air. Do not inflate if resistance is met.	Deflate balloon. Place patient on side (catheter tip down). Stop anticoagulation. Consider "wedge" angiogram. Intubate with double-lumen ET. Recommend surgery, if severe hemorrhage.
"Overwedging" or damped PAW	Overinflation of balloon. Frequent inflation of balloon.	Watch waveform during inflation; inject only enough air to obtain PAW pressure. Do not inflate 7-Fr catheter with more than 1 to 1.5 ml of air. Check inflated balloon shape before insertion.	Deflate balloon; reinflate slowly with only enough air to obtain PAW pressure. Deflate balloon; reposition and slowly reinflate.
PA balloon rupture	Overinflation of balloon. Frequent inflations of balloon. Syringe deflation, damaging wall of balloon.	Inflate slowly with only enough air to obtain a PAW pressure. Monitor PAD pressure as reflection of PAW and LVEDP. Allow passive deflation of balloon. Remove syringe after inflation.	Remove syringe to prevent further air injection. Monitor PAD pressure.
Infection	Nonsterile insertion techniques. Contamination via skin. Contamination through stopcock ports or catheter hub. Fluid contamination from transducer through cracked membrane of disposable dome. Prolonged catheter placement.	Use sterile techniques. Use sterile catheter sleeve. Prepare skin with effective antiseptic (chlorhexidine). Apply iodophor ointment and sterile gauze dressing daily. Do not use clear semipermeable dressing. Inspect site daily. Reassess need for catheter after 3 days. Avoid internal jugular approach. Use sterile dead-end caps on all stopcock ports. Change IV solution, stopcock, and tubing every 24 to 48 hours. Do not use IV solution that contains glucose. Check transducer domes for cracks. Change transducers every 48 hours. Change disposable dome after countershock. Do not use IV solution that contains glucose. Change catheter insertion site every 4 days.	Remove catheter. Use antibiotics.
Heart block during insertion of catheter	Mechanical irritation of His bundle in patients with preexisting left bundle branch block	Insert catheter expeditiously with balloon inflated. Insert transvenous pacing catheter before PA catheter insertion.	Use temporary pacemaker or flotation catheter with pacing wire.

*PAW, pulmonary artery wedge; RV, right ventricle; PA, pulmonary artery. *From:* Daily E, Schroeder J: Techniques in bedside hemodynamic monitoring, *5th ed. St. Louis, MO: CV Mosby, 1994, pp. 134–136.*

TABLE 5–8. PROBLEMS ENCOUNTERED WITH ARTERIAL CATHETERS

Problem	Cause	Prevention	Treatment
Hematoma after withdrawal of needle	Bleeding or oozing at puncture site.	Maintain firm pressure on site during withdrawal of catheter and for 5 to 15 minutes (as necessary) after withdrawal. Apply elastic tape (Elastoplast) firmly over puncture site. For femoral arterial puncture sites, leave a sandbag on site for 1 to 2 hours to prevent oozing. If patient is receiving heparin, discontinue 2 hours before catheter removal.	Continue to hold pressure to puncture site until oozing stops. Apply sandbag to femoral puncture site for 1 to 2 hours after removal of catheter.
Decreased or absent pulse distal to puncture site	Spasm of artery. Thrombosis of artery.	Introduce arterial needle cleanly, nontraumatically. Use 1 unit heparin to 1 ml IV fluid.	Inject lidocaine locally at insertion site and 10 mg into arterial catheter. Arteriotomy and Fogarty catheterization both distally and proximally from the puncture site result in return of pulse in more than 90% of cases if brachial or femoral artery is used.
Bleedback into tubing, dome, or transducer	Insufficient pressure on IV bag. Loose connections.	Maintain 300 mm Hg pressure on IV bag. Use Luer-Lock stopcocks; tighten periodically.	Replace transducer. "Fast-flush" through system. Tighten all connections.
Hemorrhage	Loose connections.	Keep all connecting sites visible. Observe connecting sites frequently. Use built-in alarm system. Use Luer-Lock stopcocks.	Tighten all connections.
Emboli	Clot from catheter tip into bloodstream.	Always aspirate and discard before flushing. Use continuous flush device. Use 1 unit heparin to 1 ml IV fluid. Gently flush <2 to 4 ml.	Remove catheter.
Local infection	Forward movement of contaminated catheter. Break in sterile technique. Prolonged catheter use.	Carefully suture catheter at insertion site. Always use aseptic technique. Remove catheter after 72 to 96 hours. Inspect and care for insertion site daily, including dressing change and antibiotic or iodophor ointment.	Remove catheter. Prescribe antibiotic.
Sepsis	Break in sterile technique. Prolonged catheter use. Bacterial growth in IV fluid.	Use percutaneous insertion. Always use aseptic technique. Remove catheter after 72 to 96 hours. Change transducer, stopcocks, and tubing every 96 hours. Do not use IV fluid containing glucose. Use sterile dead-end caps on all ports of stopcocks. Carefully flush remaining blood from stopcocks after blood sampling.	Remove catheter. Prescribe antibiotic.

From: Daily E, Schroeder J: Techniques in bedside hemodynamic monitoring, 5th ed. St. Louis, MO: CV Mosby, 1994, pp. 165–166.

mum number of stopcocks, pressure alarm system activated at all times) to prevent this bleeding and to rapidly notify clinicians of any breaks in the arterial system.

OBTAINING AND INTERPRETING HEMODYNAMIC WAVEFORMS

In order to obtain hemodynamic values, interpreting hemodynamic waveforms is necessary. The necessary equipment is a multichannel strip recorder which can give both an ECG and pressure tracing (Figure 5–12). The larger the printout, the easier is the interpretation of the wave. All waveforms are easily obtained simply by activating the record function of the bedside monitor. When obtaining waveforms for interpretation, make sure the calibration scales on the left side of the paper are properly aligned with the paper grid. Improperly aligned calibration marks will increase the difficulty in reading the waveform and increase the chance of misinterpretation.

Patient Position While Obtaining Hemodynamic Information

When obtaining hemodynamic waveforms for interpretation, the patient should be in a supine position, with the backrest elevated anywhere from 0 to 45 degrees. Gener-

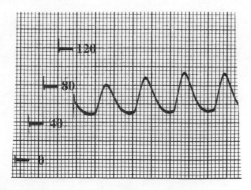

Figure 5–12. Graphic tracing of an arterial waveform preceded by calibration scale markings (0/40/80/120 mm Hg). Note how the scale markers line up with the heavy line of the tracing paper. Each 1-mm line represents 4 mm Hg in this scale.

ally, data should not be obtained if the patient is on his or her side, since it is difficult to identify the location of the catheter tip for purposes of leveling. The discrepancy in pressure readings from improper leveling can especially distort atrial and venous pressure readings.

It is important to keep in mind that patient comfort is a key issue when obtaining hemodynamic waveform readings. Do not lie a patient who is orthopneic flat for the sole reason of obtaining hemodynamic readings. It is best to obtain values in the position in which the patient is most comfortable and treat the values obtained in that position.

Interpreting Hemodynamic Waveforms

Correct interpretation of hemodynamic waveforms involves careful assessment of venous and arterial pressure waveforms for specific characteristics and location of the waveform area. Normal values for each of the hemodynamic pressures are listed in Table 5–6. In addition, Chapter 30, Hemodynamic Troubleshooting Guide, lists common problems and approaches to hemodynamic monitoring systems.

Atrial and Venous Waveforms

Pressures in the atrial and venous systems are significantly lower than in the ventricular and arterial systems. The two primary atrial/venous pressures measured in critically ill patients are the central venous pressure (CVP), also called the right atrial pressure (RAP), and the pulmonary artery capillary wedge pressure (PCWP). These pressures are used to estimate ventricular pressures since at the time of ventricular end diastole, the mitral and tricuspid valves are open (Figure 5–13). This allows a clear communication between the ventricles and the atrium, with equilibration of pressures in the two chambers. Ideally, ventricular pressures are better measures of ventricular function than atrial estimates; however, direct ventricular pressure measurement is not always available. Atrial pressures are then used

as a substitute. If ventricular waveforms are available, they should be used in place of atrial pressures. CVP and PCWP are the clinical measurements commonly performed to assess "preload" of the right and left ventricles, respectively.

CVP

The CVP is important since it is used to approximate the right ventricular end diastolic pressure (RVEDP). Ventricular end diastolic pressures, both right and left, are used to estimate the cardiac function and fluid status. The RVEDP is used to assess right ventricular function and general fluid status.

A normal CVP is between 2 and 6 mm Hg. Low CVP values typically reflect hypovolemia or decreased venous return. High CVP values reflect overhydration, increased venous return, or right-sided cardiac failure. If the CVP is low at the same time the stroke volume (SV, the amount of blood pumped from the heart with each beat) is low, hypovolemia is assumed. If the CVP is high at the same time the stroke volume is low, right ventricular dysfunction is assumed.

CVP is obtained from the proximal port of the pulmonary artery catheter or the tip of central venous catheter. Measuring the CVP needs to be done with simultaneous comparison to the ECG. Using the ECG allows the identification of the point where the CVP best correlates with the RVEDP.

The CVP is read by one of two techniques. The first technique is to take the mean (average) of the A wave of the CVP waveform (Figure 5–14). Although three waves nor-

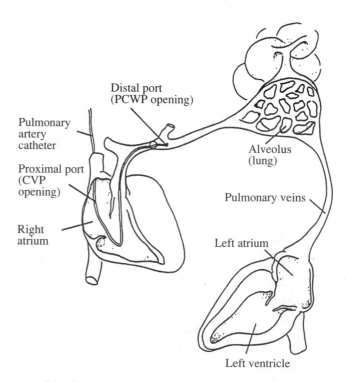

Figure 5–13. Open tricuspid and mitral valves allow atrial pressures to estimate ventricular end-diastolic pressures. *(From: Ahrens TS: Hemodynamic waveform recognition. Philadelphia: WB Saunders, 1993, p. 2.)*

mally exist on atrial waveforms (A, C, and V waves), the mean of the A wave most closely approximates ventricular end diastolic pressure. The A wave of the CVP waveform starts just after the P wave on the ECG is observed and represents atrial contraction. By taking the reading at the highest point of the A wave, adding it to the reading at the lowest point of that A wave, and dividing by 2, the average or mean CVP reading is obtained.

A second method, the Z-point technique, also can be used to estimate ventricular end diastolic pressures (Figure 5–15). The Z point is taken just before the closure of the tricuspid valve. This point is located on a CVP tracing in the mid to late QRS complex area. The Z-point technique is especially useful when an A wave does not exist, for example in atrial fibrillation when atrial contraction is absent.

By isolating the A wave or using the Z-point technique, atrial pressures can reasonably estimate ventricular end diastolic pressure. It is helpful to read these values off a multichannel strip recorder and not to always trust the digital display on the bedside monitor. Monitor values tend to be accurate in simple waveforms but become less reliable as the waveforms become more complex.

Abnormal Venous Waveforms

Two types of abnormal CVP waveforms are common. Large A waves (also called *cannon A waves*) occur when the atrium contracts against a closed tricuspid value (Figure 5–16). This occurs most commonly during arrhythmias like premature ventricular contraction (PVC) or third-degree heart block. Giant V waves are common in conditions such as tricuspid insufficiency or ventricular failure. Using the Z point for CVP readings will prevent the large A or V waves from producing incorrect values.

PCWP

Although the CVP is useful in assessing right ventricular function, the assessment of left ventricular function is generally even more important. If the left ventricle dysfunctions (e.g., with myocardial infarction or cardiomyopathies), a threat to tissue oxygenation and survival may exist due to low cardiac output. The PCWP frequently is used clinically to assess left ventricular function.

Interpreting the PCWP is very similar to interpreting a CVP waveform with the obvious exception that the PCWP assesses left ventricular end diastolic pressure (LVEDP),

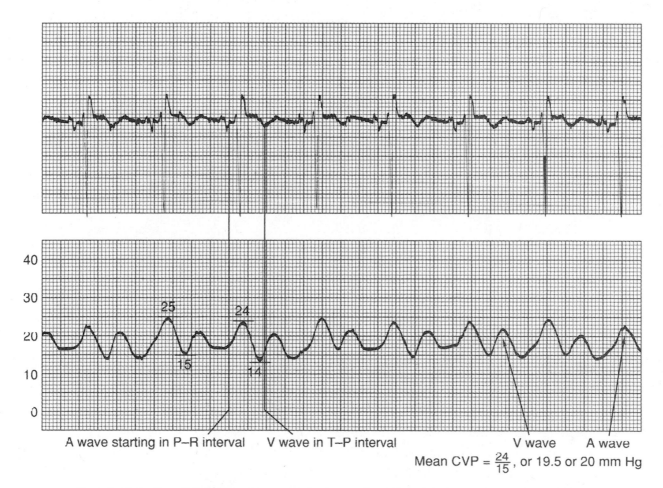

Figure 5–14. Reading a CVP waveform by averaging the A wave. *(From: Ahrens TS, Taylor L: Hemodynamic waveform analysis. Philadelphia: WB Saunders, 1992, p. 31.)*

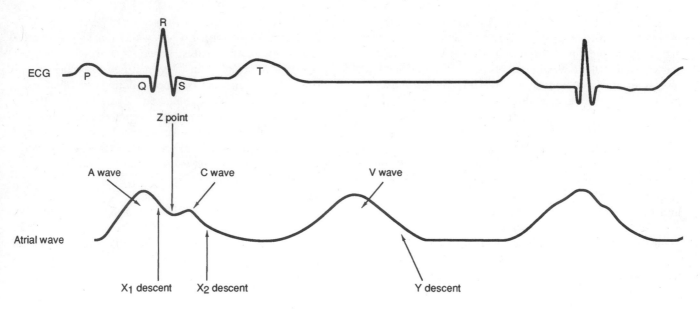

Figure 5–15. Use of the Z point to read a CVP waveform. *(From: Ahrens TS:* Hemodynamic waveform analysis. *Philadelphia: WB Saunders, 1992, p. 24.)*

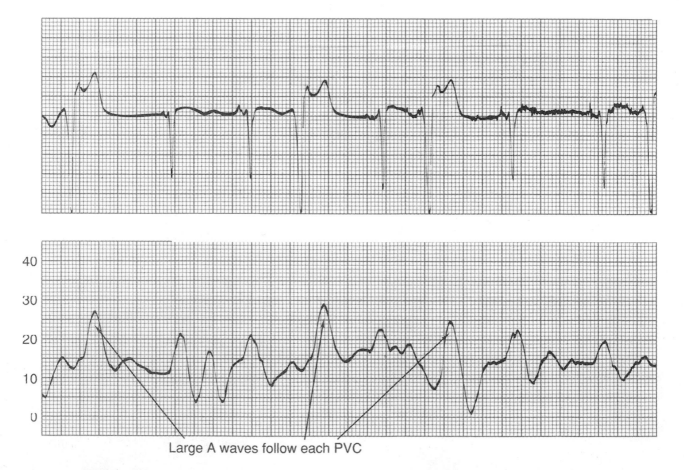

Large A waves follow each PVC

Figure 5–16. Giant A waves with loss of atrioventricular synchrony. *(From: Ahrens TS:* Hemodynamic waveform analysis. *Philadelphia: WB Saunders, 1992, p. 54.)*

not RVEDP. The LVEDP is used to assess left ventricular function and systemic fluid status.

A normal PCWP is 8 to 12 mm Hg. Low values reflect hypovolemia, with high values indicating hypervolemia and/or left ventricular failure. Mitral valve abnormalities will also cause elevations in PCWP. When the PCWP is normal at the same time stroke volume is normal, then normovolemia and acceptable left ventricular function is assumed. If the PCWP is low at the same time the stroke volume is low, hypovolemia is assumed. If the PCWP is high (usually greater than 18 mm Hg) at the same time the stroke volume is low, left ventricular dysfunction is assumed.

A PCWP waveform is obtained from the distal port of the PA catheter when the balloon on the catheter is inflated. Inflation of the balloon is performed for only a few seconds in order to avoid a disruption in pulmonary blood flow. When inflating the balloon, inflate only to the volume necessary to obtain the PCWP waveform. Record how much air it takes to inflate the balloon. If it takes less air to obtain a PCWP value than at a previous inflation, the catheter might have migrated further into the pulmonary artery. If it takes more air to obtain a PCWP, the catheter might have moved back. If no resistance is felt when the balloon is inflated and no PCWP tracing occurs, notify the physician of a possible balloon rupture.

When deflating the balloon, allow air to leave the balloon passively. Actively aspirating the air out of the balloon damages the balloon and is not necessary for complete emptying of the balloon.

The characteristics and interpretation of PCWP and CVP waveforms are similar. The difference between interpreting a CVP and a PCWP waveform mainly centers on the delay in waveform correlation with the ECG (Figure 5–17). This delay is based on the distance from the tip of the pulmonary artery catheter to the left atrium. For example, the A wave starts near the end of the QRS complex on a PCWP waveform. Averaging of the A wave's highest and lowest values, as previously described for CVP readings, is one method for obtaining the PCWP. If the Z point is to be used for a PCWP reading, this point is found at the end or immediately after (about 0.08 second) after the QRS complex (Figure 5–18).

Assessment of left ventricular function is commonly performed with the pulmonary capillary wedge pressure (PCWP). The use of the PCWP to estimate left ventricular end diastolic pressure is based on the assumption that a measurement from an obstructed pulmonary capillary will reflect an uninterrupted flow of blood to the left atrium since no valves exist in the pulmonary arterial system. A second assumption is that when the mitral valve is open, left atrial pressures reflect left ventricular end diastolic pressures. As long as these assumptions are accurate, the use of the PCWP to estimate LVEDP is acceptable.

Abnormal Venous Waveforms

Similar abnormal PCWP waveforms occur as with CVP measurements. Large A waves are observed when the left atrium contracts against a closed mitral valve. Large V waves are observed during mitral valve insufficiency and left heart failure (Figures 5–17 and 5–18).

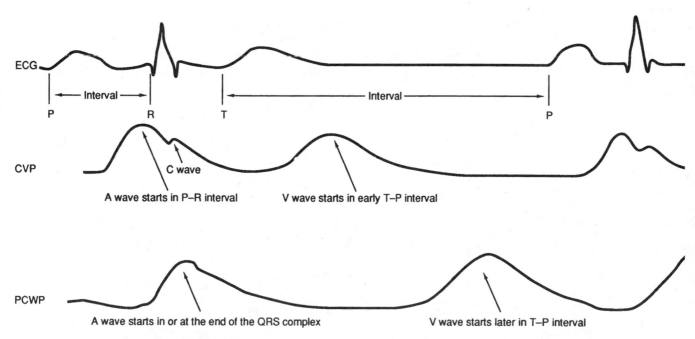

Figure 5–17. PCWP waveform with normal A waves and giant V waves. *(From: Ahrens TS:* Hemodynamic waveform analysis. *Philadelphia: WB Saunders, 1992, p. 28.)*

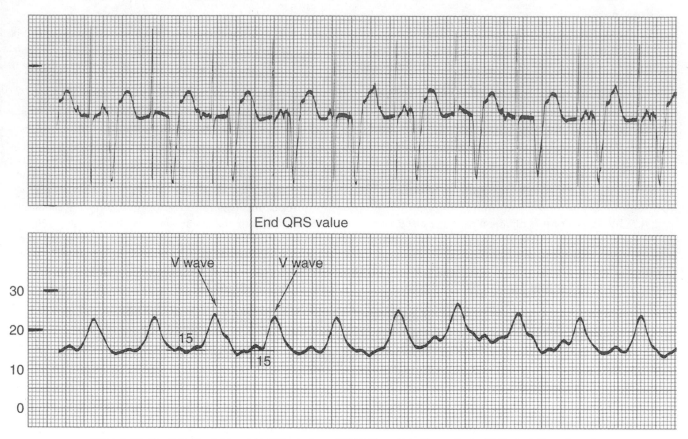

Figure 5–18. Use of the Z point to read a CVP waveform (PCWP-15 mmHg). *(From: Ahrens TS, Taylor L: Hemodynamic waveform analysis. Philadelphia: WB Saunders, 1992, p. 320.)*

Arterial and Ventricular Waveforms

An arterial waveform, such as seen in systemic and pulmonary artery tracings, has three common characteristics: (1) rapid upstroke, (2) dicrotic notch, and (3) progressive diastolic runoff (Figure 5–19). Diastole is read near the end of the QRS complex with systole read before the peak of the T wave. The mean arterial pressure can be calculated (Table 5–6) or obtained from the digital display on the bedside monitor.

A ventricular waveform also has three common characteristics: (1) rapid upstroke, (2) rapid drop in pressure, and (3) terminal diastolic rise (Figure 5–20). Systole and diastole are read in the same manner as for an arterial waveform. Left ventricular waveforms are not available in the clinical area, but can be obtained during cardiac catheterization. Normally, right ventricular waveforms are only observed during insertion of the PA catheter or if an extra lumen is present on the catheter which exists into the

Figure 5–19. Characteristics of an arterial waveform. *(From: Ahrens TS, Prentice D: Critical care: Certification preparation and review, 3rd ed. Stamford, CT: Appleton & Lange, 1993, p. 82.)*

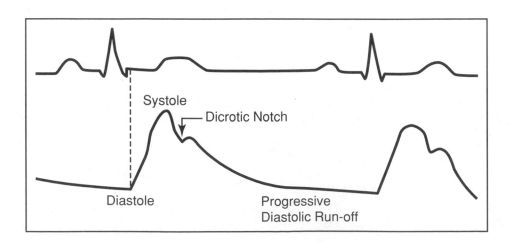

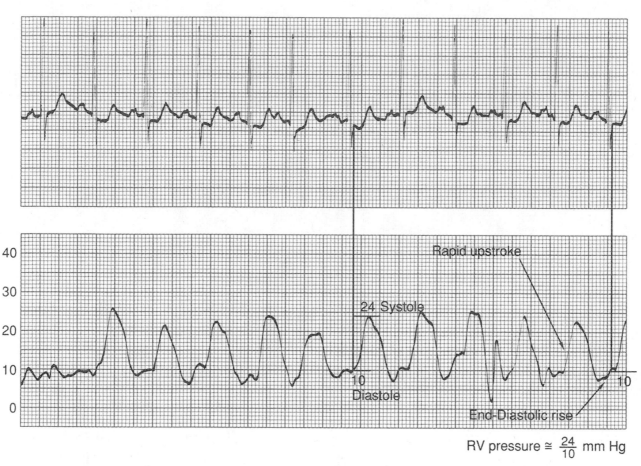

$$\text{RV pressure} \cong \frac{24}{10} \text{ mm Hg}$$

Figure 5–20. Characteristics of a ventricular waveform. *(From: Ahrens TS, Taylor L: Hemodynamic waveform analysis. Philadelphia: WB Saunders, 1992, p. 98.)*

RV (Table 5–5). If a right ventricular waveform is present during monitoring, it is important to verify the location of the catheter. The catheter may have migrated out of the PA and into the RV. A catheter which is floating free in the ventricle tends to cause ventricular ectopy (PVC) if the catheter comes into contact with the ventricular wall. In addition, assessment of PA pressures is not possible.

If the right ventricular end diastolic pressure is high (over 6 mm Hg), particularly if the stroke volume is low, some ventricular dysfunction is suspected. If the RVEDP is low (<2 mm Hg) and the stroke volume is low, hypovolemia is suspected. If the left ventricular end diastolic pressure is high (over 18 mm Hg) and stroke volume is reduced, left ventricular dysfunction is suspected. If the LVEDP is low (<8 mm Hg) and the stroke volume is reduced, hypovolemia is suspected.

PA Waveforms

Pulmonary artery pressures are obtained from a flow-directed pulmonary artery catheter (Figure 5–1). The pulmonary artery pressure is typically low in comparison to the systemic pressure. The PA pressure is determined by the right ventricular cardiac output and the pulmonary vascular resistance. Pulmonary artery blood pressure is generally in the region of 20 to 30 mm Hg systolic and 10 to 15 mm Hg diastolic (Table 5–6 and Figure 5–21). PA pressure reading is measured from the distal port of the PA catheter.

The low-pressure pulmonary system is critical to adequate gas exchange in the lungs. If the pressure in the pulmonary vasculature elevates, the capillary hydrostatic pressure exceeds capillary osmotic pressure and forces fluid out of the vessels. If the pulmonary lymphatic drainage capability is exceeded, interstitial and alveolar flooding will occur, with resulting interference in oxygen and carbon dioxide exchange.

Normally, the pulmonary artery pressure is high enough to ensure blood flow through the lungs to the left atrium. Subsequently, blood pressure in the pulmonary arteries only should be high enough to overcome the resistance in the left atrium. The mean pulmonary artery pressure must always be higher than left atrial pressure or else blood flow through the lungs would cease. As a practical guideline, the pulmonary artery diastolic pressure is higher than the mean left atrial pressure (the mean left atrial pressure is generally estimated by the pulmonary capillary wedge pressure). If the pulmonary artery diastolic value is

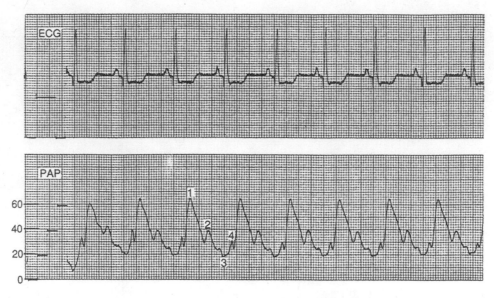

Figure 5–21. PA waveform and components. 1 = PA systole; 2 = dichrotic notch; 3 = PA end diastole; 4 = anacrotic notch of PA valve opening. *(From: Boggs R, Wooldridge-King M: AACN procedure manual for critical care, 3rd ed. Philadelphia: WB Saunders, 1993, p. 316.)*

less than the left atrial or wedge pressure, either a very low pulmonary blood flow state exists or the waveforms have been misinterpreted.

Measurement of PA pressures can be helpful in diagnosing many clinical conditions. Elevated PA pressures occur in pulmonary hypertension, chronic pulmonary disease, mitral valve disease, left ventricular failure, hypoxia, and pulmonary emboli. Below-normal PA pressures occur primarily in conditions which produce hypovolemia. If blood volumes are reduced, less resistance to ventricular ejection occurs with a resulting drop in arterial pressures. In this situation, the pulmonary artery diastolic pressure is also near the left atrial pressure.

Systemic Arterial Pressures

Direct measurement of systemic arterial pressures is obtained from the tip of an arterial catheter (Figure 5–6), with pressure waveforms interpreted as previously described. Normal pressures are generally in the region of 100 to 140 mm Hg systolic, 60 to 90 mm Hg diastolic, and 70 to 100 mm Hg mean (Table 5–6).

Systemic arterial pressures are not interpreted without other clinical information. In general, however, hypotension is assumed if the mean arterial pressure drops below 60 mm Hg. Hypertension is assumed if the systolic blood pressure (SBP) is greater than 140 to 160 mm Hg or the diastolic pressure exceeds 90 mm Hg.

The arterial pressure is one of the most commonly used parameters for assessing the adequacy of blood flow to the tissues. Blood pressure is determined by two factors, cardiac output (CO) and systemic vascular resistance (SVR). Blood pressure will not reflect early clinical changes in hemodynamics because of the interaction with cardiac output and systemic vascular resistance. Although the interaction between CO and SVR is not always perfectly predictable, the interaction generally works as follows. If the cardiac output decreases, the systemic vascular resistance will increase to maintain the blood pressure. The increase in resistance is just enough to overcome the fall in cardiac output, with blood pressure maintained at near normal levels if SVR is increased enough to overcome the drop in cardiac output. On the other hand, if the systemic vascular resistance falls, the cardiac output will increase to offset the fall in SVR. Again, the BP will be near normal if the increase in cardiac output is high enough to overcome the fall in SVR. In both circumstances the blood pressure does not change early due to the interaction of cardiac output and systemic vascular resistance.

In addition, the cardiac output is comprised of heart rate and stroke volume. These two interact with each other to keep the cardiac output normal. Subsequently, if the stroke volume begins to fall due to loss of volume (hypovolemia) or dysfunction (left ventricular failure), the heart rate will increase to offset this decrease in stroke volume. The net effect will be to maintain the cardiac output at near normal levels. If the cardiac output does not change, then there will be no change in the blood pressure.

The key aspect for the clinician to remember is that because of the above interactions, blood pressure is unable to signal early clinical changes in hemodynamic status. If a patient begins to bleed postoperatively, the blood pressure will generally not reflect this change until the heart rate and SVR increases can no longer compensate. The same situation exists for a patient who has congestive heart failure or a myocardial infarction. Blood pressure will not reflect the early changes in hemodynamics since compensatory mechanisms serve to keep the blood pressure normal.

Another major clinical consideration in assessing blood pressure is in terms of identifying what is a clinically acceptable blood pressure. Identifying what is a normal blood pressure is based on identifying that blood flow to the tissues is not below adequate levels (hypotension) and excessive pressure and damage to peripheral circulation is not occurring (hypertension).

Hypotension probably is present only if evidence of tissue oxygenation deficits exists. This means that blood pressure needs to be assessed along with measurements of tissue oxygenation, such as mixed venous oxyhemoglobin (SvO_2) and lactate levels (see Chapter 23, Advanced Respiratory Concepts, for a detailed discussion of SvO_2). The implication of the interaction between tissue oxygenation and blood pressure is that blood pressure values cannot be viewed in isolation.

Hypertension is more difficult to identify since fewer clinical parameters exist to indicate when peripheral circulatory changes are occurring. However, pressure alone is one important determinant of circulatory damage. As such, it is a little more reliable as a parameter than blood pressure reflecting hypotension. Studies of hypertension-induced injury are not clear in terms of what blood pressure produces actual injury. For a guideline, however, any SBP >140 should be considered potentially injurious to the circulation.

Artifacts in Hemodynamic Waveforms: Respiratory Influence

Respiration can physiologically change hemodynamic pressures. Spontaneous breathing augments venous return and slightly increases resistance to left ventricle filling. Mechanical ventilation does the opposite, potentially reducing venous return and reducing the resistance on the heart. The effect on pressures varies, but the effect of respiration can be noted by observing the venous and arterial waveforms (Figures 5–22).

A spontaneous breath or a triggered ventilator breath produces a drop in the waveform due to the decrease in pleural pressure (Figure 5–23). A ventilator breath will produce an upward distortion of the baseline, due to an increase in unmeasured pleural pressure (Figure 5–24). The key to reading the waveform properly is to isolate the point where pleural pressure is closest to atmospheric pressure. This point is usually at end expiration. By identifying the point before the patient begins an inspiratory effort, end expiration is relatively easy to identify (Figure 5–25).

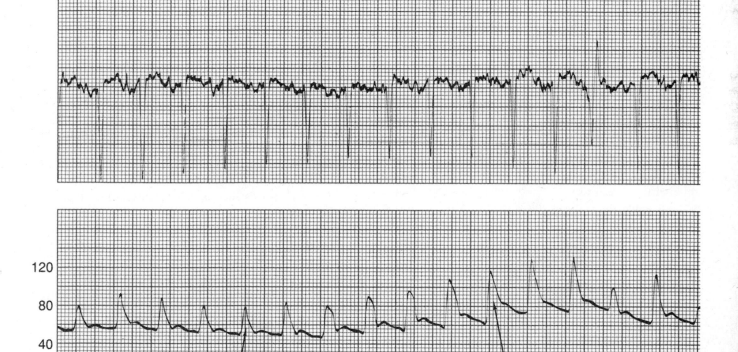

Figure 5–22. Effect of respiration on arterial pressures. *(From: Ahrens TS: Hemodynamic waveform analysis. Philadelphia: WB Saunders, 1992, p. 161.)*

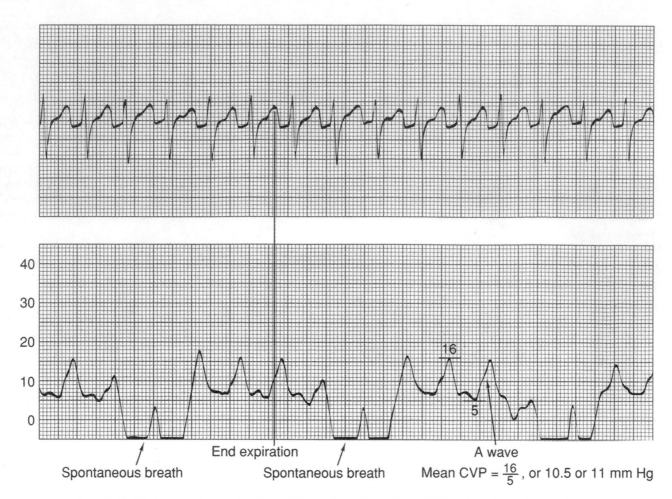

Figure 5–23. Effect of a spontaneous breath on a CVP waveform. *(From: Ahrens TS:* Hemodynamic waveform analysis. *Philadelphia: WB Saunders, 1992, p. 165.)*

DERIVED HEMODYNAMIC PARAMETERS

Several hemodynamic parameters can be calculated based on other measured variables. These parameters are usually referred to as derived values. Formulas for some common hemodynamic derived variables are listed in Table 5–6. Most bedside monitors will perform the calculations necessary to achieve these values. However, it is essential for critical care clinicians to know which variables are included in the calculation. This knowledge is essential in order to understand how hemodynamics interact and in order to interpret the derived variables.

Vascular Resistance

One of the most common derived parameters is vascular resistance. Vascular resistance is frequently assumed to represent afterload, or the resistance the ventricles face to eject blood. It is important to keep in mind that afterload is not completely measured by vascular resistance. Resistance is also influenced by blood viscosity and valvular resistance.

Although these values can change, it is helpful to use vascular resistance to estimate afterload since viscosity and valve resistance tend to change less often than blood vessel resistance.

Vascular resistance is calculated from a variation of Ohm's law. Ohm's law is commonly used in many fields in addition to health care. There are three key concepts in this estimate of resistance; one is the pressure present entering an area, a second is the pressure present resisting flow into the area, and the third is the total flow which occurs through the area. These three concepts are placed into the following formula:

$$\text{Resistance} = \frac{\text{Driving pressure} - \text{Resisting pressure}}{\text{Total flow}}$$

In clinical practice, this formula is adapted as follows:

$$\text{Vascular resistance} = \frac{\text{Mean arterial pressure} - \text{Right atrial pressure}}{\text{Cardiac output}}$$

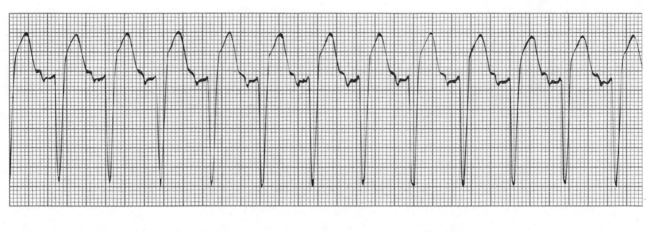

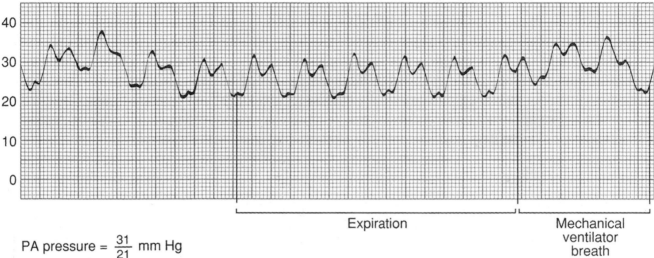

$$\text{PA pressure} = \frac{31}{21} \text{ mm Hg}$$

Figure 5–24. Effect of a mechanical ventilator breath on pulmonary artery waveform. *(From: Ahrens TS:* Hemodynamic waveform recognition. *Philadelphia: WB Saunders, 1993, p. 92.)*

The value obtained from this formula is multiplied by a factor of 80 to generate a value measured in dynes per second per centimeter to the 5th power (dynes/second/cm^5).

Two types of vascular resistance are commonly measured. Systemic vascular resistance reflects left ventricular afterload, and pulmonary vascular resistance reflects right ventricular afterload.

Systemic Vascular Resistance

Normal systemic vascular resistance (SVR) is about 900 to 1300 dynes/second/cm^5. If the SVR is elevated, the left ventricle will face an increased resistance to the ejection of blood. The SVR commonly elevates as a pathological response to hypertension or a low cardiac output, such as would occur in shock states. It is important for the clinician to know why the SVR is elevated. If the SVR is elevated due to systemic hypertension, afterload reducing agents are a critical part of the therapy. However, if the SVR is elevated secondary to a compensation for low cardiac output, therapy is directed at improving the cardiac output more than reducing SVR.

If the SVR is low, the LV faces a lower resistance to the ejection of blood. Generally, the SVR does not lower except as a pathological response to inflammatory conditions (e.g., sepsis, fever). The SVR can also be reduced in hepatic disease due to increased collateral circulation or from neurogenic induced central vasodilation. Generally, if the SVR is reduced, attempts to increase the resistance center on the administration of vasopressor drugs. A more important concept to remember, however, is the treatment of the underlying condition. If the underlying condition is not treated, the use of vasopressors will provide only short-term success.

Pulmonary Vascular Resistance

Pulmonary vascular resistance (PVR) is lower in comparison to SVR. Normal PVR is about 40 to 150 dynes/second/cm^5. Generally, the main problem with the PVR is when it elevates. An elevation of the PVR produces a strain on the right ventricle. If this strain in unrelieved, over time the right ventricle will eventually fail. Failure of the right ventricle will cause less blood to enter the lungs and the left

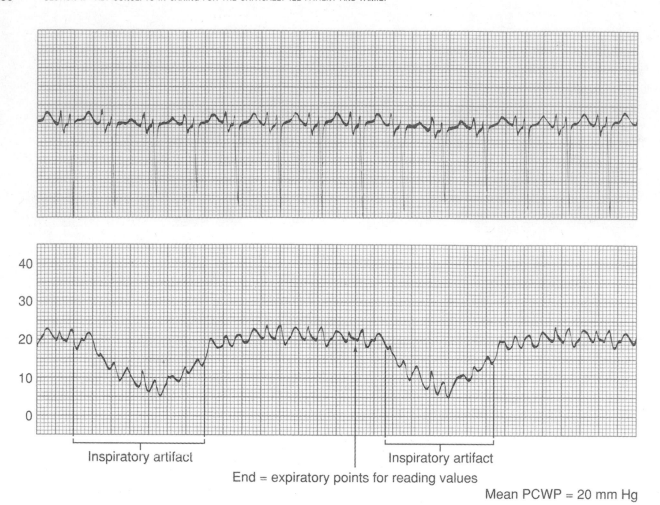

Figure 5–25. Reading end expiration before a spontaneous breath. *(From: Ahrens TS, Taylor L:* Hemodynamic waveform analysis. *Philadelphia: WB Saunders, 1992, p. 170.)*

ventricle. Systemic hypotension will eventually occur due to right ventricular dysfunction. The most common causes of an increase in PVR include pulmonary hypertension, hypoxia, and pulmonary emboli.

CARDIAC OUTPUT

Perhaps the most important information obtained from the pulmonary artery catheter is the measurement of blood flow parameters such as cardiac output and stroke volume. Understanding these parameters is critical in order to assess the adequacy of cardiac function. Flow parameters like cardiac output and stroke volume are the first parameters assessed when monitoring hemodynamic data.

If flow parameters are adequate, tissue oxygenation is generally maintained. If flow parameters are abnormal, the clinician must suspect a threat to tissue oxygenation and consider interventions aimed at improving cardiac function. Keep in mind that blood flow can fluctuate with many conditions. If hypovolemia is present (e.g., from GI bleeding or postoperative complications), blood flow will drop. If left

ventricular failure is present (e.g., from myocardial infarction or congestive heart failure), blood flow will drop. It is up to the bedside clinician to detect these changes and prevent them from causing harm to the patient. Unfortunately, there is no easy way of noninvasively identifying blood flow. At times, changes in blood flow are obvious (the patient loses pulses, changes level of consciousness, decreases urine output). However, these measures can be late and do not provide specific or quantitative information. Measurement of blood flow is generally only possible through invasive hemodynamic monitoring with a pulmonary artery catheter. Keep in mind that the most important component of delivering oxygen to the tissues is blood flow. Assessment of oxygenation begins with an assessment of blood flow. Thus, hemodynamic monitoring is the essential step for assessing the adequacy of oxygen delivery to the tissues.

Measurement of Cardiac Output

Cardiac outputs are clinically obtained by one of two methods: the intermittent thermodilution technique or the continuous technique. Both types of measures rely on measuring changes in blood temperatures. The most commonly used technique is the intermittent, thermodilution technique (Figure 5–26). This technique is based on the Stewart-Hamilton equation. This equation is based on injecting a known volume of fluid at a given temperature into the blood. As the blood temperature changes to near the injectate temperature, a sensor near the distal tip of the pulmonary artery catheter measures this change. Cardiac output is then computed based on the temperature change and the time it takes the injected volume to pass the thermistor. The calculation of cardiac index is automatically done by most cardiac output computers if body surface information is available (Table 5–6). The temperature change during injection can be graphically displayed on the cardiac output computer or bedside monitor as a cardiac output curve (Figure 5–27A). If the cardiac output is low, the curve is large, reflecting the large temperature change in the blood which occurs from the low blood flow state (Figure 5–27B). If the cardiac output is high, the curve is small, indicating the lack of temperature change from the rapid movement of blood past the thermistor (Figure 5–27C).

Key Concepts in Measuring Cardiac Output

In order to correctly measure the cardiac output, the clinician needs to program the bedside cardiac output computer with the following information:

- *Type of PA catheter.* Different companies may have different catheter configurations. This requires a slightly different computation by the computer. The manufacturer will provide the correct computation factor to be programmed into the cardiac output computer.
- *Volume of injectate.* Normally, 5 or 10 ml of D_5W or normal saline is used.
- *Temperature of the injectate.* Either cold (also called iced) or room-temperature injectate can be used. When using cold injectate, the injectate solution must be placed in a container of ice water (Figure 5–26A). Room-temperature injectate has an advantage in that it avoids the cumbersome cooling system necessary with iced injectate. Whichever technique is used, the system should be a closed system to prevent increased risk of IV nosocomial infections.
- *Computation constant.* The manufacturer of the cardiac output system will provide the correct computation constant to use based on the specific solution volume and temperature used for cardiac output measurements. This information is programmed into the cardiac output computer before performing cardiac output measurements.

Factors Affecting the Accuracy of the Cardiac Output Measurement

For the thermodilution cardiac output to be accurate, several factors should be present. These factors include a functioning tricuspid valve, no ventricular septal defect, and a stable cardiac rhythm. The presence of cardiac valve or rhythm abnormalities will cause the thermodilution cardiac output measurement to be inaccurate. Chapter 30, Hemodynamic Troubleshooting Guide, identifies common problems associated with measurement of cardiac output.

Interpreting Cardiac Output and Cardiac Index

Normal blood flow is typically defined as a cardiac output (CO) of 4 to 8 L/minute. Many clinicians prefer to use the term cardiac index (CI), which is an adjustment of cardiac output based on the size of the person (Table 5–6). A normal cardiac index is 2.5 to 4 L/minute/m^2.

Generally, the cardiac index is a better parameter to use than cardiac output. The following example will illustrate why this is so. Consider two different patients, one large (120 kg, 6 feet 2 inches, body surface area (BSA) 2.53m^2) and one is smaller (57 kg, 5 feet 0 inches, BSA 1.59 m^2). Assume they both have a cardiac output of 4.4 L/minute. A CO of 4 L/minute is within normal limits. However, if one calculates the cardiac index, the large person has a cardiac index of 1.74 L/minute/m^2, while the smaller person has a CI of 2.77 L/minute/m^2. Interpreting the CI reveals that the large person has a low blood flow for his body size, while the smaller person has an adequate blood flow.

The cardiac index is a critical parameter to monitor since blood flow is the key to adequate oxygen delivery. If a threat to blood flow occurs, tissue oxygenation is immediately placed at risk. If adequate blood flow is present, as measured through the cardiac output or index, generally one can assume the patient does not have a major disturbance in oxygenation. However, it is important to correlate CI with a tissue oxygenation parameter, such as mixed venous oxyhemoglobin (SvO_2) or lactate levels to ensure adequate tissue oxygenation is present (Table 5–9).

There is no one CI which requires intervention. However, whenever the CI is below 2.5 L/minute/m^2, the clinician should be concerned about tissue oxygenation. An investigation into why the CI might be decreasing is warranted whenever the index is below 2.5. If the CI drops below 2.2, the investigation becomes urgent. However, some patients tolerate low CIs without clinical problems. Tracking trends in CI values is generally more useful than monitoring single data points since temporary changes in values may not be clinically significant. In any event, if the CI decreases below normal, the clinician should suspect a potential problem is developing. The seriousness of the low CI is a function of the severity of tissue oxygenation disturbance. Using both CI and tissue oxygenation parameters, such as SvO_2, will increase the accuracy in identifying a clinically dangerous event.

Regulation of Cardiac Output

Cardiac output is determined by two factors, heart rate and stroke volume. Understanding heart rate and stroke volume is essential for understanding how to treat abnormal cardiac

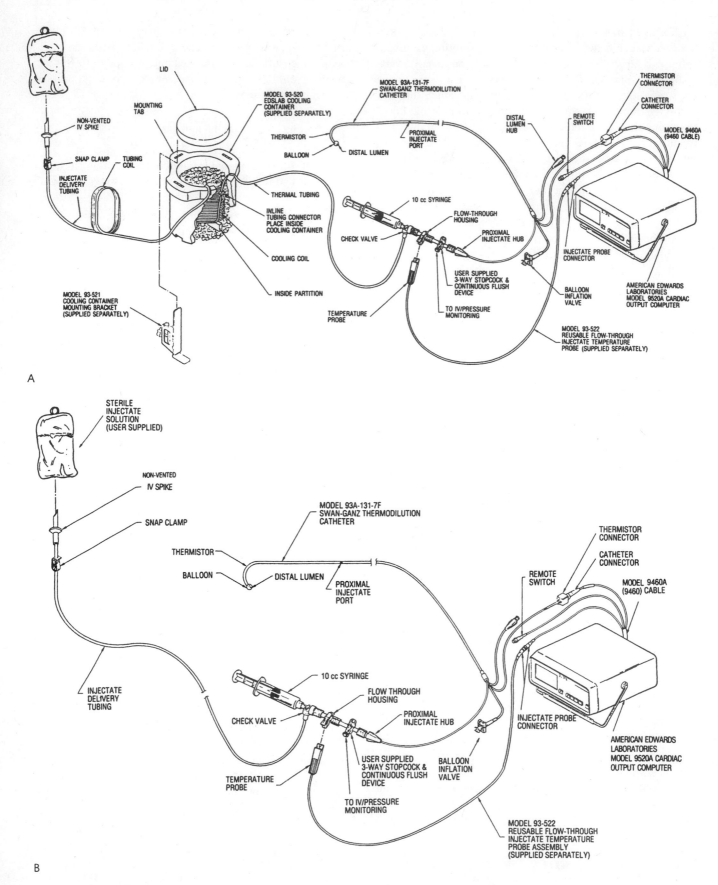

Figure 5–26. Closed thermodilution cardiac output setup. (A) Iced injectable setup. (B) Room-temperature injectate setup. *(From: Baxter Healthcare Corporation, Edwards Critical Care Division, Santa Ana, CA).*

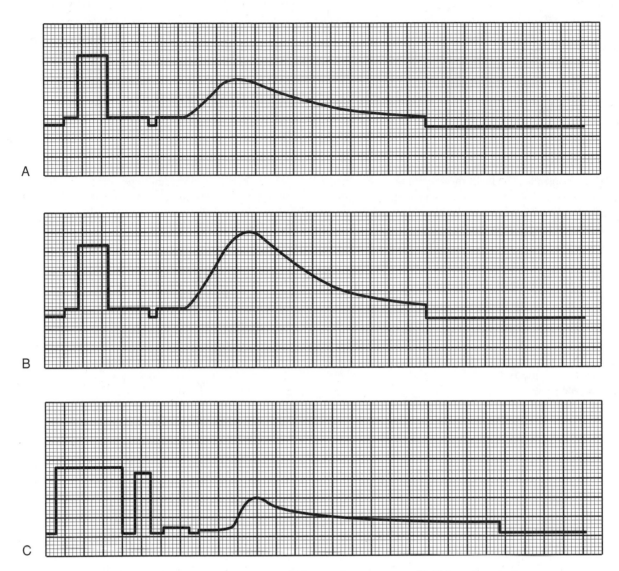

Figure 5–27. (A) Normal cardiac output curve. (B) Low cardiac output curve. (C) High cardiac output curve.

outputs. The most common problems affecting abnormal cardiac outputs are problems with stroke volumes.

Stroke Volume and Stroke Index

Stroke volume (SV) is defined as the amount of blood ejected with each heart beat. Stroke index (SI), like cardiac index, is a more useful measure for individualizing stroke volumes based on the patient size. Stroke index is obtained by dividing the stroke volume by the patient's BSA (Table 5–6).

TABLE 5–9. TISSUE OXYGENATION PARAMETERS

Sv_{O_2}	60 to 75%
Lactate	1 to 2 mEq/L
pH	7.35 to 7.45
Pyruvate	0.1 to 0.2 mEq/L
HCO_3	22 to 26 mEq/L

The amount of blood pumped with each beat is one of the key hemodynamic parameters to monitor. In any condition where the heart begins to dysfunction, the stroke volume or index will eventually decline. Initially, the stroke volume may not decline due to compensatory mechanisms which occur in the heart. One of the more important parameters to monitor for a change before a change in stroke index is ejection fraction.

Ejection Fraction

Ejection fraction (EF) is defined as how much blood is pumped with each contraction in relation to how much blood is available to be pumped. For example, assume the left ventricular end diastolic volume (LVEDV = the amount of blood left in the heart just before contraction) is about 100 ml. Also assume the stroke volume is 80 ml. This will give an ejection fraction of 80% since 80 ml of the possible 100 ml in the ventricle was ejected. A normal ejection fraction is usually over 60% (Table 5–6).

The EF can change before the stroke volume in certain conditions, such as left ventricular failure and sepsis. For example, if a patient begins to have left ventricular dysfunction from coronary artery disease, the left ventricle can start to dilate. This dilation will increase the LVEDV. The increase in LVEDV might prevent a drop in stroke volume but can be detected by monitoring the EF. For example, assume a patient starts with the following: LVEDV 110 ml, SV 70 ml, and EF 64% (70/110 ml). Over time, the same patient begins to have left ventricular dysfunction with dilation of the left ventricle. The heart muscle begins to weaken, but the SV is maintained by the increase in LVEDV: LVEDV 170 ml, SV 70 ml, and EF 41% (70/170 ml). The SV is maintained, but the EF and LVEDV reflect early left ventricular dysfunction. Because the EF and LVEDV are early warning signs for ventricular dysfunction, they are ideal monitoring parameters. Unfortunately, EF and LVEDV are not routinely available. This leaves SV and SI as the best measures to assess left and right ventricular dysfunction.

The SV or SI becomes the single most important piece of information regarding cardiac function in the absence of EF. The SV is extremely important because it will typically fall once blood volume is too low (hypovolemia) or when the left ventricle is too weak to eject blood (left ventricular dysfunction). In some cases the SV can increase, such as with exercise or in clinical conditions such as sepsis.

Regulation of SV

Three factors regulate SV. These factors are preload, afterload, and contractility. Preload is concerned with factors which affect the stretch of myocardial muscle. Factors which control the stretch of a muscle include the pressure and volume in the ventricle as well as the compliance (ability to stretch) of the muscle. Afterload is the amount of resistance the ventricle faces prior to contraction. Factors which control afterload include systemic vascular resistance (SVR), blood viscosity, and valve resistance. Contractility is the force of the muscle during activation.

According to the principle of Starling's law (Figure 5–28), the more a muscle stretches, the more forceful is the contraction. This principle is accurate only to a point, since if the muscle stretches too much, contraction becomes weaker. While this concept of Starling's law is widely accepted, it is difficult in clinical practice to actually measure preload. Clinically we estimate preload from ventricular filling pressures as measured by PCWP or CVP, an estimate which frequently is inaccurate since pressures alone do not determine preload. However, the assumption used to estimate preload is important to understand since it is widely used in critical care. Basically, estimation of preload from ventricular pressures proceeds as follows: If the ventricular filling pressures increase beyond normal [normal LVEDP (or PCWP) is about 8 to 12 mm Hg], it is assumed the left ventricle is weakening. If the pressure exceeds about 18 mm Hg, the ventricle is assumed to be at near-fail-

ure levels, the point where the muscle is stretching excessively. The other end of this concept is when the ventricular filling pressures are too low (PCWP <8 mm Hg). If the pressures are too low, it is assumed the blood volumes are low and hypovolemia exists.

Many clinicians use the above guidelines as if the preload is really measured simply by ventricular pressures. This simplistic interpretation frequently creates an inaccurate clinical impression, since it assumes pressure alone tells us about muscle stretch. Since other aspects of stretch, such as volume and compliance, are not measured with pressure, the pressure may not necessarily reflect muscle stretch. Since the ventricle changes according to different clinical conditions (e.g., hypertrophy and chamber dilation, interstitial fibrosis with cardiac remodeling), all potentially changing the volume, pressure, and compliance of the heart, assuming pressure alone reveals muscle stretch will clearly be inaccurate at times.

In order to help reduce the frequency of inaccurate assessments of muscle stretch with pressure values, pressure measurements should always be compared with blood flows, particularly SV or SI. For example, if the filling pressures elevate, they should decrease SI if they are clinically significant. If the filling pressures are low, the SI should be low as well before the clinician assumes hypovolemia exists. Combining the SI with filling pressures is essential in order to avoid misinterpreting filling pressures. Ventricular filling pressures (PCWP and CVP) should never be used in isolation because of the potential for misinterpretation.

Heart Rate

The heart rate needs to be evaluated routinely in order to detect early changes in hemodynamics. Since cardiac output is a product of SV times heart rate, any change in SV will normally produce a change in the heart rate. If the SV is elevated, the heart rate may decrease (e.g., as seen in adaptation to exercise). The exception to this guideline is during an increase in metabolic rate, where both the SV and heart rate increase.

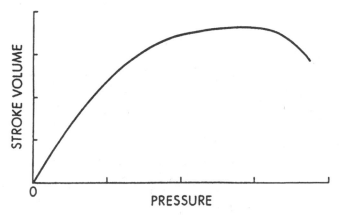

Figure 5–28. Concept of Starling's law.

If the SV falls, the heart rate normally increases. Subsequently, evaluating tachycardias becomes an essential component of hemodynamic monitoring. Generally, bradycardias and tachycardias are potentially dangerous since they may reflect an interference in cardiac output. Bradycardias which develop suddenly are almost always reflective of a threat to cardiac output. Tachycardias, a more common clinical situation, also may be a threat to cardiac output but need to be isolated as to their potential cause since tachycardias may not always reflect a low-cardiac-output state.

Several reasons exist for the development of a sinus tachycardia and include an increase in metabolic rate (e.g., with a temperature elevation); pain, anxiety, or fear; hypoxemia; and a reduction in SV. When evaluating a rapid heart rate, each of the main sources for the tachycardia must be evaluated. For example, if a patient has a heart rate of 120/minute, the clinician must assess if a temperature is present or if a source of anxiety or pain exists before assuming the heart rate is increased due to a reduced SV.

If the heart rate is increased, and a metabolic rate increase or psychological factors do not appear to be the cause, then an investigation of the cause of a low SV is necessary. The two most common reasons for a low SV are hypovolemia and left ventricular dysfunction. Both causes of low SV can produce an increased heart rate if no abnormality exists in regulation of the heart rate (such as autonomic nervous system dysfunction or use of drugs which interfere with the sympathetic or parasympathetic nervous system).

An increased heart rate can compensate for a decrease in SV, although this compensation is limited. The faster the heart rate, the less time exists for ventricular filling. As an increased heart rate reduces diastolic filling time, the potential exists to eventually reduce the SV. There is no specific heart rate where diastolic filling is reduced so severely that SV decreases. However, as the heart rate increases, it should be remembered that SV can be negatively affected.

Another important concept regarding heart rate has to do with the effect is has on myocardial oxygen consumption (MVO_2). The higher the heart rate, the more likely it is that the heart will consume more oxygen. Typically, myocardial oxygen consumption can only be estimated since direct measurement is not easy under normal clinical situations. Since heart rate is not the only determinant of oxygen consumption (contractility and vascular resistance are also determinants), heart rate alone will not predict MVO_2. Some patients are more sensitive to elevated MVO_2 than others. For example, a young person might tolerate sinus tachycardias as high as 160 for several days, while a patient with coronary artery disease might go into congestive heart failure with heart rates in the 130s. Keeping heart rates as low as possible, particularly in patients with altered myocardial blood flow, is one way of protecting myocardial function.

Low Cardiac Output States

Hemodynamic disturbances present as either a high or low blood flow state. Initially, compensatory mechanisms may present to keep blood flow normal, but eventually the output will be either too high or too low. The most common situation is the development of a low cardiac output state.

Low cardiac output states fall into one of two categories, i.e., hypovolemia or left ventricular dysfunction. While many conditions can cause either hypovolemia or LV dysfunction, all will produce a low cardiac output state. Before the cardiac output falls, however, the SV will decrease. Therefore, the SV or SI is an earlier warning sign of impending low flow states. As such, it should be examined before the cardiac output or index. When SV can no longer be compensated (by heart rate), the total blood flow (cardiac output) will decrease. From a tissue oxygenation perspective, the drop in SV will not harm oxygen delivery as long as the total blood flow (cardiac output) is maintained. Parameters such as SvO_2 will remain normal as long as total blood flow is unchanged. Since SV will decrease in both hypovolemia and LV dysfunction, without necessarily changing cardiac output or SvO_2 levels, it is important to assess SI first when examining hemodynamic parameters.

AT THE BEDSIDE
▶ *Hypovolemia*

A 67-year-old female is admitted to the unit with the diagnosis of hypotension of unknown origin. She presently is unresponsive but is breathing spontaneously and is not intubated. Breath sounds are clear, urine output is 15 ml in 8 hours, and her skin is cool. A pulmonary artery catheter is inserted to aid in the interpretation of the situation. The following data are available:

BP	86/54	SI	16 ml/m²
P	118/minute	PA	24/10
RR	30/minute	PCWP	6 mm Hg
T	37.3°C	CVP	3 mm Hg
CI	1.9 L/min/m²	SvO₂	50%

Note the low blood flow (CI and SI below normal) and low intracardiac pressures (PCWP). This combination of low flows and intracardiac pressures is consistent with hypovolemia. In addition, the SvO_2 is low, indicating that a threat to tissue oxygenation is likely.

The exact cause of the hypovolemia cannot be discerned from the hemodynamics. Further investigation to isolate the exact problem, such as GI bleeding, dehydration, or other forms of blood loss, is necessary to diagnose the underlying cause of the hypovolemia.

AT THE BEDSIDE
▶ *Left Ventricular Dysfunction*

A 76-year-old male is admitted to the unit with the diagnosis of acute inferior wall myocardial infarction and a history of chronic obstructive pulmonary disease (COPD). During the shift he begins to complain of shortness of breath. He has crackles one-third the way up his posterior lobes along with expiratory wheezing. He has an S_3 (gallop) and a II/VI systolic murmur. The following hemodynamic information was obtained on admission:

BP	100/58	PA	38/23
P	112/minute	PCWP	21 mm Hg
CI	2.1 L/min/m^2	CVP	13 mm Hg
CO	4.6 L/min	Svo_2	49%
SI	19		

In this case, the patient presents with low blood flow (CI and SI) and high intracardiac pressures (PCWP, CVP). This combination of low blood flow and high filling pressures suggests left and right ventricular dysfunction. The low Svo_2 level suggests a serious disturbance in tissue oxygenation. Intervention to support cardiac output is required. Further investigation to isolate the exact problem, such as congestive heart failure, myocardial infarction, or cardiomyopathy, is necessary.

Identifying the cause of the low flow state (e.g., hypovolemia or LV dysfunction) is done with a combination of clinical and hemodynamic information. For example, the patient's physical assessment and history might reveal the presence of a pathological clinical condition such as left ventricular failure. From a hemodynamic monitoring perspective, the use of intracardiac pressures (PCWP, CVP) is the most common method of differentiating the cause of the low blood flow state.

When intracardiac pressures are low, hypovolemia is assumed to be present. If intracardiac pressures are elevated, LV dysfunction is assumed to be present. Since intracardiac pressures are not consistent between patients, and since they do not always reflect preload accurately, they are used primarily when assessing the cause of a low blood flow state. Intracardiac pressures should not be used in isolation. If the intracardiac pressures are abnormal, but the SV or SI is normal, it may not be necessary to intervene. However, if the SV or SI is abnormal even in the presence of normal intracardiac pressures, intervention is necessary due to the potential threat to tissue oxygenation.

Many patients will present with borderline parameters. In order to safely and effectively assess low cardiac output situations, follow these guidelines:

- Examine SV first to identify if a problem exists. If SV and SI are abnormal, intervention is usually required.
- Use pressures to help guide SV interpretations. If the pressures are low in the presence of a low SV, hypovolemia is likely. If the pressures are high in the presence of a low SV, LV dysfunction is likely. If the SV is low and the filling pressures are normal, it is more likely that hypovolemia is present than LV dysfunction.
- Use Svo_2 levels to identify the significance or importance of any hemodynamic change.

Management of low cardiac output states begins by treating problems of either LV dysfunction or hypovolemia.

Left Ventricular Dysfunction

Low cardiac output states that are caused by left ventricular dysfunction are managed with a variety of therapies to decrease left ventricular work and improve performance: improvement of contractility, preload reduction, and afterload reduction. Generally, pharmacologic therapies are employed to treat the dysfunctional left ventricle. However, a few physical interventions are available, such as allowing the patient to sit up or attempting to reduce anxiety, as well as mechanical supports, such as intraaortic balloon pumping and ventricular assist devices (See Chapter 22, Advanced Cardiovascular Concepts). Improvement of LV function, however, is heavily reliant on pharmacologic support.

Improvement of Contractility

As a patient presents with symptoms of LV dysfunction, relief is obtained by improving left ventricular function. Inotropic therapy commonly is employed during an acute episode of LV dysfunction. Inotropic therapy increases the strength of the cardiac contraction, thereby increasing ejection fraction, SV, cardiac output, and tissue oxygenation.

Three common inotropic drugs are used in acute care to improve ventricular contractility: dobutamine (Dobutrex), dopamine, and amrinone (Inocor) (Table 5–10). Although other agents are used occasionally, by far the most common drug used in acute treatment is dobutamine. Dobutamine acts as a sympathetic stimulant, increasing the stimulation of beta cells of the sympathetic nervous system. This stimulation produces a positive inotropic (contractile) response, as well as a positive chronotropic (heart rate) response. Dobutamine also has a slight vasodilator effect due to B_2 stimulation, causing a slight reduction in preload and afterload. Based on these effects, dobutamine is an ideal first choice to pharmacologically increase the cardiac output and SV.

TABLE 5–10. COMMON INOTROPIC THERAPIES IN TREATING ABNORMAL HEMODYNAMICS

Drug	Dosage	Onset of Action	Route
Dobutamine (Dobutrex)	1–20 µg/kg/minute	1–2 minutes	IV
Dopamine (Intropin)	2–10 µg/kg/minute	1–2 minutes	IV
Amrinone (Inocor)	Loading 0.75 mg/kg, then 5–10 µg/kg/minute	<5 minutes	IV
Digoxin (normally not used in acute LV failure)	0.5 mg at first; then 0.25 every 6 hours until desired effect, then 0.125–0.25 mg/day	1–2 hours	IV

AT THE BEDSIDE
▶ *Inotropic Therapy*

A 71-year-old male is admitted to the ICU with hypotension of unknown origin. He presently has a fiberoptic pulmonary artery catheter in place to determine the origin of the hypotension. At 1800 hours, he is unresponsive with a Glasgow Coma Score of 4. His vital signs and pulmonary artery catheter reveal the following information:

BP	102/68
P	101/minute
CO	3.9 L/minute
CI	2.3 L/minute/m^2
SI	23
PA	42/22
PCWP	18 mm Hg
CVP	12 mm Hg
SvO$_2$	51%

Dobutamine is added to the patient's management regime. One hour after the dobutamine, a repeat set of hemodynamics reveals the following:

BP	104/66
P	106/minute
CO	4.4 L/minute
CI	2.6 L/minute/m^2
SI	25
PA	40/20
PCWP	14 mm Hg
CVP	13 mm Hg
SvO$_2$	57%

Based on the slight improvement in SI, CI, and SvO$_2$, as well as the decrease in PCWP, there has been a mild improvement in the hemodynamic parameters. Further increases of dobutamine should be considered since SvO$_2$ is not yet normal.

If dobutamine is not effective, amrinone may be used since its action is different from dobutamine. Dobutamine may not be effective in cases where sympathetic stimulation has already achieved its maximal impact. Amrinone is a phosphodiesterase inhibitor, increasing the availability of intracellular calcium. Although amrinone is associated with coagulopathic side effects, it is a logical alternative to dobutamine or dopamine.

Dopamine also can be used to improve the contractile state of the heart. Since dopamine also stimulates alpha cells of the sympathetic nervous system, afterload also will be increased, a situation which is not always desired in low cardiac output states. The net effect is an improvement in blood pressure and possibly cardiac output and SV, but the cost in terms of myocardial oxygen consumption is higher than with the other two inotropes. As such, dopamine is not a first-line drug to treat acute left ventricular dysfunction unless hypotension is present.

The potential negative effect of inotropic therapy is the increase in myocardial oxygen consumption which accompanies the increased contractile state. Unfortunately, it is not easy to measure myocardial oxygenation. Due to this potential problem, many clinicians prefer to use agents which either reduce preload or afterload, neither of which will increase myocardial oxygen consumption.

Preload Reduction in LV Dysfunction
Reduction of preload is thought to be beneficial in the patient with left ventricular dysfunction by decreasing the distention of overstretched myocardial muscle fibers. Many therapies have been designed for preload reduction, although they generally fall into one of two groups: drugs which reduce blood volume (diuretics) and those which promote vasodilation (nitrates, calcium channel blockers, beta blockers) (Table 5–11).

TABLE 5–11. COMMON PRELOAD REDUCERS FOR ABNORMAL HEMODYNAMICS

Diuretic Agents

Drug	Dose	Onset of Action	Route
Furosemide (Lasix)	20 mg or higher	<5 minutes	IV/PO
Bumetanide (Bumex)	0.5–10 mg/day	<5 minutes	IV/PO
Ethacrynic Acid (Edecrin)	50–100 mg/day	<5 minutes	IV/PO
Chlorothiazide (Diuril)	500–2000 mg/day	1–2 hours	IV/PO
Metolazone (Zaroxolyn)	2.5–20 mg/day	1 hour	PO
Mannitol	12.5–200 g/day	<5 minutes	IV
Vasodilating Agents			
Dopamine	1–2 µg/kg/minute	<5 minutes	IV
Nitroglycerine (Tridil, Nitrostat IV)	5–400 µg	1–2 minutes	IV

AT THE BEDSIDE
▶ *Preload Reduction*

A 77-year-old female is in the unit following an episode of angina which precipitated an episode of congestive heart failure. She has a pulmonary artery catheter in place which reveals her initial set of information. Also, she has a second set of hemodynamics which indicates her status following the initiation of nitroglycerine. Based on the data, was the nitroglycerine effective in improving her hemodynamics?

Initial Values		Postnitroglycerine Values
BP	114/76	112/72
P	106/minute	92/minute
CI	2.4 L/minute/m^2	2.6 L/minute/m^2
SI	23	28
PA	40/23	35/20
PCWP	22 mm Hg	17 mm Hg
CVP	12 mm Hg	9 mm Hg
Svo$_2$	56%	65%

Based on the increase in SI and Svo$_2$, as well as a decrease in PCWP, this therapy appears to have been effective. Even though the cardiac output did not change markedly, the increase was enough to improve tissue oxygenation. This example illustrates the need to evaluate more than one parameter (such as the PCWP).

The most common therapy to reduce preload is with diuretics. Diuretics are preferred since they attempt to eliminate the excess fluid buildup which has occurred as a renal compensatory mechanism for left ventricular dysfunction. As the left ventricle begins to fail, blood flow is decreased to the kidneys. This reduced blood flow is interpreted by the kidneys as insufficient blood volume. The kidneys then increase the reabsorption of water, producing an increase in intravascular volume. This increase contributes to venous engorgement and dependent edema in congestive heart failure.

The most common diuretics used to reduce preload are the loop diuretics. Loop diuretics work through their effect of blocking the reabsorption of sodium and water in the loop of Henle. The subsequent loss of sodium and water allows for a reduction in vascular volume. The reduction in vascular volume theoretically reduces the amount of blood returning to the heart and reduces the tension on myocardial muscle. The reduced tension allows the heart to return to a more normal contractile state.

Other preload reducers, such as nitroglycerine, act by promoting vasodilation. The result of vasodilation is to reduce the amount of blood returning to the heart. The net effect is to reduce preload and improve the left ventricular contractile state. In clinical practice, it is common to use either form of preload reduction or both. Preload reducers

such as nitroglycerine have the added benefit of improving myocardial blood flow. However, they do not eliminate the excess fluid which has accumulated due to left ventricular dysfunction.

Afterload Reduction in LV Dysfunction

Reduction of the resistance the heart faces to eject blood is the cornerstone of treating LV dysfunction on a long-term basis. Short-term reduction of afterload, such as one sees in the acutely ill patient with LV dysfunction, is important, but is used only after ensuring the presence of an adequate SV. When afterload reduction should be used in acute care is somewhat controversial. However, if the patient has a blood pressure or SVR which can be reduced to decrease afterload, the potential benefit is important. The benefit from reducing afterload is the reduction in left ventricular work and the subsequent improvement in LV contractile state and a reduced myocardial oxygen consumption.

AT THE BEDSIDE
▶ *High SVR*

A 73-year-old female is in the unit with the diagnosis of congestive heart failure. She presently is alert and oriented but complains of severe shortness of breath. Her pulse oximeter reveals a value of 89% on a fraction of inspired oxygen content (FIO$_2$) of 50% via a high-humidity face mask. She has crackles throughout both lungs and has 3+ pitting edema of both lower legs. She has a pulmonary artery catheter inserted to aid in the interpretation of the situation. The following data are available:

BP	202/114	SVR	2674
P	74/minute	PVR	191
RR	34/minute		
T	37.6°C		
CO	3.9 L/minute		
CI	1.8 L/minute/m^2		
SI	24		
PA	43/24		
PCWP	21 mm Hg		
CVP	13 mm Hg		
Svo$_2$	52%		

Based on this information, the best choice for management is an afterload reducer since the SVR and blood pressure are markedly elevated. A rapid-acting agent like nitroprusside would be preferable to achieve an immediate improvement in symptoms, SI, cardiac index, and Svo$_2$. Caution should be used when lowering the SVR and blood pressure to avoid too rapid a change. Patients who are used to elevated blood pressures can have a decrease in organ perfusion at higher pressures than the clinician might normally expect.

In an acutely ill patient with LV dysfunction, afterload reduction will be employed when the patient is hypertensive or has a high SVR. Generally, afterload reducers are used initially only if the blood pressure or high SVR is considered to be the cause of the LV dysfunction. Otherwise, afterload reducers are employed after inotropic therapy and preload reduction.

In acute management of an increased afterload, the most common afterload reducer is nitroprusside (Table 5–12). This arterial dilating agent works very fast (within 2 minutes) and has only a short-acting half-life (also about 2 minutes). The disadvantage of nitroprusside is that it breaks down into thiocyanate, a precursor to cyanide. Thiocyanate levels need to be monitored daily in patients on nitroprusside.

Other rapid afterload-reducing agents are available, including newer calcium channel and beta-blocking agents. Keep in mind that these agents might act as negative inotropes and actually weaken the heart. Their use in acute management of LV dysfunction is controversial, while their long-term use in managing congestive heart failure is well established.

Other common agents to reduce afterload are the angiotensin-converting enzyme (ACE) inhibitors. Generally, these drugs are used for the chronic management of afterload in an oral form, although some IV forms are available (enalapril). See Chapter 9, Critical Care, Pharmacology, for additional information on drug therapy.

Hypovolemia

If the underlying cause of the low cardiac output state is hypovolemia, two key approaches are used: preload augmentation and identification of the optimal type of preload agent. Identifying when to treat a patient who is potentially hypovolemic is greatly enhanced with hemodynamic monitoring. It is critical to use the guidelines previously outlined to avoid common errors in interpretation of hemodynamic monitoring data. For example, in the patient who is hypovolemic, the SV or SI will change when vascular volume has been significantly altered. This change in SV is frequently accompanied by reduced cardiac pressures (e.g., PCWP, CVP). However, the key parameter to monitor is SV. Keep in mind that cardiac pressures do not necessarily reflect changes in volume, due to ventricular compliance. In order to avoid errors in interpreting hypovolemia, always examine if a low SV is present before examining the cardiac pressures.

Perhaps one of the most controversial areas in the treatment of hypovolemia is the choice of the agent to use in improving vascular volume. There are three major categories of agents to be considered: blood, crystalloids, and colloids. Blood solutions such as packed cells or whole blood are in somewhat of a special category. They are not restricted to the patient who has a low SV, unlike the other categories. Blood is used when hemoglobin levels are less than 8 g/dl, frequently regardless of any other clinical sign. This approach is necessary due to the potential loss of oxygen delivery with the loss of hemoglobin.

AT THE BEDSIDE
▶ Hypovolemia

A 62-year-old male is in the unit with the diagnosis of ruptured diverticula. He presently is unresponsive and is being prepared for surgery. Breath sounds are clear, urine output is 20 ml in 9 hours, and his skin is cool and dry. A pulmonary artery catheter is inserted to aid in the interpretation of the situation. The following data are available:

BP	82/58
P	111/minute
RR	33/minute
T	38.4°C
CI	1.7 L/min/m^2
SI	15
PA	23/11
PCWP	7 mm Hg
CVP	2 mm Hg
Svo$_2$	53%

The most important parameters to treat are the low SI, CI, and Svo$_2$. A threat to tissue oxygenation clearly exists based on these parameters. Immediate supportive therapy would include a fluid bolus of normal saline or lactated Ringer's solution. Blood products (whole blood, albumin) or other colloids (hetastarch or pentastarch) could also be considered until the patient is taken to surgery.

Crystalloids are solutions such as normal saline and lactated Ringer's solution. They obtain their benefit primarily through the sodium in the solution. Sodium levels in crystalloid solutions are generally near blood levels (approximately 140 mEq). Colloids are solutions such as blood products (albumin) or synthetic solutions (hetastarch, a glucose polymer). Their fluid-retaining effect is due to the large molecules (protein or glucose polymers) in the solution.

There are several advantages of crystalloid solutions. They are inexpensive and they do not produce immunologic responses. The key clinical advantage is that they expand into all fluid compartments (vascular, interstitial, and intracellular) since most of the solution does not remain in just the vascular bed. For example, if 1000 ml of NS is given, less than 200 ml is believed to stay in the vascular bed. The rest diffuses into the other fluid compartments. This makes crystalloids ideal for treating patients who have chronic hypovolemia or dehydration. This advantage is also a limitation in some cases. If a rapid vascular expansion is required, it will take large volumes of crystalloids since most of the solution is not staying in the vascular system.

TABLE 5–12. COMMON AFTERLOAD REDUCING AGENTS

Drug	Dose	Onset of Action	Route
Smooth Muscle Relaxants and Alpha Inhibitors			
Nitroprusside (Nipride)	0.5–10 µg/kg/minute	1–2 minutes	IV
Nitroglycerine (Tridil, Nitrostat IV)	5–400 µg	1–2 minutes	IV
Diazoxide (Hyperstat IV)	50–150 mg	1–2 minutes	IV
Hydralazine (Apresoline)	10–40 mg	10–20 minutes	IV/IM
Methyldopa (Aldomet)	250 mg–1 g	2 hours	IV
Trimethaphan (Arfonad)	3–6 mg/min	1–2 minutes	IV
Phentolamine (Regitine)	0.1–2 mg/min	<1 minute	IV
Angiotension-Converting Enzyme Inhibitors			
Captopril (Capoten)	25–400 mg/day in 2–3 doses	15–30 minutes	PO
Enalapril/Enalaprilat (Vasotec/Vasotec IV)	2.5–4.0 mg/day	15 minutes	PO/IV
Lisinopril (Zestril)	10–40 mg/day	1 hour	PO

Colloids have one key advantage over crystalloids in that they rapidly expand the vascular volume. Virtually all the colloid solution infused will remain in the vascular bed, at least initially. This allows for a much more rapid treatment of hypovolemia, frequently necessary in conditions such as trauma and postoperative bleeding. One disadvantage to colloids is their expense. Controversy does exist, however, about whether colloids are any more effective than crystalloids. Concerns have been raised that colloids may potentially cause harm in conditions with capillary leak syndromes [(e.g., sepsis and adult respiratory distress syndrome (ARDS)]. In these conditions, the leakage of fluid through damaged capillaries is exacerbated if large proteins (or glucose polymers) leak through the capillaries since they will pull large amounts of fluid along with them.

While crystalloids appear to be generally as effective as colloids, the best agent is still controversial. Each has its own benefits and limitations. Regardless of which is to be used, its effect should be measured on how well it improves tissue oxygenation, SV, SI, and intracardiac pressures.

High Cardiac Output States

Cardiac output values can be elevated as well as lowered. In normal people, cardiac outputs elevate secondary to increased oxygen demand (e.g., exercise) or psychological stimulation (fear, anxiety). In clinical practice, three reasons exist for an increased cardiac output: response to a systemic inflammation (e.g., sepsis, systemic inflammatory response syndrome), hepatic disease, or neurogenic mediated vasodilation. The most common reason for the cardiac output to elevate is systemic inflammation. Inflammation, which is common in conditions such as sepsis, causes systemic vascular resistance to decrease. This decrease in resistance produces a compensatory increase in cardiac output. The increase in cardiac output might be minimal or marked. The key point to remember is that the cardiac output elevation is a symptom of a problem rather than the problem. If the problem is treated, the cardiac output will return to normal.

AT THE BEDSIDE
▶ *Low SVR*

A 65-year-old male is in the unit after developing hypotension on the floor. He had femoral-popliteal bypass surgery 4 days earlier and was doing well until yesterday. He began to complain of generalized malaise with the following vital signs:

BP	122/78	RR	27/minute
P	110/minute	T	38.1°C

His wound site is reddened but has no drainage. This morning, he was less oriented and was hypotensive (BP 88/54, P 114/minute), prompting a transfer to the unit. He does not complain of any discomfort or shortness of breath. His lung sounds are clear and he has a pulse oximeter value of 99%. A flow-directed pulmonary artery catheter is inserted to assist in the assessment of the cause of hypotension. The following data are available from the pulmonary artery catheter:

CO	10.5 L/minute	SVR	475
CI	6.0 L/minute/m²	PVR	51
PA	22/11	CVP	2 mm Hg
PCWP	8 mm Hg	SvO₂	84%

Based on the above information, a systemic inflammation appears to be developing, producing a low SVR. In addition, the vasodilation is also producing low cardiac pressures. The most likely immediate therapies are fluid therapies (normal saline or lactated Ringer's solution) and perhaps vasopressors (norepinephrine or dopamine). Obviously, none of these therapies is curative and a more definitive therapy (such as appropriate antibiotics) needs to be applied.

When a patient has high cardiac outputs in sepsis, it does not mean the heart is functioning normally. Because of the release of myocardial depressant factors, the ejection fraction normally is depressed in sepsis. The method by which the SV is maintained is through an increase in end diastolic volume. This increase in EDV allows SV to be maintained even though ejection fractions are reduced.

If the hemodynamic problem appears to be a low SVR, initial treatment centers on increasing afterload (SVR), augmenting preload, and administration of inotropic therapy. None of these therapies for managing low SVR states is curative, and the underlying cause of the low SVR (such as infection) must be corrected. The following section only addresses the management of low SVR states, since preload and inotropic therapy have been previously discussed.

Increasing the afterload/SVR is usually accomplished by administering an alpha-stimulating drug. Three common agents used for this purpose: norepinephrine (Levophed), dopamine (Intropin) and phenylephrine (Neo-synephrine). Norepinephrine and dopamine have a combination of alpha and beta stimulation, producing both vasoconstriction and increased cardiac stimulation (inotropic and chronotropic responses). This makes the heart beat both stronger and faster. These two agents have a greater likelihood of increasing blood pressure and SVR due to this combined cardiac and vascular effect. Phenylephrine is only an alpha stimulant, which has some advantages. Since it only causes alpha stimulation, there is less direct effect on the heart. Although the SVR and blood pressure might not be increased as quickly with phenylephrine, it does avoid some of the direct increase of myocardial oxygen consumption that is seen with norepinephrine and dopamine. Clinically, any of these agents could be used to increase the SVR. Since they are strong alpha stimulants, their use should be considered with a degree of caution.

Direct alpha stimulants can cause severe vasoconstriction. These agents are so strong that if they infiltrate into normal tissue, the resulting vasoconstriction might cause local tissue death. As a precaution, these drugs are only given in large, central veins. From an assessment perspective, if these drugs are effective, the SVR should increase as well as the blood pressure. However, it is critical to remember that with these drugs the clinician must assess tissue oxygenation as well as SVR and blood pressure. If the SVR or blood pressure increases, parameters such as SvO_2 must also increase to indicate tissue oxygenation is also improving. SVR and BP do not always directly correlate with blood flow, which makes the addition of tissue oxygenation parameters (like SvO_2) an essential part of assessing the effect of vasopressors like norepinephrine, dopamine, and phenylephrine.

Fluid administration with crystalloids (or colloids) is common since the low SVR produces a pseudohypovolemia from vasodilation. Fluid administration is given to the same end points as in the case of the patient with hypovolemia.

Inotropic therapy can be given to try to increase cardiac output and oxygen delivery. Administration of inotropic therapy might seem unusual in a patient with a high cardiac output. However, some investigators believe that oxygen delivery needs to be increased to supranormal levels in order to help improve patient outcome. Supranormal oxygen delivery can be achieved by such methods as fluid administration and inotropic therapy. Whether this concept is valid or not has not been clarified in the literature.

One of the reasons for suspecting that supranormal amounts of oxygen are required is the microcapillary shunting and dysoxia which occurs in low SVR states like sepsis (Figure 5–29). The result is tissue hypoxia. SvO_2 levels are paradoxically high, reflecting the regional maldistribution

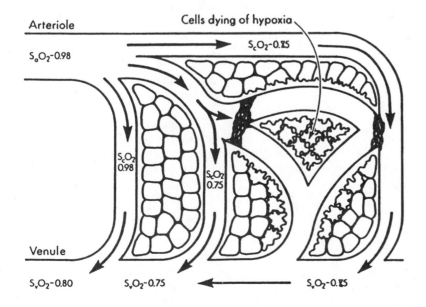

Figure 5–29. Microcapillary shunting due to obstruction at the capillary level. *(From: Ahrens TS, Rutherford KA: Essentials of oxygenation. Boston: Jones & Bartlett, 1993, p. 108.)*

of blood flow. Due to a lack of blood flow to some regions, oxygen delivery is forced to supranormal levels in an attempt to force oxygen into these threatened areas.

Whether this therapy is effective is still being investigated. If the problem is simply microcapillary shunting, increasing oxygen delivery might be sufficient. However, if the problem is cellular dysoxia or an inability to effectively use oxygen, then increased oxygen delivery alone is unlikely to be helpful.

SELECTED BIBLIOGRAPHY

Hemodynamic Monitoring

Ahrens TS: Effect of mechanical ventilation on hemodynamic waveform recognition. *Critical Care Nursing Clinics of North America.* 1991;3:629–639.

Ahrens TS: Airway pressure measurement as an aid in hemodynamic waveform interpretation. *Critical Care Nurse.* 1992;12:44–48.

Ahrens TS: *Hemodynamic waveform recognition.* Philadelphia: WB Saunders, 1993.

Ahrens TS, Taylor L: *Hemodynamic waveform analysis.* Philadelphia: WB Saunders, 1992.

Booker KJ, Arnold JS: Respiratory induced changes on the pulmonary capillary wedge pressure tracing. *Critical Care Nurse.* 1993;13:80–88.

Bridges EJ, Woods SL: Pulmonary artery pressure measurement: State of the art. *Heart and Lung.* 1993;22:99–111.

Daily EK, Schroeder JS: *Techniques in bedside hemodynamic monitoring.* St. Louis, MO: Mosby-Year Book, 1989.

Doering LV: The effect of positioning on hemodynamics and gas exchange in the critically ill: A review. *American Journal of Critical Care.* 1993;2:208–216.

Iberti TJ, Daily EK, Leibowitz AB, Schecter CB, Silverstein JH, Fischer EP. Assessment of critical care nurses' knowledge of the pulmonary artery catheter. The pulmonary artery catheter study group. *Critical Care Medicine.* 1994;22:1674–1678.

Iberti TJ, Fischer EP, Leibowitz AB, Panacek EA, Silverstein JH, Albertson TE: A multicenter study of physicians' knowledge of the pulmonary artery catheter. *Journal of the American Medical Association.* 1990;264:2928–2932.

Kee LL, Simonson JS, Stotts NA, Skov P, Schiller NB: Echocardiographic determination of valid zero reference levels in supine and lateral positions. *American Journal of Critical Care.* 1993;2:72–80.

Potger KC, Elliott D: Reproducibility of central venous pressures in supine and lateral positions. A pilot evaluation of the phlebostatic axis in critically ill patients. *Heart and Lung.* 1994;23:285–299.

Quaal SJ: Quality assurance in hemodynamic monitoring. *AACN Clinical Issues in Critical Care Nursing.* 1993;4:197–206.

Wadas TM: Pulmonary artery catheter removal. *Critical Care Nurse.* 1994;14:63–72.

Woods SL, Osguthorpe S: Cardiac output determination. *AACN Clinical Issues in Critical Care Nursing.* 1993;4:81–94.

Management of Pathological Conditions

Chanatry BJ, Gettinger A: Transfusion therapy in the critically ill patient. *International Anesthesiology Clinics.* 1993;31:73–95.

Chatterjee K, Whofe CL, DeMarco T: Nonglycoside inotropes in congestive heart failure. Are they beneficial or harmful? *Cardiology Clinics.* 1994;12:63–72.

Dahlof B: Angiotensin-converting enzyme inhibitors and effects on left ventricular hypertrophy. *Blood Pressure.* 1994;2(Suppl):35–40.

Elkayam U: Nitrates in heart failure. *Cardiology Clinics.* 1994;12:73–85.

Griffel MI, Kaufman BS: Pharmacology of colloids and crystalloids. *Critical Care Clinics.* 1992;8:235–253.

Hauser CJ, Shoemaker WC, Turpin I, et al: Oxygen transport responses to colloids and crystalloids in critically ill surgical patients. *Surgery, Gynecology, and Obstetrics.* 1980;150:811.

Greenberg B. Role of vasodilator therapy in congestive heart failure. *Cardiology Clinics.* 1994;12:87–99.

Kaminski MV, Haase TJ: Albumin and colloid osmotic pressure implications for fluid resuscitation. *Critical Care Clinics.* 1992;8:311–321.

Klaus D: The role of calcium antagonists in the treatment of hypertension. *Journal of Cardiovascular Pharmacology.* 1992;20(Suppl):S5–S14.

Lindeborg DM, Pearl RG: Inotropic therapy in the critically ill patient. *International Anesthesiology Clinics.* 1993;31:49–71.

McGhie AI, Golstein RA: Pathogenesis and management of acute heart failure and cardiogenic shock: Role of inotropic therapy. *Chest.* 1993;102:626S–632S.

Reyes AJ: Loop diuretics versus others in the treatment of congestive heart failure after myocardial infarction. *Cardiovascular Drugs and Therapy.* 1993;7:869–876.

Shoemaker WC, Appel PL, Kram HB: Oxygen transport measurements to evaluate tissue perfusion and titrate therapy: Dobutamine and dopamine effects. *Critical Care Medicine.* 1991;19:672–688.

Steltzer H, Hiesmayr M, Mayer N, Krafft P, Hammerle AF: The relationship between oxygen delivery and uptake in the critically ill: Is there a critical or optimal therapeutic value? A meta-analysis. *Anesthesia.* 1994;49:229–236.

Wagner BKJ, D'Amelio LF: Pharmacologic and clinical considerations in selecting crystalloid, colloid, and oxygen carrying resuscitation fluids, part 2. *Clinical Pharmacy.* 1993;12:415–427.

Airway and Ventilatory Management

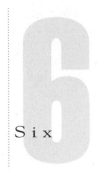

Six

► Knowledge Competencies

1. Interpret normal and abnormal arterial blood gas results and common management strategies for treatment.

2. Identify indications, complications, and management strategies for artificial airways, oxygen delivery, and monitoring devices.

3. Identify indications, principles of operation, complications, and management strategies for mechanical ventilation.

■ *What Heals: Reducing Noise Levels*

Florence Nightingale believed that the quality of the patient's environment could influence healing and recovery. Recent research investigating the effects of noise on physiologic, psychologic, and behavioral outcomes supports Nightingale's early suspicions.

Noise level in most critical care units is above Environmental Protection Agency (EPA) recommendations. Noise levels distress patients because critically ill patients have been found to have a lower threshold of tolerable sound. The physiologic effects of noise can include increased levels of adrenocorticosteroids, epinephrine, and norepinephrine; peripheral vasoconstriction; heart rate changes and dysrhythmias; elevated cerebral blood flow; increased skeletal muscle tension; and higher cholesterol levels. Exposure to noise has also been found to reduce pain thresholds and produce irritability, anxiety, sleep loss, emotional liability, and "ICU psychosis."

Despite EPA recommendations that were established in 1974, the structural, mechanical, and personnel noise levels in critical care units continue to be a problem. Although structural and acoustical factors have been altered in critical care units to reduce and deaden noise (e.g., carpets and draperies), it does not appear that we have made much progress in reducing noise generated from equipment. What can we do about mechanical noise? We can offer patients earplugs. We can turn off equipment when not in use or not needed and silence alarms when we suspect we will trigger them. Equipment such as IV pumps can be placed as far from the head of the bed as possible. Backs of ventilators can be turned away from patients.

We also need to work creatively with our bioengineering departments to insulate patients from mechanical noise. We need to establish a louder voice in transmitting this problem to the designers and manufacturers of new technology. When we evaluate new equipment for purchase, we can include the level of mechanical noise as one of our criteria for equipment selection. In addition, we can refuse to purchase new equipment that is overly noisy.

Even more striking, however, in the more than 20 years since the EPA has established environmental noise recommendations, is that we have done very little to reduce people-generated noise. It may be that some mechanical noise is an inherent reality in most critical care units. People-generated noise, however, need not be viewed with this same level of resignation. Where we talk and how loud we do it is a variable that can be changed. We can limit loud talk, close doors when suctioning patients, and make patient assignments in the conference room, with the doors closed. We can provide patients with distractors (e.g., radios with headsets, television, family visitation, reading). We can use signs to remind staff to control noise. Every critical care unit needs to formulate, follow, and reinforce guidelines and procedures to reduce people-generated noise to an acceptable day level and a lower acceptable night level.

There are also interventions, based on scientific studies, that can be used to alter human responses to environmental noise. Use of various alternative therapies can be implemented to induce relaxation, reverse the stress response, and enhance psychophysiologic measures of recovery. These alternative therapies can be used independently by the nurse and include such modalities as biofeedback, breathing and muscle relaxation techniques, music therapy exercises, and imagery, to name only a few. Patients who demonstrate high levels of stress seem to be highly responsive to these kinds of interventions. Thus, even if it is not possible to eliminate all of the environmental factors that produce noise, perhaps it is possible to change the patient's perception of them.

CEG & BMD

Adapted from: Guzzetta CE: Comments. Capsules & Comments in Critical Care Nursing. *1993;1:67–68.*

RESPIRATORY ASSESSMENT TECHNIQUES, DIAGNOSTIC TESTS, AND MONITORING SYSTEMS

Arterial Blood Gas Monitoring

Arterial blood gas (ABG) monitoring is frequently performed in critically ill patients to assess acid-base balance, ventilation, and oxygenation. An arterial blood sample is analyzed for oxygen tension (PaO_2), carbon dioxide tension ($PaCO_2$), and pH using a blood gas analyzer. From these measurements, several other parameters are calculated by the blood gas analyzer, including base excess, bicarbonate (HCO_3^-), and oxygen saturation (SaO_2). Arterial SaO_2 can be directly measured if a co-oximeter device is available on the ABG analyzer. Normal ABG values analysis are listed in Table 6–1.

ABG samples are obtained by direct puncture of an artery, usually the radial artery, or by withdrawing blood through an indwelling arterial catheter system. A heparinized syringe is used to collect the sample to prevent clotting of the blood prior to analysis. Blood gas samples are kept on ice until analyzed to prevent the continued transfer of CO_2 and O_2 in and out of the red blood cells. Arterial blood gas analysis equipment is often kept in or near the critical care unit to maximize accuracy and decrease the time for reporting of results. Regardless of the

TABLE 6–1. LABORATORY AND CALCULATED RESPIRATORY VALUES

Parameter	Value
Arterial Blood Gases	
pH	7.35 to 7.45
$PaCO_2$	35 to 45 mm Hg
HCO_3^-	22 to 26 mEq/L
Base Excess	-2 to $+2$ mEq/L
PaO_2	70 to 95 mm Hg (normals vary with age and altitude)
SaO_2	>95% (normals vary with age and altitude)
Venous Blood Gases	
pH	7.33 to 7.43
$PvCO_2$	35 to 45 mm Hg
PvO_2	35 to 40 mm Hg
SaO_2	70% to 80%
Respiratory Parameters	
Tidal volume (TV)	6 to 8 ml/kg
Respiratory rate	8 to 16/minute
Respiratory static compliance	70 to 100 ml/cm H_2O
Inspiratory force (IF)	>—20 cm H_2O
Respiratory Calculations	
Alveolar gas equation (PaO_2)	$PaO_2 = \dfrac{FiO_2(P_{ATM} - P_{H_2O}) - PaCO_2}{\text{Respiratory quotient (RQ)}}$
Static compliance	$\dfrac{TV}{(\text{Plateau pressure} - PEEP)}$

method used to obtain the ABG sample, practitioners should wear gloves to prevent exposure to blood during the sampling procedure.

New indwelling devices are available for the continuous monitoring of ABG values by insertion of special probes into arterial catheters. These probes are then connected to a bedside analysis machine which continuously displays ABG values. These devices are rarely used in critical care units at this time because of their cost.

Technique for Sampling

Indwelling Arterial Catheter

All the pressure monitoring systems which are used with indwelling arterial catheters have sites where samples of

arterial blood can be withdrawn for ABG analysis or other laboratory testing (Figure 6–1). Using the stopcock closest to the catheter insertion site, or the indwelling syringe or reservoir of the needleless systems, a 3- to 5-ml sample of blood is withdrawn to clear the catheter system of any flush system fluid. A 1-ml sample for ABG analysis is then obtained in a heparinized syringe. Any air remaining in the syringe is then removed, an airtight cap is placed on the end of the syringe, and the sample is placed on ice to ensure accuracy of the measurement. The arterial catheter system is then flushed to clear the line of any residual blood.

Complications associated with this technique for obtaining ABG samples include infection and hemorrhage. Any time an invasive system is used, the potential exists for contamination of the sterile system. The use of needleless

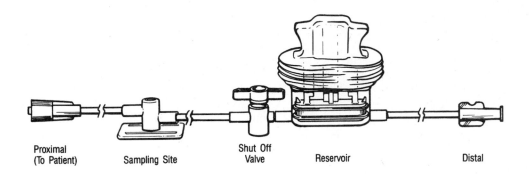

Proximal
(To Patient)   Sampling Site   Shut Off Valve   Reservoir   Distal

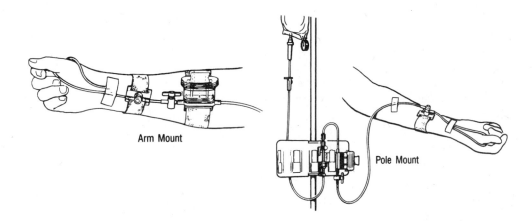

Arm Mount   Pole Mount

A

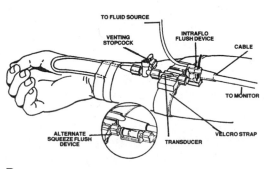

B

Figure 6–1. Examples of indwelling arterial catheter systems for blood gas analysis. (A) Closed blood withdrawal system. (B) Open blood withdrawal system. *(Courtesy of: Baxter Edwards Laboratories [A], and Abbott Critical Care Systems, North Chicago, IL [B].)*

systems on indwelling catheter systems decreases patients' risk for infection, as well as the critical care practitioners' risk for accidental needlestick injuries, and should be used whenever feasible. Hemorrhage is a rare complication, occurring when stopcocks are inadvertently left in the wrong position after blood withdrawal. This latter complication can be avoided by carefully following the proper technique during blood sampling, limiting sample withdrawal to experienced critical care practitioners, and keeping the pressure alarm system of the bedside monitoring system activated at all times.

Arterial Puncture

Occasionally, when indwelling arterial catheters are not in place, ABG samples are obtained by directly puncturing the artery with a needle and syringe. The most common sites for arterial puncture are the radial, brachial, and femoral arteries. Similar to venipuncture, the technique for obtaining an ABG sample is relatively simple, but success in obtaining the sample requires ongoing experience.

Following location of the pulsating artery and antiseptic preparation of the skin, the needle is inserted into the artery at a 45° angle with the bevel facing upward. The needle is slowly advanced until arterial blood appears in the syringe barrel or the insertion depth is below the artery location. If blood is not obtained, the needle should be pulled back to just below the skin and relocation of the pulsating artery verified prior to advancing the needle again.

As soon as the 1-ml sample of arterial blood is obtained, the syringe should be withdrawn and firm pressure quickly applied to the insertion site with a sterile gauze pad. Hand held pressure should be maintained for 5 minutes and the site inspected for bleeding or oozing of blood. If present, pressure should be reapplied until all evidence of oozing of blood at the site has stopped. Pressure dressings should not be applied if hemostasis has not been achieved.

As described above, all air must be removed from the ABG syringe and an airtight cap applied to the end (remove the needle first). Given the importance of maintaining pressure at the puncture site, it is best to have another practitioner assisting during arterial puncture to ensure appropriate handling of the blood sample.

Complications associated with arterial puncture include arterial vessel tears, air embolism, hemorrhage, arterial obstruction, loss of extremity, and infection. The incidence of these complications can be dramatically decreased by using proper technique during sampling. Damage to the artery can be decreased by the use of as small a diameter needle (21 gauge in adults) as practical and avoidance of multiple attempts at arterial puncture at the same site. After one or two failed attempts at entering the artery, a different site should be selected or a more experienced practitioner should attempt the ABG sampling.

Hemorrhage can occur easily into the surrounding tissues if adequate hemostasis is not achieved with pressure.

Bleeding into the tissue can range from small blood loss with minimal local damage to large blood loss with loss of distal circulation and even exsanguination. Large blood loss is more commonly seen with femoral punctures and is caused by the difficulty of achieving adequate pressure on the artery following needle removal. Bleeding from the femoral artery is difficult to visualize, so significant blood loss can occur before practitioners are alerted to problems. For this reason, the femoral site is the least preferred for ABG sampling and is used only when other sites are not accessible.

The need for frequent ABG sampling for ventilation and oxygenation assessment and management may require the insertion of an arterial catheter and monitoring system to decrease the risks associated with repetitive arterial punctures.

Analysis of Arterial Blood Gases

The approach to analyzing the results of ABG analysis should be a systematic one. Analysis of results is broken into two phases: analysis of acid base status and oxygenation status. Upon receipt of ABG results, the practitioner should first identify which are normal and abnormal values (Table 6–1), followed by acid base and oxygenation status analysis.

Acid-Base Analysis

Optimal cellular functioning occurs when the pH of the blood is between 7.35 and 7.45. Decreases in pH below 7.35 are termed *acidemia,* and increases in pH above 7.45 are termed *alkalemia.* When the amount of acids or bases in the body increases or decreases, the pH changes if the ratio of acids to bases is altered. For example, if acid production increases twofold, and there is no change in the amount of base production, the pH will decrease. If the base production were to increase twofold as well, then no change in pH would occur because the ratio of acids to bases was maintained. Since the body functions best at a pH in the 7.35 to 7.45 range, there are strong systems in place to maintain the balance between acids and bases, even if one of those components is functioning abnormally. Although a variety of regulatory systems are involved in acid-base balance, the bicarbonate (HCO_3^-) and carbon dioxide (CO_2) levels are the primary regulators of acid-base balance.

Metabolic Component

HCO_3^- levels are controlled primarily by the kidneys and have been termed the *metabolic component* of the acid-base system. By increasing or decreasing the amount of HCO_3^- excreted in the kidneys, the pH of the blood can be increased or decreased. Changes in HCO_3^- excretion may take up to 24 hours to accomplish, but can be maintained for prolonged periods of time.

TABLE 6–2. ACID-BASE ABNORMALITIES

Acid-Base Abnormality	Primary ABG Abnormalities			ABG Changes with Compensation (if present)	
	pH	$Paco_2$	HCO_3^-	Respiratory ($Paco_2$)	Metabolic (HCO_3^-)
Alkalemia					
Metabolic	↑		↑	↑	
Respiratory	↑	↓			↓
Acidemia					
Metabolic	↓		↓	↓	
Respiratory	↓	↑			↑

Respiratory Component

CO_2 levels are controlled primarily by the lungs and are termed the *respiratory component* of the acid-base system. By increasing or decreasing the amount of CO_2 excreted by the lungs, the pH of the blood can be increased or decreased. Changes in CO_2 excretion can occur rapidly, within a minute, by increasing or decreasing respiration (minute ventilation). Respiratory system changes, however, are difficult to maintain over long periods of time (>24 hours).

Acid-Base Abnormalities

A variety of intrinsic and extrinsic acid-base abnormalities can occur to cause a critical illness or as a result of critical illnesses (Tables 6–2 and 6–3).

Metabolic alkalemia occurs when the pH is >7.45 and the HCO_3^- is >26 mEq/L. In metabolic alkalemia there is inadequate excretion of HCO_3^- from the body by the kidneys. The respiratory system will attempt to compensate for the increased pH by decreasing the amount of CO_2 eliminated from the body (hypoventilation). This compensatory attempt by the respiratory system will result in some change in pH, but return to normal pH values is unlikely. Clinical situations or conditions which cause metabolic alkalemia include loss of body acids (nasogastric suction of HCl, vomiting, excessive diuretic therapy, steroids, hypokalemia) and ingestion of exogenous bicarbonate or citrate substances.

Management of metabolic alkalemia is directed at treating the underlying cause, decreasing or stopping the acid loss (e.g., use of antiemetic therapy for vomiting), or replacing lost acid in extreme states of alkalemia.

Metabolic acidemia occurs when the pH is <7.35 and the HCO_3^- is <22 mEq/L. In metabolic acidemia there is excessive excretion of HCO_3^- from the body by the kidneys. The respiratory system will attempt to compensate for the decreased pH by increasing the amount of CO_2 eliminated from the body (hyperventilation). This compensatory attempt by the respiratory system will result in some change in pH, but return to normal pH values is unlikely. Clinical situations or conditions which cause metabolic acidemia include increased metabolic formation of acids (diabetic ketoacidosis, uremic acidosis, lactic acidosis), loss of bicarbonate (diarrhea, renal tubular acidosis), hyperkalemia, toxins (salicylates overdose, ethylene glycol, methanol, paraldehyde), and adrenal insufficiency. Management of metabolic acidemia is directed at treating the underlying cause, decreasing acid formation (e.g., decreasing lactic acid production by improving cardiac output in shock), decreasing bicarbonate losses (e.g., treatment of diarrhea), removal of toxins through dialysis or cathartics, or administering $NaHCO_3$ in extreme metabolic acidemia states.

Respiratory alkalemia occurs when the pH is >7.45 and the $Paco_2$ is <35 mm Hg. In respiratory alkalemia there is an excessive amount of ventilation and removal of CO_2 from the body. If these ABG changes persist for 24 hours or more, the kidneys will attempt to compensate for the elevated pH by increasing the excretion of HCO_3^- until normal or near normal pH levels occur. Clinical situations or conditions which cause respiratory alkalemia include neurogenic hyperventilation, interstitial lung diseases, pulmonary embolism, asthma, acute anxiety/stress/fear, hyperventilation syndromes, excessive mechanical ventilation, and severe hypoxemia. Management of respiratory alkalemia is directed at treating the underlying cause and decreasing excessive ventilation if possible.

Respiratory acidemia occurs when the pH is <7.35 and the $Paco_2$ is >45 mm Hg. In respiratory acidemia there is an inadequate amount of ventilation (hypoventilation) and

TABLE 6–3. EXAMPLES OF ARTERIAL BLOOD GAS RESULTS

ABG Analysis	pH	$Paco_2$ (mm Hg)	HCO_3^- (mEq/L)	Base Excess	Pao_2 (mm Hg)	Sao_2
Normal ABG	7.37	38	24	−1	85	96%
Respiratory acidemia, no compensation, with hypoxemia	7.28	51	25	−1	63	89%
Metabolic acidemia, no compensation, normal oxygenation	7.23	33	14	−12	92	97%
Metabolic alkalemia, partial compensation, normal oxygenation	7.49	48	37	+11	84	95%
Respiratory acidemia, full compensation, with hypoxemia	7.35	59	33	+6	55	86%
Respiratory alkalosis, no compensation, with hypoxemia	7.52	31	24	0	60	88%
Metabolic acidemia, partial compensation, with hypoxemia	7.30	29	16	−9	54	85%
Laboratory error	7.31	32	28	0	92	96%

removal of CO_2 from the body. If these ABG changes persist for 24 hours or more, the kidneys will attempt to compensate for the decreased pH by increasing the amount of HCO_3^- in the body (decreased excretion of HCO_3^- in the urine) until normal or near normal pH levels occur. Clinical situations or conditions which cause respiratory acidemia include overall hypoventilation associated with respiratory failure [e.g., adult respiratory distress syndrome (ARDS), pneumonia, chronic pulmonary diseases], pulmonary embolism, cardiac failure, respiratory center depression and neuromuscular disturbances in the presence of normal lungs, and inadequate mechanical ventilation. Management of respiratory acidemia is directed at treating the underlying cause and improving ventilation.

Mixed (combined) disturbance is the simultaneous development of a primary respiratory and metabolic acid-base disturbance. For example, metabolic acidosis may occur from diabetic ketoacidosis, with respiratory acidosis occurring from respiratory failure associated with aspiration pneumonia. Mixed acid-base disturbances create a more complex picture when examining ABGs and are beyond the scope of this text.

Oxygenation

After determining the acid-base status from the ABG, assessment of the adequacy of oxygenation should occur. Normal values for PaO_2 are dependent on age and altitude. Lower levels of PaO_2 are acceptable as normal with increasing age and altitude levels. In general, PaO_2 levels between 75 and 95 mm Hg are considered normal.

SaO_2 levels are also affected by age and altitude, with values >95% considered normal. Hemoglobin saturation

with oxygen is primarily influenced by the level of PaO_2 (Figure 6–2). The S shape to the oxyhemoglobin curve emphasizes that as long as PaO_2 levels are >60 mm Hg, 90% or more of the hemoglobin is saturated with O_2. Factors which can shift the oxyhemoglobin curve to the right and left include temperature, pH, $PaCO_2$, and abnormal hemoglobin conditions. In general, shifting the curve to the right decreases the affinity of oxygen for hemoglobin, resulting in an increase in the amount of oxygen released to the tissues. Shifting of the curve to the left increases the affinity of oxygen for hemoglobin, resulting in a decreased amount of oxygen released to the tissues.

A decrease in PaO_2 below normal values is termed *hypoxemia*. A variety of conditions cause hypoxemia:

- *Altitude.*
- *Overall hypoventilation.* Decreases in tidal volume, respiratory rate, or both will reduce minute ventilation and cause hypoventilation. Alveoli are underventilated, leading to a fall in alveolar oxygen tension (PaO_2) and decreased PaO_2 levels. Causes of hypoventilation include respiratory center depression from drug overdose, anesthesia, excessive analgesic administration, neuromuscular disturbances, and fatigue.
- *Ventilation-perfusion mismatch.* When the balance between adequately ventilated and perfused alveoli is altered, hypoxemia develops. Perfusion of blood past underventilated alveoli decreases the availability of oxygen for gas exchange, leading to poorly oxygenated blood in the pulmonary vasculature. Examples of this include bronchospasm, atelectasis, secretion retention, pneumonia, and pulmonary edema.
- *Diffusion defect.* Thickening of the alveolar-capillary membrane decreases oxygen diffusion and leads to hypoxemia. Causes of diffusion defects are chronic disease states such as fibrosis and sarcoidosis.
- *Shunt.* When blood bypasses or shunts past the alveoli, gas exchange cannot occur and blood returns to the left side without oxygenation. Shunts that are due to anatomic origins include pulmonary arteriovenous fistulas or cardiac anomalies, such as tetralogy of Fallot. Physiologic shunts are due to a variety of conditions where blood is not allowed contact with ventilated alveoli, such as lobar atelectasis.

Venous Blood Gas Monitoring

Analysis of oxygen and carbon dioxide levels in the venous blood provides additional information about the adequacy of perfusion and oxygen use by the tissues. Venous blood gas analysis, also referred to as a mixed venous blood gas sample, is done in the same manner as an ABG analysis, but with a venous blood sample. The venous sample can be obtained from the distal tip of a pulmonary artery (PA)

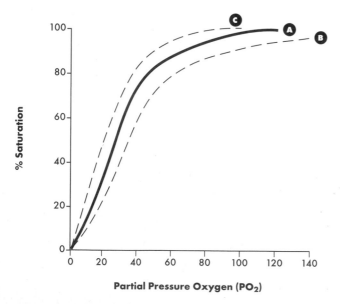

Figure 6–2. Oxyhemoglobin dissociation curve. (A) Normal. (B) Shift to the right. (C) Shift to the left.

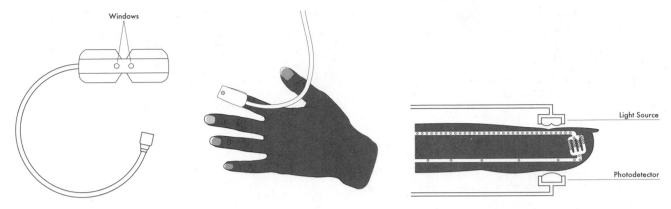

Figure 6–3. Pulse oximeter. (A) Sensor. (B) Schematic of sensor operation on finger.

catheter or from a central venous pressure (CVP) catheter. If the distal tip of the PA catheter is used, withdrawal of the blood should be done slowly over a 20-second period to avoid arterialization of the pulmonary artery blood. This approach is not important when sampling through a CVP catheter. Normal values for venous blood gas values are listed in Table 6–1.

Pulse Oximetry

Pulse oximetry is a common method for the continuous, noninvasive monitoring of SaO_2. A sensor is applied to skin over areas with high blood flow, typically one of the fingers or the bridge of the nose or ear, and is connected to a microprocessing unit (Figure 6–3). Light-emitting diodes on one side of the sensor transmit light of two different wavelengths (infrared and red) through arterial blood flowing under the sensor. Depending on the level of oxygen saturation of hemoglobin in the arterial blood, different amounts of light are detected on the other side of the sensor. This photodetection aspect of the sensor transmits information to the microprocessor for calculation and digital display of the oxygen saturation.

When blood perfusion to the sensor is adequate and SaO_2 levels are greater than 70%, there is a close correlation between the noninvasive SaO_2 from the pulse oximeter and SaO_2 directly measured from arterial blood gases. In situations where perfusion to the sensor is diminished (e.g., shock, hypoperfusion), the accuracy of pulse oximetry may be less than under normal perfusion conditions.

Pulse oximetry has several advantages for respiratory monitoring. The ability to have continuous information on the SaO_2 level of critically ill patients without the use of invasive devices decreases infection risks and blood loss from frequent ABG analysis. In addition, these monitors are easy to use, well tolerated by most patients, and portable enough to use during transport situations.

The major disadvantage of pulse oximeters for assessing oxygen status is that accuracy depends on adequate arterial blood flow beneath the sensor. Clinical situations that decrease the accuracy of the device include:

- Hypotension
- Low cardiac output states
- Vasoconstriction or vasoactive drugs
- Hypothermia
- Movement of the sensor and/or poor skin adherence

Since these conditions commonly occur in critically ill patients, caution should be exercised when using pulse oximetry in critical care units. Proper use (Table 6–4) and periodic validation of the accuracy of these devices with ABG analysis is essential to avoid erroneous patient assessment.

Assessing Pulmonary Function in Critical Care

A variety of measurements, besides ABG analysis, can assist the practitioner to further evaluate the respiratory system in the critically ill patient.

Measurement of selected long volumes can be perfused easily at the bedside. Tidal volume, minute ventila-

TABLE 6–4. TIPS TO MAXIMIZE SAFETY AND ACCURACY OF PULSE OXIMETRY

- Apply sensor to dry finger of nondominant hand according to manufacturer's directions and observe for adequate pulse wave generation on microprocessing unit.
- Avoid tension on the sensor cable.
- Rotate application sites and change sensor at least every 24 hours and whenever adherence is poor.
- In children and elderly patients, rotate application sites more often and carefully assess skin for heat damage from sensor light source.
- Verify adequacy of pulse wave generation prior to obtaining readings.
- If pulse wave generation is inadequate, check for proper adherence to skin and position. Apply a new sensor to another site, if necessary.
- Compare pulse oximeter SaO_2 values with arterial blood gases every 24 hours, when changes in the clinical condition may decrease accuracy and/or when values do not fit the clinical situation.

tion, and inspiratory force (IF) are measured with portable, handheld equipment (spirometer and IF meter, respectively). Lung compliance and alveolar oxygen content can be calculated with standard formulas (Table 6–1). Frequent trend monitoring of these parameters provides an objective evaluation of the patient's response to interventions.

AIRWAY MANAGEMENT

Maintaining an open and patent airway is an important aspect of critical care management. Patency can be ensured through conservative techniques such as coughing, head/neck positioning, and alignment. If conservative techniques fail, insertion of an oral or nasal airway or endotracheal tube will be required.

AT THE BEDSIDE
▶ *Respiratory Failure*

Mrs. L, a 73-year-old woman with a long history of asthma, was admitted to the intermediate care unit with viral pneumonia. Vital signs and laboratory tests on admission were:

Temperature	38.1°C (oral)
Heart rate	110/minute, slightly labored
BP	148/90 mm Hg

Arterial blood gases on room air were:

pH	7.33
$Paco_2$	46 mm Hg
HCO_3^-	26 mEq/L
Base excess	0 mEq/L
Pao_2	53 mm Hg

She was begun on oxygen therapy at 28% O_2, using a Venturi mask to ensure accurate O_2 delivery. Within 2 hours her BP, heart rate, and respiratory rate had decreased to normal values, with improvement in her Pao_2 level (68 mm Hg).

Two days after admission, she became progressively more dyspneic, with heart rate, BP, and respiratory rate increases. Arterial blood gases at that time revealed a respiratory acidosis with partial compensation and hypoxemia on 35% O_2 by Venturi mask:

pH	7.31
$Paco_2$	55 mm Hg
HCO_3^-	29 mEq/L
Base excess	−2 mEq/L
Pao_2	48 mm Hg

Mrs. L. was intubated with a 7.5-mm oral ET tube without difficulty, and placed on a microprocessor ventilator (Mode, SIMV; Rate, 15/minute; TV, 600 ml; FIO_2, 0.5; PEEP, 5 cm H_2O). Immediately after intubation and initiation of mechanical ventilation, Mrs. L's BP decreased to 90/64 mm Hg. Following a 500-ml bolus of IV fluids, BP returned to normal values (118/70). Arterial blood gases 15 minutes after ventilation were:

pH	7.36
$Paco_2$	50 mm Hg
HCO_3^-	29 mEq/L
Base excess	+2 mEq/L
Pao_2	65 mm Hg

Oropharyngeal Airway

The oropharyngeal airway, or oral bit block, is used to relieve upper airway obstruction caused by tongue relaxation (e.g., postanesthesia or during unconsciousness), secretions, seizures, or biting down on oral endotracheal tubes (Figure 6–4A). Oral airways are made of rigid plastic or rubber material, semicircular in shape, and available in sizes for infants to adults. The airway is inserted either right

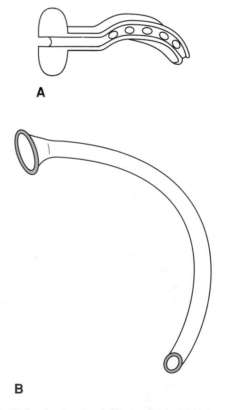

Figure 6–4. (A) Oropharyngeal and (B) nasopharyngeal airways.

side up or upside down and rotated during insertion to fit the curvature of the oral cavity and ensure the tongue is not obstructing the airway. The tip of the oropharyngeal airway rests near the posterior pharyngeal wall. For this reason, oral airways are not recommended for use in alert patients as they may trigger the gag reflex and cause vomiting. Oropharyngeal airways are temporary devices for achieving airway patency.

Management of oropharyngeal airways includes frequent assessment of the lips and tongue to identify pressure areas. The airway should be removed at least every 12 hours to check for pressure areas and to provide oral hygiene.

Nasopharyngeal Airway

The nasopharyngeal airway, or nasal trumpet, is another device to maintain airway patency, especially in the semiconscious patient (Figure 6–4B). The nasopharyngeal airway is also used to facilitate nasotracheal suctioning. Made of soft malleable rubber, the nasal airway ranges in sizes from 26 to 35 Fr. Prior to insertion, a topical anesthetic (e.g., viscous lidocaine) is applied to the nares. The nasopharyngeal airway, lubricated with a water-soluble gel, is gently inserted into one of the nares. The patency of the airway is assessed by listening for, or feeling with your hand, air movement during expiration. Complications of these airways include sinusitis and erosion of the mucous membranes.

Care of the patient with a nasal airway includes frequent assessment for pressure areas and occlusion of the airway with dried secretions. The nasal airway is changed daily and rotated from nostril to nostril. When performing nasotracheal suctioning through the nasal airway, the suction catheter should be lubricated with a water-soluble gel. Refer to the following discussion on suctioning for further standards of care.

Artificial Airways

Artificial airways (oral and nasal endotracheal tubes, tracheostomy tubes) are used when a patent airway cannot be maintained with an adjunct airway device for mechanical ventilation or to manage severe airway obstruction. The artificial airway also protects the lower airway from aspiration of oral or gastric secretions and allows for easier secretion removal.

Types of Artificial Airways and Insertion

Endotracheal tubes are made of polyvinyl chloride and are available in a variety of sizes and lengths (Figure 6–5A). Standard features include a 15-mm adapter at the end of the tube for connection to mechanical ventilation equipment or a manual resuscitation bag (MRB). Air is injected into the cuff near the distal tip of the ET tube through a small connector and lumen. Measuring markers along the side of the tube are useful for estimating tube position.

ET tubes are inserted into the patient's trachea either through the mouth or nose (Figures 6–6, 6–7). With use of the laryngoscope, the upper airway is visualized and the tube inserted through the vocal cords into the trachea, 2 to 4 cm above the carina. The presence of bilateral breath sounds, along with equal chest excursion during inspiration, preliminarily confirms proper tube placement. A portable chest x-ray will verify proper tube placement. Once proper placement is confirmed, the tube is anchored to prevent movement with either tape or a special ET fixation device (Figure 6–8). The centimeter marking of the ET tube at the

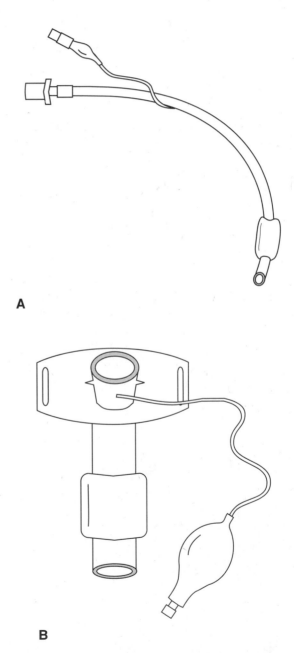

Figure 6–5. Artificial airways. (A) Endotracheal tube. (B) Tracheostomy tube.

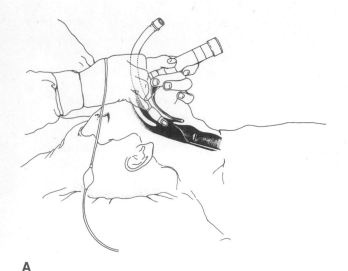

A

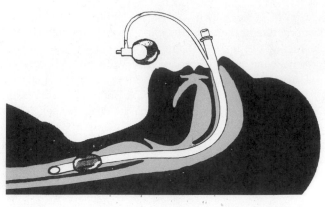

Figure 6–7. Nasal endotracheal tube. *(With permission from Mallinckrodt Medical, Inc., St. Louis, MO.)*

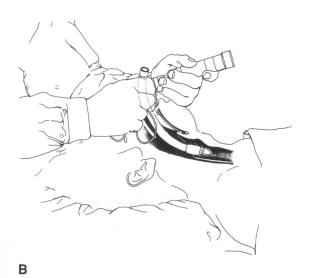

B

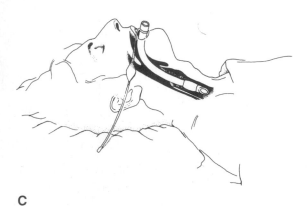

C

Figure 6–6. Oral intubation with an endotracheal (ET) tube. (A) Insertion of ET tube through the mouth with the aid of a laryngoscope. (B) ET tube advanced through the vocal cords into the trachea. (C) ET tube positioned with the cuff below the vocal cords. *(From Boggs R, Wooldridge-King M: AACN procedure manual for critical care, 3rd ed. Philadelphia: WB Saunders, 1993, p. 34–36.)*

lip is documented and checked each shift to monitor proper tube placement.

Oral ET tubes are easier to insert than other artificial airways since the upper airway and vocal cords are easily visualized. Oral ET tubes, however, can stimulate the gag reflex, cause increased salivation, and often require an oral "bite block" to prevent occlusion of the airway during biting of the mouth. Compared to nasal tubes, oral ET tubes are more difficult to secure and less stable.

The nasal ET tube often is tolerated better by an alert patient. With a nasal ET tube, the patient can "mouth" words to communicate more easily than with an oral tube. A nasal tube is usually smaller in diameter than an oral endotracheal tube since the nasal passage cannot accommodate large tubes. Smaller ET tubes can increase airway resistance, making spontaneous breathing more difficult and increasing the work of breathing. Other complications with nasal tubes include kinking of the tube at the back of the nasal pallet and the potential for sinus infections and nasal necrosis. Nasal tubes are also more difficult to insert since visualization of the nasal passage is not possible.

ET tubes are often left in place for up to 6 weeks, depending on institutional policies. If an artificial airway is needed for a longer period of time, a tracheostomy tube will be inserted electively. Complications of ET intubation are numerous and include laryngeal and tracheal damage, laryngospasm, aspiration infection, discomfort sinusitis, and subglottic injury.

The majority of tracheostomy tubes used in critically ill patients also are made of polyvinyl chloride and come in a variety of sizes (Figure 6–5B). As with ET tubes, a standard 15-mm adapter at the tip assures universal connection to MRBs and ventilator circuits. Tracheostomy tubes are usually inserted as an elective procedure in the operating room.

Tracheostomies are secured with cloth tape or special holders attached to the flange of the tube. Many tra-

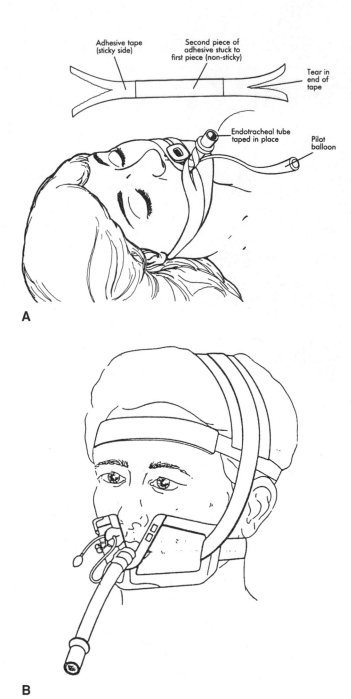

A

B

Figure 6–8. Methods for anchoring an endotracheal tube to prevent movement. (A) Taping of an oral ET tube. *(From: Boggs R, Wooldridge-King M: AACN procedure manual for critical care, 3rd ed. Philadelphia: WB Saunders, 1993, p. 108.)* B. Use of a special fixation device. *(From: Kaplow R, Bookbinder M: A comparison of four endotracheal tube holders. Heart and Lung. 1994;23(1):60.)*

cheostomies have inner cannulas which can be easily removed for periodic cleaning or replacement. Tracheostomies are often better tolerated by patients than oral or nasal ET tubes. Secretion removal and communication are easier with tracheostomy tubes.

Complications of tracheostomies include hemorrhage from erosion of the innominate artery; tracheal stenosis, malacia, or perforation; laryngeal nerve injury; infection; air leak; and mechanical problems. Most complications rarely occur with proper management.

Cuff Inflation

After insertion of an oral or nasal ET or tracheostomy tube, the cuff of the tube is inflated with just enough air to create a seal. The cuff is inflated with the lowest possible pressure that will prevent an air leak during mechanical ventilation and decrease the risk of pulmonary aspiration. Cuff pressure should be maintained under 25 cm H_2O. Excessive cuff pressures cause tracheal ischemia, necrosis, and erosion, as well as obstruction of the distal airway from cuff herniation.

There are two basic techniques to ensure proper cuff inflation without overinflation: the minimal leak and minimal occlusive volume techniques. The minimal leak technique involves listening over the larynx with a stethoscope during the inflation of the ET cuff in 0.5- to 1-ml increments. Inflation continues until only a small air leak, or rush of air, is heard over the larynx during inspiration. The minimal leak technique should result in no more than a 50- to 100-ml air loss per breath during mechanical ventilation. The amount of air instilled into the balloon should be recorded.

The minimal occlusive volume cuff inflation technique is similar to the minimal leak technique. Cuff inflation continues, however, until the air leak completely disappears. The measurement of cuff pressure should be done during cuff inflation and periodically to ensure intracuff pressure is less than 25 cm H_2O. The amount of air instilled into the balloon should be recorded.

Cuff Pressure Measurement

The connection of a stopcock to the cuff lumen allows for the simultaneous measurement of pressure during inflation or periodic checking (Figure 6–9). The need for pressures greater than 25 cm H_2O to properly seal the trachea may indicate the ET tube diameter is too small for the trachea. Cuffs should be inflated to properly seal the trachea until the appropriately sized ET tube can be electively reinserted.

Endotracheal Suctioning

Pulmonary secretion removal is normally accomplished by coughing. An effective cough requires a closed epiglottis so intrathoracic pressure can be increased prior to sudden opening of the epiglottis and secretion expulsion. The presence of an artificial airway prevents glottic closure and effective coughing, necessitating the use of endotracheal suctioning periodically to remove secretions.

Currently, two methods are commonly used for ET suctioning: the open method and the closed method. Closed suctioning means the ventilator circuit remains closed while suctioning is performed, whereas open suctioning means the ventilator circuit is opened, or removed, during suction-

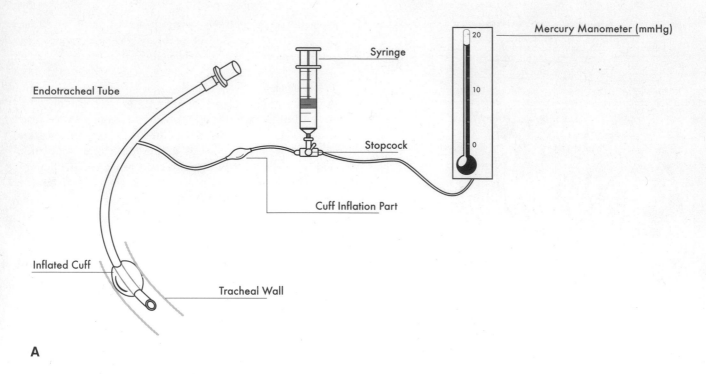

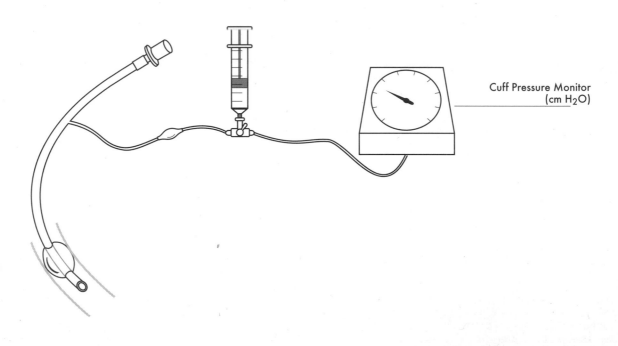

Figure 6–9. Measurement of cuff pressure with (A) bedside mercury manometer or (B) cuff pressure monitor.

ing. The open method requires disconnection of the ET tube from the mechanical ventilator or oxygen therapy source and insertion of a suction catheter each time the patient requires suctioning. The closed method refers to suctioning devices which remain attached to the ventilator circuit, allowing periodic insertion of the suction catheter through a diaphragm to suction without removing the patient from the ventilator. Following suctioning, the catheter is withdrawn into the plastic sleeve of the in-line device until the next suctioning procedure. Recommendations for use of the open and closed techniques in various clinical situations are summarized in Table 6–5.

TABLE 6–5. CLINICAL INDICATIONS FOR USE OF CLOSED AND OPEN CATHETER SUCTIONING SETUPS

Closed Method	Open Method
• Suctioning frequency every hour or less	• Intubated <24 hours
• Copious amounts of secretions	• Small to moderate secretions
• High levels of PEEP (>10 cm H_2O)	• Suctioning frequency every 2 hours
• Decreases in Sao_2 or hemodynamic compromise during suctioning	
• Highly contagious respiratory infections (TB, MRSA)	
• Blood in secretions	

Indications for Suctioning

The need for ET suctioning is determined by a variety of clinical signs and symptoms, such as coughing, increased inspiratory pressures on the ventilator, and the presence of adventitious sounds (rhonchi, gurgling) during chest auscultation. Suctioning may also be performed periodically to assess airway patency. Suctioning should only be done when there is a clinical indication and never on a routine schedule.

Procedure

Hyperoxygenation with 100% O_2 is provided with each suctioning episode, whether using an open or closed technique (Table 6–6). Hyperoxygenation prevents decreases in arterial oxygen levels after suctioning. Hyperoxygenation can be done by increasing the O_2 delivered via the mechanical ventilator or by using an MRB to deliver 100% O_2. At least two or three breaths of 100% O_2 should be given before and after each pass of the suction catheter. In spon-

TABLE 6–6. STEPS FOR SUCTIONING THROUGH AN ARTIFICIAL AIRWAY

1. Determine the need for suctioning. Clinical indicators of the need for suctioning include:
   • Coughing
   • Increase in ventilator airway pressures
   • Respiratory distress
   • Decrease in arterial oxygen levels
   • Decreased breath sounds
   • Adventitious sounds during chest auscultation or noisy respirations
   • Assessment of airway patency

2. Hyperoxygenate with 100% oxygen using MRB or ventilator before and after each suction pass.

3. Limit suction passes to two or three at most, with suction duration limited to 10 seconds or less. Use sterile technique in hospitalized patients.

4. Continuously monitor the patient's response to suctioning (cardiac rhythm, Sao_2, color, heart rate, respiratory rate, MAP, ICP, and the patient's subjective response). Stop suctioning and hyperoxygenate immediately if signs of intolerance occur.

5. Once the airway is cleared, document the patient's tolerance of the procedure along with a description of the secretions removed. Remember to compare your findings with the report from the previous shift. Changes in secretion color or volume indicate a change in the patient's pulmonary condition.

taneously breathing patients, encourage several deep breaths of 100% O_2 before and after each suction pass. The tidal volume (TV) of the breaths should be at least the usual TV, with hyperinflation breaths (1.5 times the TV) sometimes advocated. Caution should be used when giving hyperinflation breaths since large TV breaths can cause barotrauma, such as pneumothorax, as well as decreased venous return.

The number of suction passes should be limited to only those necessary to clear the airway of secretions—usually two or three suction passes. The mechanical act of inserting the suction catheter into the trachea can stimulate the vagus nerve and result in bradycardia or asystole. Each pass of the suction catheter should be 10 seconds or less.

The instillation of 5 to 10 ml of normal saline is no longer advocated during routine ET suctioning. This practice was previously thought to decrease secretion viscosity and increase secretion removal during ET suctioning. Bolus saline instillation has not been shown to be beneficial and is associated with Sao_2 decreases and bronchospasm.

Complications

A variety of complications are associated with ET suctioning. Decreases in PaO_2 have been well documented when no hyperoxygenation therapy is provided with suctioning. Serious cardiac arrhythmias occur occasionally with suctioning, and include bradycardia, asystole, ventricular tachycardia, and heart block. Less severe arrythmias frequently occur with suctioning and include premature ventricular contractions, atrial contractions, and supraventricular tachycardia. Other complications associated with suctioning include increases in arterial pressure and intracranial pressure, bronchospasm, tracheal wall damage, and nosocomial pneumonia. Many of these complications can be minimized with vigilant monitoring during and after suctioning and the use of hyperoxygenation before and after each suction pass.

Extubation

The reversal of conditions which lead to the use of artificial airways usually signals the readiness for removal of the airway. Common indicators of readiness for artificial airway removal include:

• Ability to maintain spontaneous breathing and adequate ABG values with minimal to moderate amounts of O_2 administration (<50%)
• Ability to protect the airway
• Ability to clear pulmonary secretions

Removal of an artificial airway usually occurs following weaning from mechanical ventilatory support (see the discussion on weaning later in chapter). Preparations for extubation should include an explanation to the patient and family of what to expect, medication for pain, setting up the

TABLE 6–7. COMMON INDICATIONS FOR OXYGEN THERAPY

- Decreased cardiac performance
- Increased metabolic need for O_2 (fever, burns)
- Acute changes in level of consciousness (restlessness, confusion)
- Acute shortness of breath
- Decreased O_2 saturation
- Pao_2 <60 mm Hg or Sao_2 < 90%
- Normal Pao_2 or Sao_2 with signs and symptoms of significant hypoxia
- Myocardial infarction
- Carbon monoxide (CO) poisoning
- Methemoglobinemia (a form of hemoglobin where ferrous iron is oxidized to ferric form, causing a high affinity for O_2 with decreased O_2 release at tissue level)
- Acute anemia
- Cardiopulmonary arrest
- Reduced cardiac output
- Consider in the presence of hypotension, tachycardia, cyanosis, chest pain, dyspnea, and acute neurologic dysfunction
- During stressful procedures and situations, especially in high-risk patients (e.g., endotracheal suctioning, bronchoscopy, thoracentesis, PA catheterization, travel at high altitudes)

appropriate method for delivering O_2 therapy (e.g., face mask, nasal prongs), and positioning the patient with the head of the bed elevated at 20° to 30° or higher, if possible. Suctioning of the artificial airway also should be performed prior to extubation if clinically indicated. Obtaining a baseline cardiopulmonary assessment also is important for later evaluation of the response to extubation.

Hyperoxygenation with 100% O_2 should be provided for 30 to 60 seconds prior to extubation in case respiratory distress occurs immediately after extubation and reintubation is necessary. The artificial airway is then removed following deflation of the ET or tracheostomy cuff, if present. Immediately apply the oxygen delivery method and encourage the patient to take deep breaths.

Monitor the patient's response to the extubation. Increases in heart rate, respiratory rate, and/or BP of >110% of baseline values may indicate respiratory compromise, necessitating more extensive assessment and reintubation. Pulmonary auscultation should also be performed.

Complications associated with extubation include aspiration, bronchospasm, and tracheal damage.

OXYGEN THERAPY

Oxygen is used for any number of clinical problems (Table 6–7). The overall goals for oxygen use include increasing alveolar O_2 tension (Pao_2) to treat hypoxemia, decreasing the work of breathing, and maximizing myocardial and tissue oxygen supply.

Complications

As with any drug, oxygen should be used cautiously. The hazards of oxygen misuse can be as dangerous as oxygen underuse. Alveolar hypoventilation, absorption atelectasis, and oxygen toxicity can be life threatening.

Alveolar Hypoventilation

Alveolar hypoventilation is underventilation of alveoli, and is a side effect of great concern in patients with chronic obstructive pulmonary disease (COPD). As the patient with COPD adjusts to chronically high levels of $Paco_2$, the chemoreceptors in the carotid bodies and medulla of the brain lose responsiveness to high $Paco_2$ levels. Hypoxemia, then, becomes the stimulus for ventilation. Correction of hypoxemia in the patient with COPD eliminates the hypoxic drive, and ventilation decreases or stops.

Absorption Atelectasis

The presence of high levels of nitrogen in inspired gas (normal = 79%) absorption atelectasis results when high concentrations of O_2 (>90%) are given for long periods of time and nitrogen is washed out of the lungs. Normally, the large partial pressure of nitrogen in the alveoli helps to maintain open lungs alveoli and prevents collapse. Removal of nitrogen by inspiring 90% to 100% O_2 causes alveoli to collapse when most, or all, of the alveolar O_2 diffuses into the pulmonary capillary.

Oxygen Toxicity

The toxic effects of oxygen are targeted primarily to the pulmonary and central nervous systems. CNS toxicity usually occurs with hyperbaric oxygen treatment. Signs and symptoms include nausea, anxiety, numbness, visual disturbances, muscular twitching, and grand mal seizures. The physiologic mechanism is not understood fully but is felt to be related to subtle neural and biochemical changes that alter the electric activity of the CNS.

Pulmonary oxygen toxicity is due to prolonged exposure to high Fio_2 levels that may lead to ARDS or bronchopulmonary dysplasia. Two phases of lung injury exist. The first phase occurs after 1 to 4 days of exposure to higher O_2 levels and is manifested by decreased tracheal mucosal blood flow and tracheobronchitis. Vital capacity decreases due to poor lung expansion and progressive atelectasis persists. The alveolar capillary membrane becomes progressively impaired, decreasing gas exchange. The second phase occurs after 12 days of high exposure. The alveolar septa thickens and an ARDS picture develops, with high associated mortality (See Chapter 13, Respiratory System).

Caring for the patient who requires high levels of oxygen requires astute monitoring by the critical care nurse. Monitor those patients at risk for absorption atelectasis and oxygen toxicity. Signs and symptoms include nonproductive cough, substernal chest pain, general malaise, fatigue, nausea, and vomiting.

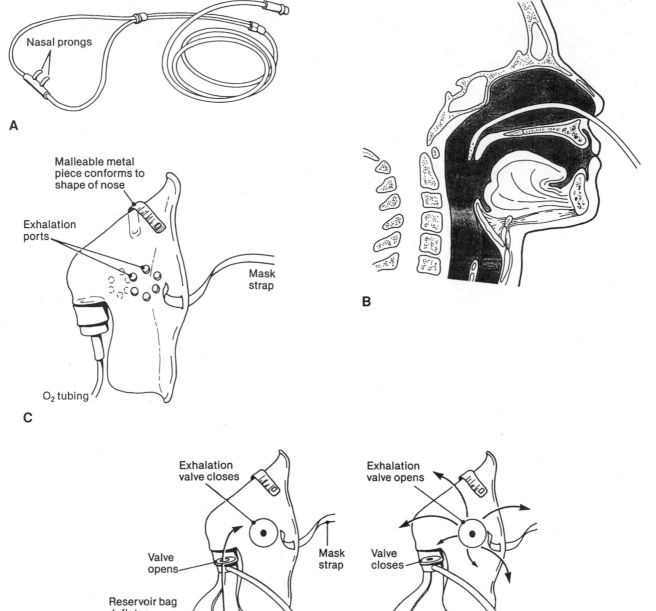

(continued)

Figure 6–10. Noninvasive and invasive methods for O$_2$ delivery. (A) Nasal prongs. (B) Nasal catheter. (C) Face mask. (D) Nonbreathing mask. *(From: Kersten L:* Comprehensive respiratory nursing. *Philadelphia: WB Saunders, 1989, pp. 608, 609.)*

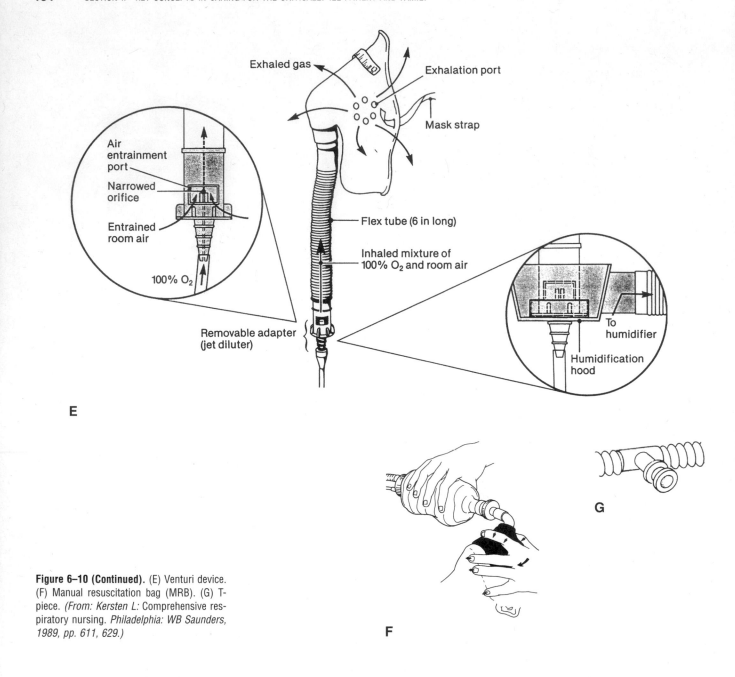

Figure 6–10 (Continued). (E) Venturi device. (F) Manual resuscitation bag (MRB). (G) T-piece. *(From: Kersten L:* Comprehensive respiratory nursing. *Philadelphia: WB Saunders, 1989, pp. 611, 629.)*

An oxygen concentration of 100% is regarded as safe for short periods of time (<24 hours). Oxygen concentrations greater than 50% for more than 24 to 48 hours may damage the lungs and worsen respiratory problems. Oxygen delivery levels should be decreased as soon as PaO_2 levels return to acceptable levels (>60 mm Hg).

Oxygen Delivery

Noninvasive O_2 Devices

Face masks and nasal cannulas are the standard fare for delivery of oxygen for the spontaneously breathing patient (Figure 6–10). Oxygen can be delivered with a high- or low-flow device, with the concentration of O_2 delivered ranging from >21% to approximately 80% (Table 6–8). An example of a high-flow device is the Venturi system with a flow of 10 L/minute. Low-flow systems include the nasal cannula, with 2- to 4-L/minute delivery rates. Noninvasive O_2 delivery devices, with the exception of Venturi masks, have the disadvantage of relatively low FIO_2 delivery, generally <0.50 (50% O_2), as well as variability in FIO_2 delivery as the patient's tidal volume and respiratory rate changes. The advantages, however, of these systems include their simple design, low cost, patient comfort during use, and low risk for causing nosocomial pneumonias.

TABLE 6–8. APPROXIMATE OXYGEN DELIVERY WITH COMMON NONINVASIVE AND INVASIVE OXYGEN DEVICES*

Device	%O_2
Nasal Prongs/Catheter	
2 L/minute	28%
4 L/minute	36%
6 L/minute	44%
Face Mask	
5 L/minute	30%
10 L/minute	50%
Nonrebreathing Mask	80% to 90%
Venturi Mask	
24%	24%
28%	28%
35%	35%
Manual Resuscitation Bag (MRB)	
PMR-2	20% to 80%
Laerdal	100%
Disposable MRB	Dependent on model

*Actual delivery dependent on minute ventilation rates except for Venturi mask.

Invasive O_2 Devices

MRB
Manual resuscitation bags provide 40% to 100% O_2 at adult TV and respiration rates to an ET or tracheostomy tube.

Mechanical ventilators
The most common method for delivering oxygen with an invasive technique is through a mechanical ventilator. Oxygen delivery can be accurately delivered from 21% to 100% O_2 with these devices. See the discussion below for further details.

Tracheal Gas Insufflation
Tracheal gas insufflation (TGI) is a new technique that may improve alveolar ventilation when used as an adjunct to conventional mechanical ventilation. A small catheter (2.2 mm) is passed down the endotracheal tube to just above the carina and low flows of oxygen (2 to 4 L/minute) are delivered. This technique is reserved for selected patients with difficult ventilation situations.

Transtracheal Oxygen Therapy
Transtracheal oxygen therapy is a method of administering continuous oxygen to patients with chronic hypoxemia. The concept involves the percutaneous placement of a small plastic catheter into the trachea. The catheter is inserted directly into the trachea above the suprasternal notch under local anesthesia in an outpatient setting. This device allows for low O_2 flow rates (<1 to 2 L/minute) to treat chronic hypoxemia. Advantages of this method for chronic O_2

delivery include improved mobility, avoidance of nasal and ear irritation from nasal cannulas, decreased O_2 requirements, and correction of refractory hypoxemia.

Typically, these patients are managed in the outpatient setting, but occasionally they may be in critical care. It is important to maintain the catheter unless specifically ordered to discontinue its use. The stoma formation process takes several weeks and if the catheter is removed, the stoma is likely to close. The catheter is cleaned daily to prevent the formation of mucous plugs. Refer to the manufacturer's guidelines for further recommendations on care of the catheter while the patient is hospitalized.

T-piece
Oxygen can also be provided directly to an ET or tracheostomy tube with a T-piece, or blow-by, in spontaneously breathing patients who do not require ventilatory support (Figure 6–10G). The T-piece is connected directly to the ET tube, providing 21% to 80% O_2.

BASIC VENTILATORY MANAGEMENT

Indications for Mechanical Ventilation
Mechanical ventilation is indicated when noninvasive management modalities fail to adequately support oxygenation and/or ventilation. The decision to initiate mechanical ventilation is based on a variety of physiologic indicators (Table 6–9). Trend monitoring of these indicators is important to differentiate stable or improving abnormal values from continuing decompensation. The need for mechanical ventilation can then be anticipated to avoid emergent use of ventilatory support.

Depending on the underlying cause of the respiratory failure, different indicators will be assessed to determine the need for mechanical ventilation. Many of the causes of respiratory failure, however, are due to inadequate alveolar ventilation and/or hypoxemia, with arterial blood gases as the primary indicator for ventilatory support. The assessment of respiratory muscle strength, by measurement of TV, vital capacity (VC), and inspiratory force, is frequently used to indicate the need for mechanical ventilation.

General Principles of Mechanical Ventilation
Mechanical ventilators are designed to partially or completely support ventilation. Two different categories of ventilators are available to provide ventilatory support. Negative pressure ventilators decrease intrathoracic pressure by applying negative pressure to the chest wall, typically with a shell placed around the chest (Figure 6–11A). The decrease in intrathoracic pressure causes atmospheric gas to be pulled into the lungs. Airway pressures during negative pressure ventilation are similar to spontaneous breathing

TABLE 6–9. INDICATIONS FOR MECHANICAL VENTILATION

Basic Physiologic Impairment	Best Available Indicators	Approximate Normal Range	Values Indicating Need for Ventilatory Support
Inadequate alveolar ventilation (acute ventilatory failure)	$Paco_2$, mm Hg	36–44	Acute increase from normal or patient's baseline
	Arterial pH	7.36–7.44	<7.25–7.30
Hypoxemia (acute oxygenation failure)	Alveolar-to-arterial Po_2 gradient breathing 100% O_2, mm Hg	25–65	>350
	Intrapulmonary right-to-left shunt fraction, percentage	<5	>20–25
	Pao_2/Fio_2, mm Hg	350–400	<200
Inadequate lung expansion	Tidal volume, ml/kg	5–8	<4–5
	Vital capacity	60–75	<10
	Respiratory rate, breaths/minute (adults)	12–20	>35
Inadequate respiratory muscle strength	Maximum inspiratory force, cm H_2O	−80−−100	<−25
	Maximum voluntary ventilation, L/minute	120–180	<2 × resting ventilatory requirement
	Vital capacity, ml/kg	60–75	<10–15
Excessive work of breathing	Minute ventilation necessary to maintain normal $Paco_2$, L/minute	5–10	>15–20
	Dead space ratio, percentage	0.25–0.40	>0.60
	Respiratory rate, breaths/minute (adults)	12–20	>35
Unstable ventilatory drive	Breathing pattern; clinical setting		

From: Luce J, Pierson D (eds.): Critical care medicine. *Philadelphia: WB Saunders, 1988, p. 219.*

patterns. Positive pressure ventilators generate high pressures to push gas into the lungs during inspiration (Figure 6–11B). Positive pressure ventilators dramatically increase airway pressures during inspiration, increasing intrathoracic pressure and potentially decreasing venous return and cardiac output.

Negative pressure ventilators are rarely used to manage acute respiratory problems in critical care. These devices are typically used for long-term ventilatory support when respiratory muscle strength is inadequate to support unassisted, spontaneous breathing. This chapter focuses only on the use of positive pressure ventilators for ventilatory support.

Patient-Ventilator System

In order to provide positive pressure ventilation, intubation of the trachea is required via an ET or tracheostomy tube. The ventilator is then connected to the artificial airway with a standard tubing circuit to maintain a closed delivery system (Figure 6–12). During the inspiratory cycle gas from the ventilator is bubbled through a heated humidifier prior to entering the lungs through the ET or tracheostomy tube. At the completion of inspiration, gas is passively exhaled through the expiratory side of the tubing circuit to the ventilator.

Ventilator Tubing Circuit

The humidifier located on the inspiratory side of the circuit is necessary to overcome two primary problems. First, the presence of an artificial airway allows gas entering the lungs to bypass the normal upper airway humidification process. Second, the high levels of oxygen typically administered during mechanical ventilation require additional humidification to avoid excessive intrapulmonary membrane drying.

Pressure within the ventilator tubing circuit is constantly measured by a probe inserted near the connection of the ventilator tubing and the ET tube attached to the side of the ventilator (Figure 6–12). Pressure measured at this location is a close reflection of the pressure within the airway and is thus termed *airway pressure*. This pressure is continuously monitored to alert clinicians to excessively high or low airway pressures. Airway pressure is dynamically displayed on the front of the ventilator control panel.

Most tubing circuits also have special water collection cups to prevent the condensation from humidified gas from obstructing the tubing. Medications, such as bronchodilators or steroids, also can be nebulized into the lungs through another cup located in the inspiratory side of the circuit.

The ventilator tubing circuit should be maintained as a closed circuit to avoid decreasing ventilation and oxygenation to the patient, as well as to decrease the potential for nosocomial pneumonias. Avoiding frequent changes of the ventilator circuit (no more frequently than every 2 to 3 days) will also decrease the risk of nosocomial pneumonias.

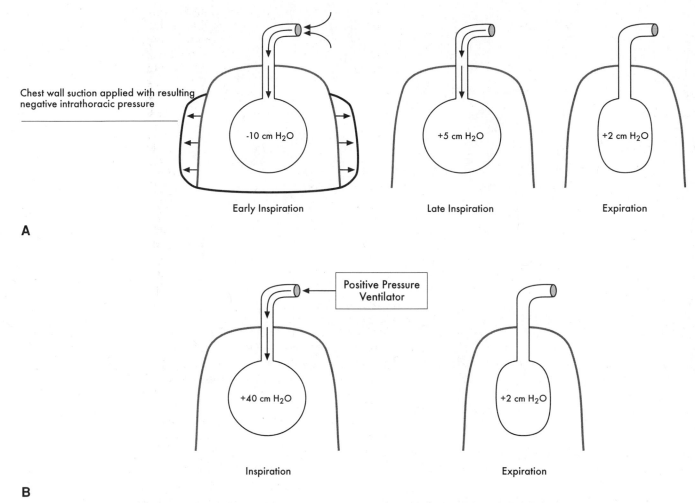

Figure 6–11. Principles of mechanical ventilation as provided by (A) negative pressure and (B) positive pressure ventilators.

Ventilator Control Panel

The front face of the ventilator includes three basic components: (1) control settings for the type and amount of ventilation and oxygen delivery, (2) alarm settings to specify high and low limits of acceptability for key ventilatory measurements, and (3) visual displays of key parameters which are measured continuously (Figure 6–13). The number and configuration of these knobs will vary from ventilator model to model, but their function and principles remain the same.

Control Settings

The control settings area of the panel contains knobs to set the mode of ventilation, TV, respiratory rate, FIO_2, positive end expiratory pressure (PEEP) level, inspiratory effort, and a variety of gas flow delivery options (e.g., inspiratory flow rate, inspiratory waveform pattern).

Alarm Settings

Alarms which continuously monitor ventilator function are essential to ensure safe and effective mechanical ventilation. Both high and low alarms are typically set to identify when critical parameters vary from the desired levels. Common alarms include exhaled tidal volume, FIO_2 delivery, respiratory rate, and airway pressures.

Visual Displays

Airway pressures, exhaled tidal volumes, and the inspiratory to expiratory (I:E) ratio are visually displayed on the control panel with each breath. The airway pressure gauge rises with inspiration, returning to baseline during exhalation. A breath delivered by the ventilator produces higher airway pressures than an unassisted, spontaneous breath by the patient (Figure 6–14). The presence of a downward deflection just prior to inspiration indicates a patient initiated breath. The presence of PEEP is identified by a positive value at the end of expiration rather than 0 cm H_2O. Careful observation of the airway pressure gauge provides the clinician with a great deal of information about the patient's respiratory effort, coordination with the ventilator, and changes in lung compliance.

The digital display of the exhaled TVs reflects the amount of gas that is returned to the ventilator via the expiratory tubing with each respiratory cycle. Each breath

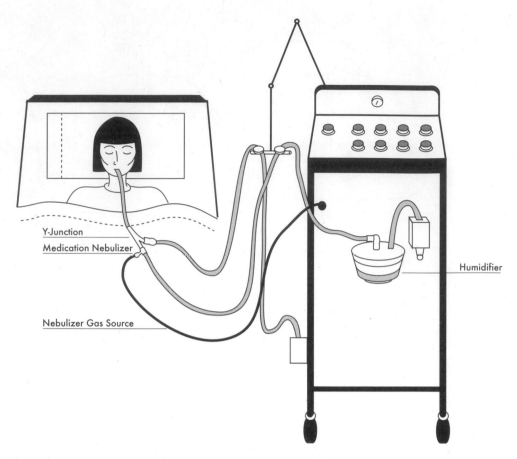

Figure 6–12. Typical setup of a ventilator, closed system tubing circuit, and humidifier connected to an endotracheal tube.

is measured and displayed on the control panel. Many ventilators also display the total ventilation over the past minute (MV) by adding together the measured TVs exhaled over the past minute. Exhaled TVs for ventilator-assisted breaths should be similar (±10%) to the desired TV setting selected on the control panel. The tidal volume of spontaneous breaths, or partially ventilator-supported breaths, however, may be different from the TV setting on the control panel.

Modes of Mechanical Ventilation

The mode of ventilation refers to one of several different methods that a ventilator uses to support ventilation. These modes generate different levels of airway pressures, volumes, and patterns of respiration and, therefore, different levels of support. The greater the level of ventilator support, the less muscle work performed by the patient. This "work of breathing" varies considerably with each of the modes of ventilation.

The different modes of ventilation used to support ventilation depend on the underlying respiratory problem and clinical preferences. As specific causes of respiratory failure are discussed in Chapter 13, Respiratory System, the mode of ventilation commonly prescribed for each is dis-

cussed there. The following discussion is a brief description of the basic modes of mechanical ventilation. Advanced modes of ventilation (e.g., pressure support, pressure control, reverse I:E ratio) are presented in Chapter 23, Advanced Respiratory Concepts.

Control Ventilation

The control mode of ventilation ensures that patients receive a predetermined number and volume of breaths each minute. No deviations from the respiratory rate or tidal volume settings are allowed with this mode of ventilation. Initiation of breaths by the patient is not allowed during control ventilation. The ventilation inspiratory valve is closed during expiration. In this mode of ventilation, all the work of breathing is performed by the ventilator.

The airway pressures, tidal volume delivery, and pattern of breathing typically observed with this mode of ventilation are shown in Figure 6–15A. The interval between each ventilator breath is similar, with high peak airway pressures generated with each breath. The lack of waveform deflections prior to inspiration indicates the breath was initiated by the ventilator and not by the patient.

The control mode of ventilation is used to support the patient with no respiratory efforts, such as in high spinal

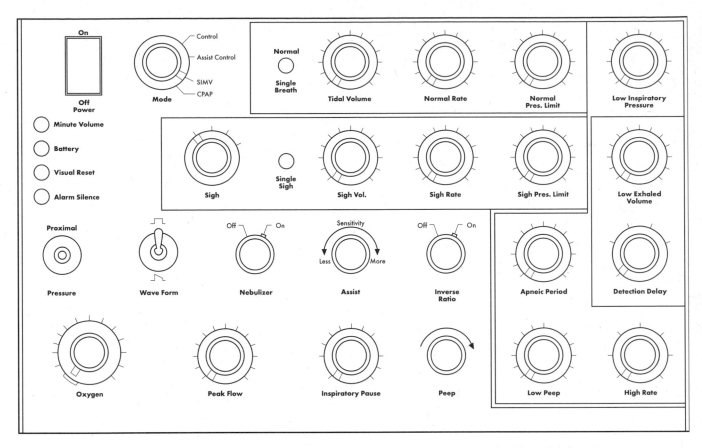

Figure 6–13. Ventilator control panel. *(From: Burton G, Hodgkin J, Ward J: Respiratory care: A guide to clinical practice. Philadelphia: JB Lippincott, 1991, p. 532.)*

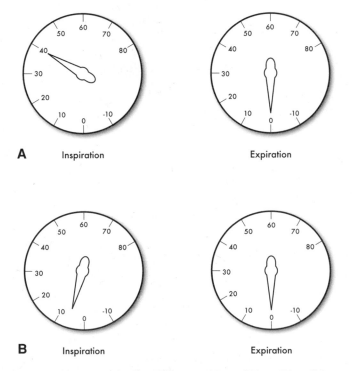

Figure 6–14. Typical airway pressure gauge changes during a (A) ventilator-assisted breath and a (B) spontaneous breath (cm H₂O).

cord injuries or drug overdoses or during neuromuscular blockade. This mode of ventilation is poorly tolerated by spontaneously breathing patients. Neuromuscular blockade is usually required to eliminate any patient-initiated respiratory effort (noted by decreases in airway pressure below baseline values) and episodes of ventilator-patient dyssynchrony, also called "bucking" or "fighting" the ventilator. Ventilator-patient dyssynchrony can have deleterious effects on MV, due to reduced TV delivery if airway pressures are high during the inspiration. For this reason, control ventilation is infrequently used today.

Assist-Control Ventilation

The assist-control mode of ventilation ensures that a predetermined number and volume of breaths will be delivered by the ventilator each minute should the patient not initiate respirations at that rate or above. If the patient attempts to initiate breaths at a rate greater than the set minimum value, the ventilator will cycle on and deliver breaths at the prescribed TV, at whatever respiratory rate desired by the patient (Figure 16–15B). While some effort is expended to initiate breaths, the work of breathing is minimal with the assist-control mode of ventilation. Increasing the work-load

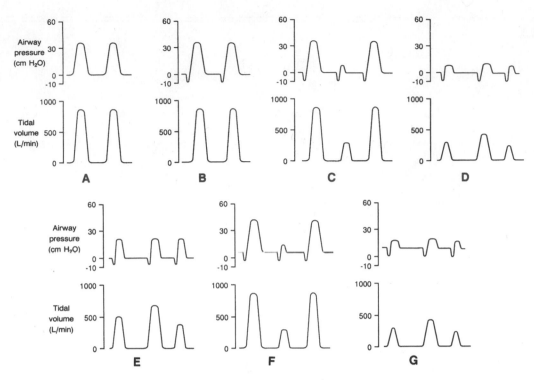

Figure 6–15. Airway pressures, tidal volumes (TV), and patterns of breathing for different modes of mechanical ventilation. (A) Controlled ventilation. (B) Assist-control ventilation. (C) SIMV (D) Spontaneous breathing. (E) Pressure support. (F) PEEP with SIMV. (G) CPAP. *(From: Dossey B, Guzzetta C, Kenner C:* Critical care nursing: Body-mind-spirit. *Philadelphia: JB Lippincott, 1992, p. 225.)*

of breathing can occur by decreasing the sensitivity setting for the initiation of a ventilator breath. This causes a greater respiratory effort to "trigger" the ventilator breath, and thus greater muscle work.

Assist-control ventilation is often used for short-term ventilatory support, such as postanesthesia and in situations where it is desired to decrease the work of breathing. Excessive ventilation can occur with this mode in situations where hyperventilation occurs for nonrespiratory reasons (e.g., pain, CNS dysfunction). Dramatic increases in MV levels can occur and result in potentially fatal respiratory alkalosis. Changing to a different mode of ventilation or blocking respiratory effort with neuromuscular blockade is necessary in these situations.

SIMV

The synchronous intermittent mandatory ventilation (SIMV) mode of ventilation ensures (or mandates) that a predetermined number and tidal volumes of breaths will be delivered each minute. Any additional breaths initiated by the patient are allowed but, in contrast to the assist-control mode, these breaths are not delivered by the ventilator. The patient is allowed to spontaneously breath at the depth and rate desired until it is time for the next ventilator-assisted breath. Ventilator-assisted breaths are synchronized with the patient's inspiratory effort, if present, to avoid delivery during the peak of inspiration of a spontaneous breath. Dur-

ing spontaneous breathing a demand valve inside the ventilator opens to allow the patient to breath gas at the same FIO_2 from a reservoir (Figure 6–15C).

The SIMV mode is a commonly used mode of mechanical ventilation. Originally designated as a ventilator mode for the gradual weaning of patients from mechanical ventilation, the SIMV use of a high rate for mandatory breaths can provide complete ventilatory support. Reduction of the number of mandatory breaths allows the patient to slowly resume greater and greater responsibility for spontaneous breathing. SIMV can be used for similar indications as the assist-control mode, as well as for weaning the patient from mechanical ventilatory support.

The work of breathing with this mode of ventilation is dependent on the TV and rate of the spontaneous breaths. When the mandated, intermittent breaths provide the majority of MV, the work of breathing by the patient will be minimal. When spontaneous breathing constitutes a large proportion of the total MV, however, the work of breathing will be higher.

While strong clinician and institutional biases exist regarding whether to use SIMV or other modes for ventilatory support, little data exist to clarify which mode of ventilation is best. Close observation of the physiologic and psychological response to the ventilatory mode is required, and consideration should be given to trials on alternative modes if warranted.

Spontaneous Breathing

Many ventilators have a mode which allows the patient to breathe spontaneously without ventilator support (Figure 6–15D). This is similar to placing the patient on a T-piece or blow-by oxygen setup, except it does have the benefit of providing continuous monitoring of exhaled volumes, airway pressures, and other important parameters. All the work of breathing is performed by the patient during spontaneous breathing. Use of the ventilator rather than the T-piece during spontaneous breathing actually may increase slightly the work of breathing. This occurs because of the additional inspiratory muscle work that is required to open the demand valve on the gas reservoir for each spontaneous breath. The amount of additional work required varies with different ventilator models. In some situations, removing the patient from the ventilator for weaning may result in a decrease in the work of breathing.

This mode of ventilation is often identified as CPAP on the selector knob rather than as spontaneous breathing. Continuous positive airway pressure (CPAP) is a spontaneous breathing setting with the addition of positive end expiratory pressure (PEEP) during the breathing cycle (see below). If no PEEP has been applied, the CPAP setting is similar to spontaneous breathing.

Pressure Support

A relatively new mode of mechanical ventilation, pressure support (PS), supplies gas to the patient throughout a spontaneous inspiration until a set pressure level is achieved (Figure 6–15E). The volume of a gas delivered by the ventilator during each inspiration varies depending on the level of pressure support. The higher the pressure support level, the higher the amount of gas delivered with each breath. Pressure support augments the spontaneous TV of the patient. At low levels of support, it is primarily used to overcome some of the airway resistance caused by breathing through the artificial airway.

Pressure support ventilation can be used in any mode of ventilation where spontaneous breaths are allowed (e.g., SIMV, CPAP). Pressure support is only applied to the spontaneous breaths. Pressure support decreases some of the work of breathing associated with spontaneous breathing.

PEEP/CPAP

Positive end expiratory pressure is used in conjunction with any of the ventilator modes to improve oxygenation (Figure 6–15F). The application of positive pressure to the airways during expiration may keep alveoli open and prevent early closure during exhalation. Lung compliance is reduced and ventilation-perfusion matching is often improved by prevention of early alveolar closure. If alveolar "recruitment" is not needed and PEEP/CPAP is applied, it may result in adverse hemodynamic or respiratory compromise.

PEEP/CPAP is indicated for hypoxemia which is secondary to diffuse lung injury (e.g., ARDS, interstitial pneumonitis). PEEP/CPAP levels of 5 cm Hg or less are often used to provide "physiologic PEEP." The presence of the artificial airway allows intrathoracic pressure to fall to zero, which is below the usual level of intrathoracic pressure at end expiration (+2 or +3 cm H_2O).

Use of PEEP increases the risk of barotrauma due to higher mean and peak airway pressures (PAPs) during ventilation, especially when PAP is greater than 50 cm H_2O. Venous return and cardiac output may also be affected by these high pressures. If cardiac output decreases with PEEP/CPAP initiation and oxygenation is improved, a fluid bolus may correct hypovolemia. Other complications from PEEP/CPAP are increases in intracranial pressure, decreased renal perfusion, hepatic congestion, and worsening of intracardiac shunts.

Complications of Mechanical Ventilation

Significant complications can arise from the use of mechanical ventilation and can be categorized as those associated with the patient's response to mechanical ventilation or those arising from ventilator malfunctions. Although the approach to minimizing and/or treating the complications of mechanical ventilation relate to the underlying cause, it is critical that frequent assessment occur routinely of the patient, ventilator equipment, and the patient's response to ventilatory management. Many clinicians participate in activities to assess the patient and ventilator, but the ultimate responsibility for ensuring continuous ventilatory support of the patient falls to the critical care nurse. Critically evaluating arterial blood gas results, in conjunction with patient status and ventilatory parameters, is essential to decrease complications associated with this highly complex technology.

Patient Response to Mechanical Ventilation

Hemodynamic Compromise

Normal intrathoracic pressure changes during inspiration and expiration fluctuate between −3 to −5 cm H_2O during inspiration and +3 to +5 cm H_2O during expiration. The use of positive pressure ventilation dramatically increases intrathoracic pressures during inspiration, commonly to +30 cm H_2O or higher. These high airway pressures impede venous return to the right atrium, thus decreasing cardiac output. In some patients, this decrease in cardiac output can be clinically significant, leading to increased heart rate and decreased blood pressure and perfusion to vital organs.

Whenever mechanical ventilation is instituted, or when ventilator changes are made, it is important to assess the patient's cardiovascular response. Approaches to managing hemodynamic compromise include increasing the preload of the heart (e.g., by fluid administration) and decreasing the airway pressures exerted during mechanical ventilation by decreasing inspiratory flow rates and TV, or using other methods to decrease airway pressures (e.g., different modes of ventilation).

Barotrauma

Barotrauma is the term used to describe damage to the pulmonary system due to alveolar rupture from excessive airway pressures and/or overdistention of alveoli. Alveolar gas enters the interstitial pulmonary structures causing pneumothorax, pneumomediastinum, pneumoperitoneum, or subcutaneous emphysema. The potential for pneumothorax and cardiovascular collapse requires prompt management of pneumothorax.

Patients with obstructive airway diseases (e.g., asthma, bronchospasm), unevenly distributed lung disease (e.g., lobar pneumonia), or hyperinflated lungs (e.g., emphysema) are at high risk for these complications. Techniques to decrease the incidence of barotrauma include the use of small TVs, cautious use of PEEP, and the avoidance of high airway pressures and development of auto-PEEP in high-risk patients.

Auto-PEEP occurs when a delivered breath is incompletely exhaled before the onset of the next inspiration. This trapping of gas increases overall lung volumes, inadvertently raising the end expiratory pressure in the alveoli. The presence of auto-PEEP increases the risk for complications from PEEP. Patients with COPD (e.g., asthma, emphysema) or high MV rates are at high risk for development of auto-PEEP.

Auto-PEEP, also termed intrinsic PEEP, is difficult to diagnose since it cannot be observed on the airway pressure gauge at end expiration. The technique for assessment for auto-PEEP varies with different ventilatory models and modes, but typically involves measuring the airway pressure close to the artificial airway during occlusion of the expiratory ventilator circuit during end expiration.

Auto-PEEP can be minimized by:

- Maximizing the length of time for expiration (e.g., increasing inspiratory flow rates)
- Decreasing obstructions to expiratory flow (e.g., using larger diameter ET tubes, eliminating bronchospasm and secretions)
- Avoiding overventilation

Nosocomial Pneumonia

The placement of invasive devices into the pulmonary airways, coupled with the immunocompromised state of many critically ill patients, dramatically increases the risk for nosocomial pneumonias during mechanical ventilation. Within 24 hours of intubation and mechanical ventilation, the trachea becomes colonized with pathological bacteria in almost all patients. Nosocomial pneumonia occurs in 20% to 60% of these patients, significantly increasing morbidity and mortality. Management strategies to prevent nosoco-

TABLE 6–10. KEY STRATEGIES TO PREVENT NOSOCOMIAL PNEUMONIA DURING MECHANICAL VENTILATION

- Avoid cross-contamination by frequent handwashing by hospital personnel.
- Decrease risk of aspiration (cuff occlusion of trachea, positioning, use of small-bore N/G tubes).
- Suction only when clinically indicated, using sterile technique.
- Maintain closed system setup on ventilator circuitry and avoid pooling of condensation in the tubing.
- Ensure adequate nutrition.
- Avoid neutralization of gastric contents with antacids and H_2 blockers.

mial pneumonia are highlighted in Table 6–10 and are discussed in detail in Chapter 13, Respiratory System.

Renal Dysfunction

Hyponatremia with total body sodium excess is a common occurrence following the institution of mechanical ventilation. Low dose dopamine therapy may decrease the impact of these changes.

Ventilator Malfunction

Problems related to the proper functioning of mechanical ventilators, while rare, can have devastating consequences for patients. Many of the alarm systems on ventilators are designed to alert clinicians to improperly functioning ventilatory systems. These alarm systems must be activated at all times if ventilator malfunction problems are to be quickly identified and corrected, and untoward patient events avoided.

Many of the "problems" identified with ventilatory equipment are actually related to inappropriate setup or use of the devices. Tubings which are not properly connected, alarm systems which are set improperly, or inadequate ventilator settings for a particular clinical condition are examples of some of these operator-related occurrences.

There are occasions, however, when ventilator systems do not operate properly. Examples of ventilator malfunctions include valve mechanisms sticking and obstructing gas flow, inadequate or excessive gas delivery, electronic circuit failures in microprocessing-based ventilators, failures with complete shutdown, and power surges in the institution.

The most important approach to ventilator malfunction is to maintain a high level of vigilance to determine if ventilators are performing properly. Ensuring that alarm systems are activated at all times, providing frequent routine assessment of ventilator functioning, and the use of experienced support personnel to maintain the ventilator systems are some of the most crucial activities necessary to avoid patient problems. In addition, whenever ventilator malfunction is suspected, the patient should be immediately removed from the device and temporary ventilation and oxygenation provided with an MRB or another ventilator until the question of proper functioning is resolved. Any sudden change in the patient's respiratory or cardiovascular status should alert the

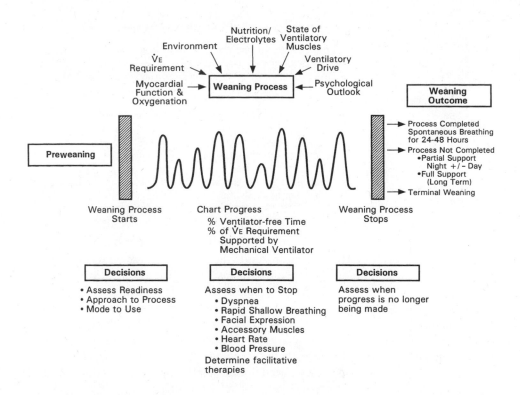

Figure 6–16. Phases of the weaning process: preweaning, weaning process, and weaning outcome. *(From: Knebel A, Shekleton M, Burns S, et al: Weaning from mechanical ventilation. American Journal of Critical Care. 1994;3(6):416–420.)*

clinician to consider potential ventilator malfunction as a cause. Chapter 31, Ventilatory Troubleshooting Guide, details common approaches to equipment and patient-related problems during mechanical ventilation.

Weaning from Short-Term Mechanical Ventilation

The process of transitioning the ventilator-dependent patient to unassisted spontaneous breathing is termed *weaning* from mechanical ventilation. This is a period of time where the level of ventilator support for oxygenation and ventilation is decreased, either gradually or abruptly, while monitoring the patient's response to the resumption of spontaneous breathing. Weaning is considered to be complete, or successful, when the patient is able to spontaneously breathe for 24 to 48 hours. Often, removal of the artificial airway occurs before that time if clinicians are optimistic that the patient's respiratory status will not deteriorate. The vast majority of patients intubated and ventilated for short periods of time (<72 hours) are successfully weaned over a 2- to 8-hour period. Approximately 20% of patients, however, will require extended time periods to successfully complete the weaning process, with some being unable to breathe without mechanical ventilation. Chapter 23, Advanced Respiratory Concepts, presents information on dealing with difficult-to-wean patients.

Weaning is usually warranted to verify that the underlying pulmonary disorder which led to mechanical ventilation has sufficiently resolved. In some cases, weaning is needed to provide reconditioning of the respiratory muscles which have weakened during the mechanical ventilation

period. The resting of respiratory muscles which occurs during mechanical ventilation rapidly leads to muscle discoordination and atrophy. This process is similar to the muscle wasting which occurs during immobilization of a fracture and the reconditioning of muscle strength which is required after removal of the cast.

Phases of Weaning

Weaning should be considered a three-phase process (Figure 6–16).

Preweaning Phase

The preweaning phase consists of activities to correct the underlying clinical disorder which led to the need for mechanical ventilation, as well as to maximize a number of clinical variables which are thought to influence weaning success (Table 6–11). Fluid and electrolyte status and arterial blood gas values should be normalized, any cardiac arrhythmias or output deficits should be corrected, meta-

TABLE 6–11. FACTORS WHICH INFLUENCE WEANING SUCCESS

- Myocardial function and oxygenation
- State of ventilatory muscles
- Ventilatory requirements and drive
- Nutrition and electrolyte balance
- Environmental factors
- Psychological outlook of the patient
- Resolution of condition which led to mechanical ventilation

From: Knebel A, Shekleton M, Burns S, et al: Weaning from mechanical ventilation. American Journal of Critical Care. 1994;3(6):416–420.

AT THE BEDSIDE

Nurse: "Just before we started to wean Mrs. L. from the ventilator, I sat down with her to explain the whole weaning process. Why weaning was necessary, how it would be done, what it might feel like for her, what she could do to facilitate the process, how I'd be there the whole time monitoring her response to weaning, and when we would stop the weaning trial. I say, 'when we would stop the weaning trial' because it's important for the patients to know they can decide it's time to stop the trial, as well as the nurse or doctor. It is important for the patients to be in control of this process. . . . After all, it's their breathing isn't it?"

bolic needs should be minimized (e.g., correcting fever or infectious processes), and nutritional status should be maximized. For most short-term ventilated patients, the correction of abnormalities, if present, is rapidly accomplished and the weaning process can begin.

Weaning Process Phase

The second phase is the weaning process phase. This phase begins with an assessment of the patient's readiness to wean, the selection and implementation of the weaning method or technique, and the monitoring of progress. Readiness to wean can be assessed with a variety of criteria (see Chapter 23, Table 23–7). However, in most institutions, assessment of readiness to wean includes just three or four criteria for most short-term ventilator patients:

- Arterial blood gases within normal limits on minimal to moderate amounts of ventilatory support ($FIO_2 \leq 0.50$, MV ≤ 10 L/minute, PEEP ≤ 10 cm H_2O)
- Negative inspiratory pressure (NIP) ≤ -20 cm H_2O
- Spontaneous TV ≥ 5 ml/kg
- Vital capacity (VC) ≥ 10 to 15 ml/kg

Following selection of the method for weaning (see the discussion below), the actual weaning trial can begin. It is important to prepare both the patient and the critical care environment properly to maximize the chances for weaning suc-

AT THE BEDSIDE

Patient: "I felt really weird about that ventilator. At first, I fought it. Then I realized it was making my breathing easier. Then, when they wanted to get me off of it, I was actually afraid that my breathing problems would start all over again."

TABLE 6–12. STRATEGIES TO FACILITATE WEANING

- Explain the weaning process to the patient/family and maintain open communication throughout weaning.
- Position to maximize ventilatory effort (sitting upright in bed or chair).
- Administer analgesics to relieve pain and sedatives to control anxiety, if appropriate.
- Remain with the patient during the weaning trial and/or provide a highly vigilant presence.
- Frequently assess the patient's response to the weaning trial.
- Avoid unnecessary physical exertion, painful procedures, and/or transports during the weaning trials.
- Maximize the physical environment to be conducive to weaning (e.g., temperature, noise, distractions).

cess (Table 6–12). Interventions include appropriate explanations of the process to the patient, positioning and medication to improve ventilatory efforts, and the avoidance of unnecessary activities during the weaning trial. Throughout the weaning time, continuous monitoring for signs and symptoms of respiratory distress or fatigue is essential (Table 6–13). Many of these indicators are subtle, but careful monitoring of baseline levels before weaning progresses and throughout the trial provides objective indicators of the need to return the patient to previous levels of ventilator support.

The need to temporarily stop the weaning trial should not be viewed as, or termed, a *failure*. The process of weaning from mechanical ventilation in some cases requires a reconditioning of the respiratory muscles, which cannot be accomplished all at one time. This process is similar to the conditioning process for running, where one does not begin to run 2 miles the first day, but progressively increases to that distance over time. When respiratory muscles have been weakened, a progressive "retraining" period may need to be undertaken. The degree of respiratory weakness depends not only on the time on ventilatory support, but also on the patient's prehospitalization status.

Weaning Outcome Phase

The third phase of the weaning process occurs when weaning is terminated. For most patients, this occurs when they can successfully breathe spontaneously for 24 to 48 hours without ventilator assistance. In a small number of patients, spontaneous breathing for 24 hours cannot be accomplished after multiple weaning trials (see Chapter 23, Advanced Respiratory Concepts). Long-term ventilator support or terminal weaning is the outcome for these patients.

TABLE 6–13. CLINICAL INDICATORS OF THE NEED TO STOP WEANING TRIAL

- Dyspnea
- Increased respiratory rate, heart rate, or BP
- Shallow breaths or decreased spontaneous TV
- Accessory muscle use
- Anxiety
- Deterioration in Pao_2 and/or $Paco_2$

Methods for Weaning

A variety of methods are available for weaning patients from mechanical ventilation. To date, research on these techniques has not clearly identified any one method as optimal for weaning from short-term mechanical ventilation. Most institutions, however, use one or two approaches routinely in their facility "because it's the best." Most experts on weaning believe that, with short-term ventilator-dependent patients, the method used to wean the patient is not an important contributor to weaning success. The vast majority of these patients need little, if any, "weaning" as long as their underlying problem has been resolved.

SIMV

One of the most popular methods of weaning patients from ventilation is the use of the SIMV mode on the ventilator. By progressively decreasing the number of mandated breaths delivered by the ventilator, the patient performs more and more of the work of breathing by increasing spontaneous breathing. Advantages to the SIMV mode are the presence of built-in alarms to alert clinicians when ventilation problems occur and the guarantee of a minimum amount of minute ventilation. The disadvantage of SIMV is that each spontaneous breath requires some additional work of breathing to open the valve of the demand reservoir for gas. Depending on the type of ventilator, this increased work of breathing is felt to be relatively minor and to not interfere with most short-term weaning attempts.

T-Piece or Blow-By

The T-piece method of weaning involves removing the patient from the mechanical ventilator and attaching an oxygen source to the artificial airway with a "T" piece (Figure 6–10G). No ventilatory support occurs with this device, with the patient completely breathing spontaneously the entire time this device is connected. Many clinicians refer to this as the "sink or swim" method of weaning, where the patients either breathe on their own or they don't. The advantage of this method of weaning is that the resistance to breathing is low, since no special valves need to be pulled open in order to breath in gas. Rapid assessment of spontaneous breathing abilities is another purported advantage. Disadvantages with the T-piece are that PEEP therapy cannot be maintained and there are no alarm systems or backup systems to support the patient should ventilation be inadequate. This system relies on the clinician to monitor for signs and symptoms of respiratory difficulty.

CPAP

The use of the ventilator to allow spontaneous breathing without mandated breaths, similar to the T-piece, can be done with the CPAP mode. With this approach, ventilator alarm systems can be used to monitor spontaneous breathing rates and volumes, and PEEP can be maintained if needed. The disadvantage of this approach, similar to the SIMV mode, is that the resistance to breathing from the need to open the demand valve for each spontaneous breath is higher than with the T-piece. For most patients, this slight additional work of breathing is not likely to be a critical factor to their weaning success or failure.

Pressure Support

A relatively new method for weaning from ventilation is the use of pressure support (PS) ventilation. With this method, patients can spontaneously breathe on the ventilator with a small amount of ventilator "support" to augment their spontaneous breaths. This technique overcomes some of the resistance to breathing associated with ET tubes and demand valves. The main disadvantage with this approach is that clinicians may underestimate the degree of support to spontaneous breathing provided with this method and prematurely stop the weaning process. See Chapter 23, Advanced Respiratory Concepts, for a more detailed explanation of PS ventilation.

Troubleshooting Ventilators

The complexity of ventilators and the dynamic state of the patient's clinical condition, as well as the patient's response to ventilation, create a variety of common problems which occur during mechanical ventilation (Table 6–14). It is crucial that critical care clinicians be expert in the prevention,

TABLE 6–14. COMMON PROBLEMS RELATED TO MECHANICAL VENTILATION

Related to Equipment Malfunction
- Patient not receiving prescribed tidal volume
- Patient receiving no tidal volume

Related to Pathological Condition from Ventilator Use
- Barotrauma (increased airway pressures, pneumothorax, tension pneumothorax)
- Aspiration
- Nosocomial pneumonia
- GI bleeding
- Inappropriate ventilation (respiratory acidosis or alkalosis)
- Thick secretions
- Pulling or jarring of tracheostomy or ET tube causing patient discomfort
- High Pao_2
- Low Pao_2
- Decreased cardiac output with hypotension
- Anxiety and fear
- Arrhythmias or vagal reactions during or after suctioning
- Incorrect PEEP setting
- Inability to tolerate ventilator mode

Normal or Exaggerated Response to Mechanical Ventilation
- Intrathoracic pressure changes leading to decrease in cardiac output and to hypotension

Adapted from: Grossbach I: Troubleshooting ventilator- and patient-related problems, Parts 1 and 2. Critical Care Nurse; 1989;6(4,5):58–70, 64–71.

identification, and management of ventilator-associated problems in critically ill patients. Chapter 31, Ventilatory Troubleshooting Guide, details specific causes and intervention and prevention strategies for common ventilator-related problems.

During mechanical ventilation sudden changes in the clinical condition of the patient, particularly respiratory distress, as well as the occurrence of ventilator alarms and/or abnormal functioning of the ventilator, require immediate assessment and intervention. A systematic approach to each of these situations will prevent or minimize untoward ventilator events (Figure 6–17).

The first step is to determine the presence of respiratory distress or hemodynamic instability. If either is present the patient should be removed from the mechanical ventilator and manually ventilated with a MRB and 100% O_2 for a few minutes. During manual ventilation, a quick assessment of the respiratory and cardiovascular system should take place, noting changes from previous status. Clinical improvement rapidly following removal from the ventilator suggests a ventilator problem. Manual ventilation should be continued while another clinician corrects the ventilator problem (e.g., tubing leaks or disconnections, inaccurate gas delivery) or connects a replacement ventilator. Continuation of respiratory distress after removal from the ventilator and during manual ventilation suggests a patient-related cause.

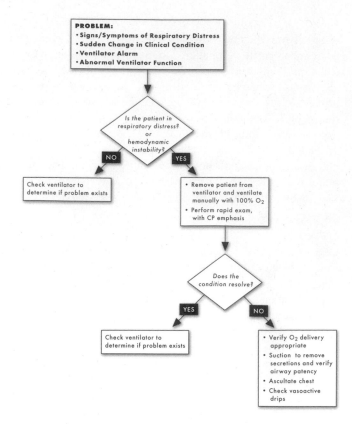

Figure 6–17. Algorithm for management of ventilator alarms and/or development of acute respiratory distress.

Patient Needs and Principles of Management

The majority of interventions related to mechanical ventilation focus on maximizing oxygenation and ventilation, prevention of complications associated with artificial airways, and/or the sequelae of assisting the patient's ventilation and oxygenation with an invasive mechanical device which does not mimic physiologic breathing.

Maximizing Oxygenation and Ventilation

1. Insure synchrony of respiratory patterns between ventilator and patient.
   - Give frequent explanations of the purpose of the ventilator and how to synchronize breathing with it.
   - Monitor the patient's response to ventilator therapy and for signs that the patient is out of phase with the ventilator respiratory pattern.
   - Consider ventilator changes to maximize synchrony (e.g., changes in flow rates, respiratory rates, sensitivities, and/or modes).

- Administer neuromuscular blockage and/or sedative agents as required to prevent asynchrony with the ventilator (see below).
2. Maintain a patent airway.
   - Suction when indicated according to standardized guidelines (Table 6–6).
   - Decrease secretion viscosity by maintaining adequate hydration, humidification of all inhaled gases, and administration of mucolytic agents as appropriate.
   - Monitor for signs and symptoms of bronchospasm and administer bronchodilator therapy as appropriate (Chapter 9, Critical Care Pharmacology; Chapter 13, Respiratory System).
   - Prevent obstruction of oral ET tubes by the use of an oral bite block.
3. Monitor oxygenation and ventilation status frequently.
   - ABG analysis as appropriate (e.g., 10 to 15 minutes after each ventilator change, with respiratory distress

or cardiovascular instability, or with significant changes in clinical condition).

- Continuous noninvasive monitoring of SaO_2. Validate noninvasive measures with periodic ABG analysis (Table 6–4).
- Observe for signs and symptoms of decreases in PaO_2, increases in $PaCO_2$, and/or respiratory distress. Development of respiratory distress requires immediate intervention (Figure 6–17).
- Reposition frequently to improve ventilation-perfusion relationships and prevent atelectasis.
- Aggressively manage pain, particularly chest and upper abdominal pain, to increase mobility, deep breathing, and coughing (Chapter 7, Pain Management).

5. Administer chest physiotherapy for selected clinical conditions (e.g., large mucous production, lobar atelectasis). Monitor oxygenation status closely during chest physiotherapy for signs and symptoms of arterial desaturation.
6. Maintain oxygenation and ventilatory support at all times.
- Ensure proper operation of the mechanical ventilator by activation of appropriately set alarms and frequent assessment of device function (usually, check every 1 to 2 hours).
- During even brief periods of removal from mechanical ventilation, maintain ventilation and oxygenation with MRB. During intrahospital transport, verify adequacy of ventilatory support equipment, particularly the maintenance of PEEP (when >10 cm H_2O is required).
- Emergency sources of portable oxygen should be readily available in the event of loss of wall oxygen capabilities.

Prevention of Complications Associated with Artificial Airways

1. Maintain ET or tracheostomy cuff pressures <5 cm H_2O.
2. Maintain artificial airway position by securing with tape or a special holder device. Frequently verify proper ET position by noting ET marking at lip or nares placed after intubation.
3. Ensure tape or devices used to secure the artificial airway are properly applied and are not causing pressure areas or skin breakdown. Periodic repositioning of ET

tubes may be required to prevent skin integrity problems.
4. Use a bite block with oral ET tubes if necessary to prevent accidental biting of the tube.
5. Provide frequent mouth care and assess for development of pressure areas from ET tubes.
6. Assess for signs and symptoms of sinusitis with nasal ET tube use (e.g., pain in sinus area with pressure, purulent drainage from nares, fever, increased WBC count).

Maximizing Communication Between the Nonverbal Patient and His or Her Family and Health Care Team Members

1. Assess communication abilities and establish at least a method for nonverbal communication (see the discussion of communication below). Assist the family members in using that approach with the patient.
2. Anticipate patient needs and concerns in the planning of care.
3. Ensure that call lights, bells, or other methods for notifying unit personnel of patient needs are in place at all times.
4. Frequently repeat information about communication limitations and how to use different nonverbal communication methods.

Reducing Anxiety and Providing Psychosocial Support

1. Maintain a calm, supportive environment to avoid unnecessary escalation of anxiety. Give brief explanations of activities and procedures. The vigilance and presence of health care providers during anxiety periods is crucial to avoid panic by patients and visiting family members.
2. Teach the patient relaxation techniques or diaphragmatic breathing to control anxiety (see Chapter 8, Alternative Therapies).
3. Administer mild doses of anxiolytics (e.g., lorazepam or diazepam) which do not depress respiration.
4. Encourage the family to stay with the patient as much as desired and to participate in caregiver activities as appropriate. Presence of a family member provides comfort, not only to the patient, but also assists the family member to better cope with the critical illness.

Neuromuscular Blockade

Neuromuscular blockade is a frequently used adjunct in critically ill patients, particularly when voluntary respiratory muscle movement needs to be abolished. Neuromuscular blocking agents are given intravenously to inhibit respiratory muscle movement in selected situations to improve oxygenation and ventilation. Use of these agents, however, is not selective to just the respiratory muscles; it leads to paralysis of all muscle groups, eliminating all voluntary muscle movement.

A variety of neuromuscular blocking agents are used in the critically ill patient, the most common of which are the nondepolarizing type of blockers (see Chapter 9, Critical Care Pharmacology, for a detailed discussion of these agents). Nondepolarizing blockers inhibit the transmission of nerve impulses by blocking cholinergic receptors in the neuromuscular junction. Muscle paralysis then results. The degree of neuromuscular blockade is determined by the number of receptors blocked, with full blockade resulting in flaccid muscles throughout the body. This level of blockade is most commonly used during thoracic and abdominal surgery. Partial blockade, most commonly used for management of critically ill patients, results in loss of most voluntary muscle movement (e.g., breathing; eye, head, and extremity movement; vocalization) with slight preservation of muscle tone.

The blocking of the neuromuscular junction does not alter pain pathways or the level of consciousness. Loss of voluntary muscle movement also eliminates the ability to respond to painful stimuli (e.g., withdrawal or verbalization). For this reason, use of neuromuscular blocking agents always requires the simultaneous administration of sedative agents and/or analgesic agents.

Management of Neuromuscular Blockade

The use of neuromuscular blockade, while a common phenomenon in critically ill patients, places a phenomenal responsibility on clinicians to safeguard the patient's physical and emotional well-being during this drastic approach to achieving improved physiologic functioning. While the focus is often on the physical safeguards, it is imperative that the importance of the patient's psychological well-being not be overlooked.

Assessment of Neuromuscular Blockade

The use of a peripheral nerve stimulator to provide a more accurate assessment of patients receiving neuromuscular blockade has been advocated to avoid the inadvertent overdosing with these agents. Reports of prolonged paralysis following neuromuscular blockade over the past decade have emphasized the importance of using the lowest possible dose to produce the desired respiratory effect.

Peripheral nerve simulators consist of an electrical device which deliver a series of electrical stimuli through electrodes applied to the skin (Figure 6–18). The electrical stimuli cause muscular contractions if the neuromuscular junction is functioning properly. Typically, peripheral nerve stimulation is performed on the ulnar nerve at the wrist. When disposable electrodes are applied to the ulnar nerve, the thumb abducts and the fingers flex during stimulation if the neuromuscular junction is intact.

The stimulator technique most commonly used to assess neuromuscular blockade is the Train of Four. With

this technique, four small electrical stimuli are given every half second. The degree of neuromuscular blockade can be assessed by observing or palpating the number of muscle twitches elicited during the series of four electrical stimuli (Figure 6–18).

When no neuromuscular blockade is present, four twitches of similar intensity, or height, will be noted. Following the administration of a nondepolarizing neuromuscular blocking agent, such as vecuronium, many of the neuromuscular junctions are blocked. This produces minimal response to the four delivered stimuli. As the level of neuromuscular block decreases over time, the number of twitches observed will increase until four strong, equal twitches are observed, indicating that no neuromuscular blockade is present.

The degree of neuromuscular blockade is approximately 90% when one small twitch is palpated, 80% with two small twitches, and about 75% with three small twitches. Typically, in critical care patients, a moderate blockade level of 75 to 80% is usually sufficient to achieve respiratory muscle relaxation and improved gas exchange. The presence of two or three twitches in response to the Train of Four stimulation indicates a reasonable level of neuromuscular blockade for most critically ill patients.

Communication

Mechanically ventilated (MV) patients are unable to speak and communicate verbally due to the presence of a cuffed

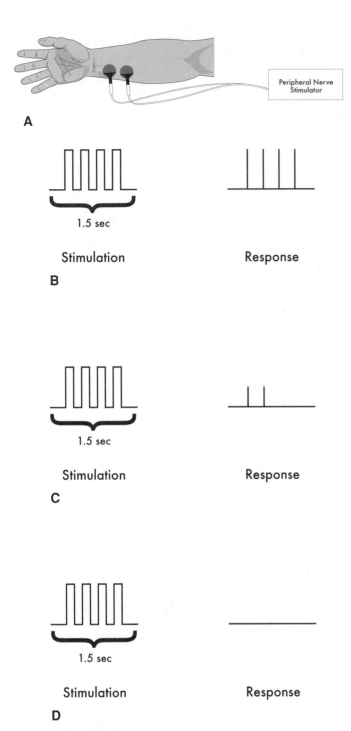

Figure 6–18. (A) Peripheral nerve stimulator and graphic display of train of four patterns for (B) no neuromuscular block, (C) moderate block (80%), and (D) complete block.

ET or tracheostomy tube. The inability to speak is frustrating for the patients, for the nurses, and for all members of the health care team. Impaired communication results in patients experiencing anxiety and fear, symptoms that can have a deleterious effect on their physical, as well as emotional, condition. Stories of patients interviewed after extu-

AT THE BEDSIDE

Nurse: "A former ventilator patient described to me how terrified she became when the ventilator connecting tubing 'popped off' the end of her endotracheal tube. She tried screaming, but no sound was produced and her call light was nowhere within her reach."

AT THE BEDSIDE

Patient: "Being on a ventilator was hell. You couldn't talk, you couldn't drink, you couldn't eat. When they pulled the tube out of my mouth, it was like being pulled out of hell in a way."

bation revealed how isolated and alone they felt because of their inability to speak.

Common Communication Problems

Patients' perceptions of communication difficulties related to mechanical ventilation include: (1) inability to communicate, (2) insufficient explanations, (3) inadequate understanding, (4) fears and dangers of not being able to speak, and (5) difficulty with communication methods. Except for the problem of inability to vocalize, all of the problems cited by ventilated patients could be resolved easily by critical care practitioners. For instance, "insufficient explanations" and "inadequate understanding" can be remedied by frequent repetition of all plans and procedures in language that is understandable to a nonmedical person and that takes into account that attention span and cognitive abilities, especially memory, are frequently diminished due to the underlying illness or injury, effects of medications and anesthesia, and the impact of the critical care environment.

Although most messages the MV patient will need to communicate lie within a narrow range ("pain," "hunger," "water," and "sleep"), communicating these basic needs is usually difficult. Most adults are accustomed to attending to their own basic needs, but in the intensive care unit, not only are they unable to physically perform certain activities, but they cannot even communicate effectively what those needs are. Basic needs include such activities as bathing, brushing teeth, combing hair, urinating and defecating, eating, drinking, and sleeping. Other examples of important basic needs which critical care nurses frequently must address are "too hot," "too cold," "turn me," "up," "down," "straighten my legs," "my arm hurts," "I can't breathe," and "moisten my lips."

Patients have described difficulties with communication methods while being mechanically ventilated. This also can be avoided by assessing the MV patient's communication abilities. Is the patient alert and oriented? Can the patient answer simple yes and no questions? Does the patient speak English? Can the patient use at least one hand to gesture? Does the patient have sufficient strength and dexterity to hold a pen and write? Is the patient's hearing and vision adequate? Knowledge of the patient's communication abilities assists the clinician to identify appropriate methods to use for communication (Figure 6–19).

Once the most successful communication methods have been identified for a particular patient, they should be written into the plan of care. Critical care units are very busy places, so it is easy to forget about the MV patient's need for communication. Continuity among health care professionals in their approach to communication with non-

vocal patients will improve the quality of care and increase patient satisfaction.

Common Methods For Communication with the Ventilator Patient

A variety of methods for augmenting communication with the temporarily voiceless MV patient are available and can be classified into two categories: nonvocal treatments (gestures, lip reading, mouthing words, paper and pen, alphabet/numeric boards, flashcards, etc.) and vocal treatments (talking tracheostomy tubes and speaking valves). The *best* way to communicate with the patient who has an artificial airway and/or is being mechanically ventilated is still largely unknown.

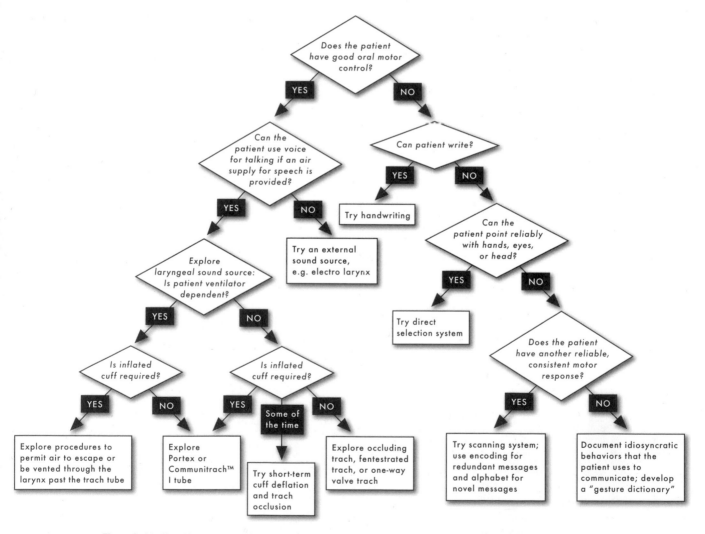

Figure 6–19. Algorithm for determining appropriate communication methods for temporarily nonvocal ventilator patients. *(Adapted from: Mitsuda PM, Baarslag-Benson R, Hazel K, Therriault TM: Augmentative communication in intensive and acute care unit settings. In Yorkston KM (ed.):* Augmentative communication in the medical setting. *Tucson, AZ: Communication Skill Builders, Inc., 1992, pp. 5–56.)*

AT THE BEDSIDE

Patient: "I'd cry because I was mad . . . angry at the whole thing . . . so they'd call a shrink, and I'd try to use the alphabet board to tell him (the psychiatrist) what was wrong, but it would take so long . . . so I'd get mad at him when he couldn't understand what I was trying to spell out."

AT THE BEDSIDE

Patient: ". . . the nurses that took more of a liking to you would take the time to try and understand me. Whereas, with some of the other ones, they just run back and forth doing their own thing. They couldn't understand me half of the time."

Nonvocal Treatments

Individual patient needs vary and it is recommended that the nurse use a variety of nonvocal treatments (e.g., gestures, alphabet board, and paper and pen). Success with communication interventions varies with the diagnosis, age, type of injury or disease, type of respiratory assist devices, and psychosocial factors. For instance, lip reading can be successful in patients who have tracheostomies since the lips and mouth are visible, but in the endotracheally intubated patient, where tape and tube holders limit lip movement and visibility, lip reading may be less successful.

Writing

Typically the easiest, most common method of communication readily available is the paper and pen. However, the supine position is not especially conducive to writing legibly. The absence of proper eyeglasses, an injured or immobilized dominant writing hand, or lack of strength also can make writing difficult for mechanically ventilated patients. Writing paper should be placed on a firm writing surface (e.g., clipboard) with an attached felt-tipped pen which will write in any position. Strength, finger flexibility and dexterity are required to grasp a pen. Many patients prefer to use a Magic Slate (Western Publishing Co., Racine, WI) or a Magna Doodle (Tyco Industries, Mount Laurel, NJ). These pressure-sensitive, inexpensive toy screens can be purchased at any department store; with them messages can be easily erased, maintaining the privacy of a written message.

A phenomenon of decoding exists between patient's written words (which often look like scribbling) and the nurse's ability to read what the patient wrote. The majority of the time, the nurse can read the writing of the patient even when it seems indistinguishable to a casual observer. This is due in part to the fact that over 65% of all communication is nonverbal and many contextual cues exist which assist in understanding and communicating effectively.

Gesturing

Another nonvocal method of communication which can be very effective is the *deliberate* use of gestures. Gestures are best suited for the short-term MV patient who is alert and can move at least one hand, even if only minimally. Generally well-understood gestures are emblematic, have a low level of symbolism, and are easily interpreted by most people.

For example, ventilated patients often indicate that they need suctioning by curving an index finger (to resemble a suction catheter), raising a hand toward the ET tube, and moving their hand back and forth. This is known as an idiosyncratic gesture, a gesture that is used by a particular community, e.g., the nurse and MV patient. Other idiosyncratic gestures include "ice chips," "moisten my mouth," "spray throat," and "doctor."

One important aspect of communicating by gesture is to "mirror" the gesture(s) back to the patient, at the same time verbalizing the message or idea conveyed by the patient's gesture. This mirroring will ensure accuracy in interpretation and will assist the clinician and patient to form a repertoire to be used successfully in future gestural conversations. When observing a patient's gestures, stand back from the bed, and watch his or her arms and hands. Most gestures are easily understood, especially those most frequently used by patients (e.g., the head nod, indicating "yes" and "no"). Practitioners should ask simple yes and no questions, but avoid playing "twenty questions" with ventilated patients because this can be very frustrating for them. Before trying to guess the needs of ventilated patients, give them the opportunity to use gestures to communicate their needs.

Alphabet Board/Picture Board

For patients who do not speak English, a picture board is sometimes useful along with well-understood gestures. Picture boards have images of common patient needs (e.g., bedpan, glass of water, medications, family, doctor, nurse) which can be pointed at by the patient. Picture boards, while commercially available, can be made easily and laminated to more uniquely meet the needs of a specific critical care population.

Another approach is the use of flash cards which can be purchased or made. Language flash cards contain common words or phrases in English or foreign languages.

Vocal Treatments

If patients with tracheostomies have intact organs of speech, they may benefit from vocal treatment strategies like pneumatic and electrical devices, fenestrated tracheostomy tubes, talking tracheostomy tubes, and tracheostomy speaking valves. Several conditions preclude use of vocalization devices, such as neurological conditions which impair vocalization (e.g., Guillain-Barré syndrome), severe upper airway obstruction (e.g., head/neck trauma), or vocal cord adduction (e.g., presence of an ET tube).

Two vocal treatments for tracheotomized patients are the Passy Muir Speaking Valve and the fenestrated tracheostomy tube (Figure 6–20). These tubes allow air to leak through fenestration points or holes in the outer cannula of the tracheostomy tube. There have been reported incidences of granuloma tissue development at the site adjacent to the fenestration, which resolves after removal of the tube. In addition, fenestrated ports often get clogged with secretions, again preventing voicing.

Another vocal treatment is the talking tracheostomy (e.g., COMMUNItrach I) which is designed to provide a means of verbal communication for the ventilator-dependent patient (Figure 6–21). It operates by gas flowing through an airflow line which has a fenestration just above the tracheostomy tube cuff. The air flows through the glottis, thus supporting vocalization. This device allows vocalization while still maintaining a closed ventilatory system. The cuff remains inflated with these tubes. However, an outside air source must be provided which is usually not humidified and the trachea can become dry and irritated. The line for this air source requires diligent cleaning and flushing of the air port to prevent it from becoming clogged. The patients must be able to shunt air through the tube with their fingers, which requires manual dexterity and coordination. The voice quality produced with this device is breathy or hoarse sounding. Patients who were otherwise considered to be "unweanable" have been reported to take a renewed interest in the weaning process and some successfully wean upon hearing their own voice.

Teaching Communication Methods

The critical care environment presents many teaching and learning challenges. Patients and families are under a considerable amount of stress, so the nurse must be a very creative teacher and offer communication techniques that are simple, effective, and easy to learn. The desire to communicate with loved ones, however, often makes the family very willing to learn. Frequently, it is the family who makes up large-lettered communication boards, or purchases a Magic Slate for the patient to use. Suggesting that families do this is usually very well received, since loved ones want so desperately to help in some way.

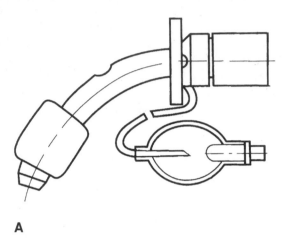

A

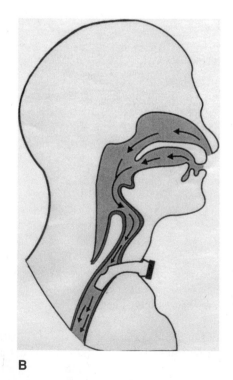

B

Figure 6–20. (A) Fenestrated tracheostomy tube. (B) Opening above the cuff site allowing gas flow past the vocal cords during inspiration and expiration. *(With permission from Mallinckrodt Medical, Inc., St Louis, MO, 1996.)*

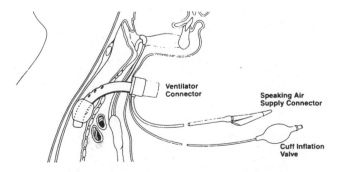

Figure 6–21. Talking tracheostomy. *(From: COMMUNItrach Product; formerly Implant Technologies, courtesy of Spectrum Medical, Irvine, CA.)*

AT THE BEDSIDE

Patient: "When I woke up and could not speak I thought it might be permanent . . . did I get scared."

All patients should be informed prior to intubation that they will be unable to speak during the intubation period. A flipchart illustrating what an endotracheal or tracheostomy tube is like, with labeling in simple words, could be shown to patients who will be electively intubated (e.g., for planned surgery). Practicing with a few nonverbal communication techniques before intubation (e.g., gestures, alphabet boards, flash cards) is also beneficial. Another important point to emphasize with patients is that being unable to speak is usually temporary, just while the breathing tube is in place. If preintubation explanations are not feasible or possible, provide these explanations to the intubated patient.

SELECTED BIBLIOGRAPHY

What Heals: Reducing Noise Levels

McCarthy DO, Ouimet ME, Daum JM: Shades of Florence Nightingale: Potential impact of noise stress on wound healing. *Hospital Nursing Practice.* 1991;5:39–48.

Williams M, Murphy JD: Noise in critical care units: A quality assurance approach. *Journal of Nursing Care Quality.* 1991;6:53–59.

General Critical Care

Burton GG, Hodgkin JE, Ward JJ: *Respiratory care: A guide to clinical practice.* Philadelphia: JB Lippincott, 1991.

Dossey BM, Guzzetta CE, Kenner, CV: *Critical care nursing: Body, mind, spirit.* Philadelphia: JB Lippincott, 1992.

DuPuis YG: *Ventilators: Theory and clinical application,* 2nd ed. St. Louis, MO: CV Mosby, 1992.

Kersten D: *Comprehensive respiratory nursing.* Philadelphia: WB Saunders, 1989.

Oakes D: *Clinical practitioners' pocket guide to respiratory care.* Old Town, ME: Health Educator Publications, 1988.

Luce J, Pierson D, Tyler M: *Intensive respiratory care,* 2nd ed. Philadelphia: WB Saunders, 1993.

McPherson S: *Respiratory therapy equipment,* 4th ed. St. Louis, MO: CV Mosby, 1990.

Tablan OC, Anderson LJ, Arden NH, Breiman RF, et al: Guideline for prevention of nosocomial pneumonia. Parts I and II. *American Journal of Infection Control.* 1994;22:247–292.

Ventilator Management

Burton GG, Hodgkin JE, Wark JJ: *Respiratory care: A guide to clinical practice,* 3rd ed. Philadelphia: JB Lippincott, 1993.

Craven D, Steger K: Nosocomial pneumonia in the intubated patient. New concepts on the pathogenesis and prevention. *Infectious Disease Clinics of North America.* 1993;3(4):843–866.

Hanneman SG, Ingersoll GL, Knebel AR, Shekleton M, Burns S, Clochesy J: Weaning from short-term mechanical ventilation: A review. *American Journal of Critical Care.* 1994;3(6):421–441.

Knebel A, Shekleton M, Burns S, et al: Weaning from mechanical ventilation. *American Journal of Critical Care.* 1994;3(6):416–420.

Pierson DJ, Kacmarek RM: *Foundations of respiratory care.* New York: Churchill Livingstone, 1992.

Shapiro B, Warren J, Egol A, Greenbaum D, Jacobi J, Nasraway S, Schein R, Spevetz A, Stone J: Practice parameters for sustained neuromuscular blockade in the adult critically ill patient: An executive summary. *Critical Care Medicine.* 1995;23(9):1601–1605.

Tablan OC, Anderson LJ, Arden NH, Breiman RF, et al: Guideline for prevention of nosocomial pneumonia. Parts I and II. *American Journal of Infection Control.* 1994;22:247–292.

Tobin M: *Principles and practice of mechanical ventilation.* New York: McGraw Hill, 1994.

Communication

Buckwalter K, Cusack D, Sidles E, Wadle K, Beaver M: Increasing communication ability in aphasic/dysarthric patients. *Western Journal of Nursing Research.* 1989;11(6):736–747.

Connolly, M: Temporarily nonvocal trauma patients and their gestures: A descriptive study. *Dissertation Abstracts International,* University Microfilm, 1992.

Connolly, M: Nonvocal treatments for short and long-term ventilator patients. In Mason M: *Speech pathology for tracheostomized and ventilator dependent patients.* Newport Beach, CA: Voicing, Inc., 1993.

Connolly M, Shekleton M: Communicating with ventilator dependent patients. *Dimensions of Critical Care Nursing.* 1991;10(2):115–122.

Dowden PA, Honsinger MJ, Beukelman DR: Serving nonspeaking patients in acute care settings: an intervention approach. *Augmentative and Alternative Communication.* 1986:25–33.

Lawless C: Helping patients with endotracheal and tracheostomy tubes communicate. *American Journal of Nursing.* 1975;75:2151–2158.

Mitsuda PM, Baarslag-Benson R, Hazel K, Therriault TM: Augmentative communication in intensive and acute care unit settings. In Yorkston, KM (ed.): *Augmentative communication in the medical setting.* Tucson, AZ: Communication Skill Builders, Inc., 1992, pp. 5–56.

Pain Management

7

■ *What Heals: Creative Pain Control*

A "hot" topic increasingly being explored (and perhaps recognized) is the amount of pain patients experience as a result of various procedures performed daily in critical care and during postoperative surgical periods. The questions go like this: How much pain do we actually inflict on patients in the course of our daily care? Why have we assumed that patients must endure this pain? What can be done about it?

Likewise, it is distressing to inspect the research findings on pain management that have accumulated in the literature recently. When examined collectively, these studies broadcast an important message—there clearly is a discrepancy between the amount of pain patients experience and the amount of analgesics patients receive.

For example, one study of 44 ICU and surgical patients found that critical care and surgical nurses gave patients an average of only one-third the maximum narcotic dose ordered. Similar findings were identified in a sample of 40 cardiac surgical patients who received approximately half the average morphine dose prescribed over their first 3 days following surgery. In another study of 150 critically ill surgical patients, nurses administered less than half the intravenous and intramuscular morphine that was ordered for pain.

While these studies did not correlate pain intensity with analgesic amount, other studies have. For example, critically ill cardiovascular surgical patients reported that their average pain intensity remained at the level of 5 (on a 0 to 10 scale) over their first 3 postoperative days in ICU. Yet, patients received significantly smaller analgesic amounts over this time (day 1, 14.4 mg morphine; day 2, 9.6 mg; day 3, 6.4 mg). There is no clear explanation as to why pain medication was reduced over the 3 days, but it is clear that a decrease in pain over time was not the reason.

When it comes to poor pain management, there is enough blame to go around. Physicians have been blamed for inadequate analgesic drug ordering habits, nurses have been blamed for inadequately assessing the intensity of the patient's pain and therefore not giving enough of the medication, and at times patients have been blamed for not complaining loudly enough. Whatever the cause (and there are probably many), we know that 43% to 90% of patients continue to report moderate to severe pain or pain-related distress, despite analgesic treatment.

The clear implications are that we need to do better. Where do we start? The first step is acknowledging that there is a problem (e.g., our patients are enduring more pain than necessary). The next step is to implement the Clinical Practice Guidelines on Acute Pain Management: Operative or Medical Procedures and Trauma developed by the Agency for Health Care Policy and Research. This federal agency has synthesized research findings on pain control and developed recommendations to implement proactive, around-the-clock pain management which includes the use of nonpharmacologic interventions. Our challenge then is to determine what is the best combination of pharmacologic and nonpharmacologic therapies to provide creative pain control for patients with various painful illnesses and surgical procedures, as well as for those undergoing assorted procedures such as venipuncture, arterial sticks, endotracheal suctioning, chest tube insertion and removal, dressing changes, range-of-motion exercises, and ambulation.

CEG & BMD

INTRODUCTION

Pain management is central to the care of the critically ill or injured patient. Patients identify physical care that promotes pain relief and comfort as an important element of their hospitalization and recovery, especially while in the critical care environment. Providing optimum pain relief for critically ill patients not only enhances their psychoemotional well-being, but also can help avert additional physiologic injury for a patient who is already physiologically compromised. This chapter explores a multilevel approach to pain management in critically ill patients that is based on the physiologic mechanisms of pain transmission and human responses to pain. Within the multilevel approach, specific pharmacologic and nonpharmacologic pain management techniques are described, including the integral relationships among relaxation, sedation, and pain relief. Strategies also are presented that promote comfort and are easy to implement into a plan of care for critically ill patients. Finally, special considerations are delineated for vulnerable populations within the critical care setting.

PHYSIOLOGIC MECHANISMS OF PAIN

Peripheral Mechanisms

The pain response is elicited with tissue injuries, whether actual or potential. Undifferentiated free nerve endings, or nociceptors, are the major receptors signaling tissue injury (Figure 7–1). Nociceptors are polymodal and can be stimulated by thermal, mechanical, and chemical stimuli. *Nociception* refers to the transmission of impulses by sensory nerves which signal tissue injury.

At the site of injury, the release of a variety of neurochemical substances potentiates the activation of peripheral nociceptors. Many of these substances are also mediators of the inflammatory response and include histamine, kinins, prostaglandins, serotonin, and leukotrienes.

The nociceptive impulse travels to the spinal cord via specialized, afferent sensory fibers. Small, myelinated A-delta fibers conduct nociceptive signals rapidly to the spinal cord. The A-delta fibers transmit sensations that are generally localized and sharp in quality. In addition to A-delta fibers, smaller, unmyelinated C fibers also transmit nociceptive signals to the spinal cord. Because C fibers are unmyelinated, their conduction speed is much slower than their A-delta counterparts. The sensory quality of signals carried by C fibers tends to be dull and unlocalized.

Spinal Cord Integration

Sensory afferent fibers enter the spinal cord via the dorsal nerve, synapsing with cell bodies of spinal cord interneurons in the dorsal horn (Figure 7–1). Most of the A-delta and C fibers synapse in laminae I through V, in an area

AT THE BEDSIDE
▶ *Epidural Catheter Pain Management*

Thomas M. is 59 years old and was admitted to the surgical ICU following a thoracotomy with wedge resection of the left lung for small-cell lung cancer. On his second postoperative day, he continued to be mechanically ventilated with extubation planned for later in the day. Thomas had two left pleural chest tubes in place with moderate amounts of drainage and a continuing air leak. He was alert, responsive, and able to communicate his needs by writing notes and gesturing. He had a thoracic epidural catheter in place (T7-8) with a bupivacaine (0.625 mg/ml) and fentanyl (5 μg/mL) combination infusing at 6 ml/hour. When asked about his pain level, he wrote that it was 4 on a scale of 0 (no pain) to 10 (worst pain imaginable).

After Thomas was extubated, his nurse noticed he was reluctant to cough and seemed to have some difficulty taking a deep breath. She also noticed his oxygen saturation was slowly drifting downward from 97% to 95%. His respiratory rate was increasing, as was his heart rate. When she listened to his breath sounds, they were bilateral and equal, but diminished throughout with scattered gurgles. When she asked him about his pain, he said his pain was still a 4 as long as he didn't move or cough. He also indicated that he tried to avoid taking a deep breath because it would make him cough and that made the pain go to an 8 or 10.

The nurse knew it would be important for Thomas to breathe deeply and cough in order to clear his lungs, but his pain and discomfort was limiting his ability to perform those maneuvers. She discussed strategies with Thomas about how to help minimize the pain associated with activity. First, she found an extra pillow for Thomas to use as a splint to support not only his incision and chest wall, but also to stabilize his chest tubes.

Next, the nurse assessed the level of sensory blockade provided by the epidural local anesthetic. When she found his sensory level to extend bilaterally from T-10 to T-6, while his incision extended to T-4, she called the anesthesiologist to confer about increasing the rate of the bupivacaine infusion to increase the distribution of the local anesthetic to cover the incisional area. She also inquired about adding ketorolac to his analgesic regimen to help with pain associated with the chest tubes.

The addition of the pillows for splinting especially helped Thomas to take deep breaths. The anesthesiologist prescribed an increase in the infusion rate to 10 ml/hr and added ketorolac, 15 mg, IV every 6 hours. Over the course of the next 2 hours, the sensory block extended from T-11 to T-4 and Thomas was able to cough more effectively, with less pain. His oxygen saturation returned to 97%.

referred to as the *substantia gelatinosa*. Numerous neurotransmitters (e.g., substance P, glutamate, and calcitonin gene-related peptide) and other receptor systems (e.g., opiate, α-adrenergic, and serotonergic receptors) modulate the processing of nociceptive inputs in the spinal cord.

Central Processing

Following spinal cord integration, nociceptive impulses travel to the brain via specialized, ascending somatosensory pathways (Figure 7–1). The spinothalamic tract conducts nociceptive signals directly from the spinal cord to the thalamus. The spinoreticulothalamic tract projects signals to the reticular formation and the mesencephalon in the midbrain, as well as to the thalamus. From the thalamus, axons project to somatosensory areas of the cerebrocortex and limbic forebrain. The unique physiologic, cognitive, and emotional responses to pain are determined and modulated by the specific areas to which the somatosensory pathways project. For example, the thalamus regulates the neurochemical response to pain, while the cortical and limbic projections are responsible for the perception of pain and aversive response to pain, respectively. Similarly, the reticular activating system regulates the heightened state of awareness that accompanies pain. The modulation of pain by activities in these specific areas of the brain is the basis of many of the analgesic therapies available to patients to treat pain.

RESPONSES TO PAIN

Human responses to pain can be both physical and emotional. The physiologic responses to pain are the result of hypothalamic activation of the sympathetic nervous system associated with the stress response. Sympathetic activation leads to:

- Blood shifts from superficial vessels to striated muscle, the heart, the lungs, and the nervous system
- Dilation of the bronchioles to increase oxygenation
- Increased cardiac contractility
- Inhibition of gastric secretions and contraction
- Increases in circulating blood glucose for energy

Signs and symptoms of sympathetic activation frequently accompany nociception and pain:

- Increased heart rate
- Increased blood pressure
- Increased respiratory rate
- Pupil dilation
- Pallor and perspiration
- Nausea and vomiting

Although patients experiencing acute pain often exhibit signs and symptoms such as these, *it is critical to note that the absence of any or all of these signs and symptoms does not negate the presence of pain.* In fact, some

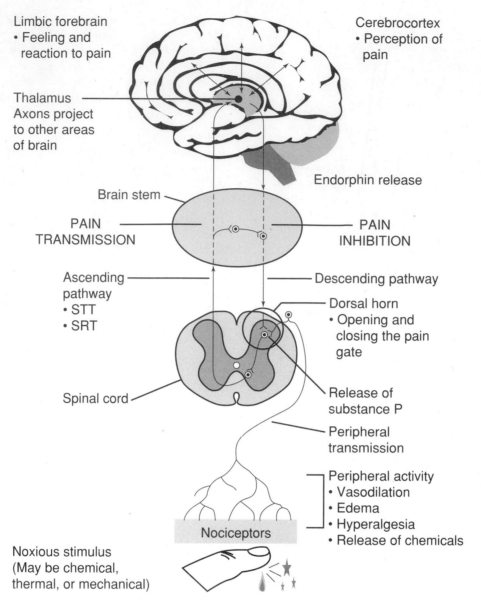

Figure 7–1. Physiologic pathway of pain transmission. *(From: Wild LR, Evans L: Pain. In Copstead L (ed.)* Perspectives on pathophysiology. *Philadelphia: WB Saunders, 1995, p. 934.)*

patients, especially those who are critically ill and with little or no compensatory reserves, may have a shock-like clinical picture in the presence of pain.

Critically ill patients also express pain both verbally and nonverbally. The expressions can take many forms, some of which are subtle cues that could easily be overlooked (Table 7–1). Any signs that may indicate pain warrant further exploration and assessment.

Although physiologic and behavioral correlates of acute pain have been described, each person's response to pain is unique. Also, it is important to remember that patients who are receiving neuromuscular blocking agents (e.g., pancuronium, vecuronium, or atracurium) may be unable to exhibit even subtle signs of discomfort because of the therapeutic paralysis. Neuromuscular blocking

agents do not affect sensory nerves and have no analgesic qualities.

PAIN ASSESSMENT

Pain assessment is a core element of ongoing surveillance of the critically ill patient. Self-report of pain intensity and distress should be used whenever possible, especially for patients who can talk or communicate effectively in other ways. Regular documentation of pain assessment not only helps monitor the efficacy of analgesic therapies, but also helps ensure communication among caregivers regarding patients' pain. A variety of tools to assess pain intensity are available. Three commonly used scales are shown in Table 7–2. With the Numeric Rating Scale (NRS), patients use

TABLE 7–1. EXAMPLES OF PAIN EXPRESSION IN CRITICALLY ILL PATIENTS

Verbal Cues	Facial Cues	Body Movements
Moaning	Grimacing	Splinting
Crying	Wincing	Rubbing
Screaming	Eye signals	Rocking
Silence		Rhythmic movement of extremity
		Shaking or tapping bed rails
		Grabbing the nurse's arm

numbers between 0 and 10 or 0 and 100 to describe their pain intensity. Some patients find it easier to use adjectives to describe their pain. The Verbal Descriptive Scale (VDS) offers patients a standardized list of adjectives to describe their pain intensity. With the Visual Analogue Scale (VAS), patients indicate their pain intensity by drawing a vertical line, bisecting a 10-cm baseline. The baseline is anchored at either end by the terms *no pain* and *worst pain imaginable*. A numeric conversion is done by measuring the line from the left anchor to the patient's mark, in centimeters.

Any of these scales can be used with patients who are intubated and unable to speak. For example, patients can be asked to use their fingers to indicate a number between 0 and 10; similarly, patients can be asked to indicate by nodding their head or pointing to the appropriate adjective or number as they either hear or read the list of choices. With the VAS, the line can be printed on a sheet of paper or marker board and the patients asked to mark the line to indicate their level of pain.

Unfortunately, some critically ill patients are unable to indicate their pain intensity either verbally or nonverbally. In these situations, nurses must use other clues to assess their patients' pain. In addition to monitoring physiologic parameters, nurses can also anticipate and recognize clinical situations where pain is likely to occur and use their knowledge of physiology and pathophysiology and experience with other patients with similar problems. By combining their knowledge and experience with well-developed interviewing and observational skills, critical care nurses can assess patients' pain effectively and intervene appropriately.

TABLE 7–2. PAIN ASSESSMENT TOOLS COMMONLY USED IN CRITICALLY ILL PATIENTS

Numeric Rating Scales (NRS)

NRS Verbal (0 to 10 scale)	NRS-101 (0 to 100 scale)
0 = no pain	0 = no pain
10 = worst pain imaginable	100 = worst pain imaginable

Verbal Descriptive Scale

None	Mild	Moderate	Severe

Visual Analogue Scale

no pain _____ worst pain imaginable

A MULTILEVEL APPROACH TO PAIN MANAGEMENT

Today there are numerous approaches and therapies available to treat acute pain. Whereas pharmacologic techniques traditionally have been the mainstay of analgesia, other complementary or nonpharmacologic methods are growing in their acceptance and use in clinical practice. Most therapies used in the treatment of acute pain can be used effectively in the critically ill. General guidelines or strategies to maximize analgesia in critically ill patients are summarized in Table 7–3.

One of the central goals of pain management is to combine therapies that target as many of the processes involved in nociception and pain transmission as possible. Analgesic therapies, both pharmacologic and nonpharmacologic, exert their effects by altering nociception at specific structures within the peripheral or central nervous system (i.e., the peripheral nociceptors, the spinal cord, or the brain) or by altering the transmission of nociceptive impulses between these structures (Figure 7–2). By understanding where analgesic therapies work, nurses can more effectively select a combination of therapies working at different sites to best treat the source or type of pain patients experience and, subsequently, help patients achieve optimal analgesia.

To assist nurses to select and maximize analgesic therapies, for each of the analgesic therapies presented here, there is a brief description of where and how the selected therapy works, clinical situations where it can be used most effectively, and strategies for titrating the therapy. Finally, because few therapies exert a singular effect, a summary of secondary or side effects commonly associated with the therapies and strategies to minimize their occurrence are also addressed.

NONSTEROIDAL ANTIINFLAMMATORY DRUGS

Nonsteroidal antiinflammatory drugs (NSAIDs) target the peripheral nociceptors. The NSAIDS exert their effect by modifying or reducing the amount of prostaglandin produced at the site of injury by inhibiting the formation of the enzyme cyclooxygenase which is responsible for the breakdown of arachidonic acid and formation of the neurotrans-

TABLE 7–3. STRATEGIES TO MAXIMIZE ANALGESIA

1. Assess pain.
2. Set realistic analgesic goals with the patient.
3. Substitute as requested with either around-the-clock dosing, continuous infusions, or PCA medication administration and titrate to desired response.
4. Set the stage for success: provide support and encouragement for patients; spend time with them.
5. Consider the broad range of therapies available; target multiple levels for intervention.
6. Document response to pain management therapies.

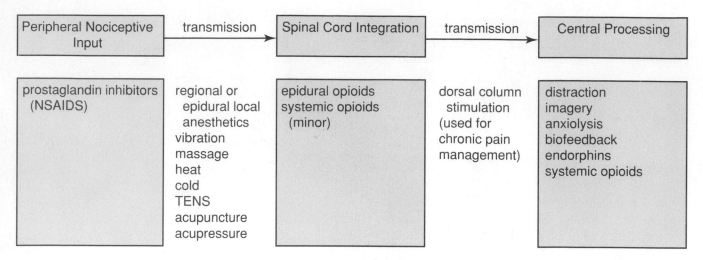

Figure 7–2. A multilevel approach to pain management.

mitter prostaglandin. As prostaglandin inhibitors, the NSAIDs have been shown to have opioid-sparing effects and are very effective in managing pain associated with inflammation, trauma to peripheral tissues (e.g., soft tissue injuries), bone pain (e.g., fractures, metastatic disease), and pain associated with indwelling tubes and drains (e.g., chest tubes).

One of the NSAIDs commonly used in the critical care setting is ketorolac tromethamine (Toradol). Ketorolac is currently the only parenteral NSAID preparation available in the United States and can be administered safely by either the intravenous (IV) or the intramuscular (IM) route. Recommended dosing for ketorolac is a 30-mg loading dose followed by 15 mg every 6 hours. Like all NSAIDs, ketorolac has a ceiling effect where administration of higher doses offers no additional therapeutic benefit yet significantly increases the risk of toxicity associated with the drug.

The side effects associated with the use of NSAIDs relate to the function of prostaglandins in physiologic processes in addition to nociception. For example, gastrointestinal (GI) irritation and bleeding may result from NSAID use because prostaglandins are necessary for maintaining the mucous lining of the stomach. Similarly, the enzyme cyclooxygenase is needed for the eventual production of thromboxane, a key substance involved in platelet function. As a result, when NSAIDs are used chronically or in high doses, platelet aggregation may be altered, leading to bleeding problems. NSAID use can also lead to renal toxicity. Cross-sensitivities with other NSAIDs have also been documented (e.g., ibuprofen, naproxen, indomethacin, piroxicam, aspirin). For these reasons, ketorolac and other NSAIDs should be avoided for patients who have a history of gastric ulceration, renal insufficiency, and coagulopathies or a documented sensitivity to aspirin or other NSAIDs. The severity of all NSAID-related side effects increases with high doses or prolonged use. For this reason, ketorolac

is designed for short-term therapy only and should not be used for more than 5 days.

OPIOIDS

The principal modality of pain management in the critical care setting continues to be opioids. Traditionally referred to as narcotics, opioids produce their analgesic effects primarily by binding with specialized opiate receptors throughout the central nervous system (CNS) and thereby altering the perception of pain. Opiate receptors are located in the brain, spinal cord, and gastrointestinal tract. Although opioids work primarily within the CNS, they also have been shown to have some local or peripheral effects.

Opioids are well tolerated by most critically ill patients and can be administered by many routes including IV, IM, oral, buccal, nasal, rectal, transdermal, and intraspinal. Morphine sulfate (MSO_4) is still the most widely used opioid and serves as the gold standard against which others are compared. Other opioids commonly used in the care of the critically ill include hydromorphone (Dilaudid), fentanyl (Sublimaze), and meperidine (Demerol). One of the key aspects of opioid therapy is that each one potentially produces the same degree of pain relief; none is inherently more likely to produce analgesia than another. Table 7–4 summarizes the equianalgesic IV doses and special considerations for commonly used opioids.

Opioid Side Effects

Patients' responses to opioids, both analgesic responses and side effects, are highly individualized. Just as all the opioid agents have similar pain-relieving potential, all opioids currently available share similar side-effect profiles. When side effects do occur, it is important to remember that they are primarily the result of opioid pharmacology, as opposed to the route of administration.

TABLE 7–4. COMMONLY USED INTRAVENOUS OPIOIDS

Drug	Equianalgesic Dose	Onset (minutes)	Duration (hours)	Special Considerations
Morphine	1 mg	2–5	4	
Hydromorphone	0.15 mg	2–5	2–4	
Fentanyl	10–25 μg	1–2	1–1.5	Highly lipid soluble; muscle rigidity has been reported with high doses
Meperidine	10 mg	2–5	2–3	Active metabolite (normeperidine) which can accumulate resulting in CNS excitation and seizures; tachyarrhythmias can result

Nausea and Vomiting

Nausea and vomiting are distressing side effects often related to opioids that, unfortunately, many patients experience. Generally, nausea and vomiting result from stimulation of the chemoreceptor trigger zone (CTZ) in the brain and/or from slowed gastrointestinal (GI) peristalsis. Nausea and vomiting often can be managed effectively with antiemetic therapy. Metoclopramide (Reglan), a procainamide derivative, works both centrally at the CTZ and at the GI level to increase gastric motility. Most patients will benefit from a 10-mg IV dose every 4 to 6 hours.

The vestibular system also sends input to the CTZ. For this reason, opioid-related nausea frequently is exacerbated by movement. If patients complain of movement-related nausea, the application of a transdermal scopolamine patch can help prevent and treat opioid-induced nausea. The use of transdermal scopolamine is best avoided, however, in patients whose age is >60 years as the drug has been reported to increase the incidence and severity of confusion in older patients.

Other antiemetics such as the phenothiazines (prochlorperazine [Compazine], 2.5 to 10 mg IV) and the butyrophenones (droperidol [Inapsine], 0.625 mg IV) treat nausea through their effects at the CTZ. The serotonin antagonist ondansetron (Zofran) is also effective for treatment of opioid-related nausea. The doses required for postoperative or opioid-related nausea are significantly smaller doses (4 mg IV) than those used with emetogenic chemotherapy.

Pruritus

Pruritus is another opioid-related side effect commonly reported by patients. The actual mechanisms producing opioid-related pruritus are unknown. Although antihistamines can provide symptomatic relief for some patients, the role of histamine in opioid-related pruritus is unclear. One of the drawbacks of using antihistamine agents, such as diphenhydramine (Benadryl), is the sedation associated with their use. Similar to other opioid side effects, the incidence and severity of pruritus is dose-related and tends to diminish with ongoing use.

Constipation

Constipation, another common side effect, results from opioid binding at opiate receptors in the GI tract and decreased peristalsis. Whereas the incidence of constipation may be low in critically ill patients, it is important to remember that it is likely to be a problem for many patients after the critical phase of their illness or injury. The best treatment for constipation is prevention by ensuring adequate hydration, as well as by administering stimulant laxatives and stool softeners, as needed.

Urinary Retention

Urinary retention can result from increased smooth muscle tone caused by opioids, especially in the detrussor muscle of the bladder. Opioids have no effect on urine production and neither cause nor worsen oliguria. Urinary retention is generally not a problem for critically ill patients since many have indwelling urinary catheters to facilitate and measure bladder drainage.

Respiratory Depression

Opioid therapy can result in respiratory depression through its effects on the respiratory centers in the brain stem. Both respiratory rate and depth of breathing can decrease as a result of opioids, usually in a dose-dependent fashion. Patients at increased risk for respiratory depression include the elderly, those with preexisting cardiopulmonary diseases, and those who receive large doses. Frequently, the earliest sign of respiratory depression is an increased level of sedation, making this an important component of patient assessment. Other signs and symptoms of respiratory depression include decreased depth of breathing, often combined with slowed respiratory rate, constriction of pupils, and hypercapnia ($PaCO_2$>45 mm Hg).

Clinically significant respiratory depression is usually treated with IV naloxone. Naloxone (Narcan) is an opioid antagonist; it binds with opiate receptors, temporarily displacing the opioid and suspending its pharmacologic effects. As with other medications, naloxone should be administered in very small doses and titrated to the desired level of alertness (Table 7–5). It should be emphasized that

TABLE 7–5. ADMINISTRATION OF NALOXONE

1. Support ventilation.
2. Dilute 0.4 mg (400 µg) ampule of naloxone with normal saline to constitute a 10-ml solution.
3. Administer in 1-ml increments, every 2 to 5 minutes, titrating to desired effect. Onset of action: approximately 2 minutes.
4. Continue to monitor patient; readminister naloxone as needed. Duration of action: approximately 45 minutes.
5. For patients requiring ongoing doses, consider naloxone infusion: administer at 50 to 250 µg/hour, titrating to desired response.

the half-life of naloxone is short—approximately 30 to 45 minutes. Because of its short half-life, additional doses of naloxone may be needed. Naloxone should be used with caution in patients with underlying cardiovascular disease; the acute onset of hypertension, pulmonary hypertension, and pulmonary edema with naloxone administration has been reported (Burke & Dunwoody, 1990). Also, naloxone should be avoided in patients who have developed a tolerance to opioids since as an opioid antagonist it can precipitate withdrawal or acute abstinence syndrome.

Intravenous Opioids

Because many critically ill patients are unable to use the oral route and pain management needs often fluctuate, the IV route is used most often. One of the advantages of IV opioids is their rapid onset of action, allowing for easy titration. Loading doses of IV opioids should be administered to achieve an adequate blood level of the drug; additional doses can then be administered intermittently to maintain analgesic levels.

Many critically ill patients can benefit from the addition of a continuous IV opioid infusion. For example, patients who may not be able to communicate their pain management needs effectively, including those who are receiving neuromuscular blocking agents, are good candidates for continuous opioid infusions. The continuous infusion not only helps achieve the appropriate blood levels, but also can be easily titrated to maintain consistent blood levels. Patients who experience significant fluctuations in analgesia or side effects related to opioid administration may also benefit from the constant blood levels provided by continuous infusions. Whenever possible, the maintenance dose for the infusion should be based on patients' previous opioid requirements.

Patient-Controlled Analgesia

Patient-controlled analgesia (PCA) pumps can also be used effectively in the critical care setting to administer opioids. With PCA, patients self-administer small doses of an opioid infusion using a programmable pump. PCA prescriptions typically include an incremental or bolus dose of the selected drug, a lockout or delay interval, and either a 1- or 4-hour limit; many of the PCA devices also can be pro-

AT THE BEDSIDE
▶ *Chemical Dependence*

Susan is a 22-year-old who was admitted to the cardiovascular ICU (CVICU) following a tricuspid valve replacement related to recurrent subacute bacterial endocarditis. She has a self-reported history of heroin use (approximately 2 g/day).

She was extubated within the first 24 hours after surgery, but remained in the CVICU for stabilization of fluid balance. During change-of-shift report the off-going nurse commented that ". . . she is a constant whine. She refuses to do anything. All she wants is to go out for a smoke and more drugs. She had 10 mg of IV morphine from the PCA pump."

When the nurse came into Susan's room to do her initial assessment, Susan said, "I can't take much more of this pain." The nurse probed further and asked Susan to use some numbers to describe her pain. Susan replied, "It's at 10!"

The nurse noticed that Susan was reluctant to move and she refused to cough. Her vital signs were:

Heart rate:	130/minute
BP:	150/85 mm Hg
Temperature:	38.5°C (orally)
Respiration rate:	26/minute, shallow

The nurse was concerned that considering Susan's preoperative use of heroin, she might not be receiving adequate doses of morphine. She consulted the clinical nurse specialist for assistance in calculating an equivalent dose of morphine based on Susan's usual heroin use. Using an estimated equivalence of heroin, 1 g = 10 to 15 mg morphine, the nurse calculated that Susan would need approximately 20 to 30 mg of morphine per day to account for her preexisting opioid tolerance; analgesic needs related to her surgery would need to be in addition to this baseline need. The primary nurse approached the surgical team to discuss the potential benefits of using a patient-controlled analgesia (PCA) pump in addition to a continuous infusion of morphine. "By doing this," the nurse explained, "Susan could receive her baseline opioid requirements that are related to her tolerance by the continuous infusion, while using the patient-controlled boluses to treat her new surgical pain. The PCA could also offer her some control during a time in her recovery when there are few avenues to maintain it." In addition to starting the PCA with a continuous infusion, the surgical team and the primary nurse also discussed using other nonopioid agents such as nonsteroidal antiinflammatory agents (NSAIDs) to augment her analgesia.

In addition to the changes in the medications, the primary nurse worked with Susan to use relaxation techniques. The nurse explained that relaxation techniques could be thought of as "boosters" to her pain medications and were something that she could do to control the pain. She and Susan also agreed to try massage in the evening to try to promote sleep and relaxation.

grammed to deliver a basal or background infusion. The incremental dose refers to the amount of the drug the patient receives following pump activation. The initial dose usually ranges between 0.5 and 2 mg of morphine, or its equivalent (refer to Table 7–4). The lockout or delay interval typically ranges between 5 and 10 minutes, which is enough time for the prescribed drug to circulate and take effect, yet allows the patient to easily titrate the medication over time. The 1- or 4-hour limit serves as an additional safety feature by regulating the amount of medication the patient can receive over this period of time.

Titrating PCA

As with nurse-administered IV opioid boluses, PCA is most effective when patients can titrate the amount of medication they receive to meet their analgesic needs by maintaining consistent blood levels. Patients will usually find a dose and frequency that balances pain relief with other medication-related side effects such as sedation. It is best to start PCA therapy after the patient has received loading doses to achieve adequate blood levels of the prescribed opioid. For patients who continue to experience pain while using the PCA pump, the first step in titration is to increase the incremental or bolus dose, usually by 50%. If patients continue to have pain in spite of the increased dose, the lockout interval or delay should then be reduced, if possible.

Patients who report problems with awakening in pain and feeling "behind" with their analgesia may benefit from the addition of a low-dose, continuous infusion. A continuous infusion is also recommended for patients who have preexisting opioid tolerance. In this way, the continuous infusion maintains their baseline opioid requirements, while the patient-controlled incremental doses are available to help manage any new pain they experience. The hourly dose of the continuous infusion should be equianalgesic to and calculated from patients' preexisting opioid requirements.

EPIDURAL ANALGESIA

Over the past decade the use of epidural analgesia has grown rapidly, especially in the critical care setting. The advantages of epidural analgesia include improved pain control with less sedation, lower overall opioid doses, and generally longer duration. Epidural analgesia has been associated with a lower morbidity and mortality in criti-

cally ill patients.[1] Both opioids and local anesthetics, either alone or in combination, commonly are administered via the epidural route. The mechanisms of action and the resultant clinical effects produced by epidurally administered opioids and local anesthetics are distinct. For this reason, these agents not only are discussed separately below, but also should be distinguished when used in clinical practice.

Epidural Opioids

When opioids are administered epidurally, they diffuse into the cerebrospinal fluid (CSF) and into the spinal cord (Figure 7–3). There, the opioids bind with opiate receptors in the substantia gelatinosa, preventing the release of the neurotransmitter, substance P, and subsequently alter the transmission of nociceptive impulses from the spinal cord to the brain. Because the opioid is concentrated in the areas of high opiate receptor density and where nociceptive impulses are entering the spinal cord, lower doses offer enhanced analgesia, with few, if any, supraspinal effects such as drowsiness.

A variety of opioids are commonly used for epidural analgesia including morphine, fentanyl, meperidine, and hydromorphone. Preservative-free (PF) preparations are usually preferred as some preservative agents can have neurotoxic effects. The opioids can be administered either by intermittent bolus or by continuous infusion depending on the pharmacokinetic activity of the selected agent. For example, fentanyl is generally administered via continuous infusion due to its high lipid solubility, resulting in a short duration of action. In contrast, the low lipid solubility of PF morphine results in a delayed onset of action (30 to 60 minutes) and a prolonged duration of action (6 to 12 hours). Because of this, PF morphine can be administered effectively as an intermittent bolus.

Side Effects of Epidural Opioids

The side effects associated with epidural opioids are the same as those described above. It is important to remember that side effects are related more closely to the drug administered than by the route of administration. For example, the incidence of nausea and vomiting with epidural morphine is similar to that associated with IV morphine. Although epidural opioids were once feared to be associated with a higher risk of respiratory depression, clinical studies and experience have not confirmed this risk. The incidence of respiratory depression has been reported as being ≤0.2%.[2] Risk factors for respiratory depression are similar to those seen with intravenous opioids: increasing age, high doses,

[1]Yeager MP, Glass DD, Neff RK, Brinck-Johnsen T: Epidural anesthesia and analgesia in high-risk surgical patients. *Anesthesiology.* 1987;66:729–736.
[2]Ready LB, Loper KA, Nessly M, Wild L: Postoperative epidural morphine is safe on surgical wards. *Anesthesiology.* 1991;75:452–456.

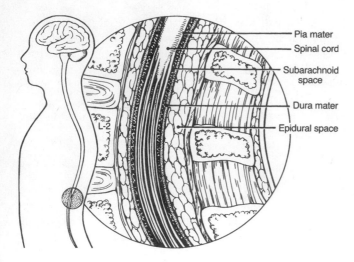

Figure 7–3. Epidural space for catheter placement.

underlying cardiopulmonary dysfunction, and the use of perioperative or supplemental parenteral opioids in addition to epidural opioids.

Epidural Local Anesthetics

Epidural opioids can also be combined with dilute concentrations of local anesthetics (LA). When administered in combination, these agents work synergistically, reducing the amount of each agent that is needed to produce analgesia. Whereas epidurally administered opioids work in the dorsal horn of the spinal cord, epidural LAs exert work primarily at the dorsal nerve root by blocking the conduction of afferent sensory fibers. The extent of the blockade is dose-related. Higher LA concentrations block more afferent fibers within a given region, resulting in an increased density of the blockade. Higher infusion rates of LA-containing solutions increase the extent or spread of the blockade since more afferent fibers will be blocked over a broader region.

Bupivacaine is the LA most commonly used for epidural analgesia and is usually administered in combination with either fentanyl or PF morphine as a continuous infusion. The concentration of bupivacaine used for epidural analgesia usually ranges between 1/16% (0.065 mg/ml) and 1/8% (1.25 mg/ml). These concentrations are significantly lower than those used for surgical anesthesia, which usually range between 1/4% and 1/2% bupivacaine. The type and concentration of opioid used in combination with bupivacaine vary by practitioner and organizational preferences, but usually range between 2 and 5 µg/ml fentanyl or between 0.02 and 0.04 mg/ml PF morphine.

Side Effects of Epidural Local Anesthetics

The side effects accompanying LAs are a direct result of the conduction blockade produced by the agents. Unfortu-

nately, the LA agents are relatively nonspecific in their capacity to block nerve conduction. That is, LAs not only block sensory afferent fibers, but also can block the conduction of motor efferent and autonomic nerve fibers within the same dermatomal regions. Side effects that can be associated with epidural LAs include hypotension—especially postural hypotension from sympathetic blockade—and functional motor deficits from varying degrees of efferent motor fiber blockade. Sensory deficits, including changes in proprioception in the joints of the lower extremities, can accompany epidural LA administration due to the blockade of nonnociceptive sensory afferents.

The extent and type of side effects that can be anticipated with epidural LAs depend on three primary factors: the location of the epidural catheter, the concentration of the LA administered, and the volume or rate of infusion. For example, if a patient has an epidural catheter placed within the midthoracic region, one could anticipate signs of sympathetic nervous blockade, such as postural hypotension, since the sympathetic nerve fibers are concentrated in the thoracic region. In contrast, a patient with a lumbar catheter may experience a mild degree of motor weakness in the lower extremities as the motor efferent and nerves exit the spine in the lumbar region. This usually presents clinically as either heaviness in a lower extremity or an inability to "lock" the knee in place when standing.

Also, as noted above, both the concentration and infusion rate of the LA will influence the severity and extent of side effects. The density of the blockade and intensity of observed side effects may be increased with high LA concentrations. With higher infusion volumes, greater spread of the LA can be anticipated which can, in turn, lead to a greater number or extent of side effects. If side effects occur, the dose of the LA often is reduced either by decreasing the concentration of the solution or by decreasing the rate.

Titrating Epidural Analgesia

To maximize epidural analgesia, doses may need to be adjusted. With opioids alone, the dose needed to produce effective analgesia is best predicted by the patient's age as opposed to body size. Older patients typically require lower doses to achieve pain relief than those who are younger. Small bolus doses of fentanyl (50 µg) can help to safely titrate the epidural dose or infusion to treat pain. Similarly, a small bolus dose of fentanyl can also help treat breakthrough pain that may occur with increased patient activity or with procedures. For patients receiving combinations of LAs and opioids, a small bolus dose of the prescribed infusate in conjunction with an increased rate can help titrate pain relief. Recall, however, that increasing the rate of the LA infusion increases the spread of the drug to additional dermatomes, whereas increasing the LA concentration increases the depth or intensity of the blockade and subsequent analgesia.

CUTANEOUS STIMULATION

One of the primary nonpharmacologic techniques for pain management used in the critical care setting is cutaneous stimulation. Cutaneous stimulation produces its analgesic effect by the altering conduction of sensory impulses as they move from the periphery to the spinal cord through the stimulation of the largest sensory afferent fibers, known as the A-alpha and A-beta fibers. The sensory information transmitted by these large fibers is conducted more rapidly than that carried by their smaller counterparts (A-delta and C fibers). As a result, nociceptive input from the A-delta and C fibers is believed to be "pre-

empted" by the sensory input from the nonnoxious cutaneous stimuli. Examples of cutaneous stimulation include the application of heat, cold, vibration, or massage. Transcutaneous electrical nerve stimulation (TENS) units produce similar effects by electrically stimulating large sensory fibers.

Cutaneous stimulation can produce potent analgesia whether used as a complementary therapy with other pharmacologic treatments or as an independent treatment modality. Nurses can integrate these therapies easily and safely into analgesic treatment plans for the critically ill, especially for patients who may be unable to tolerate higher opioid doses. To apply or administer cutaneous stimulation, one simply needs to stimulate sensory fibers anywhere between the site of injury and the spinal cord, but within the sensory dermatome (Figure 7–4). Massage, especially back massage, has additional analgesic benefits as it has been

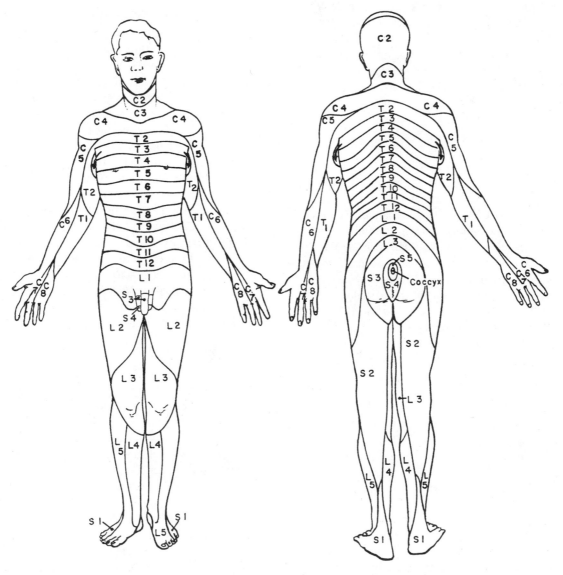

Figure 7–4. Sensory dermatomes.

shown to promote relaxation and sleep, both of which can influence patients' responses to pain.

DISTRACTION

Distraction techniques such as music, conversation, television viewing, laughter, and deep breathing for relaxation can be valuable adjuncts to pharmacologic therapies. These techniques produce their analgesic effects by sending intense stimuli through the thalamus, midbrain, and brain stem, which can increase the production of modulating substances such as endorphins. Also, since the brain can process only a limited amount of incoming signals at any given time, the input provided by distraction techniques "competes" with nociceptive inputs. This is particularly true for the reticular activating system.

When planning for and using distraction techniques, keep in mind that they are most effective when activities are interesting to the patient (e.g., their favorite type of music, television program, or video) and when they involve multiple senses such as hearing, vision, touch, and movement. Activities should be consistent with patients' energy levels and, most of all, be flexible to meet changing demands.

IMAGERY

Imagery is another technique that can be used effectively with critically ill patients, particularly during planned procedures (see also Chapter 8, Alternative Therapies). Imagery alters the perception of pain stimuli within the brain, helps promote relaxation, and can increase the production of endorphins in the brain. Patients can use imagery independently or use guided imagery where either a care provider, family member, or friend helps "guide" the patient in painting an imaginary picture. The more details that can be pictured with the image, the more effective it can be. As with distraction techniques, tapping into multiple sensations is beneficial. Some patients prefer to involve the pain in their picture and imagine it melting or fading away. Other patients may prefer to paint a picture in their mind of a favorite place or activity. Strategies to help guide patients include the use of details to describe the imaginary scene (e.g., "smell the fresh scent of the ocean air" or "see the intense red hue of the sun setting beyond the snow-capped mountains") and the use of relaxing sensory terms such as *floating, smooth, dissolving, lighter,* or *melting.* If the patients are able to talk, it can be helpful to have them describe the image they see using appropriate detail, although some patients will prefer not to talk and instead focus on their evolving image. Again, it is important to be flexible in the approach to imagery to maximize its benefits.

RELAXATION AND SEDATION TECHNIQUES

Because critically ill patients experience numerous stressors, most patients will benefit from the inclusion of relaxation or anxiolytic therapies (see also Chapter 8, Alternative Therapies). The use of relaxation techniques can help interrupt the vicious cycle involving pain, anxiety, and muscle tension that often develops when pain goes unrelieved. The physiologic response associated with relaxation includes decreased oxygen consumption, respiratory rate, heart rate, and muscle tension; blood pressure may either normalize or decrease.

A wide variety of pharmacologic and nonpharmacologic techniques can be used safely and effectively with critically ill patients to achieve relaxation and/or sedation. Relaxation techniques are simple to use and can be particularly useful in situations involving brief procedures such as turning or minor dressing changes, following coughing or endotracheal suctioning or other stressful events.

Deep Breathing and Progressive Relaxation

Guided deep breathing and progressive relaxation can be incorporated easily into a plan of care for the critically ill patient. Nurses can coach patients with deep breathing exercises by helping them focus on and guide their breathing patterns. As patients begin to control their breathing, nurses can work with them to begin progressive relaxation of their muscles. To do this, the nurse can say to the patient as he or she just begins to exhale, "Now begin to relax, from the top of your head to the tips of your toes." Change the pitch of the voice to be higher for "top of your head," lower for "tips of your toes," and be timed such that the final phrase ends as the patient completes exhalation. This procedure capitalizes on the positive aspects of normal body functions, as the body tends to relax naturally during exhalation. This process can and should be "practiced" during nonstressful periods to augment its efficacy. In fact, teaching and coaching patients to use deep breathing exercises will help equip them with a lifelong skill that can be used any time stressful or painful situations arise.

Pharmacologic Anxiolysis

A number of pharmacologic agents are also available to help manage anxiety. The agents used most commonly are the benzodiazepines, but other types of sedatives, such as propofol, are also being introduced into the critical care setting (Table 7–6). When using sedative agents in conjunction with opioid analgesics, it is important to remember that the agents potentiate each other. Doses may need to be adjusted and patients should be monitored closely for the cardiovascular and respiratory depressant effects of the medications.

Presence

Probably the single most important aspect of promoting comfort in the critically ill or injured is the underlying relationship between the patient and his or her care providers.

TABLE 7–6. COMMONLY PRESCRIBED SEDATIVES AND ANXIOLYTICS

	Midazolam	Lorazepam	Diazepam	Propofol
Type	Short-acting	Long-acting	Short-acting	Short-acting
Dose	1–4 mg Q 1–2 hours	0.5–2 mg Q 4–6 hours	2–10 mg Q 3–6 hours	10–25 µg/kg/minute
Onset	1 to 5 minutes	5 minutes (can take up to 1 hour to see effects)	1 to 5 minutes	1 to 5 minutes
Duration	1 to 6 hours	4 to 8 hours	1 to 4 hours	10 to 20 minutes
Infusions	Yes	Yes	Not recommended	Yes
Other	Administer in 0.5-mg increments when initiating therapy, especially in the elderly.	Can accumulate, especially in the elderly and those with renal insufficiency.	Half-life is 20 to 36 hours, depending on age. Can accumulate; duration increases with repeated dosing.	Suspended in lipid solution; monitor time out of refrigeration. Best if given via central line as is a vein irritant.

Presence not only refers to physically "being there," but also refers to psychologically "being with" a patient. Although presence has not been well defined as an intervention protocol, patients regularly describe the importance of the support that their nurses render simply by "being there" and "being with" them.

SPECIAL CONSIDERATIONS FOR PAIN MANAGEMENT IN THE ELDERLY

The pain experience of elderly patients has often been shadowed by myths and misperceptions. Some believe that older patients have less pain because their extensive life experiences have equipped them to cope with discomfort more effectively. Although this may be true for some individuals, to accept this generalization as truth for all elderly patients is short-sighted. In fact, the incidence of and morbidity associated with pain is higher in the elderly than in the general population.[3] Many elderly patients continue to experience chronic pain in addition to any acute pain associated with their critical illness or injury. Major sources of underlying pain in the elderly include low back pain, arthritis, headache, chest pain, and neuropathies.

Assessing Pain in the Elderly Patient

Elderly patients often report pain very differently from younger patients due to physiologic, psychologic, and cultural changes accompanying age. Some patients may fear loss of control or being labeled as a "bad patient" if they report pain-related concerns. Also, for some patients the presence of pain may be symbolic of impending death, especially in the critical care setting. In cases such as this, a patient may be reticent to report his or her pain to a care provider or family member as if to deny pain is to deny death. For reasons such as these, it is important for nurses not only to assure patients about the nature of their pain and the importance of reporting any discomfort, but also to use a variety of pain assessment strategies to incorporate behavioral or physiologic indicators of pain.

Similar strategies are often needed to assess pain in persons who are cognitively impaired. Preliminary reports from ongoing work among nursing home patients suggest that many patients with moderate to severe cognitive impairment are able to report acute pain reliably at the time they are asked. For these patients, pain recall and integration of pain experience over time may be less reliable.

Interventions

Critically ill elderly patients can benefit from any of the analgesic therapies discussed above. It is important to recall that for some elderly patients, medication requirements may be reduced due to the decreased clearance with varying degrees of renal insufficiency that accompanies aging. However, as with all patients, regardless of age, analgesic requirements are highly individualized and doses should be carefully titrated to achieve pain relief.

SELECTED BIBLIOGRAPHY

What Heals: Creative Pain Control

Maxam-Moore VA, Wilkie DJ, Woods SL: Analgesics for cardiac surgery patients in critical care: Describing current practice. *American Journal of Critical Care.* 1994;3:31–39.

Puntillo K: Advances in management of acute pain: Great strides or tiny footsteps? *Capsules and Comments in Critical Care Nursing.* 1995;3:97–100.

Puntillo K, Weiss SJ: Pain: Its mediators and associated morbidity in critically ill cardiovascular surgical patients. *Nursing Research.* 1994;43:31–36.

Sun X, Weissman C: The use of analgesics and sedatives in critically ill patients: Physicians' orders versus medications administered. *Heart and Lung.* 1994;23:169–176.

[3]Cook J, Rideout E, Browne G: The prevalence of pain complaints in a general population. *Pain.* 1984;2:49–53.

Tittle M, McMillan SC: Pain and pain-related side effects in an ICU and on a surgical unit: Nurses' management. *American Journal of Critical Care*. 1994;3:25–39.

US Department of Health and Human Services: *Acute pain management: Operative or medical procedures and trauma. Clinical practice guidelines*. Rockville, MD: Agency for Health Care Policy and Research, Public Health Service, US Department of Health and Human Services, 1992.

Pain Management

Beyer JE: *The Oucher: A user's manual and technical report*. Evanston, IL: Hospital Play Equipment, 1984.

Burke DF, Dunwoody CJ: Naloxone: A word of caution. *Orthopaedic Nursing*. 1990;9(4):44–46.

Cook J, Rideout E, Browne G: The prevalence of pain complaints in a general population. *Pain*. 1984; 2:49–53.

Faucett J: Care of the critically ill patient in pain: The importance of nursing. In Puntillo KA (ed.): *Pain in the critically ill*. Gaithersburg, MD: Aspen, 1991.

Gardner DL: Presence. In Bulechek GM, McCloskey JC (eds.): *Nursing interventions: Essential nursing treatments*. Philadelphia: WB Saunders, 1992, pp. 316–324.

Maxam-Moore VA, Wilkie DJ, Woods SL: Analgesics for cardiac surgery patients in critical care: Describing current practice. *American Journal of Critical Care*. 1994;3:31–39.

McCaffery M, Beebe A: *Pain: Clinical manual for nursing practice*. St. Louis, MO: CV Mosby, 1989.

McGrath P, Johnson G, Goodman J, Schillinger J, Dunn J, Chapman J: CHEOPS: A behavioral scale for rating postoperative pain in children. *Advances in Pain Research and Therapy*. 1985;9:395–402.

Pettigrew J: Intensive nursing care: The ministry of presence. *Critical Care Nursing Clinics of North America*. 1990;2(3):503–508.

Puntillo K: Pain experience in intensive care patients. *Heart and Lung*. 1990;19:526–533.

Puntillo K: Advances in management of acute pain: Great strides or tiny footsteps? *Capsules and Comments in Critical Care Nursing*. 1995;3:97–100.

Puntillo K, Weiss SJ: Pain: Its mediators and associated morbidity in critically ill cardiovascular surgical patients. *Nursing Research*. 1994;43:31–36.

Ready LB, Chadwick HS, Ross B: Age predicts effective epidural morphine dose after abdominal hysterectomy. *Anesthesia and Analgesia*. 1987;66:1215–1218.

Ready LB, Loper KA, Nessly M, Wild L: Postoperative epidural morphine is safe on surgical wards. *Anesthesiology*. 1991; 75:452–456.

Sun X, Weissman C: The use of analgesics and sedatives in critically ill patients: Physicians' orders versus medications administered. *Heart and Lung*. 1994;23:169–176.

Tittle M, McMillan SC: Pain and pain-related side effects in an ICU and on a surgical unit: Nurses' management. *American Journal of Critical Care*. 1994;3:25–39.

US Department of Health and Human Services: *Acute pain management: Operative or medical procedures and trauma. Clinical practice guidelines*. Rockville, MD: Agency for Health Care Policy and Research, Public Health Service, US Department of Health and Human Services, 1992.

Wong DL, Baker CM: Pain in children: Comparison of assessment scales. *Pediatric Nursing*. 1988;14(1):9–17.

Yeager MP, Glass DD, Neff RK, Brinck-Johnsen T: Epidural anesthesia and analgesia in high-risk surgical patients. *Anesthesiology*. 1987;66:729–736.

Alternative Therapies

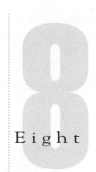

Eight

► Knowledge Competencies

1. Discuss the scientific rationale for using alternative therapies such as relaxation, imagery, music therapy, and touch in the critical care setting.

2. Describe guidelines for implementing alternative therapies with critical care patients and for personal use by critical care clinicians.

3. Compare and contrast critical care patients desired outcomes and subjective experiences with one or more alternative therapies.

■ What Heals: Preparing for a Difficult Event

Frequently, patients mentally rehearse the events surrounding their procedures, treatments, and surgery. Much of this mental rehearsal can involve negative imagery, anxiety, and fear. Patients can be taught to rehearse such situations positively, however, and to replace anxiety and fear with healthy responses. Guided imagery is one such strategy that nurses can combine with traditional teaching to help patients gain a feeling of control over the event. Patients can be guided in mentally rehearsing the experience and seeing themselves as doing well and being relaxed before, during, and after the event.

An example of this is Mr. B., a 64-year-old IBM executive who was about to undergo a cardiac catheterization. The following dialogue took place:

Nurse: *"Mr. B., how are you feeling about your cardiac catheterization?"*

Mr. B.: *"I'm scared to death. I keep having these ideas about how awful it's going to be. All I've ever seen really is stuff on television. It looks scary."*

Nurse: *"I would like to share some positive ideas with you, as well as a few skills that you can use during the procedure to help you get through it more easily. Would you be interested?"*

Mr. B.: *"You bet. What do I need to do?"*

Nurse: *"Let me ask you a few questions. Tell me about where you like to relax. What is the most perfect place which makes you feel calm and happy?"*

Mr. B.: *"That's easy. I have some property in southern Colorado with a pond, beavers, and big rainbow trout. Boy, I'd sure like to go fishing up there soon."*

Nurse: *"That's perfect. Let me guide you now in some basic relaxation skills that you can use during your cardiac catheterization. Then I'll use the information you just gave me about the beaver pond. Okay?"*

Mr. B.: *"I'm ready."*

The nurse then guided Mr. B. in a 15-minute imagery session that incorporated teaching, relaxation, and imagery. The following script was used:

Nurse: *"Mr. B., with your eyes closed and your body relaxed and lying still, travel ahead in time to the morning of your cardiac catheterization. You are awake and feeling refreshed, relaxed, and confident about this procedure. Use these first few alert, awake moments to feel the relaxation from the top of your head to the tips of your toes."*

At this point, the nurse followed a general relaxation script (See Chapter 28, Alternative Therapies Table). At the end of the general relaxation script, this is what followed:

Nurse: *"It is now time for you to get on the stretcher and go to the cardiac catheterization laboratory. You will know information soon that will help you make decisions about your continued recovery. As you ride down the hall, use this time to focus on breathing in and out and feeling very relaxed. See yourself entering the cardiac catheterization room and being greeted by two nurses. As you move onto the cardiac catheterization table, feel the security of that table as the nurses place a strap over your legs and arms to help you maintain this position. At this time, the nurses begin to prepare you for the procedure by connecting ECG leads to your chest to monitor your heart. They will wash and shave the catheter insertion sites. Continue to use this time to concentrate on your breathing and achieve a deeper state of relaxation.*

"You hear the cardiologist entering now. He greets you and makes you feel confident and cared for. Your physician begins by numbing the skin in your groin area for your comfort during the procedure. When the physician injects the contrast media to see your heart on x-ray, you may feel "hot flashes" or a burning sensation or you may feel a sense of nausea. Use this time to do your diaphragmatic deep breathing.

"At this point you feel in control of the situation. You feel confident and relaxed. Allow yourself to go to southern Colorado. It feels so good to be back. Smell the mountain air, the pine trees so fresh and strong. Look at the different trees—the aspens as their leaves quake in

the sun, the magical tall blue spruces with their unmistakable color. Look at the squirrels playing.

"Today seems special. You are walking down the path which leads to the beaver pond. You hear twigs and leaves snap and crunch as you step on them. You feel balanced while you walk. This walk is relaxed and you have nothing to do today except watch the beavers play and maybe catch some trout.

"As you get to the edge of the pond, you see the beavers playing. Neither you nor the beavers are afraid. Feel yourself with your fishing pole and bait in hand. You start to fish for the first time in a long while. Feel the excitement of that first cast. It seems perfect. You get a bite, but the trout is just playing with your line.

"As you continue your fishing, you hear the physician tell you that everything is going fine. He asks you to cough and you do so. Then you continue your image; you again bring it back into full clear, focus, adding more details—the colors, the smells, the environment, what you are doing, and what the beavers are doing. Now focus your concentration on this image for the next few minutes.

"The next thing you hear is your physician telling you that the procedure is over and it went very well. He tells you he will give you the details in a few hours.

"You feel relieved that the procedure went well. Now you are back in bed where you will remain for the next 4 to 6 hours. You remember not to move the leg where the catheter was inserted or to flex or fully extend it. You feel thirsty from the contrast media. This is normal and the nurses provide you with fluids. Also you feel the need to urinate frequently. Feel yourself successfully using the urinal while in bed. Give yourself a pat on the back for staying calm and relaxed and playing an important role in making the procedure go well.

"Now begin to feel the muscles around your eyes become less heavy as you start to move slowly and gently. And when you are ready, just open your eyes and look around."

Mr. B. was instructed to practice this exercise a few more times on his own before his cardiac catheterization. The nurse did one more session with him and was available to answer any questions.

Following his cardiac catheterization, Mr. B said that the relaxation and imagery techniques helped him tremendously in getting through the procedure. He felt relaxed during the procedure and in control of the situation. He also reported catching one of the biggest trout that he had ever caught while on the cardiac catheterization table.

CEG & BMD

Adapted from: Going fishing during a cardiac catheterization. In Guzzetta CE, Dossey BM: Cardiovascular nursing: Holistic practice. St. Louis, MO: Mosby-Year Book, 1992, pp. 542–543.

RATIONALE FOR USE OF ALTERNATIVE THERAPIES

Alternative therapies are independent nursing interventions used to treat frequently encountered problems such as anxiety, fear, ineffective coping, pain, restlessness, and sleep disturbances in critical care patients. Problems such as these have both a physiologic and a psychologic component which are responsive to alternative therapies because they are aimed at treating the body and the mind. Such interventions, when combined with the best of conventional therapies, technology, and medications, enlarge the critical care clinician's options for effective therapy in achieving optimal psychophysiologic patient outcomes.

The scientific foundation for using many of the alternative therapies is based on psychophysiologic self-regulation. Self-regulation theory focuses on the effects of parasympathetic control and the cognitive processing of information on human behavior. Many alternative therapies evoke a psychophysiologic state characterized by parasympathetic dominance in which physical, mental, and emotional tension are absent. Individuals are able to learn how to create inner calmness by evoking conscious control of the sympathetic nervous system to bring involuntary body responses (e.g., heart rate, blood pressure, respirations, muscle tension) under voluntary control.

According to self-regulation theory, perception (or imagery) elicits mental and emotional responses, generating limbic, hypothalamic, and pituitary biochemical responses. These biochemical responses bring about physiologic changes, which are again perceived and responded to, completing a cybernetic feedback loop. Any perception or image functions as a blueprint. A blueprint is a cognitive or mental device that saves and directs the retrieval of the stored information, the focus of attention, and the resulting behaviors and thoughts/images. Alternative therapies such as relaxation, imagery, and music therapy help individuals gain access to the raw material of their inner memories and internal healing resources. These new imagery patterns become new blueprints that can be reinforced or reframed into patterns that may modulate positive changes at the biochemical levels within the cells. These blueprints assist individuals in focusing their attention to influence desired psychophysiologic and behavioral responses and outcomes.

Mind Modulation and the Autonomic System

Psychoneuroimmunology is a relatively new field of research investigating the bidirectional interaction of the mind (psychologic state) on the immune, central nervous, and endocrine systems. This research has demonstrated that the mind modulates the biochemical functions within the major organ systems throughout the autonomic nervous system. The psychophysiologic stress response causes the stress hormones (e.g., cortisol, epinephrine, and norepinephrine) to mediate changes in physiologic and pathologic events which simultaneously produce corresponding psychologic and spiritual events. The process of mind modulation of cellular activities by the autonomic nervous system has three stages:

- Images, thoughts, attitudes, and feelings are generated in the frontal cortex.
- Images and thoughts are transmitted through state-dependent memory, learning, and emotional areas of the limbic-hypothalamic system by the neurotransmitters that regulate the organ systems of the autonomic nervous system branches.
- Neurotransmitters—norepinephrine (sympathetic branch) and acetylcholine (parasympathetic branch)—initiate the information transduction that activates the biochemical changes in the different tissues down to the cellular level. Neurotransmitters act as messenger molecules. They cross the nerve cell junction and fit into receptor sites found in cell walls, thus changing the receptor molecule structure. This causes a change in cell wall permeability and a shift of such ions as sodium, potassium, and calcium. The

basic metabolism of each cell is also changed by the hundreds of complex activations of cell enzymes that comprise the second messenger system.

These three stages provide an understanding of the way in which alternative therapies work. When patients are taught how to use relaxation, imagery, or music therapy, their sympathetic response to stress is reduced and the calming effect of the parasympathetic system takes over, leading to body-mind healing. These responses serve to "retune" the nervous system by dampening the production of catecholamines which stimulate limbic activity. Such changes are literally connections of patients' images, feelings, emotions, and spirit with their physiology or pathophysiology. If the actual anatomical locations were traced from the limbic system where a person's images and feelings are formed, they can be shown to correlate with physiologic changes in the brain which follow those nerve pathways down the spinal cord to then emerge to innervate every organ in the body. There are no exceptions. And all these nerves also flow from the organ systems back up to the imagery and feeling center in the limbic brain.

The newly recognized neuropeptides also have advanced our understanding of how the mind and body communicate. Neuropeptides are amino acids that open the lock to receptor sites to facilitate or block specific cellular responses. Because the autonomic, endocrine, and immune systems all make and use these messenger molecules, these systems are able to "talk" to each other. As a result, the autonomic, immune, and endocrine systems are all integrated by the neuropeptides which are responsible for connecting the body and emotions. Thus, from the research in the field of psychoneuroimmunology, we now know that what an individual feels and thinks can actually change his or her physiology.

Recognizing Anxiety and Helping Patients Cope

Patients admitted to the critical care unit get anxious for a variety of reasons because of symptoms, illness, or new diagnoses; from discomfort or pain related to tests, complications, procedures, or surgery; or because of the emotional stressors caused by medical costs and interrupted work and home routines, as well as unresolved or ongoing family crises. Just waiting for test results or anticipating painful or major procedures causes anxiety in most people. Therefore, assessing anxiety and coping is essential.

Anxiety is a vague, uneasy feeling of worry or apprehension, the source of which is often nonspecific or unknown to the individual. Anxiety is a normal reaction when a person experiences a threat to his or her physical body, loved ones, lifestyle, or values. Anxiety can stimulate a person toward purposeful action while excessive anxiety interferes with efficient functioning, causing a state of disequilibrium or tension. Anxiety can be assessed by evaluating the subjective and objective characteristics (Table 8–1)

TABLE 8–1. SUBJECTIVE AND OBJECTIVE CHARACTERISTICS OF ANXIETY

Subjective Characteristics	Objective Characteristics
• Verbalizes increased muscle tension	• Wrinkled brow and/or strained facial expression
• Verbalizes tight breathing	• Sweaty palms
• Preoccupation with a sense of impending doom	• Changes in speech pattern
• Verbalizes difficulty falling asleep	• Interrupted sleep patterns
• Feelings of tingling in hands and feet	• Tachypnea and/or tachycardia
• Expresses continuous feeling of apprehension	• Psychomotor agitation: startles easily, restlessness, jitteriness, fidgeting
• Feelings of "butterflies" in stomach	• Meaningless gestures
• Repeated expressions of concern about changes in health status and outcome of illness	• Hypervigilance (scans environment)
• Verbalizes restlessness	• Crying
• Expresses worry about complications	• May be cool, calm, self-contained

to identify whether the patient has mild, moderate, or severe anxiety or is having panic attacks (Table 8–2).

Anxiety prompts attempts at coping. Coping is a strategy to reduce tension and promote a sense of well-being between patients and their internal or external environment, as listed in Table 8–3. Ineffective coping increases tension states, requiring increased demand for energy and resulting in greater anxiety. Effective coping decreases tension states, however, and frees up energy to be used to enhance healing and well-being. Thus, the goal of care is to enhance the patient's physiologic and emotional equilibrium by implementing body-mind therapies along with effective coping strategies.

Anxiety involves changes in the patient's internal environment and external environment. The patient's subjective experience about his or her internal environment is assessed by the feelings that the patient verbalizes. These feelings might include an inability to cope; a sense of loss

TABLE 8–2. DEGREES OF ANXIETY

Mild Anxiety	Moderate Anxiety	Severe Anxiety	Panic Attacks
• Increased alertness • Increased perceptual field	• Selective inattention • Can focus on only one thing • Narrowed perceptual field	• Scattered, reduced perceptual field • Irrelevant things become the focus	• Unexpected attack of intense fear, discomfort, physiological sensations (smothering, choking, dyspnea, dizziness, faintness, tachycardia, trembling, numbness, chills, chest pain, sense of going crazy, losing control, or dying)

TABLE 8–3. EFFECTIVE AND INEFFECTIVE COPING

Effective Coping		Ineffective Coping	
Physiologic Responses	*Psychological Responses*	*Patient's Internal Environment*	*Patient's External Environment:*
• Normal heart rate • Normal blood pressure • Normal respirations • Normal peripheral skin temperature • Relaxed facial and body muscles	• Awareness that increased anxiety affects personal behavior • Understands inner anxiety response • Recognizes contributing factors to anxiety • Evaluates personal coping style • Appropriate defense mechanisms • Can select more effective coping mechanisms when needed • Realistic personal expectations • Realistic perception of current situation • Willingness to try new coping skills	• Loss of control • Helplessness • Loss of function • Loss of self-esteem • Sense of isolation • Failure of previous coping strategies • Fear of complications or fear of dying	• Noxious stimuli • Invasions of privacy • Medical/nursing jargon related to tests, procedures, or disease/illness

of control, self-esteem, and isolation; feelings of helplessness and dependence; or fear of dying. The external environment that increases anxiety includes noxious stimuli, numerous interruptions that prevent rest and sleep, invasions of personal privacy, and jargon about treatments, procedures, and disease/illness.

When either the internal or the external environment is in disequilibrium, the resulting anxiety and ineffective coping amplify sympathetic nervous system responses, producing rapid heart rates, increased blood pressure and respirations, peripheral vasoconstriction, and dry mouth. Often, despite these physiologic responses, patients may appear to be cool, calm, and self-contained. Both ranges of responses, from control to panic, require an enormous amount of energy.

Evaluate what is known about the patient's situation. Determine whether the patient is effectively or ineffectively coping by assessing his or her physiologic and psychologic coping responses and perception of his or her internal and external environments. Based on the patient problems and desired outcomes identified for anxiety and ineffective coping (Table 8-4), select one or more alternative therapies presented in Chapter 28, Alternative Therapies Table:

- Coping and stress tolerance
- Cognitive and perceptual impairments
- Self-care
- Role and relationships

INTEGRATING ALTERNATIVE THERAPIES INTO PRACTICE

Relaxation

Relaxation is a body-mind-spirit state characterized by the absence of physical, mental, and emotional tension characteristic of parasympathetic dominance or a hypometabolic

response that is the opposite of the "fight or flight" response. Relaxation allows individuals to achieve states of inner calmness and an ability to focus inward. With relaxation, individuals learn to untighten tense muscles, use relaxed abdominal breathing, decrease worried thoughts, and retreat from the stressful events of the day. Regardless of the relaxation intervention(s) used, the end result is a movement toward balance and harmony. Retreating from one's surroundings and learning conscious control of one's body-mind is a skill that requires practice. It is an effective way to increase sensitivity and awareness of being in the present moment.

Relaxation interventions can be used by patients for a few minutes or, for best results, for a period of 20 minutes several times a day. Patients can be encouraged to practice these skills throughout the day, particularly prior to or during a procedure, treatment, or surgery (if awake). The most effective way to achieve an inward or body-centered relaxation response is by focusing attention on slow, relaxed breathing. Key words or phrases to use in relaxation exercises are *clear, release, calm, open, loosen, peace,* or *smooth out.* Encourage patients to choose a comfortable word, phrase, or favorite prayer and say it slowly over and over again until relaxation is experienced. The most frequently used relaxation interventions are rhythmic breathing exercises, body scanning, autogenics, the relaxation response, prayer, and biofeedback.

Rhythmic Breathing Exercises

Rhythmic, abdominal breathing exercises are essential to achieving relaxation. To teach patients how to correctly use relaxed breathing, take a few minutes and practice the three exercises in Figure 8–1. It is important for the clinician to feel comfortable using these techniques and to learn to evoke a relaxation state in herself or himself before attempting to implement them with patients.

With stress, tension, anxiety, and ineffective coping, it is common to use the shoulders and upper chest to breath.

TABLE 8–4. PATIENT NEEDS/PROBLEMS, DESIRED OUTCOMES, AND INTERVENTIONS

Patient Problems/Needs	Patient Outcomes	Interventions	Evaluation

• Anxiety
• Ineffective coping
	• Patient will demonstrate decreased anxiety as evidenced by decreased tension and restlessness and normal heart rate, blood pressure, respirations, and muscle tension.
	• Patient will talk about anxiety.
	• Patient will demonstrate effective use of relaxation, imagery, touch and music intervention.
	• Patient will demonstrate effective use of coping skills as evidenced by effective use of cognitive, physical, and emotional strategies.
	• Patient will experience increased restful sleep.
		1. Address coping-stress tolerance.
		  • Listen to the patient's subjective experience and attend to both subjective and objective responses to anxiety.
		  • Teach patient relaxation, imagery, music therapy, and touch interventions.
		  • Give medication if indicated and monitor results.
		2. Address cognitive-perceptual impairments
		  • Help patient identify stressors.
		  • Help patient identify worry, fear, and negative thoughts.
		  • Assist patient to enhance internal healing resources by developing positive self-dialogue messages of positive outcome, increased confidence, sense of control, more effective coping, optimism, and increased speed of recovery.
		3. Address self-care and sleep-rest.
		  • Encourage diversional activity and exercise as tolerated.
		  • Reinforce active participation in healthy eating, bathing, etc.
		  • Encourage rest.
		  • Offer quiet, comfortable environment and relaxation, imagery, music therapy, and touch interventions.
		4. Address role-relationships.
		  • Have patient identify family, friend, or staff to share worries with to help enhance effective coping.
		  • Help patient delegate responsibilities which he or she is unable to complete.
		  • Encourage sharing of stressors with family or others so that they can help patient identify past effective coping strategies that have been used.
			• Patient demonstrated decreased anxiety as evidenced by decreased tension, and restlessness and normal heart rate, blood pressure, respirations, and muscle tension.
			• Patient talked about anxiety.
			• Patient demonstrated decreased anxiety.
			• Patient demonstrated effective use of relaxation, imagery, music therapy, and touch interventions.
			• Patient demonstrated effective use of coping skills as evidenced by effective use of cognitive, physical, and emotional strategies (list specifics).
			• Patient experienced increased, restful sleep.

Such breathing is usually shallow and increases tension. To learn the proper mechanics of abdominal breathing, place yourself in front of a mirror (Figure 8–1A). Sit in an armless chair with your feet flat on the floor. Let your arms drop below the seat of the chair. To hold your shoulders still, focus on pressing your elbows in with your inhale. Notice the motion of your abdomen moving out with the inhale and back to your spine with the exhale as you keep your shoulders and upper chest motionless. Modify these exercises for use with critically ill patients. The patient's bedside table mirror can be used while the patient is in the bed or sitting in a chair to help visualize still shoulders and upper chest.

In the next exercise, lie down and support your lower back by placing a pillow under your knees (Figure 8–1B). Place your palms on your abdomen and let your fingers loosely cross just above your navel. Take a slow, deep breath in to the count of 4 and feel your abdomen push your fingers towards the ceiling. As you breath out to the count of 4, lightly press your palms against your abdomen for a complete exhalation.

Next, sit in a straight-back chair with your hands relaxed in your lap and take in a rhythmic abdominal breath (Figure 8–1C). Then, with a rocking motion, let your arms fold loosely across your abdomen on the inhale and gently rock forward just enough to leave the support of the chair back. On the exhale return to the resting position. Feel the relaxed breathing as well as the stretching and tension release of the upper back muscles.

Body Scanning
Body scanning involves focusing on various parts of the body to detect areas of accumulated tension. With the help of the clinician, patients can be guided to scan various body parts such as the forehead, jaw, neck, back, and upper

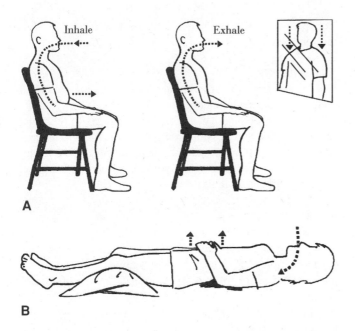

Inhale Exhale

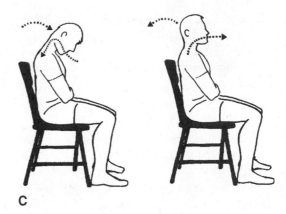

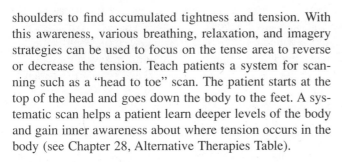

A

B

C

Figure 8–1. Abdominal breathing exercises (see text for explanation). (A) Seated position, in front of mirror. (B) Lying position. (C) Rocking position. *(Reproduced with permission from: Dossey BM, Keegan L, Guzzetta CE: The art of caring: Holistic healing using relaxation, imagery, music therapy, and touch. Boulder, CO: Sounds True, 1996.)*

shoulders to find accumulated tightness and tension. With this awareness, various breathing, relaxation, and imagery strategies can be used to focus on the tense area to reverse or decrease the tension. Teach patients a system for scanning such as a "head to toe" scan. The patient starts at the top of the head and goes down the body to the feet. A systematic scan helps a patient learn deeper levels of the body and gain inner awareness about where tension occurs in the body (see Chapter 28, Alternative Therapies Table).

Autogenics

Autogenics is a self (auto)-generated (genic) therapy that includes repetition of suggestions or positive inner phrases or dialogue in the first person, using the present tense to create a desired state of the body (e.g., heaviness and warmth). Pause for 15 seconds between phrases and repeat each phrase three times. Start with a few relaxed abdominal breaths. Have patients repeat this exercise for 10 minutes or longer. When using autogenics, the clinician says the words as the patient repeats silently:

- "My right arm is warm and heavy."
- "My right leg is warm and heavy."
- "Heaviness and warmth are flowing through my body."
- "My body breathes freely and easily."
- "My heartbeat is calm and regular."
- "My breathing is calm and relaxed."
- "My mind is quiet and still."
- "I am at peace."

Relaxation Response

The relaxation response is a hypometabolic state of decreased sympathetic nervous system arousal. It is achieved by passive concentration, slowly repeating a sin-

gle, neutral word, such as *one* or *relax,* on the exhale. The four elements of the relaxation response include:

- Quiet environment
- Comfortable position
- Passive attitude (e.g., just letting relaxation happen, neither forcing nor resisting it)
- Focused concentration on the word and breath.

The technique works best when used for 15 to 20 minutes twice a day to achieve a deep relaxed state (see Chapter 28, Alternative Therapies Table).

Prayer

Prayer is a fundamental, primordial, and important "language" spoken by humans and used as a way to connect to the spiritual core of healing. It is a unique individual experience where words or short phrases are repeated silently or aloud as a focusing device that can evoke deep states of relaxation. Prayer also may be used to enter a state of prayerfulness where stress, crisis, and illness are experienced and accepted as a natural part of life which transcends passivity. Prayer may be either directed (to someone or for something) or nondirected (simply saying, "Thy will be done").

Biofeedback

Biofeedback is another way to teach as well as evoke states of relaxation. Biofeedback uses specific instrumentation to mirror psychophysiologic processes of which the patient is normally unaware. As the patient thinks and feels relaxed and shifts towards these states, this transduction of information is registered via biofeedback electrodes attached to a patient's body. Electrodes and thermometers can measure biologic energy in terms of muscle tension and hand and foot temperatures which are then transduced into a measurement displayed on a digital meter or alarm. The patient receives validation of relaxation that is characterized by reduced muscle tension and increased hand or foot temperatures after shifting to a dominant parasympathetic response.

To enhance the effective use of relaxation, follow these steps (see also Chapter 28, Alternative Therapy Table):

1. Assess the presence of negative body-mind responses to stressful events.
2. Guide patients in a relaxation session. Encourage patients to practice relaxation skills for 20 minutes several times a day. Integrate the relaxation practice with imagery, music, and touch to evoke relaxation states and inner calmness.
3. At the end of 20 minutes (or longer) gradually bring the patient back into full awareness of the room. Encourage the patient to enjoy the state of inner calm and to reflect on how this experience feels at the end of the relaxation session.
4. Explore the patient's subjective experience with relaxation (Table 8–5).
5. Integrate relaxation with daily activities to decrease anxiety and increase effective coping skills that lead to inner calmness and more effective choices and actions.

Imagery

Imagery is a powerful, dynamic, and therapeutic intervention. It involves all of the senses—hearing, seeing, touching, tasting, and feeling. Imagery empowers individuals to use their own consciousness in the healing process.

Patients are imaging at all times. The clinician needs to listen with attention to the patients' stories about their disease/illness, life, anxiety, and pain. The clinician also needs to help patients explore their inner healing resources (e.g., inner strengths, use of prayers, affirmations, and effective coping skills) as well as their external healing resources (e.g., treatments, technology, and medications). Embedded in these stories are the patients' own individual images. Using these unique images, the clinician can then help patients reframe images towards healing rather than reinforcing complications of disease, anxiety, or pain.

Types of Imagery

It is important to differentiate the different types of imagery. Individuals unconsciously and consciously create images of well-being. They also create images of their disease, disability, and possible complications. Imagery awareness helps the clinician guide patients in integrating receptive, active, correct biologic, symbolic, process, end state, and general healing images.

Receptive Imagery

Receptive imagery is common when daydreaming, falling asleep (hypnagogic), and immediately upon awakening (hypnopompic). Receptive images appear in conscious thought and seem to just "bubble up." These are experienced as an inner knowing received without effort. Receptive imagery can be experienced. For example, take a few minutes to focus on where your body accumulates tension, such as the back of the neck or shoulders. If this can be felt, what happens for you? Can you recognize your dominant sensory modality? Common imagery expressions characterizing tension are tightness, tingling, or warmth. With this imagery, it is important for clinicians to trust the patients' imagery processes and stay out of the way as the patients tell their stories and explore their images.

Active Imagery

Active imagery occurs as a person focuses on the conscious formation of an image. Notice an image which comes from your neck or shoulders as you focus on this area once again. Common expressions that come from persons with active images are popping or grinding of muscles, or knots in muscles. A person can "literally speak to a body part" by sending a message to see, feel, hear, or touch tight muscles to release the tension.

Correct Biologic Imagery

Correct biologic imagery implies images of the body that are accurate, such as one might see if looking under a microscope. Patients can be taught how to use the imagery process to reverse or stabilize the disease/dysfunction. Patients need to be educated, however, about correct biologic images because often such images are inaccurate and can block a person's inner healing resources. For example, following an acute myocardial infarction, patients can be assisted in creating positive and correct biologic images by reinforcing concepts of normal blood flow, healthy collateral blood flow and scar formation, and the use of natural healing processes to assist in recovery.

Symbolic Imagery

Symbolic imagery is the emergence of personal symbols from an individual's unconscious and conscious awareness.

TABLE 8–5. SUBJECTIVE EXPERIENCE WITH RELAXATION

1. Was this a new experience for you? Can you describe it?
2. Did you have any physical or emotional responses to the relaxation exercises? If so, can you describe them?
3. Do you feel different after this experience? How?
4. How does your body-mind communicate with you when your stress level is at an uncomfortable point?
5. Would you like to experience this relaxation technique again?
6. Were there any distractions to your relaxation?
7. What would make the relaxation experience more pleasant for you?
8. What is your next step (or your plan) to integrate relaxation skills into your daily life?

Reprinted with permission from: Dossey BM, Keegan L, Guzzetta CE, Kolkmeier L: Holistic nursing: A handbook for practice. Gaithersburg, MD: Aspen, 1995.

It is a unique and unfolding process for each patient that cannot be forced. As patients enter into deep relaxation, their innate inner wisdom is more likely to release symbolic images. These images may or may not have healing qualities. Thus, the clinician must assess with each individual the kinds of images that emerge. When a person develops negative images, the clinician can help the individual explore the meaning of the negative images and continue to guide the person in developing positive healing images.

An example of symbolic imagery is from a 46-year-old engineer recovering from acute myocardial infarction but experiencing frequent multifocal premature ventricular contractions (PVCs). He was introduced to rhythmic breathing exercises and taught how to create symbolic images of a normal, calm conduction system. He developed his images from his work, choosing a huge computer to symbolized his body-mind communication center. He imagined an elaborate SA (sinoatrial) control panel where he could push a button to send impulses correctly down his heart's conduction pathways. This example demonstrates how he was able to integrate the correct biologic images of normal conduction with the symbolic images of the computer. Both types of images are important.

Process Imagery

Process imagery is a guided imagery process involving a step-by-step rehearsal of a procedure, treatment, surgery, or other event related to health problems prior to the event. It also involves helping individuals integrate correct biologic images of healing in their imagination. For example, in teaching patients about their upcoming cardiac catheterization, process imagery would include a rehearsal of the events the patients will experience during the procedure as a means of walking them positively through the event to prepare better for the experience (see also What Heals: Preparing for a Difficult Event, at the beginning of this chapter).

End State Imagery

End state imagery involves teaching a person to rehearse being in a final, healed state. For example, an end state image for an acute myocardial infarction patient would be first to focus on a healed heart. Later on in the rehabilitation process, end state images would be created to include success in exercising, returning to work, and engaging in healthy sexual activity.

General Healing Imagery

General healing imagery includes events rather than a process. General healing images frequently appear as colors or sounds, or as an inner guide, such as a wise person, animal, or totem. These images also may come in the form of a felt sense of unity, universal power, spirit, or God. General images are those that emerge for each person and that have personal healing significance. An example expressed by a posttrauma patient with both legs in traction was "being bathed with relaxation and the warmth of the sun, and being surrounded by a gold bubble."

Facilitating the Imagery Process

The imagery process can be facilitated by using packaged or customized imagery sessions. Packaged imagery involves using another person's images, such as those found on self-hypnosis, relaxation, and imagery scripts recorded on commercial tapes. Commercial tapes as well as tapes prepared by the clinician can be therapeutic and serve as general guides. They can facilitate the patient's healing and learning of the skills when a clinician cannot be present. The clinician also can assist patients to record their own voices using specific imagery scripts for later replay.

Customized imagery involves images that are specific to each individual. An example of customized images is from a patient who used a packaged, commercial tape containing general healing images prior to open heart surgery. Following open heart surgery, the patient customized her images by visualizing her new jump grafts as violet cylinders through which blood flowed without obstruction. As she continued to integrate her relaxation and imagery practice, she also learned to let the healing violet color fill her whole body.

Concrete Objective Preparatory Information

Concrete objective preparatory information describes both the subjective and objective experiences of health care encountered by patients during diagnostic tests, procedures, surgery, treatments, or recovery. Previously referred to as preparatory sensory information, concrete objective preparatory information reflects the accumulated research findings on the importance of describing both the subjective and objective experiences that patients encounter using concrete and objective terminology.

For a surgical patient, the subjective concrete experiences would include what is felt, heard, seen, or tasted before, during, or after a procedure. It also would include the sensory experiences of a postsurgical healing incision such as pressure, burning, and tingling. Objective experiences for a surgical patient would include those that can be observed and verified by someone other than the person going through the procedure. For the surgical patient, objective experiences may include when and where the surgeon, anesthesiologist, and presurgical nurse will visit; what information will be discussed in the visit; how and when the preoperative skin preparation is done; how the patient will be placed on the stretcher to go to surgery; what to expect when awakening in the recovery room or critical care unit; and what kinds of tubes and equipment to expect postoperatively. Information about the timing of events, the environment of the procedure, and the procedure for family visits also is included. Using such images, the clinician conveys a clear, positive picture of both the subjective and objective experience and what sensations the person may anticipate from a particular event. To assist patients create these images:

- Identify the sensory features of the procedure to be used.
- Identify the individual's perception of the procedure/treatment/test to be experienced.
- Choose words that have meaning for the person.
- Use synonyms that have less emotional impact, such as *discomfort* instead of *pain*.
- Select specific experiences rather than abstract experiences when giving examples.
- Help individuals reframe negative imagery if it is elicited in the previous steps.

Individual Differences

It also is important to understand individual differences with the imagery process. These differences include images, colors, symbols, and meanings in relationship to the cultural diversity of individuals. As clinicians learn to recognize these individual differences, facilitating patients in the imagery process becomes more effective because patients discover their own unique imagery patterns.

It is important to provide continuous suggestions for novices and less vivid imagers by including positive statements that can guide the patients in positive self-talk following the session. In contrast, if patients are vivid imagers, continuous encouragement is not needed and may be distracting. A vivid imager may find it intrusive if the guide is talking too much. The patients should be encouraged to use imagery skills 20 minutes several times a day on their own. To enhance the effective use of imagery, follow these steps (see also Chapter 28, Alternative Therapies Table):

1. Identify the problem or disease or goal of imagery. If imagery is to focus on specific physiology, teach the patient the basic physiology involved in the normal healing process.
2. Begin with several minutes of general relaxation or focused attention on the breath.
3. Develop images of:
   - The problem or disease
   - Inner healing resources (strengths, belief systems, and coping strategies)
   - External healing resources (treatments, medications, tests, and surgery).
4. End with images of the final healed state or the desired state of well-being.
5. At the end of the session, assess the imagery process (Table 8–6).
6. Also explore the patient's subjective experience with imagery (Table 8–7).
7. At this time, the patient can be given crayons and paper and encouraged to draw free-form the different images or feelings that came during or at the end of the session. This exercise has nothing to do with how well someone can draw, but is another way to experience images in a more concrete fashion.

Music Therapy

Music therapy involves the systematic use of music to evoke states of relaxation and to enhance the imagery process. Music has measurable psychophysiologic effects on patients. At the Institute for Music, Health, and Education, research has been done in the following four areas: music to (1) alter time and space relationships, (2) modify environment, (3) evoke integration and grounding, and (4) facilitate the imagery process.

TABLE 8–6. IMAGERY ASSESSMENT TOOL

Clarity of imagery: How vivid, cohesive, and complete is the imagery overall? Does the story make some sense to you?

0	1	2	3	4
not clear at all		moderately clear		extremely clear

Clarity Score_____

Imagery of disease/problem: How serious and curable is the disease or problem? Or is it incurable, vulnerable, and weak?

0	1	2	3	4
very serious		moderately serious		curable/no problem

Imagery of Disease Score_____

Imagery of inner healing forces: How powerful, righteous, pure, directed, and intense are the internal healing forces? How active and controllable are they?

0	1	2	3	4
none		moderately strong		extremely powerful

Imagery of Healing Score_____

Imagery of external healing forces: How effective, comprehensive, curable, positive, and helpful is your treatment? Do the images depict a powerful therapy or one that is destructive? If several types of external healing forces are used, evaluate them separately.

0	1	2	3	4
harmful		helpful		curative

Imagery of Treatment Score_____

Symbolism of imagery: How symbolic is the imagery? Is it more factual or concrete? High amounts of symbolism are usually associated with a personal or mythic story.

0	1	2	3	4
no symbols		mixed or some		highly symbolic

Imagery Symbolism Score_____

How to use your scores:
- Evaluate each score independently. Do not add them up.
- Identify areas where you had the highest scores. These are your strengths.
- Identify what could be strengthened or clarified—the areas where you had low scores.
- Think about your emotional response to each component.
- Modify your imagery, if you wish. Take the IAT again after you've experienced your new imagery for about a week.
- If any of the IAT areas are unclear to you, you might benefit by gaining more information about the actual nature of the component—such as details about how your external healing forces are supposed to work.

Reproduced with permission from: Achterberg J, Dossey B, Kolkmeier L: Rituals of healing. New York: Bantam, 1994.

TABLE 8–7. SUBJECTIVE EXPERIENCE WITH IMAGERY

1. Was this a new kind of imagery experience for you? Can you describe it?
2. Did you have a visual experience? Of people, places, or objects? Can you describe them?
3. Did you see colors while being guided? Did you see colors change as the guided imagery continued?
4. Were you aware of your surroundings? Were you able to let the imagery flow?
5. Did you like the imagery? Can you describe it? What is your dominant sensory mode?
6. Did the imagery produce any feelings or emotions? Can you describe them?
7. Did you notice any textures, smells, movements, or tastes while experiencing the imagery?
8. What is your next step (or your plan) to integrate imagery into your life?

Reprinted with permission from: Dossey BM, Keegan L, Guzzetta CE, Kolkmeier L: Holistic nursing: A handbook for practice. Gaithersburg, MD: Aspen, 1995.

Time and space are influenced and modified by the vertical and horizontal position of a patient's ears. Blood flow to the ear's vestibular system, which is affected by posture, is different when a patient's body is in a standing, sitting, or lying position. Thus, the message to the brain also is changed. In the relaxed, reclining position, slow music can facilitate more images and associations than in other positions because the body is not constantly working to determine its exact position and actions. This more relaxed position allows the body-mind to slow its internal clock, which also slows the "sense of time." Music also alters the sense of time and space because it changes physiologic states as a result of vibrational resonance. The choice of music can create peace, calmness, safety, or spaciousness, or it can manifest as tension, clutter, or heaviness. Music must be chosen carefully for hallways, waiting rooms, and patient units.

To achieve optimal patient outcomes with music, the patient, not the clinician, should choose the music. If patients are not capable of choosing music because they are comatose or heavily sedated, the clinician can query the family about what type of music the patient enjoys.

No "best" music exists. Music that one patient considers relaxing might make another patient tense. For the purposes of achieving relaxation, patients should be encouraged to experiment with listening to slow, soothing solo instruments such as the harp, flute, and piano; nature sounds such as ocean waves, rain, and wind; or different relaxing musical arrangements such as classical, jazz, contemporary, and choral to determine their response to a variety of selections. Musical selections without words are recommended to facilitate concentration on the music rather than focusing on the words and their meaning. Music frequently evokes different feelings and images depending on the length of time that a patient listens to a selection and the extent to which the patient releases the need to analyze the

musical arrangement and instruments. Rapid and intense music selections, on the other hand, are also important in the imagery process. When music selections with faster rhythms are selected, the notes come closer together. As a result, individuals do not have time to relax or come to resolution between the notes. Therefore, the images are intensified, and the types of images and breakthroughs experienced are different than when using slow music.

Music should be chosen based on the iso-principle, that is, matching music to the mood of the patient and then slowly changing it to the mood that a patient wants to evoke. When a patient is experiencing acute or chronic pain or is grieving, moods vary from mild discouragement to depression. If the goal of the music is to reduce the depression, the patient might start out listening to a musical selection that helps him or her to relax for several minutes and then change to music that evokes a lighter, yet related response. Patients can be encouraged to create their own music tapes to produce the kinds of feelings and experiences they wish to achieve. Certain kinds of music evoke calmness and peace; other types can help a patient work through grief, depression, worry, fear, or death imagery. Music selections stimulate images (mind modulation) that assist a person in connecting with emotions.

Clinicians can help integrate the use of relaxation, imagery, and music therapy in conventional health care settings by establishing an audio- and videocassette library (Table 8–8). In addition, personal experience with relaxation and music therapy enhances the clinician's ability to serve as an effective guide in the experience with patients. As the clinician masters relaxation and imagery skills, a deeper personal level of healing, integration, and grounding is gained.

TABLE 8–8. AUDIOCASSETTE AND VIDEOCASSETTE RESOURCE LIBRARY

- Have a variety of music tapes available—easy listening, jazz, classical, chants, popular, operatic, folk, country, hymns, chorals, and nontraditional. Commercial tapes are relatively inexpensive.
- Include relaxation, imagery, and stress management tapes and specific tapes for behavior changes as needed (e.g., weight management, smoking cessation, anxiety reduction, insomnia, pain management, and pre/post rehearsals for procedures, tests, and surgery).
- You can make your own tapes or purchase them in bookstores or through catalogues.
- Any time you hear music that you like, write the name down for later purchase. Radio stations keep a log of what they play. Note the time you heard a pleasant musical recording and call the radio station to get the name of the music selection and the musician.
- Have an audiocassette recorder and headset ready for patient session. If using a battery-operated player, check the batteries before a session begins. Have a VCR and television ready if you are using a video for the session. Adjust the volume before the session begins.
- Have a specific check-in procedure and check-out procedure for all equipment.

Reprinted with permission from: Dossey BM, Keegan L, Guzzetta CE, Kolkmeier L: Holistic nursing: A handbook for practice. Gaithersburg, MD: Aspen, 1995.

To enhance effective use of music therapy, follow these steps (see also Chapter 28, Alternative Therapies Table):

1. First, guide the patient in a general relaxation session and then begin the music.
2. Instruct the patient to let the music relax his or her body-mind-spirit even more. Ask the patient to focus all attention on the music, letting the music suggest what to think and feel. Instruct the patient not to analyze the music or melody but to flow with the sounds. If the patient finds distracting thoughts occurring, tell him or her simply to let go of the thoughts and come back to concentrating on the music.
3. Allow 20 minutes for the patient to sit or lie in a quiet, comfortable position listening to the music of the patient's choice. Leave the room.
4. Return at the end of 20 minutes and gradually bring the patient back into full awareness of the room. If you are unable to return after 20 minutes, let the patient know in advance. Give him or her instructions to enjoy the state of inner calm and reflect on how this experience feels at the end of the music tape.
5. Explore the patient's subjective experience with music therapy (Table 8–9).

Touch

Cultures throughout history have developed touch therapies that include such techniques as rubbing, pressing, massaging, and holding. These therapies are natural manifestations of the desire to heal and care for one another. Touch therapies have direct and indirect body-mind-spirit healing effects through the body's largest sense organ, the skin.

The modern-day renaissance of body therapies is probably a response to the fast-paced technologic revolution that has swept our culture. A blending of Eastern and West-

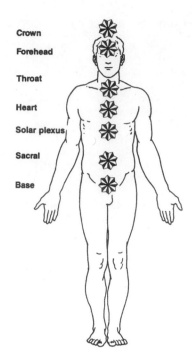

Figure 8–2. Chakras—seven main energy centers in Eastern medicine. *Crown Center* (located at the top of the head); Brow Center (located between the eyebrows at the center of the brows); Throat Center (located at the center and base of throat); Heart Center (located between the shoulder blades at the heart level); Solar Plexus (located at the solar plexus); Sacral Center (located midsacral lower abdomen, below navel); Base Center (located at the base of spine and perineal floor).

Crown
Forehead
Throat
Heart
Solar plexus
Sacral
Base

ern techniques has resulted in an explosion of new and widely practiced modalities that use the principles of chakras and energy meridian lines. Chakra locations are seen in Figure 8–2. *Chakra* is the Sanskrit word meaning wheel or disk-like spinning vortex of energy. Eastern theories explain energy meridian lines as an energy circuit or line of force following vertically through the body with culminating points on the feet, hands, and ears. Different types of touch strategies that can be successfully used in the critical care setting are foot reflexology, acupressure, shiatzu, therapeutic massage, therapeutic touch, and healing touch. When these techniques are used in critical care, explore the patient's subjective experience with touch (Table 8–10).

Foot reflexology is the application of pressure to points on the feet that correspond to other parts of the body (Figure 8–3). *Acupressure* is the application of finger and/or thumb pressure to specific sites along the body's energy meridians for the purpose of relieving tension and reestablishing the flow of energy along the meridian lines (Figure 8–4). *Shiatzu* is the use of the thumb and/or heel of the hand for deep pressure work along the energy meridian lines. *Procedural touch* is touch done to diagnose, monitor, or treat the symptoms or illness itself. It focuses on the end result of curing, decreas-

TABLE 8–9. SUBJECTIVE EXPERIENCE WITH MUSIC THERAPY

1. Was this a new kind of music experience for you? Can you describe it?
2. Did you have any visual experiences? Of people, places, or objects? Can you describe them?
3. Did you see any colors while listening? Did the colors change as the music changed? Can you describe them?
4. Did you notice any textures, smells, movements, or tastes while experiencing the music? Can you describe them?
5. Were you less aware of your surroundings? Were you able to flow with the music?
6. Did you like the music?
7. Did the music produce any feelings or emotions?
8. What would be helpful to make this a better experience for you?
9. What is your next step (or your plan) to integrate music into your daily life?

Reprinted with permission from: Dossey BM, Keegan L, Guzzetta CE, Kolkmeier L: Holistic nursing: A handbook for practice. Gaithersburg, MD: Aspen, 1995.

TABLE 8–10. SUBJECTIVE EXPERIENCES OF TOUCH THERAPIES

1. Was this a new kind of experience for you? Can you describe it?
2. Did this feel like a comforting, stimulating, or tactile sensation?
3. Was it pleasurable on all planes—physical, mental, emotional, and spiritual—or more focused in one area than another?
4. Were you aware of your surroundings during the experience or did you sink into a sense of timelessness?
5. Did emotions surface during the experience? If so, what were they? Can you focus on them now?
6. Did you experience any imagery during the touch session?
7. Did you feel comfortable with the therapist? Is there anything that you want to do to increase your comfort level with the touch therapist?
8. Did you feel relaxed and refreshed after the experience?
9. Would you like to try this again?
10. What would be helpful to make this a better experience for you?
11. Can you develop a plan or strategy to integrate more of the touch therapies into your life on a regular basis?

Reprinted with permission from: Dossey BM, Keegan L, Guzzetta CE, Kolkmeier L: Holistic nursing: A handbook for practice. Gaithersburg, MD: Aspen, 1995.

ing, or stabilizing symptoms or illness, or preventing further complications. *Therapeutic massage* involves the use of the hands to apply deep pressure and motion on the skin and underlying muscles for the purposes of physical and psychologic relaxation, improved circulation, relief of sore muscles, and other therapeutic effects, such as in giving or receiving a therapeutic back rub/massage.

Therapeutic touch is a contemporary interpretation of several combined ancient healing modalities. *Healing touch* combines principles of therapeutic touch with additional techniques. Both types of touch use the specific techniques of centering and intention while the practitioner moves the hands through the recipient's energy field for the purposes of assessing and treating energy field imbalance. *Centering*

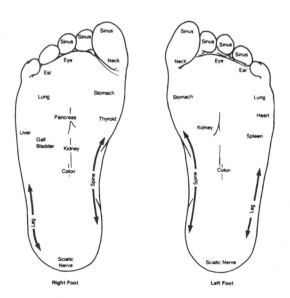

Figure 8–3. Foot reflexology chart. *(From: Dossey BM, Keegan L, Guzzetta CE, Kolkmeier L: Holistic nursing: A handbook for practice. Gaithersburg, MD: Aspen, 1995, p. 559.)*

refers to an inner calm and quietude within oneself where one can feel truly integrated, unified, and focused. *Intention* is a focused state of calmness, inner peace, and healing awareness during the therapeutic touch session.

Therapeutic touch and healing touch are used with the intent of enabling individuals to repattern their energy in the direction of health. Uses of therapeutic touch or healing touch are pain and anxiety reduction, relaxation, and enhancing the body's natural restorative processes. These techniques can be used alone or with other healing modalities. They are autonomous nursing interventions performed within professional practice guidelines. They may be used by any clinician who has successfully completed a minimum of a 2-day beginning workshop that addresses the theory and experiential components of therapeutic touch and healing touch.[1]

Creating Rituals of Healing

Healing rituals are essential to caring and healing in critical care. They are used to lessen feelings of anxiety and helplessness and assist a patient to deal with crisis, trauma, pain, and daily events. Rituals may include the way we hold a patient's hand with intention to be present in the moment, active listening to a family member, or the prayer or mantra we say to ourselves to be more empowered. If we are to evoke healing successfully in others, we must first know how to incorporate rituals in our daily lives.

An important aspect of inner work in our fast-paced lives is to create a time for rituals that have specific meaning and to assist others in the art of ritual in daily living. Critically ill patients and their families are faced with dilemmas regarding symptoms, tests, and procedures and are confronted with decisions about medical or surgical intervention or end-of-life questions. Although we never can make a decision for others, we can introduce them to ways of recognizing the inner wisdom that will enable them to make better decisions themselves.

In creating a ritual, there are no absolute rules that should be followed. One guideline is that a ritual should have a structure—a beginning, a middle, and an end. It helps to plan the details carefully in advance much like you do in anticipation of a special house guest. You give attention to details in a guest room by adding fresh flowers and books of art or poetry at a bedside, so that a special, sacred space is created. This also happens when we create a sacred space to be alone and reflect on healing awareness. We deepen our

---

[1]For information on *Therapeutic Touch Guidelines, Policy and Procedure for the Health Professional, 1991* (Krieger and Kunz method) contact: Nurse Healers-Professional Associates, Inc., 207 W. 14th Street, New York, NY 10011, (212) 741-3126.

For information on workshops and the Healing Touch Certificate Program, contact: American Holistic Nurses' Association, 4101 Lake Boone Trail, Suite 201, Raleigh, NC, 27607, (800) 278-AHNA.

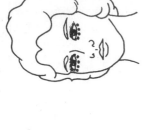

Apply deep pressure below the base of the skull to release head and neck tension. Hold for 3 seconds, pause, repeat several times and let go.

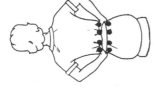

To release tight neck muscles, again with deep pressure move down the muscle lines approximately two finger widths. Let your fingers feel the muscle bands. Hold for 3 or 4 seconds, pause and move on down the neck.

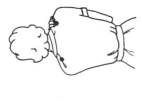

At the top of the head use your index, middle and third fingers of both hands. With moderate pressure press at the three points shown for 3 or 4 seconds, pause and move to the next two positions using the same technique.

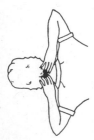

Relieve shoulder tension by placing your left hand on the back of your right shoulder. Locate what is called the "yipe" point, a key point where tension builds up. It is halfway between the base of the neck edge of the shoulders. This point may be tender. Apply deep pressure for 3 or 4 seconds, pause and repeat the sequence again on your opposite side.

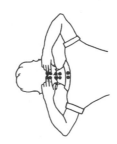

Stretch your left hand to your right shoulder to give yourself shiatzu to your upper back. Touch your index, middle and third fingers to your spine. With deep pressure find the pressure points as shown. Move two finger widths up on a line toward your shoulder, pressing in each position for 3 seconds; pause and repeat the pressure at each point.

To give self-shiatzu to your lower back, sit forward slightly in your chair. Place your fingertips above your hip bones, and extend your thumbs in toward your spine. Give deep pressure in each spot for 3 seconds, pause and repeat.

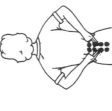
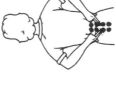
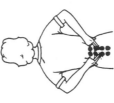

To give self-shiatzu to your spine, stand up, locate your coccyx. With your index and middle fingers apply moderate pressure for 3 seconds, pause and move up at two finger widths until you reach your waist.

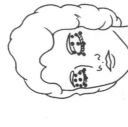

To apply self-shiatzu to your cheeks, with your index and middle fingers side by side, apply moderate pressure at the outside of the bridge of the nose. Hold for 3 seconds, pause and move one finger width across the cheeks.

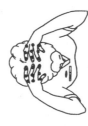

Apply self-shiatzu to your eyes. If you wear contact lenses, take them out first. The pressure points are on the inside edge of the eye sockets. With your index, middle and third fingers of each hand, press on the points shown with light pressure for 3 seconds; pause and repeat.

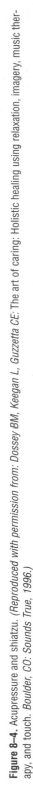

Figure 8–4. Acupressure and shiatzu. (Reproduced with permission from: Dossey BM, Keegan L, Guzzetta CE: The art of caring: Holistic healing using relaxation, imagery, music therapy, and touch. Boulder, CO: Sounds True, 1996.)

understanding of being connected with self, others, and a Higher Self. This special time is what helps us with healing our own lives so that we are available for others.

The first phase of a ritual, the *separation phase,* is a symbolic act of breaking away from life's busy activities (Table 8–11). It is done with intention and a conscious awareness to become engaged in a healing activity using relaxation, imagery, music therapy, or touch. For example, it might involve going to a quiet room for 15 to 20 minutes, taking shoes off, sitting on a pillow on the floor, putting on the answering machine, and listening to a relaxation, music, or imagery tape.

As we enter the second phase of ritual, the *transition phase,* we can more easily identify areas in our life that need

---

TABLE 8–11. HEALING RITUALS FOR RELAXATION, MUSIC THERAPY, IMAGERY, AND TOUCH

Separation Phase
Before the Session
- Turn the radio and television off. To avoid interruptions, place a sign on the door stating that a session is in progress. (If other family members or significant others are around, invite them to join in and experience the intervention being taught to the patient.)
- Prepare the room to ensure as much comfort and quietness as possible.
- Have the patient tend to basic comfort needs, such as urinating, before the session begins.
- Ask the patient to sit, recline, or lie down, depending on preference and/or the situation.
- Have a light blanket available in case the patient should feel cool.
- Become calm and centered. Let your body-mind release any tension and tightness.
- Select a relaxation, imagery, music, or touch exercise (or combine these interventions) for the session.
- Ask the patient to notice baseline feelings/emotions before the session begins.

Beginning the Session
- Discuss the purpose of the session, reinforcing the intent of developing a positive expectation of what is to occur. This explanation helps individuals to focus and organize inner experiences towards calmness, inner harmony, and healing.
- Instruct the patient to focus on the present moment in order to facilitate the best relaxation, imagery, music, or touch experience.
- Encourage spontaneous images to emerge from the inner self without analyzing them. Should participants begin to analyze the images, instruct them to let the images just float on, and to release any logical process of resolving conflicts, establishing goals, and so forth. These steps will come, but not in a logical manner.
- Ask the patient to concentrate fully on the guided relaxation, imagery, music, and touch suggestions and instructions. Different images will emerge. If any image appears that is uncomfortable or that the patient is not ready to explore, provide instruction to let go of these images and flow with the next image that appears.
- Encourage the use of positive imagery that can evoke healing and healthy expectations.
- As you begin guiding the patient in a relaxation, imagery, music therapy, or touch experience, begin the experience with "You can let your eyes close to be fully awake or you can find a spot in front of you to focus on to begin to explore this experience of inner calmness. Allow the images to emerge from this relaxed state."

Transition Phase
During the Session
- Ask the patient to follow the suggestions that you give (or that are given on the tape that he or she will use for a session). Tell the patient to add his or her own suggestions that can allow more personal images to emerge. (If relaxation and different imagery states have been previously experienced, the individual will find it easier to clear the mind of distracting thoughts than if the individual is a beginner.)
- Inform the participant that with relaxation a decreased tension in the face, chest, torso, and legs will be experienced. The changes can be subtle or dramatic. Respirations become deeper with more space between the breaths. Eyelids may flicker especially if the patient is a vivid imager. Legs and feet will also turn outward with increased relaxation.
- If the mind cannot be cleared, suggest that the patient focus on slow, rhythmic, abdominal breathing. If the mind continues to wander, focus once again on the breathing pattern. It is natural for the mind to wander, and when aware of this, return to the relaxation, imagery, music therapy, or touch experience.
- The length of a session is based on the patient's needs, body responses, and session outcomes. The sessions can be 20 minutes or as long as needed. During the day encourage patients to incorporate relaxation, imagery, music, and touch skills in mini-sessions (3 to 5 minutes).

Return Phase
Closing the Session
- Gradually bring the patient back into full alertness by counting back from 5 to 1.
- Encourage the participant to become immersed in the healing silence and relaxed state even if only for a few minutes. The immediate period following a session can be a time for personal insight. This opportunity may be lost if patients begin talking or move into daily activities too soon.
- Instruction may be given to finish the session by drawing some images or writing some thoughts that occurred during the session.
- Ask the patient to interpret the experience. Refer to the open-ended questions about the *subjective experience* of relaxation, imagery, music therapy, and touch for further meaning or more personal insight about the current situation or other important issues.
- Encourage monitoring of tension during the day to replace tension patterns with relaxation and positive imagery. This is the body-mind communication process to enhance healing and recovery.
- Encourage awareness of the constant self-talk, and focus on creating positive images that lead to healthy outcomes.
- Recommend using "constant instant practice." This is a reminder to take a moment to practice, thereby integrating the practice into daily life.
- Explore the importance of trusting intuition and images that come forth from inner awareness.
- Encourage *practice.* This is the key to developing the deep levels of insight that can be gained from these healing strategies and rituals. Each day establish a scheduled time to practice. Just as one takes medication on a schedule, a scheduled relaxation, imagery, touch or music session increases personal skills.
- Alternate between short and long practice sessions.

attention (Table 8–11). It is a time of facing the shadow where we recognize the dark and the difficult, and we search for self and for what is real and worthy and in need of healing in the deepest sense. It is the time to go into an unknown terrain, the *limen,* the meaning threshold, where we leave one way of being to enter into another way of participating. Individuals progress through the transition phase with an awareness of being changed through the 20 minutes taken to use one or more of the healing strategies discussed.

Finally, in the last phase of the ritual, the *return phase,* we reenter into real life (Table 8–11). This phase allows for a formal release, putting aside or leaving behind old ways of fears, anger, or memories that no longer serve us. It involves being renewed and changed when returning to life's activities as a result of the relaxation, imagery, music, or touch session. This phase challenges us to integrate a new way of acting, choosing, and relating, to "walk our talk" of healing awareness.

Enhancing Skills as a Guide

Clinicians can integrate the following six techniques to empower the spoken words during relaxation, imagery, music therapy, or touch sessions as well as during other interventions and patient education sessions:

1. Increase the use of metaphors, that is, implied comparisons. For example, after giving a pain medication, follow it with the suggestion "The pain medicine is in your body and working. You might imagine . . . relaxation flowing like a gentle, warm waterfall . . . relaxing you and decreasing the tension and pain." The metaphor here is relaxation and it is implied to be a gentle, warm waterfall. Metaphors work because the intuitive self deepens the experience of the words used. Also, such suggestion may evoke the placebo response to further facilitate healing (see What Heals: The Powerful Placebo at the beginning of Chapter 9).

2. Be aware of changing voice intonation, pitch, volume, tone, and speed of the spoken words and letting short phrases stand out with different words. For example, "Allow yourself . . . to relax into the pain with the next breath . . . feel . . . as you breathe into the pain." When imagery suggestions incorporate unusual grammatical structures, a person's logical thought process is occupied, allowing the intuitive, creative self to go with the suggestion.

3. Learn to divert a person's intellectual thoughts by connecting certain statements, behaviors, and actions with suggestions. For the patient in pain suggest "[insert the patient's name] . . . relax into the surface under your body . . . sink deeply into the surface . . . feeling yourself being supported by this surface . . . and let it be a reminder to take a deep breath . . . relaxing more deeply."

4. Also enhance the imagery process by providing choices such as "As you are relaxing . . . you might scan your body and see if you might want to change your position . . . or let your arms rest more deeply . . . or release the muscles of your back a little more . . . to go deeper into relaxation . . . getting more comfortable . . . until you find just the right position." A person's body-mind will relax more quickly when a person is occupied with the intellectual process involved in making several different choices.

5. Learn to help a patient to cross-sense (synesthesia—that is, combining and crossing several senses simultaneously) to become more aware of using different sensory modalities to enhance the experience. For example, "Can you see the sounds around you? Can you hear the color of your relaxation?"

6. During interactions, help the patient reframe negative thoughts and images as appropriate. Consider, for example, a patient who states, "My pain has hard walls around it." These negative images serve only to increase the discomfort and anxiety. However, patients can be assisted to reframe their images toward more comfort by the following: "Let yourself see that pain in your mind . . . focus for a moment on one side of the wall of pain . . . and begin to open and soften . . . ever so gently . . . the hardness of the wall . . . opening . . . softening . . . letting go . . . releasing . . .."

AT THE BEDSIDE
■*Thinking Critically*

Case 1: Mr. S. J., age 54, who is in the coronary care unit to rule out acute myocardial infarction, is anxious that his syncopal episode and bradycardia may signal severe illness. His thoughts are scattered and his gestures are meaningless; he has a reduced perceptual field, focusing on irrelevant ideas.

Case 2: Mrs. L. R., age 62, was resting comfortably before her daughter's visit. She is now visibly upset. She is in the critical care unit after developing a pulmonary embolus on her first postoperative day following a knee replacement. As you walk into her room, you find her crying although she tells you she is just fine. However, her facial expression is strained and she appears extremely restless.

- How do you determine if these patients are anxious or having trouble coping?
- What are the most helpful independent nursing interventions that can be used to decrease a patient's anxiety and enhance effective coping?

SELECTED BIBLIOGRAPHY

General Alternative Therapies

Birney M: Psychoneuroimmunology: A holistic framework for the study of stress and illness. *Holistic Nursing Practice.* 1991; 5:32–39.

Christman NJ, Kirchhoff KT, Oakley MG: Concrete objective information. In Bulechek GM, McCloskey JC: *Nursing interventions: Essential nursing treatments.* Philadelphia: JB Lippincott, 1992, pp. 140–150.

Dossey, B: The Psychophysiology of bodymind healing. In Dossey B, Keegan L, Guzzetta C, Kolkmeier L: *Holistic nursing: A handbook for practice,* 2nd ed. Gaithersburg, MD: Aspen, 1995, pp. 87–109.

Moye LA, Richardson MA, Post-White J, Justice B: Research methodology in psychoneuroimmunology: Rationale and design of the Images-P clinical trial. *Alternative Therapies in Health and Medicine.* 1995;1:34–39.

Rossi E: *The psychophysiology of mind-body healing.* New York: Norton, 1993.

Relaxation

Dossey B, Keegan L, Guzzetta C: *The art of caring: Using relaxation, imagery, music therapy, and touch* (four-part audiocassette-booklet program). Boulder, CO: Sounds True, 1996.

Green R et al: Feedback technique for deep relaxation. *Psychophysiology.* 1969;6:371–377.

Kolkmeier L: Relaxation: opening the door to change. In Dossey B, Keegan L, Guzzetta C, Kolkmeier L: *Holistic nursing: A handbook for practice,* 2nd ed. Gaithersburg, MD: Aspen, 1995, pp. 573–605.

Imagery

Achterberg J, Dossey B, Kolkmeier L: *Rituals of healing*: *Using imagery for health and wellness.* New York: Bantam, 1994.

Dossey B: Imagery: Awakening the inner healer. In Dossey B, Keegan L, Guzzetta C, Kolkmeier L: *Holistic nursing: A handbook for practice,* 2nd ed. Gaithersburg, MD: Aspen, 1995, pp. 609–666.

Music Therapy

Allen K, Blasoovich J: Effect of music on cardiovascular reactivity among surgeons. *Journal of the American Medical Association.* 1994;272:882–884.

Campbell D: *Music: Physician for times to come.* Wheaton, IL: Theosophical Publishing, 1991.

Elliott D: The effects of music and muscle relaxation on patient anxiety in a coronary care unit. *Heart and Lung.* 1994;23:27–35.

Good M: A comparison of the effects of jaw relaxation and music on postoperative pain. *Nursing Research.* 1995;44:52–58.

Guzzetta C: Soothing the ischemic heart. *American Journal of Nursing.* 1994;94:24.

Guzzetta C: Music therapy: Hearing the melody of the soul. In Dossey B, Keegan L, Guzzetta C, Kolkmeier L: *Holistic nursing: A handbook for practice,* 2nd ed. Gaithersburg, MD: Aspen, 1995, pp. 669–698.

White JM: Music therapy: An intervention to reduce anxiety in myocardial infarction patients. *Clinical Nurse Specialist.* 1992;6:58–63.

Winter MJ, Paskin S, Baker T: Music reduces stress and anxiety of patients in the surgical holding area. *Journal of Post Anesthesia Nursing.* 1994;9:340–343.

Touch

Hover-Kramer D: *Healing touch.* Albany, NY: Delmar, 1996.

Keegan L: Touch: Connecting with the healing power. In Dossey B, Keegan L, Guzzetta C, Kolkmeier L: *Holistic nursing: A handbook for practice,* 2nd ed. Gaithersburg, MD: Aspen, 1995, pp. 539–569.

SOURCES FOR RELAXATION, IMAGERY, MUSIC AND TOUCH TAPES

Relaxation, Imagery, Music, and Touch Tapes

The art of caring: Holistic healing using relaxation, imagery, touch and music (set of four tapes). Aspen Publishers, Inc, 7201 McKinney Circle, Frederick, MD 21701 (800-638-8437)

Awakening Productions, 4123 Tuller Ave., Culcer, CA 90230

Bodymind Systems, 910 Dakota Drive, Temple, TX 76504 (817-773-2337)

Catalog Services, PO Box 1244, Boulder, CO 80306

Conscious Living Foundation, PO Box 9, Crain, OR 97435 (800-752-CALM)

Institute for Music, Health and Education, PO Box 1244, Boulder, CO 80306 (303-443-8484)

Magna Music, 10370 Page Industrial Blvd., St. Louis, MO 63132 (800-543-3771)

Mind/Body Health Sciences, 393 Dixon Road, Goldhill, Salina Star Route, Boulder, CO 80302 (303-440-8460)

Music Design, 4650 N. Port Washington Road, Milwaukee, WI 53212 (800-862-7232)

New Era Media, 425 Alabama Street, San Francisco, CA 94110 (415-863-3555)

Sounds True, 725 Walnut, Boulder, CO 80302 (800-333-9185)

Sources Cassette, Dept 99, PO Box W, Stanford, CA 94304 (415-328-7171)

Steve Halpern Sound Rx, PO Box 1439, San Rafael, CA 94915 (415-491-1930)

Windham Hill Records, PO Box 9388, Stanford, CA 94305

Music Therapy Tapes Designed for Hospital Use

Music Rx, PO Box 173, Port Townsend, WA 98368 (206-385-6160)

Steven Halpern (Hospital Suite), PO Box 1439, San Rafael, CA 94915 (415-491-1930)

Additional Resources

American Association of Music Therapy, PO Box 80012, Valley Forge, PA 19484 (215-265-4006)

Institute for Consciousness and Music, 7027 Bellona Ave., Baltimore, MD

International Society for Music in Medicine, Sportkrankenhaus Hellersen, D-5880 Lundenscheid, Germany

Mid-Atlantic Institute for Guided Imagery and Music, Box 4655, Virginia Beach, VA 23454

National Association of Music Therapy, 8455 Colesville Road, Suite 930, Silver Spring, MD 20910 (301-589-3300)

Nine

Pharmacology

> ► Knowledge Competencies

1. Discuss advantages and disadvantages of various routes for medication delivery in critically ill patients.

2. Identify indications for use, mechanism of action, administration guidelines, side effects, and contraindications for drugs commonly administered in critical illness.

■ *What Heals: The Powerful Placebo*

Placebo means "I will please." It refers to a medically inert preparation or treatment that has no specific effects on the body and yet can evoke pain relief or dramatically affect the patient's symptoms or disease. The placebo effect always has been a nuisance and an unreliable factor in medicine. It has been assumed to work only in illnesses that somehow were not real. Those who really understand the placebo effect know this is not so. For example, why is it that the worse the pain or the more stressful the situation, the more effective is the placebo pill?

We are beginning to understand the mechanism involved. Recent evidence has shown that the placebo effect can activate the production of endorphins, which are peptide hormones produced and secreted by the brain with opiate properties that are astonishingly powerful and exponentially more potent than morphine. The placebo effect may also work by conditioning responses and by reducing anxiety and fear.

Placebo medications have been found to be effective in pain relief for some patients with postoperative pain. The placebo response is not restricted to pain medications. It has been found to

be present in many illnesses and therapeutic procedures, implicating the mind's ability to produce neurohormonal messenger molecules that alter the autonomic, endocrine, and immune systems. Examples include hypertension, stress, cardiac pain, blood cell counts, headaches, diabetes mellitus, ulcers, colitis, menstrual pain, thyrotoxicosis, the common cold, fever, asthma, rheumatoid arthritis, and cancer.

Isolating the effects of an active drug from the effects of a placebo has been the basis of many double-blind research studies investigating the efficacy of new drugs. Because some patients will respond positively to placebos alone, this baseline efficacy must be subtracted from the effectiveness of the active investigational drug. Thus, some patients respond not only to active drug, but also to the placebo effect, thereby making the active drug even more effective (e.g., the power of morphine is due to its drug effect *plus* its placebo effect). This placebo response augmenting the therapeutic effectiveness for pain medications is very common. For example, although morphine is a far more potent analgesic than aspirin, about half of the effectiveness of both aspirin and morphine is due to the placebo response. Likewise, regardless of the problem or symptom, about half of the effectiveness ratio may be due to the placebo response in many, if not all, drugs and therapeutic procedures. Thus, the placebo response is believed to be a common general mechanism that may occur in all clinical situations. It is thought to occur because of a communication link between the body and the mind that is mediated by the patient's right cerebral hemisphere.

CEG & BMD

Adapted from: Guzzetta CE: Nursing process and standards of care. In Dossey BM, Keegan L, Guzzetta CE, Kolkmeier L: Holistic nursing: A handbook for practice. Gaithersburg, MD: Aspen, 1995; and Guzzetta CE: Research in critical care nursing. In Guzzetta CE, Dossey BM: Cardiovascular nursing: Holistic practice. St. Louis, MO: Mosby-Year Book, 1992.

INTRODUCTION

Critically ill patients often receive multiple medications during their admissions to an intensive care unit. These patients may be at risk for increased pharmacologic or adverse effects from their medications because of altered metabolism and elimination. Decreased organ function or drug interactions may produce increased serum drug concentrations resulting in enhanced or adverse pharmacologic effects. Therefore, it is important to be familiar with each patient's medications, including the drug's metabolic profile, drug interactions, and adverse effect profile. This chapter reviews medications commonly used in intensive care units and discusses their mechanisms of action, indications for use, common adverse effects, contraindications, and usual doses. A summary of intravenous medications information is provided in Chapter 26, Pharmacology Tables.

MEDICATION ADMINISTRATION METHODS

Intravenous

Intravenous (IV) administration is the preferred route for medications in critically ill patients because it permits complete and reliable delivery. Depending on the indication and the therapy, medications may be administered by IV push, intermittent infusion, or continuous infusion. Typically, IV push refers to administration of a drug over 3 to 5 minutes, with intermittent infusion referring to 15-minute to 2-hour drug administration several times per day and continuous infusion administration occurring over a prolonged period of time.

Intramuscular/subcutaneous

Intramuscular (IM) or subcutaneous (SC) administration of medications should be restricted in critically ill patients because the onset of drug action may be prolonged, lack of adequate muscle or subcutaneous fat tissue may not permit these injections, hypotensive or hypovolemic patients may exhibit inadequate or altered peripheral perfusion, or inadequate perfusion may occur in areas of the body where medications have been injected in patients who are medically paralyzed. These routes of administration may result in incomplete, unpredictable, or erratic drug absorption. If medication is not absorbed from the injection site, a depot of medication can develop. Once perfusion is restored, allowing drug absorption, a supratherapeutic or toxic effect may occur from the absorption of the accumulated stores of the drug. In patients with thrombocytopenia, hematomas and bleeding complications can occur. This is also true in patients receiving thrombolytic agents or anticoagulants. Finally, administering frequent intramuscular injections may be inconvenient and painful for patients.

Oral

Oral (PO) administration of medication can also result in incomplete, unpredictable, or erratic absorption. This may be due to the presence of an ileus impairing drug absorption, or to diarrhea decreasing gastrointestinal tract transit time and thus the time for drug absorption. Diarrhea may have a pronounced effect on the absorption of sustained-release preparations such as theophylline, procainamide, or calcium channel blocking agents, resulting in a suboptimal serum drug concentration or clinical response.

In patients unable to swallow, tablets are often crushed and capsules opened for administration through nasogastric tubes. This practice is time-consuming and often results in blockage of the tube, necessitating removal of the clogged tube and insertion of a new tube. If enteral nutrition is being administered through the tube, it often has to be stopped for medication administration, resulting in inadequate nutrition for patients. Also, several medications (e.g., phenytoin, carbamazepine, warfarin) have been shown to compete, or interact, with enteral nutrition solutions. This interaction results in decreased absorption of these agents, or complex formation with the nutrition solution leading to precipitation and clogging of the feeding tube.

Liquid medications may circumvent the need to crush tablets or open capsules, but have their own limitations. Many liquid dosage forms contain sorbitol as a flavoring agent or as the primary delivery vehicle. Sorbitol's hyperosmolarity is a frequent cause of diarrhea in critically ill patients, especially in patients receiving enteral nutrition. Potassium chloride elixir is extremely hyperosmolar and requires dilution with 120 to 160 mls of water before administration. Administering undiluted potassium chloride elixir can result in osmotic diarrhea.

Lastly, sustained-release or enteric-coated preparations are difficult to administer to critically ill patients. When sustained-release products are crushed, the patient absorbs the whole dose immediately as opposed to gradually over a period of 6, 8, 12, or 24 hours. This results in supratherapeutic or toxic effects soon after the administration of the medication, with subtherapeutic effects at the end of the dosing interval. Sustained-release preparations must be converted to equivalent daily doses of immediate-release dosing forms and administered at more frequent dosing intervals. Enteric-coated dosage forms that are crushed may be inactivated by gastric juices or may cause stomach irritation. Enteric-coated tablets are specifically formulated to pass through the stomach intact so that they can enter the small intestine before they begin to dissolve.

Sublingual

Because of the high degree of vascularity of the sublingual mucosa, sublingual administration of medication often produces serum concentrations of medication that parallel intravenous administration, and an onset of action that is often faster than orally administered medications.

Traditionally, nitroglycerin has been one of the few medications administered sublingually (SL) to critically ill patients. However, several oral and intravenous medications have been shown to produce therapeutic effects after sublingual administration. Captopril and nifedipine have been shown to reliably and predictably lower blood pressure in patients with hypertensive urgency. Oral lorazepam tablets have been administered sublingually to treat patients in status epilepticus, while preparations of oral triazolam and intravenous midazolam have been shown to produce sedation after sublingual administration.

Intranasal

Intranasal administration is becoming a popular way to effectively administer sedative and analgesic agents. The high degree of vascularity of the nasal mucosa results in rapid, complete absorption of medication. Agents that have been administered successfully intranasally include meperi-

dine, fentanyl, sufentanil, butorphanol, ketamine, and midazolam.

Transdermal

Transdermal administration of medication is of limited value in critically ill patients. Although nitroglycerin ointment is extremely effective in the acute management of patients with angina, congestive heart failure, pulmonary edema, or hypertension as a temporizing measure before intravenous access is established, nitroglycerin transdermal patches are of limited benefit. Transdermal patches are limited by their slow onset of activity and their inability for dose titration. Also, patients with decreased peripheral perfusion may not sufficiently absorb transdermally administered medications in order to produce the desired therapeutic effect. Transdermal preparations of clonidine, nitroglycerin, or fentanyl may be beneficial in patients who have been stabilized on intravenous or oral doses but require chronic administration of these agents. Chronic use of nitroglycerin transdermal patches is further complicated by the development of tolerance. However, the development of tolerance can be avoided by removing the patch at bedtime, allowing for an 8- to 10-hour "nitrate-free" period.

A eutectic mixture of local anesthetic (EMLA) is a combination of lidocaine and prilocaine. This local anesthetic mixture can be used to anesthetize the skin before insertion of intravenous catheters or the injection of local anesthetics that may be required to produce deeper levels of topical anesthesia.

Although transdermal administration of medications is an infrequent method of drug administration in critically ill patients, its use should not be overlooked as a potential cause of adverse effects in this patient population. Extensive application to burned, abraided, or denuded skin can result in significant systemic absorption of topically applied medications. Excessive use of viscous lidocaine products or mouthwashes containing lidocaine to provide local anesthesia for mucositis or esophagitis also can result in significant systemic absorption of lidocaine. Lidocaine administered topically to the oral mucosa has resulted in serum concentrations capable of producing seizures. The diffuse application of topical glucocorticosteroid preparations also can lead to absorption capable of producing adrenal suppression. This is especially true with the high-potency fluorinated steroid preparations such as betamethasone dipropionate, clobetasol propionate, desoximetasone, or fluocinonide.

CENTRAL NERVOUS SYSTEM PHARMACOLOGY

Sedatives

Sedatives can be divided into four main categories: benzodiazepines, barbiturates, neuroleptics, and miscellaneous agents. Benzodiazepines are the most commonly used sedatives in critically ill patients. Neuroleptics typically are used in patients who manifest a psychological or behavioral component to their sedative needs, while barbiturates are reserved for patients with head injuries and increased intracranial pressure. A new agent, propofol, is a short-acting intravenous general anesthetic that was recently approved for use as a sedative for mechanically ventilated critically ill patients.

Benzodiazepines

Benzodiazepines are the most frequently used agents for sedation in critically ill patients. These agents provide sedation, decrease anxiety, have anticonvulsant properties, possess indirect muscle relaxant properties, and induce anterograde amnesia. Benzodiazepines bind to gamma-aminobutyric acid (GABA) receptors located in the central nervous system, modulating this inhibitory neurotransmitter. These agents have a wide margin of safety as well as flexibility in their routes of administration.

Benzodiazepines are frequently used to provide short-term sedation and amnesia during imaging procedures, other diagnostic procedures, and invasive procedures such as central venous catheter placement or bronchoscopy. A common long-term indication for using benzodiazepines is sedation and amnesia during mechanical ventilation.

Benzodiazepines are associated with minimal adverse effects. Excessive sedation and confusion can occur with initial doses, but these effects diminish as tolerance develops during therapy. Elderly and pediatric patients may exhibit a paradoxical effect manifested by irritability, agitation, hostility, hallucinations, and anxiety. Respiratory depression may be seen in patients receiving concurrent narcotics, as well as in elderly patients and patients with chronic obstructive pulmonary disease.

- *Monitoring parameters:* Mental status, level of consciousness, respiratory rate, and level of comfort should be monitored in any patient receiving a benzodiazepine. Signs and symptoms of withdrawal reactions should be monitored for patients receiving short-acting agents (i.e., midazolam).

Midazolam

Midazolam is a short-acting water-soluble benzodiazepine that may be administered intravenously, intramuscularly, sublingually, orally, intranasally, or rectally.

Midazolam's clearance is reduced in critically ill patients, and patients with liver disease, shock, or who are concurrently receiving enzyme-inhibiting drugs such as cimetidine or ciprofloxacin. Elimination half-life increases due to the inability of the liver to metabolize the drug to its primary active metabolite, 1-hydroxy midazolam. In geriatric patients, midazolam demonstrates prolonged half-lives secondary to age-related reduction in liver function.

- *Dose:* IV bolus: 0.025 to 0.035 mg/kg
  Continuous infusion: 0.5 to 5.0 μg/kg/minute

Lorazepam

Lorazepam is an intermediate-acting benzodiazepine that offers the advantage of not having its metabolism affected by impaired hepatic function, age, or interacting drugs. Glucuronidation in the liver is the route of elimination of lorazepam. Because lorazepam is relatively water insoluble, it must be diluted in propylene glycol, and it is propylene glycol that is responsible for the hypotension that may be seen after bolus intravenous administration. Recently, administration of lorazepam by continuous intravenous infusion has been advocated. However, this method of administration is hampered by the relative water insolubility of lorazepam. Large volumes of fluid are required to maintain the drug in solution, so that only 20 to 40 mg can be safely dissolved in 250 ml of dextrose-5%-water. In-line filters are recommended when administering lorazepam by continuous infusion because of the potential for the drug to precipitate. Finally, lorazepam's long elimination half-life of 10 to 20 hours limits its dosing flexibility by continuous infusion.

- *Dose:* IV bolus: 0.04 mg/kg
  Continuous infusion: 0.06 mg/kg/hour

Diazepam

Diazepam is a long-acting benzodiazepine with a faster onset of action than lorazepam or midazolam. Although its duration of action is 4 to 6 hours after a single dose, it displays cumulative effects because the activities of its metabolites (temazepam, oxazepam, and desmethyldiazepam) contribute to its pharmacologic effect. Desmethyldiazepam has a half-life of approximately 150 to 200 hours, so it accumulates slowly and then is slowly eliminated from the body after discontinuation of diazepam. Diazepam metabolism is reduced in patients with hepatic failure and in patients receiving drugs that inhibit hepatic microsomal enzymes.

- *Dose:* IV bolus: 0.1 to 0.2 mg/kg
  Continuous infusion: Not recommended

Flumazenil

Flumazenil is a specific benzodiazepine antagonist indicated for the reversal of benzodiazepine-induced conscious sedation, recurrent sedation, and benzodiazepine overdose. It should be used with caution in patients who have received benzodiazepines for an extended period of time in order to prevent the precipitation of withdrawal reactions.

- *Dose: Reversal of conscious sedation:* 0.2 mg IV over 2 minutes, followed in 45 seconds by 0.2 mg repeated every minute as needed to a maximum dose of 1 mg. Reversal of recurrent sedation is the same as for conscious sedation, except doses may be repeated every 20 minutes as needed. *Benzodiazepine overdose:* 0.2 mg over 30 seconds followed by 0.3 mg over 30 seconds; repeated doses of 0.5 mg can be administered over 30 seconds at 1-minute intervals up to a cumulative dose of 3 mg. With a partial response after 3 mg, additional doses up to a total dose of 5 mg may be administered. In all of the above-mentioned scenarios, no more than 1 mg should be administered at any one time, and no more than 3 mg in any 1 hour. Continuous infusion: 0.1 to 0.5 mg/hour (for the reversal of long-acting benzodiazepines or massive overdoses).

- *Monitoring parameters:* Level of consciousness, resedation, and signs and symptoms of withdrawal reactions.

Neuroleptics

Haloperidol and droperidol are major tranquilizers commonly used for the management of agitated, delirious patients who fail to respond adequately to nonpharmacologic interventions or other sedatives. These agents have the advantage of limited respiratory depression and little potential for the development of tolerance or dependence. Although their exact mechanisms of action are unknown, they probably involve dopaminergic receptor blockade in the central nervous system, resulting in central nervous system depression at the subcortical level of the brain.

The major side effect of these agents is their extrapyramidal reactions, such as akathisia and dystonia. These reactions usually occur early in therapy and may resolve with dose reduction or discontinuation of the drug. However, in more severe cases, diphenhydramine, 25 to 50 mg IV, or benztropine, 1 to 2 mg IV, may be required to relieve the symptoms. Extrapyramidal reactions appear to be more common after oral haloperidol than after intravenous haloperidol administration. Neuroleptic malignant syndrome may be seen with these agents, manifested by hyperthermia, severe extrapyramidal reactions, altered mental status, and autonomic instability. Treatment involves supportive care and the administration of dantrolene. Cardiovascular side effects include hypotension, especially with droperidol because of its greater alpha-adrenergic antagonistic effects. High doses of haloperidol may prolong the QT_c interval in patients, especially those patients receiving haloperidol via continuous infusion. Monitoring the QT_c interval is mandatory for all patients receiving haloperidol by continuous infusion.

- *Monitoring parameters:* Mental status, blood pressure, electrocardiogram, and electrolytes (especially with haloperidol infusions).

Haloperidol

Intravenous haloperidol is the most frequently used neuroleptic for controlling agitation in critically ill patients.

Initial doses of 2 to 5 mg may be doubled every 15 to 20 minutes until the patient is adequately sedated. Single intravenous doses as large as 150 mg have been safely administered to patients, as well as total daily doses of approximately 1000 mg. As soon as the patient's symptoms are controlled, the total dose required to calm the patient should be divided into four equal doses and administered every 6 hours on a regularly scheduled basis. When the patient's symptoms are stable, the daily dose should be rapidly tapered to the smallest dose that controls the patient's symptoms. Continuous intravenous infusions have also been advocated to allow flexible dosing in order to control patient's symptoms.

- *Dose:* IV bolus: 1 to 10 mg
  Continuous infusion: 10 mg/hour
  (not generally recommended)

Droperidol

Droperidol is similar to haloperidol but is shorter acting and produces more sedation and more adverse effects such as hypotension.

- *Dose:* IV bolus: 0.625 to 10 mg
  Continuous infusion: Not recommended

Barbiturates

Barbiturates are primarily used to reduce intracranial pressure in head injury patients after conservative therapy has failed. Barbiturates decrease cerebral oxygen consumption, decrease cerebral blood flow, and potentially scavenge free oxygen radicals.

The general central nervous system depression associated with the use of barbiturates may cause excessive sedation as well as respiratory depression. Barbiturates produce direct myocardial depression, reducing cardiac output as well as increasing venous capacitance. Rapid IV administration can result in arrhythmias and hypotension.

Pentobarbital

Pentobarbital continuous infusions are commonly used to induce barbiturate coma. The infusion should be titrated to maintain intracranial pressure < 20 mm Hg and cerebral perfusion pressure > 60 mm Hg. The mean arterial pressure should be maintained in a range that provides an adequate cerebral perfusion pressure. Therapeutic serum pentobarbital concentrations are 20 to 50 mg/L.

- *Dose:* IV bolus: 20 mg/kg infused over 2 hours
  Continuous infusion: 1 mg/kg/hour
- *Monitoring parameters:* Level of consciousness, intracranial pressure, cerebral perfusion pressure, blood pressure, and serum pentobarbital concentration.

Miscellaneous Agents

Propofol

Propofol is an intravenous general anesthetic that has become popular for sedation of mechanically ventilated patients. The advantages of propofol are its rapid onset and short duration of action compared to the benzodiazepines. Propofol has been associated with hypotension in critically ill patients, especially patients who are hypotensive or hypovolemic. Hypotension can be avoided by limiting bolus doses to 0.25 to 0.5 mg/kg and the initial infusion rate to 5 µg/kg/minute. The fat emulsion vehicle of propofol has been shown to support the growth of microorganisms so the manufacturer recommends that extemporaneously prepared infusions and the IV tubing be changed every 6 hours. If the manufacturer's infusion bottles are used, these containers, along with the IV tubing, should be changed every 12 hours. Also, since propofol is formulated in a fat emulsion vehicle that serves as a source of calories providing 1.1 calories/ml, its infusion rate must be accounted for when determining a patient's nutrition support regimen.

- *Dose:* IV bolus: 0.25 to 0.5 mg/kg
  Continuous infusion: 5 to 50 µg/kg/minute
- *Monitoring parameters:* Level of consciousness, blood pressure, and serum triglyceride level, especially at high infusion rates.

Ketamine

Ketamine is an analogue of phencyclidine that is commonly used as an intravenous general anesthetic. It is an agent that produces analgesia, anesthesia, and amnesia without the loss of consciousness. The onset of anesthesia after a single 0.5- to 1-mg/kg bolus dose is within 1 to 2 minutes and lasts approximately 5 to 10 minutes. Ketamine causes sympathetic stimulation that normally increases blood pressure and heart rate while maintaining cardiac output. This may be important in patients with hypovolemia. Ketamine is useful in patients who require repeated painful procedures such as wound debridement. The bronchodilatory effects of ketamine may be beneficial in patients experiencing status asthmaticus. However, ketamine increases intracranial pressure and should be avoided in patients with head injuries, space-occupying lesions, or any other conditions that may cause an increase in intracranial pressure. Emergence reactions or hallucinations, commonly seen after ketamine anesthesia, may be prevented with the concurrent use of benzodiazepines.

- *Dose:* IV bolus: 0.5 to 1 mg/kg
  Continuous infusion: 9 to 45 µg/kg/minute
  Oral: 10 mg/kg diluted in 1 to 2 ounces of juice
  Intranasal: 5 mg/kg
- *Monitoring parameters:* Levels of sedation and analgesia, heart rate, blood pressure, and mental status.

Analgesics

Narcotics

Narcotics produce their effects by reversibly binding to the mu, delta, kappa, and sigma opiate receptors located in the central nervous system. Mu-1 receptors are associated with analgesia, and mu-2 receptors are associated with respiratory depression, bradycardia, euphoria, and dependence. Delta receptors have no selective agonist and modulate mu receptor activity. Kappa receptors function at the spinal and supraspinal levels and are associated with sedation. Sigma receptors are associated with dysphoria and psychotomimetic effects.

- *Monitoring parameters:* Level of pain or comfort, blood pressure, renal function, and respiratory rate.

Morphine

Morphine is the most commonly used narcotic analgesic. Morphine is hepatically metabolized to several metabolites, including morphine-6-glucuronide (M6G) which is approximately 5 to 10 times more potent than morphine. M6G is renally eliminated and after repeated dosing can accumulate in patients with reduced renal function, producing enhanced pharmacologic effects. Morphine possesses vasodilatory properties due to either direct effects on the vasculature or histamine release.

- *Dose:* IV bolus: 2 to 5 mg
  Continuous infusion: 2 to 5 mg/hour
  Patient-controlled analgesia (PCA): IV bolus: 0.5 to 3 mg; lockout interval: 5 to 20 minutes

Meperidine

Meperidine is a short-acting opioid that is one-seventh the potency of morphine. It is hepatically metabolized to normeperidine, which is renally eliminated, and is also a neurotoxin. Normeperidine can accumulate in patients with reduced renal function, resulting in seizures. Meperidine should be avoided in patients taking monoamine oxidase inhibitors due to the potential for development of a hypertensive crisis when these agents are administered concurrently.

- *Dose:* IV bolus: 25 to 100 mg
  Continuous infusion: 5 to 35 mg/hour
  PCA: IV bolus: 5 to 30 mg; lockout interval: 5 to 15 minutes

Fentanyl

Fentanyl is an analog of meperidine that is 100 times more potent than morphine. After single doses, its duration of action is limited by its rapid distribution into fat tissue. However, after repeated dosing or continuous infusion administration, fat stores become saturated, thereby prolonging its terminal elimination half-life to more than 24 hours. Unlike morphine, fentanyl does not cause histamine release.

- *Dose:* IV bolus: 25 to 100 µg
  Continuous infusion: 50 to 100 µg/hour
  PCA: IV bolus: 25 to 100 µg; lockout interval: 5 to 10 minutes
  Transdermal: Patients not previously on opioids: 25 µg/hour
  Opioid-tolerant patients: 25 to 100 µg/hour

Naloxone

Naloxone is a pure opiate antagonist that displaces opioid agonists from the mu, delta, and kappa receptor binding sites. Naloxone reverses narcotic-induced respiratory depression, producing an increase in respiratory rate and minute ventilation, a decrease in arterial PCO_2, and normalization of blood pressure if reduced. Narcotic-induced sedation or sleep is also reversed by naloxone. Naloxone reverses analgesia, increases sympathetic nervous system activity, and may result in tachycardia, hypertension, pulmonary edema, and cardiac arrhythmias. Because its duration of action is generally shorter than that of opiates, the effect of opiates may return after the effects of naloxone dissipate. Naloxone administration produces withdrawal symptoms in patients who have been taking chronic narcotic analgesics. Diluting and slowly administering naloxone in incremental doses can prevent the precipitation of acute withdrawal reactions as well as prevent the increase in sympathetic stimulation that may accompany the reversal of analgesia. One 0.4-mg ampule should be diluted with 0.9% NaCl (saline) to 10 ml to produce a concentration of 0.04 mg/ml. Sequential doses of 0.04 to 0.08 mg should be administered slowly until the desired response is obtained.

- *Dose: Postoperative opiate depression:* Initial dose: 0.1 to 0.2 mg given at 2- to 3-minute intervals until the desired response is obtained. Additional doses may be necessary depending on the response of the patient and the dose and duration of the opiate administered. Continuous infusion: 0.0037 mg/kg/hour. *Known or suspected opiate overdose:* Initial dose: 0.4 to 2 mg administered at 2- to 3-minute intervals if necessary. If no response is observed after a total of 10 mg has been administered, other causes of the depressive state should be determined. Continuous infusion: Loading dose: 0.4 mg, followed by 0.0025 mg/kg/hour and titrated to the patient's response.
- *Monitoring parameters:* Signs and symptoms of withdrawal reactions, respiratory rate, blood pressure, mental status, level of consciousness, and pupil size.

Nonsteroidal Antiinflammatory Drugs

Ketorolac

Ketorolac is a nonsteroidal antiinflammatory drug (NSAID) that is indicated for the short-term treatment of moderately severe, acute pain that requires analgesia at the opioid level. The drug exhibits antiinflammatory, analgesic, and antipyretic activities. Its mechanism of action is thought to be due to inhibition of prostaglandin synthesis by inhibiting cyclooxygenase, an enzyme that catalyzes the formation of endoperoxidases from arachidonic acid. NSAIDs are more efficacious in the treatment of prostaglandin-mediated pain. Ketorolac is the only currently available NSAID approved for IM, IV, and oral administration, and it is often used in combination with other analgesics or as a sole analgesic agent because pain often involves multiple mechanisms. Combination therapy may be more efficacious than single-drug regimens, and combinations with narcotics can decrease narcotic requirements, minimizing narcotic side effects.

Ketorolac is associated with the same adverse effects as orally administered NSAIDs, such as reversible platelet effects, gastrointestinal bleeding, and reduced renal function. Ketorolac is contraindicated in patients with advanced renal failure and in patients at risk for renal failure due to volume depletion. Therefore, volume depletion should be corrected before administering ketorolac. Because of the potential for significant adverse effects, the maximum combined duration of parenteral and oral use is limited to 5 days.

- *Dose:* Loading dose: < 65 yrs: 60 mg, > 65 yrs or < 50 kg: 30 mg; maintenance dose: < 65 yrs: 30 mg q6h, > 65 yrs or < 50 kg: 15 mg q6h
- *Monitoring parameters:* Renal function and volume status.

Neuromuscular Blocking Agents

Neuromuscular blocking agents are primarily used to obtain, protect, and maintain a safe secure airway and to assist with mechanical ventilation. These agents have no sedative, amnestic, anesthetic, or analgesic properties. Neuromuscular blocking agents are categorized as either depolarizing or nondepolarizing agents.

Depolarizing

Succinylcholine

Succinylcholine is the only depolarizing agent available for clinical use and is the agent of choice for rapid intubation of the trachea. Succinylcholine binds to acetylcholine receptors causing an initial depolarizing of the muscle membrane followed by a persistent depolarization of the muscle endplate, resulting in paralysis.

Succinylcholine may increase serum potassium approximately 0.5 mEq/L after a standard intubating dose of 1 to 2 mg/kg. Critically ill patients with burns, spinal cord injury, trauma with extensive skeletal muscle damage, upper and lower motor neuron disease, and prolonged bed rest are predisposed to the development of hyperkalemia after a dose of succinylcholine due to the development of nonfunctional extrajunctional acetycholine receptors. These receptors bind succinylcholine without causing paralysis, but depolarize the muscle cells, releasing potassium and increasing serum potassium concentrations into the supratherapeutic or toxic range. Although hyperkalemia can occur within the first 24 hours after injury, patients are most at risk during the period from 7 days up to 9 months after injury. Therefore, succinylcholine is contraindicated in these patients. In situations where succinylcholine is contraindicated, a short-acting or intermediate-acting nondepolarizing agent may be used. Succinylcholine is rapidly hydrolyzed by pseudocholinesterase; however, patients with atypical pseudocholinesterase may experience prolonged blockade. Other conditions associated with prolonged blockade resulting from reduced cholinesterase activity include pregnancy, liver disease, acute infections, carcinomas, uremia, and burns.

- *Dose:* See Chapter 26, Table 26–2.
- *Monitoring parameters:* Renal function, electrolytes (especially potassium), acid-base status, and level of paralysis.

Nondepolarizing

Nondepolarizing agents are competitive antagonists of acetylcholine at the acetylcholine receptor. Nondepolarizing agents are subdivided according to chemical class: either aminosteroid (pancuronium, pipecuronium, rocuronium, vecuronium) or benzylisoquinolinium (atracurium, doxacurium, mivacurium). These agents are further classified according to duration of action: short-acting (mivacurium), intermediate-acting (atracurium, rocuronium, vecuronium), and long-acting (doxacurium, pancuronium, pipecuronium).

Nondepolarizing agents can be used for short- or long-term indications in critically ill patients. Short-term indications include intubation, stability during intrahospital transport, and immobility during procedures. Long-term indications include mechanical ventilation after optimal doses of sedatives and analgesics have not been able to prevent a patient from "fighting the ventilator."

Although adverse effects are minimal, several of them can be significant. Atracurium and mivacurium can cause histamine release after rapid intravenous bolus injection, resulting in hypotension and flushing. This adverse effect can be prevented by injecting each agent over at least 60 seconds. Laudanosine, atracurium's primary metabolite, has been shown to produce seizures in dogs after it achieves high concentrations in the cerebral spinal fluid. However, there are no reports of critically ill patients experiencing adverse central nervous system events from the accumulation of laudanosine. Mivacurium is hydrolyzed by pseudocholinesterase, and prolonged neuromuscular blockade may be seen in patients with reduced pseudocholinesterase levels.

The steroid-based agents pancuronium, pipecuronium, and vecuronium are metabolized to 3-hydroxy metabolites that have 50% of the activity of the parent compounds. These metabolites are renally eliminated and have been shown to accumulate in patients with renal dysfunction, producing prolonged periods of paralysis. Monitoring patients and adjusting doses, dosing intervals, or continuous infusion rates with the aid of a peripheral nerve stimulator to maintain one or two twitches of a Train-of-Four stimulation can usually prevent this adverse effect from occurring (see Chapter 6, Airway and Ventilatory Management).

A more serious complication associated with the use of nondepolarizing agents is the development of a prolonged disuse atrophy syndrome. This syndrome has been shown to occur after the extended administration of steroid-based and benzylisoquinolinium agents and is characterized by diffuse proximal and distal muscle weakness, normal nerve conduction and sensory function, increases in creatinine kinase, and a prolonged clinical recovery. This complication cannot be prevented by monitoring patients with peripheral nerve stimulation. Patients receiving steroids may be predisposed to developing this complication; however, this association remains to be conclusively proven.

Finally, tolerance or the need to increase doses to maintain a stable level of paralysis is often encountered in patients receiving these agents for an extended duration. Tolerance may be attributed to (1) the proliferation of nonfunctional extrajunctional receptors which bind the drug but do not cause paralysis, (2) the increased volume of distribution resulting in lower serum concentrations at the neuromuscular junction, and (3) binding to acute phase reactant proteins, decreasing the free, pharmacologically active fraction.

- *Dose:* See Chapter 26, Table 26–2.
- *Monitoring parameters:* Level of paralysis (peripheral nerve stimulation), renal function, and liver function.

Anticonvulsants

Hydantoins

Phenytoin

Phenytoin is the primary anticonvulsant used for the acute control of generalized tonic-clonic seizures. Phenytoin stabilizes neuronal cell membranes and decreases the spread of seizure activity. Phenytoin exhibits capacity-limited metabolism such that proportional increases in the dose may result in greater than proportional increases in the serum concentration. As the dose is increased, the time it takes to achieve steady-state serum concentrations also increases. Phenytoin is highly bound to albumin, and conditions resulting in hypoalbuminemia, as well as liver or renal disease, may result in increased concentrations of the pharmacologically active free fraction. In this setting free phenytoin serum concentrations should be monitored to adjust doses appropriately.

Phenytoin should not be administered intravenously at a rate faster than 50 mg/minute. Faster rates of administration may produce hypotension which is attributed to propylene glycol, the vehicle used to solubilize phenytoin. Phenytoin will precipitate in dextrose-containing solutions and only should be mixed in saline solutions.

Oral absorption may be impaired by concomitant administration with enteral nutrition solutions. When phenytoin is administered through enteral feeding tubes, enteral nutrition solutions must be stopped and the feeding tube flushed before administration of the phenytoin suspension. The phenytoin dose must be followed by a flush before restarting enteral nutritional solutions.

- *Dose:* Loading dose: 20 mg/kg IV; maintenance dose: 5 mg/kg/day IV/PO
- *Monitoring parameters:* Seizure activity, electroencephalogram, serum phenytoin concentration (free phenytoin concentration if applicable), albumin, liver function, infusion rate, blood pressure, electrocardiogram with intravenous administration, and intravenous injection site.

Barbiturates

Phenobarbital

Phenobarbital may be administered to patients with seizures who have not responded to both phenytoin and intravenous benzodiazepines. Phenobarbital depresses excitatory postsynaptic seizure discharge and increases the convulsive threshold for electrical and chemical stimulation. Phenobarbital should be administered intravenously at a rate less than 50 mg/minute to avoid propylene-glycol–induced hypotension.

- *Dose:* Loading dose: 20 mg/kg IV (1 mg/kg increases the serum concentration 1 mg/L); maintenance dose: 3 to 5 mg/kg/day IV/PO
- *Monitoring parameters:* Seizure activity, electroencephalogram, serum phenobarbital concentration, infusion rate, blood pressure, and electrocardiogram with intravenous administration.

Benzodiazepines

Benzodiazepines are the primary agents in the management of status epilepticus. These agents suppress the spread of seizure activity but do not abolish the abnormal discharge from a seizure focus. Although intravenous diazepam has the fastest onset of action, lorazepam or midazolam are equally efficacious in controlling seizure activity.

- *Monitoring parameters:* Seizure activity, electroencephalogram, and respiratory rate and quality.

CARDIOVASCULAR SYSTEM PHARMACOLOGY

Parenteral Vasodilators (Chapter 26, Table 26–3.)

Nitrates

Sodium nitroprusside

Sodium nitroprusside is a balanced vasodilator affecting the arterial and venous systems. Blood pressure reduction occurs within seconds after an infusion is started, with a duration of action of less than 10 minutes once the infusion is discontinued. Sodium nitroprusside is considered the agent of choice in acute hypertensive conditions such as hypertensive encephalopathy, intracerebral infarction, subarachnoid hemorrhage, carotid endarterectomy, malignant hypertension, microangiopathic anemia, and aortic dissection, and after general surgical procedures, major vascular procedures, or renal transplantation.

If sodium nitroprusside is used for longer than 48 hours, there is the risk of thiocyanate toxicity. However, this may only be a concern in patients with renal dysfunction. In this setting, thiocyanate serum concentrations should be monitored to ensure that they remain less than 10 mg/dl. Other potential side effects include methemoglobinemia and cyanide toxicity. Nitroprusside should be used with caution in the setting of increased intracranial pressure, such as head trauma or postcraniotomy, where it may cause an increase in cerebral blood flow. Nitroprusside's effects on intracranial pressure may be attenuated by a lowered Pa_{CO_2} and raised Pa_{O_2}. In pregnant women, nitroprusside should be reserved only for refractory hypertension associated with eclampsia, due to the potential risk to the fetus.

- *Dose:* Continuous infusion: 0.5 to 10 µg/kg/minute
- *Monitoring parameters:* Blood pressure, renal function, thiocyanate concentration (prolonged infusions), acid-base status, and hemodynamic parameters.

Nitroglycerin

Nitroglycerin is a preferential venous dilator affecting the venous system at low doses, but relaxing arterial smooth muscle at higher doses. The onset of blood pressure reduction after starting a nitroglycerin infusion is similar to sodium nitroprusside, approximately 1 to 3 minutes, with a duration of action of less than 10 minutes. Headaches are a common adverse effect that may occur with nitroglycerin therapy and can be treated with acetaminophen. Tachyphylaxis can be seen with the intravenous infusion, similar to what is seen after the chronic use of topical nitroglycerin preparations. In patients receiving heparin in addition to nitroglycerin, increased doses of heparin may be required to maintain a therapeutic partial thromboplastin time (PTT). The mechanism by which nitroglycerin causes heparin resistance is unknown. However, the PTT should be closely monitored in patients receiving nitroglycerin and heparin concurrently.

Nitroglycerin is the preferred agent in the setting of hypertension associated with myocardial ischemia or infarction because its net effect is a reduction in oxygen consumption.

- *Dose:* Continuous infusion: 10 to 300 µg/minute
- *Monitoring parameters:* Blood pressure, heart rate, signs and symptoms of ischemia, hemodynamic parameters (if applicable), and PTT (in patients receiving heparin concurrently).

Arterial Vasodilating Agents

Hydralazine

Hydralazine reduces peripheral vascular resistance by directly relaxing arterial smooth muscle. Blood pressure reduction occurs within 5 to 20 minutes after an intravenous dose and lasts approximately 2 to 6 hours.

Common adverse effects include headache, nausea, vomiting, palpitations, and tachycardia. Reflex tachycardia may precipitate anginal attacks.

- *Dose:* 10 to 25 mg IV q2-4h
- *Monitoring parameters:* Blood pressure and heart rate.

Diazoxide

Diazoxide is a nondiuretic that reduces peripheral vascular resistance by directly relaxing arterial smooth muscle. Side effects such as hypotension, nausea and vomiting, dizziness, weakness, hyperglycemia, and reflex tachycardia have been associated with the use of the higher 300-mg dosing regimen. Using lower dose regimens produces similar but less severe side effects. Caution should be used when diazoxide is administered with other antihypertensive agents since excessive hypotension may result.

Blood pressure reduction occurs within 1 to 2 minutes and lasts 3 to 12 hours after a dose. Therefore, blood pressure should be monitored frequently until stable, and then monitored hourly.

- *Dose:* IV bolus: 50 to 150 mg q5 min; continuous infusion: 7.5 to 30 mg/minute
- *Monitoring parameters:* Blood pressure, heart rate, and serum glucose.

Ganglionic Blocking Agents

Trimethaphan

Trimethaphan is the only available intravenous ganglionic blocking agent. The onset of blood pressure reduction is within minutes after starting an infusion, with a duration of action of up to 20 minutes after stopping the infusion. However, hypotension may persist for several hours after the administration of higher doses. Adverse effects that have been associated with the use of trimethaphan include ileus, urinary retention, and mydriasis.

Trimethaphan in combination with a beta blocker may be used as an alternative to nitroprusside in the setting of an acute aortic dissection. Trimethaphan should be avoided in hypertension associated with eclampsia and renal vasculature disorders.

- *Dose:* Continuous infusion: 0.5 to 5 mg/minute
- *Monitoring parameters:* Blood pressure, heart rate, bowel sounds, gastrointestinal tract function, and bladder function.

Alpha- and Beta-Adrenergic Blocking Agents

Labetalol

Labetalol is a combined alpha- and beta-adrenergic blocking agent with a specificity of beta receptors to alpha receptors of approximately 7:1. Labetalol may be administered parenterally by escalating bolus doses or by continuous infusion. The onset of action after the administration of labetalol is within 5 minutes with a duration of effect from 2 to 12 hours. Since labetalol possesses beta-blocking properties, it may produce bronchospasm in individuals with asthma or reactive airway disease. It also may produce conduction system disturbances or bradycardia in susceptible individuals, and its negative inotropic properties may exacerbate symptoms of congestive heart failure.

Labetalol may be considered as an alternative to sodium nitroprusside in the setting of hypertension associated with head trauma or postcraniotomy, spinal cord syndromes, transverse lesions of the spinal cord, Guillain-Barré syndrome, or autonomic hyperreflexia, as well as hypertension associated with sympathomimetics (e.g., cocaine, amphetamines, phencyclidine, nasal decongestants, or certain diet pills) or withdrawal of centrally acting antihypertensive agents (e.g., beta blockers, clonidine, or methyldopa). It also may be used as an alternative to phentolamine in the setting of pheochromocytoma because of its alpha- and beta-blocking properties.

- *Dose:* IV bolus: 20 mg over 2 minutes, then 40 to 80 mg IV q10 min to a total of 300 mg; continuous infusion: 2 mg/minute and titrate to effect.
- *Monitoring parameters:* Blood pressure, heart rate, ECG, and signs and symptoms of heart failure or bronchospasm (if applicable).

Alpha-Adrenergic Blocking Agents

Phentolamine

Phentolamine is an alpha-adrenergic blocking agent that may be administered parenterally by bolus injection or continuous infusion. Onset of action is within 1 to 2 minutes, with a duration of action of 3 to 10 minutes. Potential adverse effects that may occur with phentolamine include tachycardia, gastrointestinal stimulation, and hypoglycemia.

Phentolamine is considered the drug of choice for the treatment of hypertension associated with pheochromocytoma because of its ability to block alpha-adrenergic receptors. Also, it is the primary agent used to treat acute hypertensive episodes in patients receiving monoamine oxidase inhibitors.

- *Dose:* IV bolus: 5 to 10 mg q 5-15 min; continuous infusion: 1 to 10 mg/minute
- *Monitoring parameters:* Blood pressure and heart rate.

Beta-Adrenergic Blocking Agents

Beta-adrenergic blocking agents available for intravenous delivery include propranolol, esmolol, metoprolol, and atenolol. Propranolol and metoprolol may be administered by bolus injection or continuous infusion. Atenolol typically is administered by bolus injection, while esmolol is administered by continuous infusion. A continuous infusion of esmolol may or may not be preceded by an initial bolus injection.

Esmolol has the fastest onset and shortest duration of action, approximately 1 to 3 minutes and 20 to 30 minutes, respectively. Propranolol and metoprolol have similar onset times, but durations of action vary between 1 and 6 hours. The duration of action after a bolus dose of atenolol is approximately 12 hours.

All agents may produce bronchospasm in individuals with asthma or reactive airways disease and may produce conduction system disturbances or bradycardia in susceptible individuals. Also, because of their negative inotropic properties, they may exacerbate symptoms of congestive heart failure.

Beta-blocking agents typically are used as adjuncts with other agents in the treatment of acute hypertension. They may be used with sodium nitroprusside or trimethaphan in the treatment of acute aortic dissections. They should be administered to patients with hypertension associated with pheochromocytoma only after phentolamine has been given. Also, they are the agents of choice in patients who have been maintained on beta-blocking agents for the chronic management of hypertension but who have abruptly stopped therapy.

Beta-blocking agents should be avoided in patients with hypertensive encephalopathy, intracranial infarctions, or subarachnoid hemorrhages because of their central nervous system depressant effects. They also should be avoided in patients with acute pulmonary edema because of their negative inotropic properties. Finally, beta-blocking agents should be avoided in hypertension associated with eclampsia and renal vasculature disorders.

- *Dose:* Atenolol: IV bolus: 5 mg over 5 minutes, followed by 5 mg IV 10 minutes later; esmolol: IV bolus 500 µg/kg; continuous infusion: 50 to 400 µg/kg/minute; metoprolol: IV bolus: 5 mg IV q2min × 3 doses; propranolol: IV bolus: 0.2 to 1 mg q5-15 min; continuous infusion: 1 to 4 mg/hour

- *Monitoring parameters:* Blood pressure, heart rate, electrocardiogram, and signs and symptoms of heart failure or bronchospasm (if applicable).

Angiotensin-Converting Enzyme Inhibitors

Angiotensin-converting enzyme (ACE) inhibitors competitively inhibit angiotensin-converting enzyme, which is responsible for the conversion of angiotensin I to angiotensin II. In addition, these agents inactivate bradykinin and other vasodilatory prostaglandins, resulting in an increase in plasma renin concentrations and a reduction in plasma aldosterone concentrations. The net effect is a reduction in blood pressure in hypertensive patients and a reduction in afterload in patients with congestive heart failure.

ACE inhibitors are indicated in the management of hypertension and congestive heart failure. Adverse effects associated with ACE inhibitors include rash, taste disturbances, and cough. Initial dose hypotension may occur in patients who are hypovolemic, hyponatremic, or who have been aggressively diuresed. Hypotension may be avoided or minimized by starting with low doses or withholding diuretics for 24 to 48 hours. Worsening of renal function may occur in patients with bilateral renal artery stenosis.

Captopril

Captopril is a short-acting ACE inhibitor with an onset of action of approximately 15 to 45 minutes and a duration of action between 6 and 8 hours.

- *Dose:* 6.25 to 50 mg PO, SL q6-8h

Enalapril

Enalapril is a prodrug that is converted in the liver to its active moiety, enalaprilat, a long-acting ACE inhibitor. Enalapril is available in an oral dosage form, while enalaprilat is available in the intravenous form. Following an intravenous dose of enalaprilat, blood pressure lowering occurs within 15 minutes and lasts 4 to 6 hours.

- *Dose:* Enalaprilat: IV bolus: 0.625 to 1.25 mg over 5 minutes q6h; continuous infusion: not recommended; enalapril: oral: 2.5 to 40 mg qd.
- *Monitoring parameters:* Blood pressure, heart rate, renal function, and electrolytes.

Calcium Channel Blocking Agents

Calcium channel blocking agents may be used as alternative therapy in the treatment of hypertension resulting from hypertensive encephalopathy, myocardial ischemia, malignant hypertension, or eclampsia, or after renal transplantation.

Nicardipine

Nicardipine is an intravenous calcium channel blocking agent that is primarily indicated for the treatment of hypertension. Onset is within 5 minutes with a duration of approximately 30 minutes. Nicardipine also is available in an oral dosage form so that patients started on intravenous therapy can convert to oral therapy when indicated.

- *Dose:* Continuous infusion: 5 mg/hour, increase every 15 minutes to a maximum of 15 mg/hour; oral: 20 to 40 mg q8h

Nifedipine

Nifedipine is an oral calcium channel blocking agent that is effective in lowering blood pressure after either oral or sublingual administration. Absorption is reliable after oral administration and produces a reduction in blood pressure within 30 minutes with a duration of action ranging from 3 to 6 hours. When nifedipine is administered sublingually, the capsule may be punctured and chewed, expelling the liquid contents of the capsule. The liquid may be absorbed sublingually or swallowed and absorbed. The capsule also may be punctured by a needle attached to a syringe and the contents aspirated into the syringe. The needle is removed from the syringe and the contents of the syringe can be "expelled" into the sublingual space. Although sublingual absorption is quite variable, onset of action is typically within 15 to 30 minutes with a duration of action of approximately 3 to 6 hours.

- *Dose:* 10 to 20 mg PO, SL, buccal q3-8h
- *Monitoring parameters:* Blood pressure and heart rate.

Central Sympatholytic Agents

Methyldopa

Methyldopa is decarboxylated in the central nervous system to α-methylnorepinephrine, which lowers blood pressure by stimulation of central inhibitory alpha-adrenergic receptors. Methyldopa should not be used in settings that require rapid blood pressure reduction because its onset may not occur for 4 to 6 hours. The duration of blood pressure reduction is quite variable and ranges from 10 to 16 hours. Methyldopa is available as the oral dosage form, while methyldopate is available as the parenteral dosage form. Methyldopa therapy may be associated with sedation or excessive central nervous depression. Intravenous methyldopate may be used in the setting in which patients have been maintained on oral methyldopa or clonidine but are unable to take oral medications.

- *Dose:* Oral: methyldopa 250 to 1000 mg q6h; IV: methyldopate 250 to 1000 mg q6h
- *Monitoring parameters:* Blood pressure, heart rate, and mental status.

Clonidine

Clonidine is an oral agent that stimulates alpha$_2$-adrenergic receptors in the medulla oblongata, causing inhibition of sympathetic vasomotor centers. Although clonidine typically is used as maintenance antihypertensive therapy, it can be used in the setting of hypertensive urgencies or emergencies. Its antihypertensive effects may be seen within 30 min-

utes and last 8 to 12 hours. Once blood pressure is controlled, oral maintenance clonidine therapy may be started.

Centrally acting sympatholytics rarely are indicated as first-line agents except when hypertension may be due to the abrupt withdrawal of one of these agents.

- *Dose:* Hypertensive urgency: 0.2 mg PO initially, then 0.1 mg/hour PO (to a maximum of 0.8 mg); transdermal: TTS-1 (0.1 mg/day) to TTS-3 (0.3 mg/day) topically q1week
- *Monitoring parameters:* Blood pressure, heart rate, and mental status.

Antiarrhythmics (Chapter 26, Table 26–4).

Antiarrhythmic agents are divided into five classes. Dosage information for individual antiarrhythmic agents are listed in Chapter 26, Table 26-4.

Class I

Class I agents are further divided into four subclasses: Ia (procainamide, quinidine, disopyramide), Ib (lidocaine, tocainide, mexiletine), Ic (flecainide, propafenone), and others (moricizine). All class I agents block sodium channels in the myocardium and inhibit potassium repolarizing currents to prolong repolarization.

Class Ia

Class Ia agents inhibit the fast sodium channel (phase 0 of the action potential), slow conduction at elevated serum drug concentrations, and prolong action potential duration and repolarization. Class Ia agents can cause proarrhythmic complications by prolonging the QT interval or by depressing conduction and promoting reentry.

- *Monitoring parameters:* ECG (QRS complex, QT interval, arrhythmia frequency).

Class Ib

Class Ib agents have little effect on phase 0 depolarization and conduction velocity, but shorten the action potential duration and repolarization. QT prolongation typically does not occur with class Ib agents. Class Ib agents act selectively on diseased or ischemic tissue where they block conduction and interrupt reentry circuits.

- *Monitoring parameters:* ECG (QT interval, arrhythmia frequency).

Class Ic

Class Ic agents inhibit the fast sodium channel and cause a marked depression of phase 0 of the action potential and slow conduction profoundly, but have minimal effects on repolarization. The dramatic effects of these agents on conduction may account for their significant proarrhythmic effects, which limit their use in patients with supraventricular arrhythmias and structural heart disease.

- *Monitoring parameters:* ECG (PR interval and QRS complex, arrhythmia frequency).

Class Ib/Ic

Morizicine is a phenothiazine derivative that possesses electrophysiologic effects similar to class Ib and Ic agents. It slows atrioventricular nodal and intraventricular conduction without affecting the action potential duration or repolarization. Its use is limited to patients with life-threatening ventricular arrhythmias resistant to other agents.

- *Monitoring parameters:* ECG (PR interval and QRS complex, arrhythmia frequency).

Class II

Beta-blocking agents inactivate sodium channels and depress phase 4 depolarization and increase the refractory period of the atrioventricular node. These agents have no effect on repolarization. Beta blockers competitively antagonize catecholamine binding at beta-adrenergic receptors.

Beta-blocking agents can be classified as selective or nonselective agents. Nonselective agents bind to beta-1 receptors located on myocardial cells and beta-2 receptors located on bronchial and skeletal smooth muscle. Stimulation of beta-1 receptors causes an increase in heart rate and contractility, while stimulation of beta-2 receptors results in bronchodilation and vasodilation. Selective beta-blocking agents block beta-1 receptors in the heart at low or moderate doses, but they become less selective with increasing doses.

Class II agents are used for the prophylaxis and treatment of both supraventricular arrhythmias and arrhythmias associated with catecholamine excess or stimulation, slowing the ventricular response in atrial fibrillation, lowering blood pressure, decreasing heart rate, and decreasing ischemia. Esmolol is useful especially for the rapid, short-term control of ventricular response in atrial fibrillation or flutter.

Nonselective beta-blocking agents should be avoided or used with caution in patients with congestive heart failure, atrioventricular nodal blockade, asthma, chronic obstructive pulmonary disease, peripheral vascular disease, Raynaud's phenomenon, and diabetes. Beta-1 selective beta-blocking agents should be used with caution in the above populations.

- *Monitoring parameters:* ECG (heart rate, PR interval, arrhythmia frequency).

Class III

Class III agents (amiodarone, bretylium, and sotalol) lengthen the action potential duration and effective refractory period and prolong repolarization. Additionally, amiodarone possesses alpha- and beta-blocking effects and calcium channel blocking properties and inhibits the fast sodium channel. Bretylium is taken up into sympathetic nerve endings, causing a release of norepinephrine followed by a depletion of norepinephrine in the nerve ending. Sotalol possesses nonselective beta-blocking properties. These agents usually are reserved for arrhythmias refractory to other antiarrhythmic agents. Although torsades de pointes is relatively rare with amiodarone, precautions should be taken to prevent hypokalemia- or digitalis-toxicity–induced arrhythmias. Sotalol may be associated with proarrhythmic effects in the setting of hypokalemia, bradycardia, high sotalol dose, and QT-interval prolongation, and in patients with preexisting congestive heart failure.

- *Monitoring parameters:* Amiodarone: ECG (PR and QT intervals, arrhythmia frequency); sotalol: ECG (QT interval, QRS complex, arrhythmia frequency).

Class IV

Calcium channel blocking agents inhibit calcium channels within the atrioventricular node and sinoatrial node, prolong conduction through the atrioventricular and sinoatrial nodes, and prolong the functional refractory period of the nodes, as well as depress phase 4 depolarization. Class IV agents are used for the prophylaxis and treatment of supraventricular arrhythmias and to slow the ventricular response in atrial fibrillation, flutter, and multifocal atrial tachycardia.

- *Monitoring parameters:* ECG (PR interval, arrhythmia frequency).

Class V

Adenosine, digoxin, and atropine possess different pharmacologic properties but ultimately affect the sinoatrial node or atrioventricular node. Adenosine decreases conduction through the atrioventricular node by increasing potassium conductance, causing hyperpolarization and a decrease in calcium channel conduction in myocardial cells within the atrioventricular node. Digoxin slows the sinoatrial node rate of depolarization and conduction through the atrioventricular node primarily through vagal stimulating effects.

Adenosine

Adenosine depresses sinus node automaticity and atrioventricular nodal conduction. Adenosine is indicated for the acute termination of atrioventricular nodal and reentrant tachycardia, and for supraventricular tachycardias, including Wolff-Parkinson-White syndrome.

Atropine

Atropine increases the sinus rate and decreases atrioventricular nodal conduction time and effective refractory period by decreasing vagal tone. The major indications for the use of atropine include symptomatic sinus bradycardia, sinus arrest, sinoatrial block, and type I second-degree atrioventricular block.

Digoxin

Digoxin is indicated for the treatment of supraventricular tachycardia and for controlling ventricular response associated with supraventricular tachycardia.

- *Monitoring parameters:* ECG (heart rate, PR interval, ST segment, T wave, arrhythmia frequency).

Thrombolytic Agents

Thrombolytic agents are beneficial in all types of myocardial infarctions, including in patients with previous myocardial infarctions and regardless of age. Indications for thrombolytic agents for the treatment of acute myocardial infarction include elapsed time from onset of infarctive symptoms > 30 minutes but < 6 hours, possibly effective when elapsed time > 6 hours and < 12 hours, ST segment elevation > 1 mm in two contiguous leads, or a new bundle branch block.

Major contraindications to the use of thrombolytic agents include any active or recent bleeding, intracranial or intraspinal neoplasm, arteriovenous malformation or aneurysm, neurosurgery or head injury within the previous 6 weeks, stroke within the previous 2 months, or prolonged or traumatic cardiopulmonary resuscitation.

Relative contraindications include menstruation, neurosurgery or head injury in the preceding 6 weeks, stroke in the preceding 2 months, transient ischemic attacks, major surgery or trauma in the preceding 10 days to 2 months, pregnancy, disorders of hemostasis, and brief atraumatic cardiopulmonary resuscitation.

Adverse effects include bleeding from the gastrointestinal or genitourinary tract, as well as gingival bleeding and epistaxis. Superficial bleeding may occur from trauma sites such as those for intravenous access or invasive procedures. Intramuscular injections, as well as noncompressible arterial punctures, should be avoided during thrombolytic therapy.

- *Monitoring parameters:* For short-term thrombolytic therapy of myocardial infarction: ECG, signs and symptoms of ischemia, and signs and symptoms of bleeding at intravenous injection sites (laboratory monitoring is of little value); continuous infusion therapy: thrombin time, activated partial thromboplastin time, and fibrinogen, in addition to above-mentioned monitoring parameters.

Streptokinase

Streptokinase is indicated in the treatment of acute myocardial infarction, deep venous thrombosis, and pulmonary embolism. Streptokinase works indirectly by forming a streptokinase-plasminogen activator complex, thus activating other plasminogen and converting it to the proteolytic enzyme plasmin. Plasmin hydrolyzes fibrin, fibrinogen, factors II, V, VIII, complement, and kallikreinogen. The duration of action is immediate after IV administration and lasts approximately 6 to 8 hours after the infusion is discontinued. Occasional allergic reactions may occur including fever, urticaria, itching, flushing, and musculoskeletal pain. Although anaphylaxis is rare, transient hypotension may occur.

- *Dose:* Acute myocardial infarction: 1.5 million units IV over 1 hour; deep venous thrombosis: 250,000-unit IV bolus over 30 to 60 minutes, followed by 100,000 units/hour for 2 to 3 days; pulmonary embolism: 250,000-unit IV bolus over 30 to 60 minutes, followed by 100,000 units/hour for 12 to 24 hours

Alteplase

Alteplase (recombinant tissue-type plasminogen activator—rtPA) has a high affinity for fibrin-bound plasminogen, allowing activation on the fibrin surface. Most plasmin formed remains bound to the fibrin clot, minimizing systemic effects. Alteplase is nonantigenic and should be considered in patients who have received streptokinase or anistreplase in the previous 6 to 9 months. The risk of an intracerebral bleed is approximately 0.5%.

- *Dose:* Acute myocardial infarction: 100 mg IV over 3 hours (10 mg IV over 2 minutes, then 50 mg over 1 hour, and then 40 mg over 2 hours); pulmonary embolism: 100 mg IV over 2 hours

Eminase

Eminase [anisoylated plasminogen-streptokinase activator complex (APSAC)] is an acylated form of streptokinase-plasminogen complex which is temporarily inactive. After deacylation, the complex promotes thrombolysis by converting plasminogen to the proteolytic enzyme plasmin. Thrombolysis occurs through the action of plasmin on fibrin. APSAC is antigenic, and hypotension and anaphylaxis occur in an incidence similar to streptokinase.

- *Dose:* 30 units IV over 5 minutes

Vasoconstricting Agents (Chapter 26, Table 26-3)

Dopamine is both an indirect-acting and a direct-acting agent. Dopamine works indirectly by causing the release of norepinephrine from nerve terminal storage vesicles as well as directly by stimulating alpha and beta receptors. Dopamine is unique in that it produces different pharmacologic responses based on the dose infused. At doses less than 5 µg/kg/minute, dopamine stimulates dopaminergic receptors in the kidneys, increasing urine output without affecting creatinine clearance. Doses between 5 and 10 µg/kg/minute are typically associated with an increase in inotropy resulting from stimulation of beta receptors in the heart, while doses above 10 µg/kg/minute stimulate peripheral alpha-adrenergic receptors, producing vasoconstriction and an increase in blood pressure. Doses above 20 to 30 µg/kg/minute usually produce no added response, so that if doses in this range do not produce the desired increase in blood pressure, alternative agents such as norepinephrine, phenylephrine, or epinephrine should be instituted.

Renal-dose dopamine, doses less than 5 µg/kg/minute, is commonly used with other vasoactive agents (i.e., norepinephrine, phenylephrine, dobutamine) to improve or maintain urine output. The benefit of this practice remains to be proven in humans.

Norepinephrine is a direct-acting vasoactive agent. It possesses alpha- and beta-adrenergic agonist properties producing mixed vasoconstrictor and inotropic effects. As a vasoconstrictor it is useful when dopamine has produced an inadequate increase in blood pressure. Norepinephrine's effect on the heart includes a more pronounced effect on inotropy than on heart rate.

Phenylephrine is a pure alpha-adrenergic agonist. It produces vasoconstriction without a direct effect on the heart, although it may cause a reflex bradycardia. Phenylephrine may be useful when dopamine, dobutamine, norepinephrine, or epinephrine cause tachyarrhythmias and when a vasoconstrictor is required.

Epinephrine possesses both alpha- and beta-adrenergic effects, increasing heart rate, contractility, and vasoconstriction with higher doses. Epinephrine's use is reserved for when other, less potent, vasoconstrictors are inadequate. Adverse effects include tachyarrhythmias; myocardial, mesenteric, renal, and extremity ischemia; and hyperglycemia.

- Dose: See Table 26-3
- *Monitoring parameters:* Blood pressure, heart rate, electrocardiogram, urine output, and hemodynamic parameters.

Inotropic Agents (Chapter 26, Table 26-3)

Catecholamines

Dobutamine
Dobutamine produces pronounced beta-adrenergic effects such as increases in inotropy and chronotropy along with vasodilation. Dobutamine is useful especially for the acute management of low cardiac output states. Adverse effects that are associated with the use of dobutamine include tachyarrhythmias and ischemia.

Dopamine
Dopamine in the range of 5 to 10 µg/kg/minute typically produces an increase in inotropy and chronotropy. Doses above 10 µg/kg/minute typically produce alpha-adrenergic effects.

Isoproterenol
Isoproterenol is a potent pure beta receptor agonist. It has potent inotropic, chronotropic, and vasodilatory properties. Its use typically is reserved for temporizing life-threatening bradycardia. Adverse effects associated with isoproterenol include tachyarrhythmias, myocardial ischemia, and hypotension.

Epinephrine
Epinephrine produces pronounced effects on heart rate and contractility and is used when other inotropic agents have not

resulted in the desired pharmacologic response. Epinephrine is associated with tachyarrhythmias; myocardial, mesenteric, renal, and extremity ischemia; and hyperglycemia.

- Dose: See Table 26-3
- *Monitoring parameters:* Blood pressure, heart rate, electrocardiogram, urine output, and hemodynamic parameters.

Phosphodiesterase Inhibitors

Amrinone and milrinone
Amrinone and milrinone produce increases in contractility and heart rate, as well as vasodilation. The mechanism of action of these agents is thought to be due to the inhibition of myocardial cyclic adenosine monophosphate phosphodiesterase (AMP) activity resulting in increased cellular concentrations of cyclic AMP. Increased tissue concentrations of cyclic AMP may result in the alteration of extracellular and intracellular calcium concentrations, thereby affecting the availability of calcium to contractile proteins by prolonging the release of calcium into the sarcoplasmic reticulum and increasing the rate of calcium sequestration. These agents are useful in the setting of low-output heart failure and can be combined with dobutamine to increase cardiac output. Amrinone has been associated with thrombocytopenia as well as a flulike syndrome. Both agents can produce tachyarrhythmias, ischemia, and hypotension.

- *Dose:* Amrinone: loading dose: 0.75 to 3 mg/kg; maintenance dose: 5 to 20 µg/kg/minute; milrinone: loading dose: 50 µg/kg; maintenance dose: 0.375 to 0.75 µg/kg/minute
- *Monitoring parameters:* Blood pressure, heart rate, electrocardiogram, urine output, hemodynamic parameters, and platelet count (especially amrinone).

PULMONARY PHARMACOLOGY

Phosphodiesterase Inhibitors

Theophylline
Theophylline is a bronchodilator that can be administered intravenously or orally. Theophylline should be used with caution in critically ill patients for several reasons. First, theophylline is metabolized in the liver, and illnesses such as low-output heart failure or hepatic failure impair the ability of the liver to metabolize theophylline, resulting in increased serum theophylline concentrations. Second, many agents routinely administered to critically ill patients are known to impair the metabolism of theophylline. Antibiotics such as erythromycin and ciprofloxacin can decrease the clearance of theophylline, producing supratherapeutic or toxic serum concentrations. Cimetidine, an agent used for both the prevention of stress gastritis and the treatment of gastrointestinal bleeding, also inhibits the metabolism of

theophylline. Inhibition of theophylline metabolism results in increased serum theophylline concentrations and predisposes patients to adverse effects such as arrhythmias and seizures. In patients receiving theophylline who develop supraventricular tachycardia, increased doses of adenosine are needed to treat the dysrhythmia.

- *Dose:* Loading dose: 6 mg/kg IV/PO (each 1.2 mg/kg aminophylline increases the theophylline serum concentration 2 mg/L); continuous infusion: smokers: 0.9 mg/kg/hour; nonsmokers: 0.6 mg/kg/hour; liver failure, congestive heart failure: 0.3 mg/kg/hour
- *Monitoring parameters:* Serum theophylline concentration, signs and symptoms of toxicity such as tachycardia, arrhythmias, nausea, vomiting, and seizures.

GASTROINTESTINAL PHARMACOLOGY

Antacids

Antacids once were considered the primary agents for the prevention of stress gastritis. Their main attributes were their effectiveness and low cost. However, this was offset by the need to administer 30 to 120 ml doses every 1 to 2 hours. Large doses of antacids had the potential to produce large gastric residual volumes, resulting in gastric distention and bloating, as well as increasing the risk for aspiration. Magnesium-containing antacids are associated with diarrhea and can produce hypermagnesemia in patients with renal failure. Aluminum-containing antacids are associated with constipation and hypophosphatemia. Large, frequent doses of antacids prevent the effective delivery of enteral nutrition. Finally, antacids are known to impair the absorption of digoxin, ciprofloxacin, and captopril. Also, alkalinization of the gastrointestinal tract may predispose patients to nosocomial pneumonias with gram-negative organisms that originate in the gastrointestinal tract.

- *Dose:* 30 to 120 ml PO, NG q1-4h
- *Monitoring parameters:* Nasogastric aspirate pH, serum electrolytes, bowel function (diarrhea, constipation, bloating), hemoglobin, hematocrit, and nasogastric aspirate and stool guaiac.

H₂ Antagonists

Ranitidine, cimetidine, and famotidine essentially have replaced antacids as therapy for the prevention of stress gastritis. These agents have the benefit of requiring administration only every 6 to 12 hours or may be delivered by continuous infusion. When they are administered by continuous infusion, they may be added to parenteral nutrition solutions, decreasing the need for multiple daily doses. Each agent has been associated with thrombocytopenia and mental status changes. Mental status changes typically occur in elderly patients or in patients with reduced renal function in whom the doses have not been adjusted to account for the reduction in renal function. Cimetidine also has been shown to inhibit hepatic microsomal enzymes, thus impairing the metabolism of agents such as theophylline and lidocaine. Also, similar to antacids, alkalinization of the gastrointestinal tract with H_2 antagonists may predispose patients to nosocomial pneumonias with gram-negative organisms that originate in the gastrointestinal tract.

- *Dose:* Ranitidine: intermittent IV: 50 mg q8h; continuous infusion 6.25 mg/hour; cimetidine: intermittent IV: 300 mg q6h; continuous infusion: 37.5 mg/hour; famotidine: intermittent IV: 20 mg q12h; continuous infusion: not recommended
- *Monitoring parameters:* Nasogastric aspirate pH, platelet count, hemoglobin, hematocrit, and nasogastric aspirate and stool guaiac.

Other Agents

Sucralfate

Sucralfate is an aluminum disaccharide compound that has been shown to be safe and effective for the prophylaxis of stress gastritis. Sucralfate may work by increasing bicarbonate secretion, mucus secretion, or prostaglandin synthesis to prevent the formation of stress ulcers. Sucralfate has no effect on gastric pH. It can be administered either as a suspension or as a tablet that can be partially dissolved in 10 to 30 ml of water and administered orally or through a nasogastric tube. Although sucralfate is free from systemic side effects, it has been reported to cause hypophosphatemia, constipation, and the formation of bezoars. Since sucralfate does not increase gastric pH, it lacks the ability to alkalinize the gastric environment and may decrease the development of gram-negative nosocomial pneumonias. Sucralfate is an effective alternative to H_2 antagonists in patients with thrombocytopenia or mental status changes. Also, it may be a useful alternative in patients receiving medications whose metabolism may be inhibited by cimetidine.

- *Dose:* 1 g PO, NG q6h
- *Monitoring parameters:* Hemoglobin, hematocrit, and nasogastric aspirate and stool guaiac.

Omeprazole

Omeprazole is a proton pump inhibitor that completely shuts down gastric acid secretion. Several reports have documented its ability to prevent stress gastritis. Omeprazole is only available as a sustained release capsule; therefore, it cannot be crushed. The capsule may be opened and the contents emptied into 10 to 30 ml of water for administration through a nasogastric tube. Omeprazole also inhibits hepatic microsomal enzymes; thus the metabolism of agents such as theophylline may be reduced when omeprazole is coadministered.

- *Dose:* 20 mg PO, NG q24h
- *Monitoring parameters:* Nasogastric aspirate pH, hemoglobin, hematocrit, and nasogastric aspirate and stool guaiac.

Vasopressin

Vasopressin is a peptide produced by the posterior pituitary gland that causes splanchnic vasoconstriction, reducing portal blood flow and portal pressure. Although vasopressin has been administered intraarterially and intravenously, intravenous administration is the preferred route of administration because of the ease in obtaining and maintaining vascular access. Vasopressin has the potential to produce serious adverse effects including abdominal cramps, diarrhea, bowel ischemia and necrosis, increased cardiac afterload with a reflex bradycardia, decreased coronary perfusion, and arrhythmias. Vasopressin also causes plasminogen activator and factor VIII release, which may aggravate coagulopathy. In patients with ischemic heart disease, nitroglycerin often is administered concomitantly to reduce arterial vasoconstriction and decrease portal pressures.

- *Dose:* 0.3 to 0.9 units/hour
- *Monitoring parameters:* Hemoglobin, hematocrit, nasogastric aspirate and stool guaiac, electrocardiogram, signs and symptoms of ischemia, blood pressure, and heart rate.

Octreotide

Octreotide is a long-acting somatostatin analogue. Octreotide reduces intravariceal pressure and azygos and hepatic blood flow, and has uncertain effects on portal pressure. Octreotide appears to be at least as efficacious as, if not superior to, vasopressin in controlling acute esophageal bleeding. Additionally, adverse effects such as headache, abdominal pain, and chest pain appear to be significantly lower with octreotide. Although octreotide may be more effective than vasopressin in initially controlling acute esophageal bleeding until an elective endoscopic procedure can be performed, there does not appear to be any difference in the reduction in mortality between octreotide and vasopressin.

- *Dose:* Initial bolus dose: 100 µg, followed by 50-µg/hour continuous infusion
- *Monitoring parameters:* Hemoglobin, hematocrit, and nasogastric aspirate and stool guaiac.

Propranolol

Propranolol has been shown to reduce portal pressure both acutely and chronically in patients with portal hypertension by reducing splanchnic blood flow. The primary use of propranolol has been in the prevention of variceal bleeding.

Propranolol or other betablockers should be avoided in patients experiencing acute gastrointestinal bleeding, as beta-blocking agents may prevent the compensatory tachycardia needed to maintain cardiac output and blood pressure in the setting of hemorrhage.

- *Monitoring parameters:* Hemoglobin, hematocrit, heart rate, and blood pressure.

RENAL PHARMACOLOGY

Diuretics

Diuretics may be categorized in a number of ways, including site of action, chemical structure, and potency. Although many diuretics are available for oral and intravenous administration, intravenously administered agents typically are given to critically ill patients because of their guaranteed absorption and more predictable responses. Therefore, the primary agents used in intensive care units are the intravenously administered loop diuretics, thiazide diuretics, and osmotic agents. However, the oral thiazide-like agent, metolazone, is used commonly in combination with loop diuretics to maintain urine output for patients with diuretic resistance.

- *Monitoring parameters:* Urine output, blood pressure, renal function, electrolytes, weight, fluid balance, and hemodynamic parameters (if applicable).

Loop Diuretics

Loop diuretics (furosemide, bumetanide, torsemide) act by inhibiting active transport of chloride and possibly sodium in the thick ascending loop of Henle. Administration of loop diuretics results in enhanced excretion of sodium, potassium, hydrogen, magnesium, ammonium, and bicarbonate. Chloride excretion exceeds sodium excretion. Maximum electrolyte loss is greater with loop diuretics than with thiazide diuretics. Furosemide, bumetanide, and torsemide have some renal vasodilator properties that reduce renal vascular resistance and increase renal blood flow. Additionally, these three agents decrease peripheral vascular resistance and increase venous capacitance. These effects may account for the decrease in left ventricular filling pressure that occurs before the onset of diuresis in patients with congestive heart failure.

Loop diuretics typically are used for the treatment of edema associated with congestive heart failure, the management of hypertension complicated by congestive heart failure or renal failure, in combination with hypotensive agents in the treatment of hypertensive crisis, especially when associated with acute pulmonary edema or renal failure, and in combination with 0.9% sodium chloride to increase calcium excretion in patients with hypercalcemia.

Common adverse effects associated with loop diuretic administration include hypotension from excessive reduction in plasma volume, hypokalemia and hypochloremia resulting in metabolic alkalosis, and hypomagnesia. Reduction in these electrolytes may predispose patients to the development of supraventricular and ventricular ectopy. Tinnitus, with reversible or permanent hearing impairment, may occur with the rapid administration of large intravenous doses. Typically, intravenous bolus doses of furosemide should not be administered faster than 40 mg/minute.

- *Dose:* Furosemide: IV bolus: 10 to 100 mg q1-6h; continuous infusion: 1 to 15 mg/hour; bumetanide: IV bolus: 0.5 to 2.5 mg q1-2h; continuous infusion: 0.08 to 0.3 mg/hour; torsemide: IV bolus: 5 to 20 mg qd

Thiazide Diuretics

Thiazide (IV chlorothiazide) and thiazidelike (PO metolazone) diuretics enhance excretion of sodium, chloride, and water by inhibiting the transport of sodium across the renal tubular epithelium in the cortical diluting segment of the nephron. Thiazides also increase the excretion of potassium and bicarbonate.

Thiazide diuretics are used in the management of edema and hypertension as monotherapy or in combination with other agents. They have less potent diuretic and antihypertensive effects than loop diuretics. Intravenously administered chlorothiazide or oral metolazone is often used in combination with loop diuretics in patients with diuretic resistance. By acting at a different site in the nephron, this combination of agents may restore diuretic responsiveness. Thiazide diuretics decrease glomerular filtration rate, and this effect may contribute to their decreased efficacy is patients with reduced renal function (i.e., GFR < 20 ml/minute). Metolazone, unlike thiazide diuretics, does not substantially decrease glomerular filtration rate or renal plasma flow and often produces a diuretic effect even in patients with glomerular filtration rates less than 20 ml/minute.

Adverse effects that may occur with the administration of thiazide diuretics include hypovolemia and hypotension, hypochloremia and hypokalemia resulting in a metabolic alkalosis, hypercalcemia, hyperuricemia, and the precipitation of acute gouty attacks.

- *Dose:* Chlorothiazide: 500 to 1000 mg IV q12h; metolazone: 2.5 to 20 mg PO qd

Osmotic Diuretics

Mannitol

Mannitol is an osmotic diuretic commonly used in patients with increased intracranial pressure. Mannitol produces a diuretic effect by increasing the osmotic pressure of the glomerular filtrate and preventing the tubular reabsorption of water and solutes. Mannitol increases the excretion of sodium, water, potassium, and chloride, as well as other electrolytes.

Mannitol is used to treat acute oliguric renal failure, reduce intracranial pressure, and reduce intraocular pressure. The renal protective effects of mannitol may be due to its ability to prevent nephrotoxins from becoming concentrated in the tubular fluid. However, its ability to prevent or reverse acute renal failure may be due to restoring renal blood flow, glomerular filtration rate, urine flow, and sodium excretion. In order to be effective in preventing or reversing renal failure, mannitol must be administered before reductions in glomerular filtration rate or renal blood flow have resulted in acute tubular damage. Mannitol is useful in the treatment of cerebral edema, especially when there is evidence of herniation or the development of cord compression.

The most severe adverse effect of mannitol is overexpansion of extracellular fluid and circulatory overload, producing acute congestive heart failure and pulmonary edema. This effect typically occurs in patients with severely impaired renal function. Therefore, mannitol should not be administered to individuals in whom adequate renal function and urine flow has not been established.

- *Dose:* 0.25 to 0.5 g/kg, then 0.25 to 0.5 g/kg q4h
- *Monitoring parameters:* Urine output, blood pressure, renal function, electrolytes, weight, fluid balance, hemodynamic parameters (if applicable), serum osmolarity, and intracranial pressure (if applicable).

HEMATOLOGIC PHARMACOLOGY

Anticoagulants

Heparin

Heparin is a mixture of mucopolysaccharides derived from the mast cells of beef lung and porcine intestinal tissues. It binds with antithrombin III, accelerating the rate at which antithrombin III neutralizes coagulation factors XII, XI, IX, X, VII, and II. Heparin is used for prophylaxis and treatment of venous thrombosis, pulmonary embolism, and atrial fibrillation with embolization, and for the treatment of acute disseminated intravascular coagulation.

The main adverse effects may be attributed to excessive anticoagulation. Bleeding occurs in 3% to 20% of patients receiving short-term, high-dose therapy. Bleeding is increased threefold when the partial thromboplastin time (PTT) is 2 to 2.9 times above control and eightfold when the PTT is more than 3 times the control value. Heparin-induced thrombocytopenia may occur in 1% to 5% of patients receiving the drug.

- *Dose:* Full therapy: standard 5000-unit bolus, followed by a continuous infusion of 1000 units/hour; individualized dosing: bolus: 80 units/kg followed by a continuous infusion of 18 units/kg/hour; infusion rates should be adjusted to maintain a PTT between 1.5 to 2 times the control value

- *Monitoring parameters:* PTT, hemoglobin, hematocrit, and signs of active bleeding.

Warfarin

Warfarin prevents the conversion of vitamin K back to its active form from the vitamin K epoxide, impairing the formation of vitamin-K–dependent clotting factors VII, IX, X, prothrombin, and protein C. Warfarin is indicated in the treatment of venous thrombosis or pulmonary embolism following full-dose heparin therapy. Warfarin is also used to reduce the risk of thromboembolic episodes in patients with chronic atrial fibrillation.

Bleeding is the major complication associated with warfarin, occurring in 6% to 29% of patients receiving the drug. Bleeding complications include ecchymoses, hemoptysis, and epistaxis, as well as fatal or life-threatening hemorrhage.

- *Dose:* 10 mg po qd × 3 days, then adjusted to maintain the International Normalized Ratio (INR) between 2 and 3; to prevent thromboembolism associated with prosthetic heart valves, the dose should be adjusted to maintain an INR between 2.5 and 3.5
- *Monitoring parameters:* INR, hemoglobin, hematocrit, and signs of active bleeding.

THERAPEUTIC DRUG MONITORING (CHAPTER 26, TABLE 26–5).

Therapeutic drug monitoring may be defined as the process of using drug concentrations, pharmacokinetic principles, and pharmacodynamics to optimize drug therapy. The goal of therapeutic drug monitoring is to maximize the therapeutic effect while avoiding toxicity. Drugs that produce toxicity at serum concentrations close to those required for therapeutic effect are the drugs most commonly monitored. The indications for therapeutic drug monitoring include narrow therapeutic range, no clinically observable endpoint, unpredictable dose-response relationship, serious consequences of toxicity or lack of efficacy, correlation between serum concentration and efficacy or toxicity, and the availability of serum drug concentrations.

There are multiple indications for obtaining serum drug concentrations. The specific indication is important as it will affect the timing of the sample. Timing of sample collection depends on the question being asked. The indications for obtaining serum drug concentrations include therapeutic confirmation, limited objective monitoring parameters, poor patient response, suspected toxicity, identification of drug interactions, determination of individual pharmacokinetic parameters, and changes in patient pathophysiology or disease state.

The timing of serum drug concentrations is critical for the interpretation of the results. The timing of peak serum drug concentrations is dependent on the route of administration and the drug product. Peak serum drug concentrations occur soon after an intravenous bolus dose, whereas they are delayed after intramuscular, subcutaneous, or oral doses. Oral medications can be administered as either liquid or rapid- or slow-release dosage forms (e.g., theophylline). The absorption and distribution phases must be considered when obtaining a peak serum drug concentration. The peak serum concentration may be much higher and occur earlier after a liquid or rapid-release dosage form compared to a sustained-release dosage form. Trough concentrations usually are obtained just prior to the next dose. Drugs with long half-lives (e.g., phenobarbital) or sustained-release dosage forms (e.g., theophylline) have minimal variation between their peak and trough concentrations. The timing of the determination of serum concentrations may be less critical in patients taking these dosage forms. Serum drug concentrations may be drawn at any time after achieving a steady state in a patient who is receiving a drug by continuous intravenous infusion. However, in patients receiving drug by continuous infusion, the serum specimen should be drawn from a site away from where the drug is infusing. If toxicity is suspected, serum drug concentrations can be obtained at any time during the dosing interval.

Appropriate interpretation of serum concentrations is the step that requires an understanding of relevant patient factors, pharmacokinetics of the drug, and dosing regimen. Misinterpretation of serum drug concentrations can result in ineffective and, at worst, harmful dosage adjustments. Interpreting serum concentrations includes an assessment of whether the patient's dose is appropriate, if the patient is at a steady state, the timing of the blood samples, an assessment of whether the time of blood sampling is appropriate for the indication, and an evaluation of the method of delivery to assess the completeness of drug delivery. Serum drug concentrations should be interpreted within the context of the individual patient's condition. Therapeutic ranges serve as guidelines for each patient. Doses should not be adjusted on the basis of laboratory results alone. Individual dosage ranges should be developed for each patient as various patients may experience either therapeutic efficacy, failure, or toxicity within a given therapeutic range.

AT THE BEDSIDE

▶ *Tips for Calculating Intravenous Medication Infusion Rates*

Information required to calculate intravenous infusion rates to deliver specific medication doses:

1. Dose to be infused (e.g., mg/kg/minute, mg/minute, mg/hour)
2. Concentration of intravenous solution (e.g., dopamine 400 mg in D5W 250 ml = 1.6 mg/ml; nitroglycerin 50 mg in D5W 250 ml = 200 µg/ml)
3. Patient's weight

A. Calculate the intravenous infusion rate in milliliters per hour for a 70-kg patient requiring dobutamine 5 µg/kg/minute using a dobutamine admixture of 500 mg in D5W 250 ml.

  1. Dose to be infused: 5 µg/kg/minute
  2. Dobutamine concentration: 500 mg/250 ml = 2 mg/ml or 2000 µg/ml
  3. Patient weight: 70 kg

Calculation: 5 µg/kg/minute × 70 kg = 350 µg/minute
350 µg/minute × 60 minutes/hour = 21,000 µg/hour
21,000 µg/hour ÷ 2000µg/ml = 10.5 ml/hour
Answer: Setting the infusion pump at 10.5 ml/hour will deliver dobutamine at a dose of 5 µg/kg/minute.

B. Calculate the intravenous infusion rate in milliliters per hour for a 70-kg patient requiring nitroglycerin 50 µg/minute using a nitroglycerin admixture of 50 mg in D5W 250 ml.

  1. Dose to be infused: 50 µg/minute
  2. Nitroglycerin concentration: 50 mg/250 ml = 0.2 mg/ml or 200 µg/ml
  3. Patient weight: 70 kg

Calculation: 50 µg/minute × 60 minutes/hour = 3000 µg/hour
3000 µg/hour ÷ 200 µg/ml = 15 ml/hour
Answer: Setting the infusion pump at 15 ml/hour will deliver nitroglycerin at a dose of 50 µg/minute.

C. Calculate the intravenous loading dose and infusion rate in milliliters per hour for a 70-kg patient requiring aminophylline 0.6 mg/kg/hour using an aminophylline admixture of 1 g in D5W 500 ml. The loading dose should be diluted in D5W 100 ml and infused over 30 minutes.

  1. Desired dose: Loading dose: 6 mg/kg
                Maintenance infusion: 0.6 mg/kg/hour
  2. Aminophylline concentration:
                Aminophylline vial: 500 mg/20 ml = 25 mg/ml
                Aminophylline infusion: 1 g/500 ml = 2 mg/ml
  3. Patient weight: 70 kg

Calculation:
Loading dose: 6 mg/kg × 70 kg = 420 mg
420 mg ÷ 25 mg/ml = 16.8 ml

Infusion rate: Aminophylline 16.8 ml + D5W 100 ml = 116.8 ml
116.8 ml ÷ 0.5/hours = 233.6 ml/hour
Answer: Setting the infusion pump at 234 ml/hour will infuse the aminophylline loading dose over 1/2 hour
Maintenance dose: 0.6 mg/kg/hour × 70 kg = 42 mg/hour
42 mg/hour ÷ 2 mg/ml = 21 ml/hour
Answer: Setting the infusion pump at 21 ml/hour will deliver the aminophylline maintenance dose at 42 mg/hour, or 0.6 mg/kg/hour.

SELECTED BIBLIOGRAPHY

What Heals: The Powerful Placebo

Beecher H: The powerful placebo. *Journal of the American Medical Association.* 1955;159:1602.
Dossey L: *Healing words: The power of prayer and the practice of medicine.* San Francisco: Harper Collins, 1993, pp. 134–135.
Evans F: Expectancy, therapeutic instructions, and the placebo response. In White L, Tursky B, Schwartz G (eds.): *Placebo: Theory, research, and mechanism.* New York: Guilford Press, 1985.
Frank J: Mind-body relationships in illness and healing. *Journal of the International Academy of Preventive Medicine.* 1975; 2:46.
Roberts A: Placebo therapies spark 'improvement' for 7 of 10. *Brain Mind Bulletin.* 1993;18(12):1.
Rossi EL: *The psychobiology of mind-body healing.* New York: WW Norton, 1993.
Sandroff R: The potent placebo. *RN.* 1980; April:35.

General

Chernow B (ed.): *The pharmacologic approach to the critically ill patient,* 3rd ed. Baltimore: Williams & Wilkins, 1994.
Townsend P (ed.): Applied pharmacokinetics. In Rippe JM, Irwin RS, Alpert JS, Fink MP (eds.): *Intensive care medicine,* 2nd ed. Boston: Little Brown, 1991.

Handbooks

Susla GM, Masur H, Cunnion RE, Suffredini AF, Ognibene FP, Hoffman WD, Shelhamer JH: *Handbook of critical care drug therapy.* New York: Churchill Livingston, 1994.
Knoben JE, Anderson PO (eds.): *Handbook of clinical drug data.* Hamilton, IL: Drug Intelligence Publications, 1993.

Intravenous Therapy Guidelines

Trujillo MH, Bellorin-Font E: Drugs commonly administered by intravenous infusion in intensive care units: A practical guide. *Critical Care Medicine.* 1990;18:232–238.

Ethical and Legal Considerations

► Knowledge Competencies

1. Characterize the nurse's role as patient advocate in upholding the doctrine of informed consent.

2. Describe the elements that determine decision-making capacity.

3. Identify the purpose and use of advance directives in guiding care for the incompetent patient.

■ *What Heals: Values Clarification*

Values are affective dispositions about the worth, truth, or beauty of a person, behavior, thought, or object. Values influence our decisions and our nursing practice. They give direction and meaning to life and guide our behaviors and conduct. They give us a personal and professional framework by which to integrate, explain, and evaluate new thoughts, experiences, and relationships.

Values possess cognitive, affective, and behavioral components, as well as motivation characteristics. Frequently, when confronted with a situation that requires an action, we have a variety of alternative approaches. It is important to focus on values to choose the best alternative.

Values clarification is a process that employs our capacity for intelligent, independent thought. By using critical thinking, answers to a variety of questions or dilemmas can be found. Values clarification involves three steps: choosing, prizing, and acting. During choosing, after evaluating each alternative choice and its consequences, the individual freely and willingly embraces the value. Prizing involves cherishing the decision and professing the choice to others. Acting entails finding ways to incorporate the value in what we do. These steps transform values into behavior and actions that become consistent and reproducible over time.

As nurses help patients clarify their values, a closer fit is established between what patients say they want and what they actually do (i.e., the behaviors or actions they choose). Nurses can help patients explore their values by pointing out alternative choices and consequences. From this exploration, they can assist patients to choose an alternative behavior or action that is consistent with their values. When nurses spend time clarifying their own values, they are better able to help patients in this process. Values clarification is a critical process for both the patient and the nurse because values greatly influence the decisions we all make and the types of behaviors and health care interventions we choose.

As new ethical issues in critical care continue to emerge, it is essential that practitioners in critical care develop skills in moral reasoning. Competence in moral decision-making abilities evolves throughout one's professional career. However, there are general moral principles and guidelines that direct ethical reasoning and provide a standard to which professional nurses are held. Beginning clinicians, as well as more experienced nurses, should be familiar with the moral expectations and ethical accountability embedded in the nursing profession. This chapter introduces the elements that serve as a foundation for moral decision making. Ethical principles and rules, the ethic of care, patient advocacy, and other issues of ethical concern to critical care nurses are discussed.

THE FOUNDATION FOR ETHICAL DECISION MAKING

Professional Codes and Standards

The purpose of professional codes is to identify the moral requirements of the relationships they oversee. The Code for Nurses developed by the American Nurses' Association (ANA) articulates the essential values, principles, and obligations that guide nursing actions. The ANA Code suggests proper professional conduct in ethical matters and proposes actions to guide the nursing profession. In other words, the code identifies common moral themes that arise in nursing practice and provides a framework for moral inquiry.

In addition to a code of ethics, nurses function in accordance with particular standards of practice. Standards of nursing practice are delineated by professional organizations and statutory bodies that govern the practice of nursing in various jurisdictions. Derived from nursing's contract with society, professional nursing standards define the criteria for the assessment and evaluation of nursing practice. External bodies, such as state boards of nursing, impose certain regulations for licensure, regulate the practice of nursing, and evaluate and monitor the actions of professional nurses. Many organizations also delineate standards of practice for registered nurses practicing in a defined area of specialty. For example, the American Association of Critical-Care Nurses (AACN) has established standards and expectations of performance for nurses practicing in critical care.

Standards of practice outlined by statutory bodies and specialty organizations are not confined to clinical skills and knowledge. Nurses are expected to function within the profession's code of ethics and are held morally and legally accountable for unethical practice. When allegations of unsafe, illegal, or unethical practice arise, the regulatory body serves to protect the public by investigating and disciplining the culpable professional. Although specialty organizations do not have authority to retract professional licensure, issues of professional misconduct are reviewed and may result in revocation of certification and notification of external parties.

AT THE BEDSIDE
▶ *Making the Right Decision*

Mary Whitson is a 72-year-old grandmother who has been in the coronary care unit for 4 weeks following a large anterolateral myocardial infarction. She has suffered from CHF, pulmonary edema, and hypotension, and now has developed ARDS. Mrs. Whitson's family is very supportive and visits her often. The physicians caring for Mrs. Whitson have communicated with the family, and the family has entrusted the physicians with making the "right decisions" for Mrs. Whitson.

Currently, Mrs. Whitson requires maximal ventilatory support to maintain adequate oxygenation. Her cardiac output and blood pressure are maintained at an adequate level with IV vasopressors and inotropic agents. Attempts to keep her pain-free are sometimes thwarted by a drop in her blood pressure when she receives morphine and other medications. The nurses caring for Mrs. Whitson believe that it is inappropriate to continue treating her aggressively and that the patient does not want such extensive treatment. They believe that Mrs. Whitson is able to make decisions regarding her life, even though she cannot speak. She appropriately gestures to the nurses and maintains eye contact when the nurses talk to her. She is weak, and her writing is often difficult to read.

When the nurse asks the physician to please ask Mrs. Whitson what she wants before they begin new treatments, the physician responds that the patient is "not competent because of her illness and prolonged stay in the CCU." The physician states that the family told him to make the "right decisions" and that gives him the authority to decide what is best for Mrs. Whitson. The nurse is uncomfortable providing aggressive care based on the physician's perspective rather than a clear understanding of the patient's values and goals regarding continued treatment.

Position Statements and Guidelines

In an effort to address specific issues in clinical practice, many professional organizations develop position statements or guidelines. The purpose of position statements is to apply the values, principles, and rules described in the Code for Nurses to particular contemporary ethical issues. Familiarity with the AACN and ANA position statements will help the critical care nurse clarify and articulate a position consistent with the professional values of nursing.

AT THE BEDSIDE
▶ *Refusing Further Treatment*

Mr G., 68 years old, is admitted to the coronary care unit following exacerbation of heart failure secondary to dilated cardiomyopathy. Despite aggressive treatment, Mr. G.'s cardiac index remained at 1.9 with an SVR of 600. His ABGs were pH 7.30, Paco₂ 56 mm Hg, and Pao₂ 60 mm Hg on 100% nonrebreather. Mr. G. refused intubation and any further treatments. He openly discussed his fear of prolonged suffering and asked the nurse to accelerate his death with a lethal dose of morphine.

In the above case example, the critical care nurse was asked to intentionally hasten a patient's death. Both the Code for Nurses and ANA position statements on assisted suicide and active euthanasia clarify the nurse's role when such requests are made. In addition, the AACN position statement on withholding and withdrawing life-sustaining treatments provides guidance for structuring end-of-life discussions (Table 10–1). In this case, the nurse and physician should explore Mr. G.'s request for an accelerated death and explain the legal and moral boundaries of his request. The option to withdraw treatment and provide aggressive palliative care should be offered and examined with the patient. A treatment plan that reflects the patient's underlying needs (a comfortable death) should be developed so that compassionate and humane care is provided.

Institutional Policies

Because critical care nurses practice within organizations, institutional policies and procedures affect and direct their practice. Institutional guidelines for assessing decision-making capacity or policies for the determination of brain death prescribe the expected actions by individuals employed by, or practicing within, the organization. These policies usually reflect ethical expectations congruent with the professional codes of ethics. However, in some circumstances, organizations may assume a particular position or value and therefore expect the employees to uphold this position. For example, some hospitals endorse particular religious positions and may prohibit professional practices that violate the institutional tenets. It is most desirable for the nurse and institution to have complementary values and beliefs about professional responsibilities and obligations.

Institutions often provide internal resources to help clinicians resolve difficult ethical issues. Institutional ethics committees have been formed in many institutions to provide consultation on ethical situations. Institutional policies

outlining the procedures of case review and access to the ethics committee should be available to all employees.

Legal Standards

Public policies and state and federal laws directed at health care influence the practice of health care professionals. Policies from agencies such as the Centers for Disease Control (CDC) or the Department of Health and Human Services (DHHS) generate changes in practice and in the actions of health professionals. For example, the DHHS has established regulations for institutional review boards regarding the protection of human research subjects. State and federal laws often complement public policies and reinforce the position set forth. Additionally, state and federal laws outline expected behaviors or actions, such as the federal recommendations in the Patient Self-Determination Act.

It is important for critical care nurses to understand legislation that directly influences clinical practice, such as state laws influencing advance directives. Beyond this

AT THE BEDSIDE
▶ *The Patient's Wishes*

Mr. Johnson is a 86-year-old widower who resides in an elderly care facility. He has one adult daughter who lives out of town and regularly visits him twice a month. One morning the care providers at the geriatric facility find him unresponsive with shallow respirations and a bradycardic pulse. A note, written by Mr. Johnson, is attached to his body and states that he intentionally took a lethal overdose and that he does not wish to be resuscitated. Empty bottles of levodopa and amitriptyline are found in his room next to a glass partially filled with alcohol. Residents of the geriatric facility said that Mr. Johnson had continued to express sadness over the loss of his wife 2 years ago and that progression of the Parkinson's disease also was troubling to him. The providers at the geriatric facility call the rescue squad, and he is rapidly transported to the hospital.

Mr. Johnson is hypotensive and unresponsive upon admission to the medical intensive care unit. Laboratory tests reflecting his renal and hepatic function are grossly abnormal. Gastric lavage and activated charcoal are initiated to remove the drugs.

Mr. Johnson's daughter requests that everything be done to save her father. The health care team respects the daughter's wishes as surrogate, but are concerned that this is not what Mr. Johnson wanted. They believe that the likelihood of a full recovery for Mr. Johnson is remote and he should be allowed a peaceful death.

TABLE 10–1. AMERICAN ASSOCIATION OF CRITICAL-CARE NURSES (AACN) POSITION STATEMENT ON WITHHOLDING AND/OR WITHDRAWING LIFE-SUSTAINING TREATMENT

Advances in health care technology have dramatically increased the ability to prolong life. Because of these advances, ethical and legal dilemmas arise when complex therapy is instituted to sustain vital functions, even when there is no hope of reversing the disease processes.

The American Association of Critical-Care Nurses recognizes that critical care nurses have a significant role in supporting a patient's preferences and beliefs about ending treatments of this type.

Therefore, AACN resolves that when choices about withholding and/or withdrawing life-sustaining treatments are being considered, critical care nurses should collaborate with individual patients or their surrogates, physicians and other healthcare providers. This should happen in an atmosphere that promotes reasoned deliberation and communication of a patient's preferences and best interests.

To support this resolution, AACN believes that the following elements are essential for nursing practice:
- Critical care nurses will participate in ongoing assessment of a patient's ability to make decisions about their own healthcare.
- Critical care nurses will participate in discussions exploring the patient's beliefs about end of life care at the earliest appropriate time. The best time for discussions and decision-making about withholding and/or withdrawal of life-sustaining treatment is before entry into the healthcare system.
- When patients cannot make decisions for themselves, their preferences may be determined from advanced directives (such as living wills or durable power of attorney for health care), previous spoken or written information and personal lifestyle.
- Critical care nurses, as patient advocates, will initiate and promote the decision-making process and assure that nursing care goals are consistent with patient preferences or best interests.
- In the event that life-sustaining treatment is withheld or withdrawn, critical care nurses will participate in planning, implementing, and evaluating supportive care. Supportive care includes providing comfort, hygiene, safe surroundings, and emotional support for patients and the family.

Thus AACN believes that healthcare institutions must have policies that direct a process to withhold and/or withdraw life-sustaining treatment. These policies should include:
- A process for ongoing review of treatment goals and interventions. The scope of the care the patient will receive should be specified in writing.
- A process for designating a surrogate when the patient does not have decision-making capacity.
- A process for dispute resolution among patients, surrogates, and health care team members when there is disagreement about the decision-making process.
- A process for transferring care of a patient to another qualified critical care nurse, when a decision to withhold and/or withdraw life-sustaining treatment conflicts with the nurse's personal beliefs and values.

This position on withholding and/or withdrawing life-sustaining treatment is based on these beliefs and ethical principles:
1. Individuals have a moral and legal right and responsibility to make decisions about their healthcare and the use of life-sustaining treatment.
2. There is no moral or legal difference between withholding and withdrawing treatment. Considerations that justify not initiating treatment also justify withdrawing treatment.
3. A person's capacity to make decisions is shown by their ability to understand relevant information, reason and deliberate about choices, reflect on information according to their individual values and preferences, and communicate their decision to healthcare providers.
4. The process for decision-making on behalf of incapacitated patients should be directed by the established standards of substituted judgment or best interests.

Definitions

Advance Directives: A document in which a person gives advance directions about medical care or designates who should make medical decisions on their behalf if they should lose decision-making capacity. There are two types of advance directives; treatment directives, such as living wills, and proxy directives, such as durable power of attorney for health care.

Best Interest Standard: This standard gives priority to the protection of the patient's welfare. In these cases the designated surrogate tries to make a choice on the patient's behalf that seeks to implement what is in the patient's best interests by reference to more objective, societally shared criteria.

Substituted Judgment: The doctrine of substituted judgment requires that the surrogate attempt to reach the decision that the incapacitated person would make if he/she were able to choose. This standard preserves the patient's interest in self-determination.

Bibliography

American Association of Critical-Care Nurses (1989). *Role of the critical care nurse as a patient advocate.* Newport Beach, CA.

American Nurses' Association (1985). *Code for nurses with interpretive statements.* Kansas City, MO.

President's Commission for the Study of Ethical Problems in Medicine and Biomedical and Behavioral Research (March 1983). Washington, DC: Government Printing Office.

The Hastings Center (1987). *Guidelines on the termination of life-sustaining treatment and the care of the dying.* Briarcliff Manor, NY.

American Association of Critical-Care Nurses: Position statement: Withholding or withdrawing life-sustaining treatment. *Aliso Viejo, CA: AACN, 1990.*

immediate need, clinicians should rely on resources within the institution and professional organizations to interpret and clarify relevant policies and laws affecting practice.

PRINCIPLES OF ETHICS

One of the dominant and most influential perspectives in biomedical ethics is that of principle ethics. Inherent in this viewpoint is the belief that some basic moral principles serve to define, describe, and interpret the essence of ethical dilemmas. These basic principles, and derivative principles or rules, are considered prima facie or binding. Therefore, it is considered wrong to breach a principle unless there are prevailing and compelling reasons that outweigh the necessary infringement. The principles and rules are binding, but not absolute.

Because many approaches to ethics integrate the rules and principles outlined by the principle-oriented approach, it is important for the critical care nurse to understand the fundamental concepts of principle ethics. The primary principles used to describe and define most moral dilemmas are nonmaleficence, beneficence, utility, justice, and respect for personal autonomy. The derivative principles or rules include privacy, confidentiality, veracity, and fidelity.

The principles are not ordered in a particular hierarchy, with application and interpretation based on the specific features of the dilemma. In other words, once the underlying principles in conflict are identified, values of the decision makers influence which principle takes precedence over other moral claims.

Nonmaleficence

The principle of nonmaleficence imposes the duty to do no harm. This injunction suggests that the nurse should not knowingly inflict harm and is responsible if negligent actions result in detrimental consequences. In general, a critical care nurse preserves the principle of nonmaleficence by maintaining competence and practicing within the accepted standards of care.

Although the principle of nonmaleficence appears rather straightforward and easily preserved, there are some situations in which it is necessary for the nurse to inflict harm in order for a greater good to be realized. For example, some of the harmful consequences of pain medication, such as respiratory depression, may be outweighed by the greater good of easing a terminally ill patient's pain at the end of life. The use of pain medication in this case is justified because a greater good, that of comfort, is recognized by the patient and caregivers as more desirable than the avoidance of respiratory depression. The concept that supports this reasoning is called the principle of double effect (see the pain management discussion, page 219).

Beneficence

The ethical principle of beneficence affirms an obligation to prevent harm, remove harm, and promote good by actively helping others advance and realize their interests. Intrinsic to this principle is action. The nurse moves beyond the concept of not inflicting harm (nonmaleficence) by actively preventing and removing harm, as well as by promoting the well-being of others.

When the patient's safety or well-being is threatened by the actions of others, the nurse is obligated to remove and prevent harm. Knowledge of unsafe, illegal, or unethical practice by any health care provider obligates the nurse both morally and legally to intervene. The nurse must remove the immediate danger and communicate the infringement to the appropriate sources to prevent further harm. The nurse should turn to institutional policies and state nurse practice acts for guidance in the appropriate process of reporting.

To optimize the patient's well-being and prevent harm, nurses must practice with the essential knowledge and skills required of the clinical setting. Nurses are expected to practice according to established standards of practice and to continue professional learning to improve clinical practice.

Although clinical competence is essential, the patient's well-being is upheld when the patient's perspective is known and valued. Therefore, the nurse must gain an understanding of the patient's underlying value structure to ensure that actions are consistent with the patient's wishes. The duty to do good requires that the health care team understand the patient's interpretation of a desirable outcome or goal.

The need to balance the patient's beliefs with the duty to promote good is difficult and confusing for critical care nurses. In the critical care setting it is often unclear what actions or course of treatment will most benefit the patient physiologically and which plan best reflects the patient's values. This lack of certainty may result in fragmented discussions with the patient or surrogate and a treatment plan that reflects the values of the health care team rather than the patient. The nurse's moral obligation is to continue to promote the patient's interests by pursuing an accurate representation of the patient's beliefs and values, and to raise concerns of conflicting interpretations to appropriate members of the health care team.

Utility

As any critical care nurse knows, it often is not possible to avoid all harms and produce only good effects. The principle of utility or proportionality advocates for a positive balance of benefits over burdens. Benefits contribute to the patient's well-being by improving the patient's health, such as through eradication of disease or symptom management. Benefits also are realized when the patient's quality of life is enhanced. Burdens, on the other hand, produce no measurable improvement in health or quality of life and may increase the patient's suffering or debilitation.

The benefit-burden analysis is advanced as a morally appropriate process to delineate and evaluate treatment choices. When provided with complete, comprehensive information regarding approaches to treatment, patients weigh the benefits and burdens of the proposed plans. Although a proposed course of treatment may be recommended, the patient's analysis of the risks and benefits guides the interventions. However, if the patient is incapable of participating in the decision-making process, the designated surrogate examines the options and determines the course of treatment based on an understanding of the patient's underlying values and beliefs.

Respect for Personal Autonomy

The principle of respect for personal autonomy affirms the freedom and right of an individual to make decisions and choose actions based on that individual's personal values and beliefs. In other words, an autonomous choice is an informed decision made without coercion that reflects the individual's underlying interests and values.

To respect a person's autonomy is to recognize that patients may hold certain views and take particular actions that are not congruent with the values of the health care providers. Often this concept is difficult for health care providers to accept and endorse, particularly when the patient's choice may result in a less desirable outcome as viewed by the caregivers. As an advocate, the nurse appreciates this diversity and continues to provide care as long as the patient's choice is an informed decision and does not infringe on the autonomous actions of others.

The problem most frequently encountered in the critical care setting is that patients have varying degrees of autonomy. The capacity of critically ill patients to participate in the decision-making process often is compromised and constrained by internal factors such as the effects of pharmacologic agents, the emotional elements associated with a sudden acute illness, and the physiologic factors related to the underlying illness. External factors, such as the ICU environment, also influence the patient's potential to make autonomous choices. The critical care nurse advocates for the patient by eliminating and containing, as much as possible, the factors that constrain the patient's freedom to make autonomous choices. In this way the nurse is supporting the principle of respect for personal autonomy and upholding the ethical duty of beneficence.

Justice

The principle of justice requires that similar cases be treated in similar ways and that all persons are to be treated according to their needs. Patients are to be treated equally regardless of disease state, socioeconomic status, gender, age, religious beliefs, or moral convictions. Treating patients equally does not mean treating all patients in the same manner. Instead, the health care needs of the patient, rather than other nonrelevant factors, determine the amount of health care resources received. For example, individuals in a community may have equal access to a critical care unit when they are critically ill. However, once patients are admitted to critical care, essential resources are allocated to patients based on individual needs. For example, a patient with a myocardial infarction receives antiarrhythmic therapy, while a patient with respiratory distress is supported by mechanical ventilation.

The principle of justice is complex, includes several characteristics, and is interpreted in divergent and controversial manners. One concept underlying the principle of justice that is important to nursing is that of fair distribution. When resources are limited, the benefits and burdens of health care must be distributed fairly within society. This theory is evident in discussions encompassing issues of organ transplantation. The manner in which patients are placed on waiting lists, the limited availability of organs, the cost of transplantation, and the responsibility of society to meet the health care requirements of patients in need of transplantation are several issues involving fair distribution.

Critical care nurses allocate nursing resources to patients and other members of the health care team, and within the institution. The complex and competing demands of individuals and groups in need of nursing resources often leads to chaotic and random decisions. The principle of justice argues for a comprehensive, thoughtful plan that outlines a decision-making process in times of opposing claims.

Privacy and Confidentiality

Privacy and confidentiality are associated, but distinct, concepts that are derived from the principles of respect for autonomy, beneficence, and nonmaleficence. Privacy refers to the right of an individual to be free from unjustified access by others. It is considered a negative right because it is a right of noninterference, or the right to be left alone, not listened to, and not touched.

In the critical care setting the patient's privacy often is disregarded. The design of many critical care units includes easy visualization of patients from the nurses' station, and open access to the patient is presumed by most care givers. This suggests a limiting of an individual's privacy. Critical care practitioners should be particularly attentive to requesting permission from the patient for any bodily intrusion or physical exposure. The casual infringement of an individual's privacy erodes the foundation for establishing a trusting and caring practitioner-patient relationship.

Confidentiality is described in terms of the protection of information. When the patient shares information with the nurse or a member of the health care team, the information should be treated as confidential and discussed only with those directly involved in the patient's care. Exceptions to confidentiality include quality improvement activities, mandatory disclosures to public health agencies, reporting child abuse, or required disclosure in a judicial setting. When an exception exists, the individual should be informed that the required reporting will occur. Most other disclosures of information obtained in a confidential manner should be shared with appropriate persons only when strong and compelling reasons to do so exist. Again, the patient should be informed of the impending disclosure, and ideally the patient should authorize the disclosure.

Violations of patient confidentiality occur in many subtle ways. The computerization of medical records and the use of facsimile distribution of personal medical information is common practice in many institutions. Persons unrelated to the patient's medical care who have access to the computers or facsimile may view confidential information without the individual's permission. Other ways in which confidentiality is unprotected include casual conversations in hallways or elevators in which patient information is shared within earshot of strangers, the unauthorized release of patient information to friends or the media, and health care professionals within the institution taking the liberty to view a coworker's medical record.

Nurses may feel conflicted when a patient discloses confidential information. The profession of nursing strongly values the principle of respect for persons and highly regards the concept of protecting confidential information. Therefore, decisions to break a patient's confidentiality must be well considered and require balancing competing obligations and claims. For example, a nurse may consider breaking a patient's confidentiality if there is a clear indication that, without doing so, harm may come to another individual or identifiable others. Clearly, this decision should not be made in isolation, and the nurse should seek advice when confronted with this difficult situation.

Veracity

The rule of veracity simply means that one should tell the truth and not lie or deceive others. Derived from the principle of respect for persons and the concept of fidelity, veracity is fundamental to relationships and society. The nurse-patient relationship is based on truthful communication and the expectation that each party will adhere to the rules of veracity. Deception, misrepresentation, or inadequate disclosure of information undermines and erodes the patient's trust in health care providers.

Patients expect that information about their condition will be relayed in an open, honest, and sensitive manner. Without truthful communication, patients are unable to assess the options available and make fully informed decisions. However, the complex nature of critical illness does not always manifest as a single truth with clear boundaries. Uncertainty about the course of the illness, the appropriate treatment, or the plan of care is common in critical care and a single "truth" may not exist. As emphasized in a model of shared decision making, patients or surrogate decision makers must be kept informed of the plan of care and areas of uncertainty should be openly acknowledged. Disclosure of uncertainty enables the patient or surrogate to realistically examine the proposed plan of care and reduces the likelihood that the health care team will proceed in a paternalistic manner.

Fidelity

Fidelity is defined as the obligation to keep promises and uphold the implicit and explicit commitments associated with a trusting nurse-patient relationship. The nurse portrays this concept by maintaining a loyal and faithful moral relationship with the patient. Fidelity also means that the patient's best interests and welfare will be pursued, preserved, and protected.

The concept of fidelity is particularly important in critical care. Because many critically ill patients are unable to adequately communicate their wishes or direct their care, they are prone to control and dominance by others. This vulnerability underscores the importance of a dependable and dedicated relationship between the nurse and patient.

The implicit and explicit commitments, such as the provision of competent care and the promise to advocate for the patient's welfare, are comforting and encouraging to patients and families. Nurses are expected to protect the patient's safety, promote quality care, restore health, and alleviate suffering. These expectations reflect the fundamental nursing responsibilities in a relationship based on fidelity.

CARE

The ethic of care is viewed as an alternative to the principled approach in bioethics. Rather than distinguish the ethical problem as a conflict of principles, the ethic of care invites the analysis of relationships and the associated obligations.

The ethic of care begins from an attached, involved, and interdependent position. From this standpoint, morality is viewed as caring about others, developing relationships, and maintaining connection. Moral problems result from disturbances in interpersonal relationships and disruptions in the perceived responsibilities within relationships. The resolution of moral issues emerges as the involved parties examine the contextual features and embrace the relevance of the relationship and the related responsibilities.

In contrast, a principle-oriented or justice approach originates from a position of detachment and individuality. The justice approach recognizes the concepts of fairness, rights, and equality as the core of morality. Therefore, dilemmas arise when these elements are compromised. From this perspective, the approach to moral resolution is a reliance on formal logic, deductive reasoning, and a hierarchy of principles.

For nursing the ethic of care provides a useful approach to moral analysis. Traditionally, nursing is a profession that necessitates attachment, caring, attention to context, and the development of relationships. To maintain this position, nurses develop proficiency in nurturing and sustaining relationships with patients and within families. The ethic of care legitimizes and values the emotional, intuitive, and informal interpretation of moral issues. This perspective expands the sphere of inquiry and promotes the understanding and resolution of moral issues.

PATIENT ADVOCACY

The ethic of care and the ethical principles and rules support the intrinsic values found in models of patient advocacy. Although there are many models for defining and interpreting the relationship between the nurse and patient, the most familiar image is that of the nurse as a patient advocate. The AACN developed a position statement that endorsed patient advocacy as a fundamental model for critical care nursing practice (Table 10–2). This position state-

TABLE 10–2. AMERICAN ASSOCIATION OF CRITICAL-CARE NURSES (AACN) POSITION STATEMENT ON THE ROLE OF THE CRITICAL CARE NURSE AS PATIENT ADVOCATE

The American Association of Critical-Care Nurses believes that patient advocacy is an integral component of critical care nursing practice. Therefore, definitions of advocacy and the behaviors that typify advocacy are essential.

Whereas, the *Code for Nurses* (American Nurses' Association, 1985) requires that nurses safeguard the patient and the public when health care and safety are affected by the incompetent, unethical, or illegal practice of any person and

Whereas, many definitions of advocacy exist, and

Whereas, critical care nurses are confronted with situations that require them to act immediately on the patient's behalf, and

Whereas, personal and professional risks are associated with being a patient advocate, and

Whereas, state nurse practice acts may require the nurse to be a patient advocate, and

Whereas, the process of informed consent mandates that the patient or the patient's surrogate be informed fully and give consent freely, and

Whereas, the continuum of advocacy is not limited to the individual but may extend to societal concerns.

Therefore, be it resolved that the American Association of Critical-Care Nurses believes the critical care nurse is a patient advocate.

And that the American Association of Critical-Care Nurses defines advocacy as respecting and supporting the basic values, rights, and beliefs of the critically ill patient.

Be it further resolved that the American Association of Critical-Care Nurses believes that as a patient advocate, the critical care nurse shall do the following:

1. Respect and support the right of the patient or the patient's designated surrogate to autonomous informed decision making.
2. Intervene when the best interest of the patient is in question.
3. Help the patient obtain necessary care.
4. Respect the values, beliefs and rights of the patient.
5. Provide education and support to help the patient or the patient's designated surrogate make decisions.
6. Represent the patient in accordance with the patient's choices.
7. Support the decisions of the patient or the patient's designated surrogate or transfer care to an equally qualified critical care nurse.
8. Intercede for patients who cannot speak for themselves in situations that require immediate action.
9. Monitor and safeguard the quality of care the patient receives.
10. Act as liaison between the patient, the patient's family, and health care professionals.

Be it resolved that the American Association of Critical-Care Nurses recognizes that health care institutions are instrumental in providing an environment in which patient advocacy is expected and supported.

Also, be it further resolved that as patient advocate, critical care nurses initiate and promote actions to improve the health care of the critically ill through social change.

Reference
American Nurses' Association (1985). Code for nurses with interpretive statements. Kansas City, MO.

American Association of Critical-Care Nurses: Position statement: Role of the critical care nurse as patient advocate. *Aliso Viejo, CA: AACN, 1989.*

ment guides and directs the critical care nurse in activities that support and advance the rights of patients and their surrogates.

The role of patient advocate often is a difficult and confusing position to assume. Questions raised regarding this model are numerous and, in reality, no single model thoroughly describes the complexity and uniqueness of the nurse-patient relationship. Instead, the characteristics of the advocacy model are offered as a typical, but not exclusive description of the moral relationship between the nurse and patient.

The description of the advocacy role embraced by the AACN reflects a model in which the nurse acknowledges and encourages an equal relationship with the patient. The patient's values, beliefs, and rights are respected and endorsed as significant and central to the decision-making process. This interpretation is a blend of the value-based decision model and the respect-for-persons model. In the value-based decisions model, the nurse helps the patient gain the necessary information to make an informed choice. The nurse may guide the patient or surrogate through value clarification, the identification of interests, and the process of communicating decisions. The nurse does not speak for

the patient, or impose particular values or preferences. Instead, the patient or surrogate is empowered to guide and direct the health care plan.

The respect-for-persons model augments the value-based model by including the expectation that nurses uphold and protect the basic human rights of patients. In this model, the nurse acts to sustain the patient's welfare by seeking the appropriate information or support for the patient. In the event the patient is unable to speak for himself or herself and no surrogate is available, the nurse protects the patient's best interests. The principle of fidelity plays an important role in this model of advocacy because the nurse's actions reflect the underlying commitment and loyalty to advancing the patient's welfare.

Assuming the role of patient advocate is not without risk. Nurses may find that obligations to oneself, the patient, the patient's family, other members of the health care team, or the institution are in conflict and have competing claims on nursing resources. These situations are intensely troubling to nurses, and it is imperative to have the support of colleagues when engaging in the analysis of difficult moral issues. In circumstances of conflict, nurses should clarify the nature and significance of the moral problem, engage in a systematic process of moral decision making, communicate concerns openly, and seek mutually acceptable resolutions. A framework within which to identify and compare options provides the necessary structure to begin the process of moral resolution.

THE PROCESS OF ETHICAL ANALYSIS

When faced with an ethical problem, the nurse is expected to implement an intellectual and reasonable process that promotes resolution. Approaching ethical dilemmas in a structured way provides consistency, eliminates the risks of overlooking relevant contextual features, and invites thoughtful reflection on moral problems. A stepwise method that mirrors the nursing process provides the necessary elements for a comprehensive evaluation. The following steps are involved in case analysis:

Assessment
- Identify the problem. Clarify the competing ethical claims, the conflicting obligations, and the personal and professional values in contention. Acknowledge the emotional components and communication issues.
- Gather the data. Distinguish the morally relevant facts. Identify the medical, nursing, legal, social, and psychological facts. Clarify the patient's religious and philosophical beliefs.
- Identify the individuals involved in the dilemma. Clarify who is involved in the problem development and who should be involved in the decision-making process. Identify who should make the decision, and discern what factors may impede that individual's ability to make the decision.

Plan
- Consider all options, and don't restrict choices to the most obvious.
- Identify the harms and goods likely to arise from each option.
- Analyze each plan according to ethical theories and principles.
- Search for institutional procedures or guidelines that address this issue.

Implementation
- Choose a plan and act.
- Anticipate objections.

Evaluation
- Outline the results of the plan. Identify what harm or good occurred as a result of the action.
- Identify the necessary changes in institutional policy or other strategies to avoid similar conflicts in the future.

This stepwise process of ethical analysis incorporates ethical principles and rules, relevant medical and nursing facts, and specific contextual features, and reflects a model of shared decision making. This ideology is essential if current and future moral issues are to be addressed and negotiated.

CONTEMPORARY ETHICAL ISSUES

Informed Consent

As a patient advocate, the critical care nurse recognizes the patient's or surrogate's central role in decision making. It is imperative that patients make informed decisions based on accurate and appropriate information. By uncovering the patient's primary values and beliefs, the nurse empowers patients and surrogates to articulate their preferences. Therefore, the nurse does not speak for the patient, but instead maintains an environment in which the patient's autonomy and right to self-determination are respected and preserved.

The doctrine of informed consent encompasses four elements: disclosure, comprehension, voluntariness, and competence. Information must be provided so patients understand their current medical status, the proposed interventions (including the nature of the therapy and its purpose, risks, and benefits), and the reasonable alternatives to the proposed treatment.

What is told to the patient often is understood based on *how* it is told. The overriding goal of the treatment, rather than just the procedure, should be discussed with the patient and the goals should reflect the desirable and likely outcomes for this individual. The nurse can contribute significantly to the comprehension portion of the consent process by clarifying the patient's or surrogate's perception of the situation. Questions such as "What additional information do you need to help you make this decision?" or "What do you understand are the goals of this treatment?" will help highlight the patient's interests and comprehension of the situation.

Decisions must be reached voluntarily, and any threat of coercion, manipulation, duress, or deceit is unacceptable. Voluntariness upholds the principle of respect for persons and supports the concept of self-determination.

The term *competence* generally refers to the individual's capacity to participate in the decision-making process. However, competence is a legal term and reflects judicial involvement. On the other hand, the term *capacity* reflects a medical decision regarding the patient's functional ability to participate in the decision-making process. The components of decisional capacity are discussed in the section on determining capacity on page 216.

The intent of the informed consent process is based on the principles of respect for personal autonomy, nonmaleficence, and beneficence. In theory, the consent process provides an individual with the necessary information to compare options and make a reasoned choice. In reality, the consent process is handled more as an event than a process. The focus is to "get consent" rather than to help the patient gain an understanding of the proposed treatment. The critical care nurse must be sensitive to the timing of such discussions and should attempt to optimize the environment and enhance the patient's ability to participate in the decision-making process. Interactions should be uninterrupted, free from distractions, during intervals when the patient is fully awake, and if desired by the patient, in the presence of loved ones.

Nurses have both a moral and a legal duty in the consent process. Incorrect information given with the intent to deceive or mislead the patient must be reported according to institutional guidelines and in some states may qualify as professional misconduct to be reported to the profession's state board. The Code for Nurses portrays the nurse's role during the consent process as a patient advocate upholding the patient's right to self-determination. Therefore, the nurse must respect the competent patient's choice and support the patient's decisions.

Determining Capacity

Patients are presumed to possess decision-making capacity unless there are clear indications that the individual's choices are harmful or inconsistent with previously stated wishes. Questioning another's ability to engage in the decision-making process should be executed with caution. Value-laden judgements of an individual's competence, such as restricting involvement based on mental illness or advanced age, should be prohibited. In addition, evaluations of capacity based on the presumed outcome of the decision are equally unjust. Determining rationality based on what the caregivers or family believe, rather than on the patient's values, should not be tolerated. Instead, a functional standard to evaluate decision-making capacity is recommended.

The functional standard of determining capacity focuses on the patient's abilities as a decision maker rather than on the condition of the patient or the projected outcome of the decision. The three elements necessary for a patient to meet the functional standard are the abilities to comprehend, to communicate, and to form and express a preference.

The ability to comprehend infers that the patient understands the information relevant to the decision. A patient must exhibit abilities sufficient to understand only the facts pertinent to the prevailing issue. Therefore, orientation to person, place, and time does not guarantee nor preclude the patient's ability to understand and comprehend the relevant information.

Decision-making capacity requires a communication of the decision between the patient and health care team. Communication with critically ill patients often is compromised by pharmacologic or technological interventions. The critical care nurse should attempt to remove barriers to communication and advance the patient's opportunity to engage in the decision-making process.

The final component essential for evaluating functional capacity is evidence of the patient's ability to reason about his or her choices. An individual's choices should reflect the person's own goals, values, and preferences. To evaluate this aspect, comments such as "Tell me about some of the most difficult health care decisions that you had to make in the past" or "Describe how you reached the decision you did" are useful. The patient should recount a pattern of reasoning that is consistent with personal goals and that reflects an accurate understanding of the consequences of the decision.

When the patient lacks decision-making capacity, and attempts to control factors and return the patient to an autonomous state are unsuccessful, the health care team must rely on other sources for direction in approximating the patient's preferences. Advance directives and surrogate decision makers are two ways in which the patient's choices can be understood.

Advance Directives

The Patient Self-Determination Act (PSDA), effective December 1, 1991, is a federal law that requires health care institutions receiving Medicare or Medicaid funds to inform patients of their legal rights to make health care decisions and execute advance directives. The purpose of the PSDA is to preserve and protect the rights of adult patients to make choices regarding their medical care. The PSDA also requires institutions to inform individuals of relevant state laws surrounding the preparation and execution of advance directives.

Advance directives are statements provided by an individual with decision-making capacity that describe the care or treatment he or she wishes to receive when no longer competent. Most states recognize two forms of advance directives, the treatment directive, or living will, and the proxy directive. The treatment directive enables the individual to specify in advance his or her treatment choices and which interventions are desired. Usually treatment directives focus on cardiopulmonary resuscitation, mechanical ventilation, nutrition and hydration, and other life-sustaining technologies.

Proxy directives expand the sphere of decision making by identifying an individual to make treatment decisions when the patient is unable to do so. The appointed individual, a relative or close friend, assumes responsibility for health care decisions as soon as the patient loses the capacity to participate in the decision-making process. Treatment decisions by the health care proxy are based on a knowledge and understanding of the patient's values and wishes regarding medical care. Most states have statutory provisions that recognize the legal authority of the health care proxy, and this individual is given complete authority to accept or refuse any procedure or treatment.

Although it is recommended that most adults complete both a treatment and proxy directive, the proxy directive has some important advantages over a treatment directive. Many treatment directives are valid only under certain conditions. Terminal illness or an imminent death are common limitations required before the patient's treatment directive is enacted. Such restrictions are not relevant in proxy directives, and the sole requirement before the proxy assumes responsibility on the individual's behalf is that the patient lack decisional capacity. Furthermore, the proxy directive enables the authorized decision maker to consider the contextual and unique features of the specific situation before arriving at a decision. In this way, the benefits and burdens of proposed interventions are considered in partnership with the knowledge and understanding of the patient's preferences and values.

If a patient lacks decision-making capacity and has not previously designated a proxy decision maker in an advance directive, the health care team must identify an appropriate surrogate to make decisions on the patient's behalf. Generally, family members have the patient's best interests in mind, and many state statutes identify a hierarchy of relatives as appropriate surrogate decision makers.

Regardless of whether the decision maker is a designated proxy or family member, the process of making decisions on behalf of the incapacitated patient is difficult and arduous. If the patient left no written treatment directive, the surrogate decision maker and the designated proxy follow the same guidelines for making decisions. The decisions are made based on either the substituted judgement standard or the best interest standard.

Substituted Judgement

When a patient previously has expressed his or her wishes regarding medical care, the surrogate decision maker invokes the standard of substituted judgement. The patient's goals, beliefs, and values serve to guide the surrogate in constructing and shaping a decision that is congruous with the patient's expressed wishes. An ideal interpretation of substituted judgement is that the patient, if competent, would arrive at the same decision as the surrogate. This standard originates in the belief that when we know someone well enough, we often are able to determine how he or she would have reacted to a particular situation, and therefore can make decisions in that person's behalf.

Best Interests

The best interest standard is used when the patient's values, ideals, attitudes, or philosophy are not known. For example, if a patient never gained decision-making capacity and lacked competence throughout his or her life, it would be unlikely that another individual could articulate

the patient's wishes and beliefs about health care. Using the best interest standard, the surrogate decision maker determines the course of treatment based on what would be in the patient's best interests, considering the needs, risks, and benefits to the affected person. This burden-benefit analysis includes considering the relief of suffering, restoration of function, likelihood of regaining capacity, and quality of an extended life.

Although neither the best interest standard nor the substituted judgement standard is problem-free, when possible the decision maker for an incapacitated patient should follow the principles of substituted judgement. Knowledge of the patient's underlying values should guide the surrogate and will most likely result in a decision reflective of the patient's interests and well-being.

Decisions to Forego Life-Sustaining Treatments

Decisions to forego life-sustaining treatments are made almost daily in the hospital setting. The prevalence of these decisions does not diminish the difficulty that patients, families, nurses, and physicians face when considering to forego treatment. The model for this decision-making process should reflect a collaborative and enduring approach that promotes the patient's interests and well-being (Table 10–1).

The patient's interests are best served when information is shared among the caregivers, patient, and family in an open and honest manner. Through this process, a plan of care that reflects the patient's goals, values, and interests is developed. Continued collaboration is essential to ensure that the plan promotes the patient's well-being and reflects the patient's preferences. However, the patient may determine that the current plan imposes treatments that are more burdensome than beneficial, and may choose to forego new or continued therapies.

Grounded in the right to noninterference, patients with capacity have the moral and legal right to choose to forego life-sustaining treatments. The right of a capable patient to refuse treatment, even beneficial treatment, must be upheld if the elements of informed consent are met and innocent or third parties are not injured by the refusal. Ongoing dialogue among the health care team, family, and patient is appropriate so that mutually satisfactory goals are adopted. Patients must understand that refusal of treatment will not lead to inadequate care or abandonment by members of the health care team.

In patients without decisional capacity, the determination to withdraw or withhold treatments is made by the identified surrogate. If the wishes and values of the patient are known, the surrogate makes treatment decisions based on this framework. If, however, the patient's values or wishes are unknown, or the patient never had capacity to express underlying beliefs, the decision maker must consider and weigh the benefits and burdens imposed by the particular treatments. The concept of a benefit-burden analysis was introduced by the President's Commission for the Study of Ethical Problems in Medicine and Biomedical and Behavioral Research in 1983. Any treatment that inflicts undue burdens on the patient without overriding benefits or that provides no benefit may be justifiably withdrawn or withheld. If the benefits outweigh the burdens, the obligation is to provide the treatment to the patient.

In cases where the identified surrogate is not acting in the patient's best interests, health care professionals have a moral obligation to negotiate an acceptable resolution to the problem. As defined in AACN's position statement on the nurse as a patient advocate (Table 10–2), critical care nurses should intervene when the best interest of the patient is in question. If extensive attempts to resolve the differences through the use of internal and external resources are unsuccessful in facilitating an acceptable solution, the health care professional should seek the appointment of an alternative surrogate. Often, the burden of proof will be upon the health care professional to justify the need for an alternative decision maker. In situations in which the patient's life is threatened and the refusal of treatment by the surrogate would jeopardize the patient's safety, the health care team must seek an alternative surrogate without prolonged discussion with the identified surrogate. This situation arises when parents who are Jehovah's Witnesses refuse a life-saving blood transfusion for their child. The health care team can rapidly acquire court approval to transfuse the minor. In less emergent situations, attempts to convince the surrogate of the need for treatment and to reach a satisfactory settlement may take more time.

In the case of Mr. Johnson (the third case study at the beginning of this chapter), members of the health care team interpreted the patient's actions as a decision made by a competent individual. They realized that even after aggressive treatment Mr. Johnson would most likely be dependent on hemodialysis, and therefore his independence and living environment would change. On the other hand, Mr. Johnson's daughter saw her father's act as a reflection of his depression from Parkinson's disease and the loss of his wife. The daughter believed that additional antidepressant medications and more frequent psychiatric evaluations would renew her father's desire to live. In this case, both parties believe they are advancing the patient's best interests. Reflection on the patient's life, work, actions, religion, and beliefs will help all parties clarify the patient's values, and may help in the development of an acceptable resolution.

Conflicts regarding the withdrawal of life-sustaining treatments often reflect differences in values and beliefs. Typically, health care professionals value life and health. When patients or surrogates choose to forego treatments that have minimal benefit, it is difficult to relinquish the original goal of restoring health. This delemma is particularly apparent in the ICU setting, where actions and interventions are aggressive, dramatic, and often life-saving. Shifting from this model to a paradigm that advocates for a calm and peaceful death requires the critical care nurse and health care team to relinquish control and move into the provision of aggressive comfort care. The intensity required to support the patient and family during the process of withdrawal of treatment must also be valued and appreciated by health care professionals in critical care.

In some circumstances, surrogate decision makers will insist on treatment that members of the health care team believe is burdensome and nonbeneficial for the patient. Frequently, the request for futile treatment reflects the surrogate or patient's desire to be assured that "everything" is being done to eradicate the disease or restore health. Fears of abandonment, impending death, pain, discomfort, and suffering may motivate individuals to pursue nonbeneficial, and even harmful, treatments. If patients and surrogates are kept fully informed of the goals and the successes and failures throughout the course of treatment, the request for futile therapies is unlikely. If, after numerous discussions, the patient or surrogate continues to request futile treatment, it is useful to elicit help from an uninvolved party, such as an ethics committee, to facilitate discussions. Health care institutions should have policies that delineate the responsibilities of the caregiver and the resources within the institution to resolve these unusual situations. In rare circumstances, judicial involvement is necessary to determine the outcome of the case.

Nutrition and Hydration

To many nurses, the provision of nutrition and hydration exemplifies compassion and comfort and is fundamental to patient care. Therefore, it is quite unsettling to nurses when the withdrawal of nutrition and hydration are considered. However, any treatment or therapy, including the provision of nutrition and hydration, may in some circumstances be judged to be more burdensome than beneficial. Medical nutrition and hydration are administered through intravenous access, nasogastric and duodenal feeding tubes, or via gastrostomy. The image of gently spoon feeding a dying patient is replaced with the reality of meeting the nutritional requirements through invasive and uncomfortable technologies. Often, patients require physical restraint to ensure stability of the medical therapy, and iatrogenic consequences, such as infection, pulmonary edema, or aspiration pneumonia, are prevalent.

The determination to provide medical nutrition and hydration should be based on a careful burden-benefit analysis. If medical nutrition and hydration will support and expedite the patient's return to an acceptable level of functioning (as defined by the patient or surrogate), then continued provision of the therapy is considered beneficial. When uncertainty exists, the presumption should be to provide nutrition and hydration. On the other hand, when continued provision of nutrition and hydration is futile and will not restore an adequate nutritional status, the treatment may be discontinued. If the patient's underlying condition will not change by the provision of nutrition and hydration (as is the case with patients in persistent vegetative states or irreversible coma), or the treatment is more burdensome than beneficial to the patient, the treatment justifiably may be withheld or withdrawn.

Because the provision of food and fluids imparts important symbolic images, decisions to withdraw or withhold nutrition and hydration are difficult for caregivers and families. The presumption to prolong life infers continued nutritional support. However, it is important to acknowledge that in some situations the provision of nutrition and hydration may be more harmful than good.

Pain Management

When decisions to forego life-sustaining treatments in a critically ill patient arise, issues regarding the aggressive management of pain and comfort develop. In some circumstances patients receive inadequate amounts of pain medication to manage the symptoms of their illness. Whether the inadequate management is due to the practitioner's lack of knowledge in determining appropriate treatments or an unwillingness to prescribe the necessary medication, it is unethical for insufficient amounts of pain medication to be ordered. Nurses are obligated to ensure that patients receive care and treatments that are consistent with their choices. There are few patients in whom adequate pain management cannot be achieved. The ANA Position Statement on Promotion of Comfort and Relief of Pain in Dying Patients delineates the role of the nurse in the assessment and management of pain.

When sufficient amounts of pain medication are ordered, nurses may raise concerns about administering a symptom-relieving medication, such as morphine, knowing that it may hasten or cause the patient's death. The dilemma, as constructed by the nurse, is that although the death is unintended, it is a direct consequence of the medication. Therefore, is the nurse responsible for killing the patient?

The simple answer to this question is no. Although actively killing patients is prohibited, the appropriate administration of pain medication for the relief of suffering is considered acceptable practice. The distinction in this case is one of intended consequences versus unintended, but foreseeable, consequences. The nurse intends to relieve pain and suffering and not deliberately hasten death. The moral issue is whether or not the decision makers have considered the foreseeable consequences, that the risk is justified in light of other options, and they have knowingly accepted the risk involved. The principle of double effect delineates the necessary conditions for an act that causes harm to be morally justifiable.

The Principle of Double Effect

The principle of double effect is invoked when an act that causes indirect and unintended harmful effects is morally justified. Four conditions must be present to justify the undesirable consequences of the act. These conditions are: (1) the action itself must be good or morally neutral; (2) only the good effect is intended, although the harmful effect may be foreseeable, but unintended; (3) the harmful effect cannot be a means to the good effect; and (4) the resulting good effect sufficiently produces a greater good than the harm that is incurred.

All these conditions must be present for the principle of double effect to be applied. In the case of administering pain medication to the terminally ill patient, the nurse first must be certain that the patient or identified surrogate understands that the purpose of the pain medication is to alleviate suffering, but that the unintended but foreseeable consequence of respiratory depression and possibly the hastening of death may occur. The act of medicating the patient for pain is at least morally neutral, and the good effect is the intended and desired outcome. The harmful effect of respiratory depression is not the means to alleviating suffering and is not intended. Finally, the relief of pain is determined by the patient and caregivers to be the greater good rather than a prolonged, but painful existence. In this case, the nurse's actions are justified by the principle of double effect and upheld in the Code for Nurses.

Resuscitation Decisions

Critically ill patients are susceptible to sudden and unpredictable changes in cardiopulmonary status. Most hospitalized patients presume that, unless discussed otherwise, resuscitation efforts will be instituted immediately upon cardiopulmonary arrest. In-hospital resuscitation is moderately successful, and delay in efforts significantly reduces the chance of the victim's survival. The emergent nature, the questionable effectiveness, and the presumed provision of cardiopulmonary resuscitation (CPR) contribute to the ethical dilemmas that surround this intervention.

Do Not Resuscitate Orders

"Do not resuscitate" (DNR) or "no code" are considered to be orders to withhold CPR. Other medical or nursing interventions are not influenced directly by a DNR order. In other words, the decision to forego CPR is not a decision to forego all other interventions to sustain life. The communication surrounding this decision is one of the most important elements in designing a mutually acceptable goal (Table 10–3).

Appropriate discussions with the patient or surrogate must occur before a resuscitation decision is made. Conversations about resuscitation status and the overall treatment goals should occur with the patient or surrogate, physician, nurse, and other appropriate members of the health care

TABLE 10–3. AMERICAN ASSOCIATION OF CRITICAL-CARE NURSES (AACN) POSITION STATEMENT ON CLARIFICATION OF RESUSCITATION STATUS IN CRITICAL CARE SETTINGS

Critical care nurses practice in an environment where life and death are becoming less clearly defined. As 24-hour bedside practitioners, critical care nurses need clear medical treatment goals to facilitate decision making. Frequently there are no written resuscitation orders or those written may be ambiguous. As a result, nurses are often confronted by a lack of or confusing directions in resuscitation efforts when time is of the essence.

Therefore, guidelines must be written denoting levels of resuscitation efforts for each patient within the critical care setting.

Therefore, development and uniform implementation of the guidelines must be a collaborative effort between medicine and nursing (AACN, 1981). Nursing administrators of critical care units are responsible and accountable for responding to the critical care nurses' need to develop such guidelines when guidelines do not already exist.

Thus, guidelines must include, but are not limited to, the following components:
- a system and process for classification of patient resuscitation status.
- a mechanism for documentation and review of resuscitation status and the process used to arrive at this decision.
- a mechanism for assurance of patient and family rights.
- use of clearly defined terminology.

And thus, the critical care nurse will:
- assure quality of patient care regardless of resuscitation status.
- review daily with the physician the current resuscitation status of the patient.
- reflect the resuscitation status in the patient's plan of care.

References
American Association of Critical-Care Nurses. Standards for Nursing Care of the Critically Ill. Reston, Virginia: Reston Publishing Company, Inc., 1981, p. 37.
Pontoppidan, H. Optimal care for the hopelessly ill patient. New England Journal of Medicine 295(7):362–364, 1976.
Powner, D.J., and A. Grenvik. Triage in patient care: from expected recovery to brain death. Heart & Lung 8(6):1103–1108, 1979.

American Association of Critical-Care Nurses: Position statement on clarification of resuscitation status in critical care settings. *Aliso Viejo, CA: AACN, 1985.*

team. Open communication and a shared understanding of the treatment plan is essential to understanding and responding to the patient's interests and preferences.

Once a decision is made regarding DNR status, the physician must document the discussion and decision in the medical record. When the issue of resuscitation status is not addressed with the patient or surrogate or the decision is not documented or communicated with caregivers, issues such as partial codes or slow codes result.

Slow Codes or Partial Codes
The failure to define the DNR status and other treatment or nontreatment decisions often reflects the absence of an overall treatment goal. This terminology (slow code, partial code) leads to confusion, misunderstanding, inconsistencies, or worse among members of the health care team and the patient's family. The underlying message of a slow code directive is for the caregivers to perform an intervention somewhere between an all-out effort and no effort at all. If a successful resuscitation is desired, then the appropriate attempt should be instituted. If members of the health care team are knowledgeable about the treatment goal, the communication is strengthened and the overall treatment is enhanced. If the resuscitation is not appropriate, then no attempt should be made. To do so only confuses the family and forces caregivers to perform aggressive interventions that are not beneficial and even harmful.

Institutions should develop policies that address the process of writing and implementing a DNR order. In addition to documenting the decision, physicians also should document the process of arriving at the decision. The critical care nurse should document his or her participation in the discussion and understanding of the patient's or surrogate's comprehension. In addition, the nurse must continue ongoing dialogue with the patient or surrogate, answering any questions that arise and communicating any misunderstandings with the health care team.

It is essential that patients or their surrogates be involved in decisions surrounding resuscitation decisions. Although some individuals believe that patients or surrogates need not be informed of medical decisions to withhold CPR, the President's Commission rejects this approach. Because patients or surrogates consent to the plan of care, including decisions to omit particular treatments, the provision of CPR should be treated in the same manner.

BUILDING AN ETHICAL ENVIRONMENT

Values Clarification

One of the most useful and essential skills offered by nurses is that of assisting the patient and family in value clarification. This process helps families in the burdens and benefits assessment and provides them with a framework of the patient's preferences and interests. Additionally, families are less encumbered during the bereavement process, when reflecting on the patient's hospitalization, if they feel the decisions they made for the patient reflected the patient's values.

Provide Information and Clarify Issues

Patients and families rely on nurses to provide clarity to medical discussions and explore the meaning of the treatments. The trusting relationship that develops is based on the nurse's abilities to communicate and understand the patient's needs. Questions that help unveil patients' families' perceptions of the situation include: "What information do you need to make this decision?", "What do you understand of your (or your loved one's) condition?", or "What are your fears about being sick?"

The information provided to patients and surrogates must be more than simply disclosing facts. The dialogue must be ongoing, open, honest, and expressed with concern. Because the understanding of new knowledge is often based on old knowledge, it is helpful for the nurse to assess the patient's or surrogate's experience with the health care system. Patients and families often draw conclusions or create relationships based on incomplete or inaccurate interpretations of information. Nurses play a key role is facilitating communication and translating discrepancies in perceptions.

Engage in Collaborative Decision Making

Nursing offers a distinct perspective that is grounded in humanistic and caring values. Nurses recognize, interpret, and react to the patient's and the family's response to health problems. Factors such as the patient's ability to adapt to changes in health, cope with a diagnosis, or adjust to a treatment are valuable contributions to a model of shared decision making. It is nursing that embraces this viewpoint, and therefore, nurses must have a consistent presence in the health care team. Patients and families expect and need nurses to be actively involved in planning and implementing the plan of care.

In a collaborative model, nursing's contributions and perspectives are valued, pursued, and acknowledged. When nurses are absent from the circle of decision making, clinical and moral dilemmas arise and communication falters. It is essential that every critical care nurse remain involved, attached, and committed to the process of shared decision making and collaborative interaction.

SELECTED BIBLIOGRAPHY

General Ethics

Beachamp TL, Childress JF: *Principles of biomedical ethics,* 4th ed. New York: Oxford University Press, 1994.

Carse AL: The 'voice of care': Implications for bioethical education. *The Journal of Medicine and Philosophy.* 1991;16:5–28.

Cooper MC: Principle oriented ethics and the ethic of care: A creative tension. *Advances in Nursing Science.* 1991;14(2):22–31.

Fowler MDM, Levine-Ariff J (eds.): *Ethics at the bedside.* Philadelphia: JB Lippincott, 1987.

Fry ST: *Ethics in nursing practice: A guide to ethical decision making.* Geneva: International Council of Nurses, 1994.

President's Commission for the Study of Ethical Problems in Medicine and Biomedical and Behavioral Research: *Deciding to forego life-sustaining treatment.* Washington DC: U.S. Government Printing Office, 1983.

Purtilo R: *Ethical dimensions in the health professions.* Philadelphia: WB Saunders, 1993.

Withdrawal and Withholding of Life Support

Ahronheim JC, Moreno J, Zuckerman C: *Ethics in clinical practice.* Boston: Little, Brown, 1994.

Fowler MDM: Ethical decision making in clinical practice. *Nursing Clinics of North America.* 1989;24(4):955–965.

The Hastings Center: *Guidelines on the termination of life-sustaining treatment and the care of the dying.* Bloomington, IN: Indiana University Press, 1987.

Jonsen AR, Toulmin S: *The abuse of casuistry: A history of moral reasoning.* Berkeley, CA: University of California Press, 1988.

Miles SH, August A: Courts, gender, and the "right to die." *Law, Medicine and Health Care.* 1990;18(1–2):85–95.

Rushton CH: Ethical decision making in critical care, Part 1: The role of the pediatric nurse. *Pediatric Nursing.* 1988;14(5): 411–412.

Rushton CH, Reigle J: Ethical issues in critical care. In Kinney MR, Packa DR, Dunbar SB (eds.): *AACN's clinical reference for critical-care nursing,* 3rd ed. St. Louis, MO: Mosby-Year Book, 1993, pp. 8–43.

Solomon MZ, O'Donnell L, Jennings B, Guilfoy V, Wolf SM, Nolan K, Jackson R, Koch-Weser D, Donnelley S: Decisions near the end of life: Professional views on life-sustaining treatments. *American Journal of Public Health.* 1993;83(1):14–25.

Veatch RM, Fry ST: *Case studies in nursing ethics.* Philadelphia: JB Lippincott, 1987.

Zaner RM: *Ethics and the clinical encounter.* Englewood Cliffs, NJ: Prentice Hall, 1988.

Values Clarification and Values History

Doukas DJ, McCullough LB: The values history. *The Journal of Family Practice.* 1991;32(2):145–150.

Kielstein R, Sass HM: Using stories to assess values and establish medical directives. *Kennedy Institute of Ethics Journal.* 1993;3(3):303–325.

Uustal D: Values: The cornerstone of nursing's moral art. In Fowler MDM, Levine-Ariff J, (eds.): *Ethics at the bedside.* Philadelphia: JB Lippincott, 1987.

The Ethic of Care

Benner P: The role of experience, narrative, and community in skilled ethical comportment. *Advances in Nursing Science.* 1991;14(2):1–21.

Carse AL: The 'voice of care': Implications for bioethical education. *The Journal of Medicine and Philosophy.* 1991;16:5–28.

Cooper MC: Principle oriented ethics and the ethic of care: A creative tension. *Advances in Nursing Science*. 1991;14(2):22–31.

Fry ST: The ethic of caring: Can it survive in nursing? *Nursing Outlook*. 1988;36(1):17.

President's Commission for the Study of Ethical Problems in Medicine and Biomedical and Behavioral Research. *Deciding to forego life-sustaining treatment*. Washington, DC: U.S. Government Printing Office, 1983.

Professional Codes, Standards, and Position Statements

American Association of Critical-Care Nurses: *Position statement: Ethics in critical care research*. Aliso Viejo, CA: AACN, 1984.

American Association of Critical-Care Nurses: *Position statement on clarification of resuscitation status in critical care settings*. Aliso Viejo, CA: AACN, 1985.

American Association of Critical-Care Nurses: *Position statement: Role of the critical care nurse as patient advocate*. Aliso Viejo, CA: AACN; 1989.

American Association of Critical-Care Nurses: *Position statement: Withholding or withdrawing life-sustaining treatment*. Aliso Viejo, CA: AACN; 1990.

American Nurses' Association: *Code for nurses with interpretive statements*. Washington, DC: ANA, 1986.

American Nurses' Association: *Position statement on promotion of comfort and relief of pain in dying patients*. Washington, DC: ANA, 1991.

American Nurses' Association: *Position statement on nursing and the patient self-determination act*. Washington, DC: ANA, 1991.

American Nurses' Association: *Position statement on nursing care and do-not-resuscitate decisions*. Washington, DC: ANA, 1992.

American Nurses' Association: *Position statement on foregoing artificial nutrition and hydration*. Washington, DC: ANA, 1992.

American Nurses' Association: *Position statement on active euthanasia*. Washington, DC: ANA, 1994.

American Nurses' Association: *Position statement on assisted suicide*. Washington, DC: ANA, 1994.

Sanford S, Disch J: *Standards of nursing care of the critically ill*. Stamford, CT: Appleton & Lange, 1989.

Advance Directives

Emanual L: Appropriate and inappropriate use of advance directives. *The Journal of Clinical Ethics*. 1994;5(4):357–359.

Marsden C: Making patient self-determination a reality in critical care. *American Journal of Critical Care*. 1992;1(1):122–124.

Reigle J: Preserving patient self-determination through advance directives. *Heart and Lung*. 1992;21(2):196–198.

Safety Issues

11

Transportation of the Critically Ill Patient

1. Identify equipment and personnel supports required to safely transport the critically ill patient within the hospital

2. Describe transfer-related complications and preventive measures to be taken before and during transport.

Infection Control

1. Identify routes of transmission and methods of control of nosocomial infections in the critical care unit.

2. Identify organisms of significance in the critical care unit and describe methods for control.

3. Describe the biological hazards present in the critical care unit and discuss methods for control.

■ *What Heals: Humanizing Technology*

How does one integrate healing into technologic environments and critical care units? Planetree, a 13-bed medical-surgical unit in San Francisco Pacific Presbyterian Medical Center, sets a dramatic example for us all in terms of its philosophy, design, and day-to-day activities. Planetree's philosophy is one of changing the way hospitals do business to make it more humanized and consumer-oriented. At Planetree, the staff is selected carefully to ensure that their values and beliefs are consistent with the Planetree philosophy. The nurses' station is open to all patients, and patients can read their own medical charts and add their own observations, responses, and feelings. The staff is committed to answering patient and family questions and dispelling the mysteries of hospitalization and illness. Patients can read and learn about their illness by requesting pertinent medical literature from the Planetree library.

At Planetree, a nurturing environment has been created using carefully selected colors, lighting, fabrics, carpet, furniture, art, and curved walls. There is a piano and an art program available, and patients may select pictures for the wall of their room from an "art cart." Intrusive hospital clutter such as chart racks, linen carts, and technologic equipment are kept in storage and brought out only when needed.

Visiting hours for families and friends are determined by the patient. A patient lounge and comfortable surroundings encourage family and friends to stay near. Family and friends are taught how to participate in care before, during, and after the patient's hospitalization. Patients and families can cook for themselves in the unit's kitchen, and a nutritionist is available to assist them in selecting the most beneficial foods for recovery.

More than 20 hospitals currently have affiliated with Planetree, named after the sycamore tree where Hippocrates taught his students about body-mind connections. These hospitals have the commitment to humanize health care for patients and their families. They do so in a variety of ways such as redesigning the environment and grounds, integrating alternative therapies such as massage, yoga, and meditation together with conventional treatments, and incorporating an extensive patient education program into the system. Planetree exemplifies how changes can be created within a technologic health care system by modeling a philosophy, an environment, and a health care team approach that facilitates the healing and well-being of patients, families, and the staff.

The next time you walk into a patient's room, look around. What is healing about the environment? What takes your energy away? How could healing be brought into this environment?

CEG & BMD

Adapted from: Bringing healing into technology. In Guzzetta CE, Dossey BM: Cardiovascular nursing: Holistic practice. St. Louis, MO: Mosby-Year Book, 1992, pp. 628–629.

TRANSPORT OF THE CRITICALLY ILL PATIENT[1]

Transporting the critically ill patient to other areas of the hospital is often necessary for diagnostic and therapeutic purposes. The decision to transport the critically ill patient out of the well-controlled environment of the critical care unit elicits a variety of responses from clinicians. It's not uncommon to hear phrases like these: "She's too sick to leave the unit!" "What if something happens in route?" "Who'll take care of my other patients while I'm gone?" Responses like these underscore the clinicians' understanding of the risks involved in transporting critically ill patients.

Transportation of a critically ill patient involves more than putting the patient on a stretcher and rolling him or her down the hall. Safe patient transport requires thoughtful planning, organization, and interdisciplinary communication and cooperation. The goal during transport is to maintain the same level of care to the patient, regardless of the location in the hospital. The transfer of critically ill patients always involves some degree of risk to the patient. The decision to transfer, therefore, should be based on an assessment of the potential benefits of transfer and be weighed against the potential risks.

The reason for moving a critically ill patient is typically the need for care, technology, or specialists not available in the critical care unit. Whenever feasible, diagnostic testing or simple procedures should be performed at the patient's bedside within the critical care unit. If the diagnostic test or procedural intervention under consideration is unlikely to alter management or outcome of the patient, then the risk of transfer may outweigh the benefit. It is imperative that every member of the health care team assist in clarifying what, if any, benefit may be derived from transport.

Assessment of Risk for Complications During Transportation

Prior to initiating transport, a patient's risk for development of complications during transport should be systematically assessed. Switching of life support technologies in the critical care unit to portable devices may lead to undesired physiologic changes. In addition, complications may arise from environmental conditions outside the critical care unit which are difficult to control, resulting in body temperature fluctuations or inadvertent movement of invasive devices (e.g., endotracheal tube, chest tubes, intravenous devices). Common complications associated with transportation are summarized in Table 11–1.

Respiratory Complications

Maintaining adequate ventilation and oxygenation during transport is a challenge. Patients who are not intubated prior to their transfer are at risk for developing airway obstruction. This is particularly a problem in patients with decreased levels of consciousness. Continuous monitoring of airway patency is critical to ensure rapid implementation of airway strategies, if necessary. Elective intubation prior to transport may need to be considered for patients at high risk for airway problems.

For patients who are intubated, ventilation is often maintained manually. Delivery of the appropriate minute ventilation is difficult, since tidal volume delivery must be estimated. Hypoventilation or hyperventilation rapidly will result in pH changes which can lead to tissue perfusion and oxygenation deficits. Therefore, respiratory and nursing personnel who are trained properly in the mechanisms of manual ventilation need to provide ventilation during trans-

---

[1]Adapted from: American Association of Critical-Care Nurses: *Guidelines for the transfer of critically ill patients*. Aliso Viejo, CA: AACN, 1993.

TABLE 11–1. POTENTIAL COMPLICATIONS DURING TRANSPORT

Neurological
Increased intracranial pressure
Cerebral hypoxia
Cerebral hypercarbia
Paralysis

Pulmonary
Hyperventilation
Hypoventilation
Airway obstruction
Aspiration
Recurrent pneumothorax
Arterial blood gas changes

Cardiovascular
Hypotension
Hypertension
Arrhythmias
Decreased tissue perfusion
Cardiac ischemia
Peripheral ischemia

Gastrointestinal
Nausea
Vomiting

port. Some facilities may have a portable ventilator which delivers an appropriate tidal volume during the transfer. If the patient currently is requiring positive end expiratory pressure (PEEP), the percentage of inspired oxygen (FIO_2) may need to be increased during transport to balance the loss of PEEP. Increasing the FIO_2 for any patient requiring transfer may help to avoid other complications from hypoxia.

Cardiovascular Complications

Whether related to their underlying disease processes or the anxiety of being taken out of a controlled environment, the potential for cardiovascular complications exists in all patients being transported. These complications include hypotension, hypertension, arrhythmias, tachycardia, ischemia, and acute pulmonary edema (heart failure). Many of these complications can be avoided by adequate patient preparation with pharmacologic agents to maintain hemodynamic stability and manage pain and/or anxiety. Continuous infusions should be carefully maintained during transport, with special attention given to IV lines during movement of the patient from one surface to another.

Neurological Complications

The potential for respiratory and/or cardiovascular changes during transport increases the risk for cerebral hypoxia, hypercarbia, and intracranial pressure (ICP) changes. Patients with high baseline ICP may require additional interventions to stabilize cerebral perfusion and oxygenation prior to transport (e.g., hyperventilation, increased PaO_2, blood pressure control). In addition, patients with suspected cranial or vertebral fractures are at high risk for neu-

rologic damage during repositioning from bed to transport carts or diagnostic tables. Proper immobilization of the spine is imperative in these situations, as is the avoidance of unnecessary repositioning of the patient. Positioning the head in the midline position with the head of the bed elevated, when not contraindicated, may decrease the risk of increases in ICP.

AT THE BEDSIDE
▶ *Risk Factors During Transport*

Mr. W., a 45-year-old, was involved in a motor vehicle accident when he fell asleep on his way home from work. Mr. W. was not wearing a seat belt, and there were no air bags in the car. His injuries included chest contusions and broken ribs from the steering wheel and lacerations of his scalp from the windshield.

He was stabilized in the emergency department with the insertion of a chest tube to relieve his left pneumothorax and placement of a pulmonary artery (PA) catheter to monitor for possible cardiac tamponade. He was then admitted to the intensive care unit. Mr. W. was assigned to one of the critical care nurses, Nancy, who had two other patients. One of these patients was mechanically ventilated, having undergone repair of an abdominal aortic aneurysm yesterday, and the other was recovering from a large anterior MI suffered after a total hip replacement.

Nancy was aware of the possible complications Mr. W. might experience during transport: respiratory, cardiovascular, or safety compromises. Possible respiratory complications included upper airway obstruction, respiratory depression, hypoxia, or hypercarbia, especially in a patient who has head and chest trauma and whose oxygenation is already compromised. Cardiovascular risks included hypotension, tachycardia due to cardiac tamponade, and decreased tissue perfusion due to decreased cardiac output and increased tissue oxygen demand during the transfer. Anxiety was another potential complication that Nancy considered, both from the activity of transfer and the uncertainty of Mr. W.'s future.

Anticipating complications, Nancy planned ahead. She asked that Mr. W. be intubated and mechanically ventilated prior to the transport. With his respiratory status under control, Mr. W. could be safely medicated for pain and anxiety, and ultimately decrease his oxygen demand. Intubating Mr. W. electively in the controlled environment of the ICU prevented an emergency situation by eliminating the possible complications of respiratory arrest and emergency intubation.

Gastrointestinal Complications

Gastrointestinal complications may include nausea and/or vomiting, which can threaten the patient's airway, as well as cause discomfort. Premedicating patients at risk for GI upset with an H_2 blocker or an antiemetic may be helpful. For patients with large nasogastric drainage, preparations to continue NG drainage during transportation and/or in the destination location may be necessary.

Pain

The level of pain experienced by the patient is likely to be increased during transport. Many of the diagnostic tests and therapeutic interventions in other hospital departments are uncomfortable and/or painful. Anxiety associated with transport may also increase the level of pain. Additional pain medication and/or anxiolytic drugs may be required to ensure adequate pain management during the transport process. Keeping the patient and family members well informed is also helpful in decreasing anxiety levels.

Level of Care Required During Transport

During transport, there should be no interruption in the monitoring or maintenance of the patient's vital functions. The equipment used during transport, as well as the skill level of accompanying personnel, must be equivalent with the interventions required or anticipated for the patient while in the critical care unit (Table 11–2). Intermittent and continuous monitoring of physiologic status (e.g., cardiac output and rhythm, blood pressure, oxygenation, ventilation) should continue during transport and while the patient is away from the critical care unit (Table 11–3).

Questions which need to be answered to prepare for transfer include:

- What is the current level of care (equipment, personnel)?
- What will be needed during the transfer to maintain that level of care?
- What additional resources may be required during transport?

Preparations for Transport

Before transfer, the plan of care for the patient during and after transfer should be coordinated to ensure continuity of care and availability of appropriate resources (Table 11–4). Receiving units should be contacted to confirm that all preparations for the patient's arrival have been completed. Communication, both written and verbal, between team members should delineate the current status of the patient, management priorities, and the process to follow in the event of untoward events (e.g., unexpected hemodynamic instability or airway problems).

After you have assessed the patient's risk for transport complications, the patient should be prepared for transfer, both physically and mentally. As you are organizing the

TABLE 11–2. TRANSPORT PERSONNEL AND EQUIPMENT REQUIREMENTS

Personnel

A minimum of two people should accompany the patient.

One of the accompanying personnel should be the critical care nurse assigned to the patient or a specifically trained critical care transfer nurse. This critical care nurse should have completed a competency-based orientation and meet the described standards for critical care nurses.

Additional personnel may include a respiratory therapist, registered nurse, critical care technician, or physician. A respiratory therapist should accompany all patients requiring mechanical ventilation.

Equipment

The following minimal equipment should be available.

- Cardiac monitor/defibrillator.
- Airway management equipment and resuscitation bag of proper size and fit for the patient.
- Oxygen source of ample volume to support the patient's needs for the projected time out of the ICU, with an additional 30-minute reserve.
- Standard resuscitation drugs: epinephrine, lidocaine, atropine.
- Blood pressure cuff (sphygmomanometer) and stethoscope.
- Ample supply of the IV fluids and continuous drip medications (regulated by battery-operated infusion pumps) being administered to the patient.
- Additional medications to provide the patient's scheduled intermittent medication doses and to meet anticipated needs (e.g., sedation) with appropriate orders to allow their administration if a physician is not present.
- For patients receiving mechanical support of ventilation, a device capable of delivering the same volume, pressure, and PEEP and an FIO_2 equal to or greater than that the patient is receiving in the ICU. For practical reasons, in adults an FIO_2 of 1.0 is most feasible during transfer because this eliminates the need for an air tank and air-oxygen blender. During neonatal transfer, FIO_2 should be precisely controlled.
- Resuscitation cart and suction equipment need not accompany each patient being transferred, but such equipment should be stationed in areas used by critically ill patients and be readily available (within 4 minutes) by a predetermined mechanism for emergencies that may occur en route.

(From: American Association of Critical-Care Nurses: Guidelines for the transfer of critically ill patients. *Aliso Viejo, CA: AACN, 1993.)*

equipment and monitors, explain the transfer process to the patient and his or her family. The explanation should include a description of the sensations the patient may expect, how long the procedure should last, and the role of members of the transport team. It's important to allay any patient or family anxiety by identifying current caregivers who will accompany the patient during transport. The availability of emergency equipment and drugs and how communication is handled during transportation also may be information that will reassure the patient and family.

Transport

Once preparations are complete, the actual transfer can begin. Connect each of the portable monitoring devices prior to disconnection from the bedside equipment, if possible. This will enable a comparison of hemodynamic values with the portable equipment.

TABLE 11–3. MONITORING DURING TRANSFER

- If technologically possible, patients being transferred should receive the same physiological monitoring during transfer that they were receiving in the ICU.
- Minimally, all critically ill patients being transferred must have continuous monitoring of ECG and pulse oximetry and intermittent measurement and documentation of blood pressure, respiratory rate, and pulse rate.
- In addition, selected patients, based on clinical status, may benefit from monitoring by capnography; continuous measurement of blood pressure, PAP, and ICP; and intermittent measurement of CVP, Pao, and CO.
- Intubated patients receiving mechanical support of ventilation should have airway pressure monitored. If a transfer ventilator is used, it should have alarms to indicate disconnects or excessively high airway pressures.

From: American Association of Critical-Care Nurses: Guidelines for the transfer of critically ill patients. *Aliso Viejo, CA: AACN, 1993.*

Once hemodynamic pressure and noninvasive oxygenation monitors are in place and values verified, disconnect the patient from the mechanical ventilator or bedside oxygen source, and begin portable ventilation and oxygenation. Assess for clinical signs and symptoms of respiratory distress and changes in ventilation and oxygenation. Obtaining an arterial blood gas a few minutes after initiating portable/manual ventilation prior to transport may be appropriate in patients with severe respiratory compromise. If it is necessary to move the patient onto a stretcher, have plenty of help. It may be easier to transfer the patient on the bed if it will fit in elevators and spaces in the receiving area. Check IV lines, pressure lines, monitor cables, nasogastric tubes, chest tubes, Foley catheters, or drains of any sort to ensure proper placement during transport and to guard against accidental removal during transport.

TABLE 11–4. PRETRANSFER COORDINATION AND COMMUNICATION

- Physician-to-physician and/or nurse-to-nurse communication regarding the patient's condition and treatment preceding and following the transfer should be documented in the medical record when the management of the patient will be assumed by a different team while the patient is away from the ICU.
- The area to which the patient is being transferred (X-ray, operating room, nuclear medicine, etc.) must confirm that it is ready to receive the patient and immediately begin the procedure or test for which the patient is being transferred.
- Ancillary services (e.g., security, respiratory therapy, escort) must be notified as to the timing of the transfer and the equipment and support needed.
- The responsible physician must be notified either to accompany the patient or to be aware that the patient is out of the ICU at this time and may have an acute event requiring the physician's response to provide emergency care in another area of the hospital.
- Documentation in the medical record must include the indication for transfer, the patient's status during transfer, and whether the patient is expected to return to the ICU.

From: American Association of Critical-Care Nurses: Guidelines for the transfer of critically ill patients. *Aliso Viejo, CA: AACN, 1993.*

AT THE BEDSIDE
▶ *Preparing For Transport*

Having recognized and addressed Mr. W.'s risk factors, his nurse Nancy organized the team for the transport of Mr. W. to CT scan, making sure another nurse was able to care for her other patients while she was off the unit. Mr. W. needed a respiratory therapist during the transport. Other members of the transport team included two transporters to help manage the equipment, open doors, and hold elevators. Nancy gathered the portable equipment and connected it to Mr. W. This included a cardiac monitor, a blood pressure monitor, a pulse oximeter, and a monitor for the PA pressures. IV lines were organized so that only essential infusions were transported with Mr. W.

Other concerns which Nancy considered included: Is there a nurse in the CT suite who can care for Mr. W. once he arrives there? How long should she expect him to be gone? Are there electrical outlets for all this equipment in CT? How long will the batteries last? Is there oxygen available in CT? Will the water seal for the chest tube hang on the bed? Will he need suction? Is there suction in the CT suite? What medicines does Mr. W. need? Does he need something for pain or his next dose of antibiotic? Will he need new IV fluids while he's gone? If he is able, does he understand the procedure that he's going to have? Where is his family? Do they know what is going on?

Fortunately for Nancy, one battery-operated machine was able to monitor pressures, cardiac rhythm, and pulse oximetry. The respiratory therapist used a portable ventilator to provide ventilation and oxygenation. A ventilator was set up in the CT suite for Mr. W. The chest tube drain fit over the rail around the bed, maintaining the water seal without suction. The Foley catheter also had a special hook on the side of the bed.

Mr. W. was understandably anxious about what was going on, as was his wife. While Nancy got all the equipment together, she talked to both of them about what to expect during the transport, as well as in the CT suite. She explained how long the procedure should last, and where Mrs. W. could wait while the procedure was in progress. She allowed Mrs. W. to stay with her husband as long as possible during the transfer.

During transport, the critical care nurse is responsible for continuous assessment of cardiopulmonary status (ECG, blood pressures, respiration, oxygenation, etc.) and interventions as required to ensure stability. Throughout the time away from the critical care environment, it is imperative that vigilant monitoring occur of the patient's response not only to the transport, but also to the procedure or therapeutic intervention taking place. Alterations in drug administration, particularly analgesics, sedatives, and vasoactive drugs, are frequently needed during the time away from the critical care unit to maintain physiologic stability. Documentation of assessment findings, interventions, and the patient's responses should continue throughout the transport process.

Following return to the critical care unit, monitoring systems and interventions are reestablished and the patient is completely reassessed. Often, some adjustment in pharmacologic therapy or ventilator support is required following transport. Allowing for some uninterrupted time for the family to be at the patient's bedside and for rest is another important priority following return to the unit. Documentation of the patient's overall response to the transport situation should be included in the medical record.

Interhospital Transfers

Interhospital patient transfers, while similar to transfers within a hospital, frequently can be more challenging. The biggest differences between the two are the isolation of the patient in the transfer vehicle, limited equipment and personnel, and a high complication rate due to longer transport periods and inability to control environmental conditions (e.g., temperature, atmospheric pressure, sudden movements) which may cause physiologic instability.

The primary consideration in interfacility transfer is maintaining the same level of care provided in the critical care unit. Accordingly, the mode of transfer should be selected with this in mind. The resources available in the sending facility must be made as portable as possible and must accompany the patient. For example, intraaortic balloon pump therapy and ventilation must be continued without interruption. This requirement often challenges critical care practitioners' skills and abilities, as well as the equipment resources necessary to ensure a safe transport.

Detailed information regarding the planning for interfacility transfer has been developed by multidisciplinary professional groups and is summarized in Chapter 29, Guidelines for the Transfer of Critically Ill Patients.

INFECTION CONTROL

Critically ill patients are especially vulnerable to infection during their stay in the critical care unit. It is estimated that 20% to 60% of critically ill patients acquire some form of infection during their critical illness period, with significant increases in their morbidity and mortality rates from these infections. It is imperative for critical care practioners to understand the processes that contribute to these potentially lethal infections and their role in preventing these untoward events.

Chain of Infection

To describe the mechanism of infectious disease transmission, the concept of a chain of infection is frequently used (Figure 11–1). Each link in the chain represents a critical component of disease transmission. If one link is broken, the chain is interrupted and no disease transmission can occur. All infection control efforts are aimed at breaking at least one of the links in the chain.

Reservoir

The reservoir is the first link in the chain. Every infectious organism, whether it is bacterial, viral, or fungal, has a reservoir, or a place where it lives and thrives. There are many reservoirs for pathogenic microorganisms in the intensive care unit. Careful control and monitoring of these reservoirs can prevent nosocomial transmission of these organisms.

Water is a very significant reservoir for microorganisms in the health care setting. Many pathogenic organisms, such as *Pseudomonas, Serratia marcescens, Legionella* and

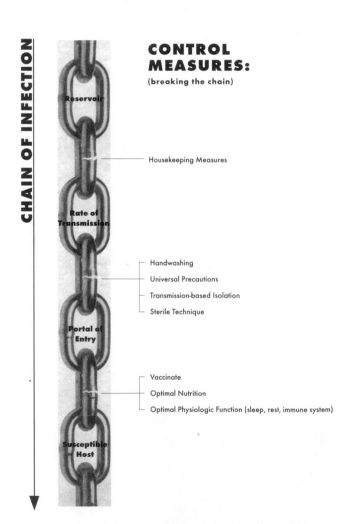

Figure 11–1. Chain of infection with infection control methods to break the chain.

some species of *Mycobacteria,* flourish in water. Although one might expect to find these pathogens in any wet area, special attention should be paid to certain areas. Taps, drains, and sinks all most likely are contaminated with these pathogens; however, their significance in the transmission of nosocomial infection has not been demonstrated. Clearly, they are contaminated areas and should be considered in the case of an infection outbreak.

Tap water, or portable water, may be contaminated with gram-negative microorganisms such as *Pseudomonas* and *Serratia.* These organisms actually multiply in water, so a small number of bacteria can rapidly proliferate. For this reason tap water should never be used to irrigate sterile body areas or to rinse equipment that may be used in respiratory therapy procedures.

Route of Transmission

All organisms have a specific route of transmission—either direct or indirect (Table 11–5). Direct transmission is the immediate transfer of the infectious agent from the infected host to the portal of entry. This can be through direct contact, as with sexually transmitted diseases, or through droplet contact by sneezing or coughing into the mucous membranes of others.

Indirect contact can happen in one of three ways. Vehicleborne transmission, the most common way infectious diseases are transmitted in the health care setting, is contact through inanimate objects (fomites) such as bedding, contaminated food, surgical instruments, or a health care worker's hands.

Vectorborne transmission occurs when the infectious agent is transferred by an arthropod to a host. Examples of vectorborne infectious diseases are Rocky Mountain spotted fever, transmitted by the dog tick, and Lyme disease, transmitted by the deer tick.

The third route of indirect transmission is airborne, either through dusts or droplet nuclei. Some fungal and viral infections can be transmitted through the generation of dusts that are inhaled by a susceptible host. *Aspergillus* is a fungus that is found in decaying wood and soil. It can be transmitted

TABLE 11–5. SUMMARY OF MECHANISMS OF DISEASE TRANSMISSION

Direct
The immediate transfer of infectious agent from the infected host to a portal of entry.
Direct contact: kissing, sexually transmitted diseases.
Droplet: sneezing and coughing into the mucous membranes of others.

Indirect
Vehicleborne: direct contact through inanimate objects (fomites) such as bedding, surgical instruments, contaminated food, or health care workers' hands.
Vectorborne: the infectious agent is transferred by an arthropod to a susceptible host.
Airborne: dusts and droplet nuclei.

via construction dust in hospitals and can cause life-threatening pneumonia in immunocompromised hosts. *Mycobacterium tuberculosis* is another infectious agent that is transmitted by droplet nuclei. These tiny particles are formed from the evaporation of respiratory droplets that have been coughed or sneezed into the air. These infectious droplet nuclei may remain airborne for long periods of time, perhaps as long as 30 to 60 minutes. If they are inhaled, they can be carried into the alveoli in the lungs and cause infection.

Transmission-Based Isolation

Specific control measures are aimed at specific routes of transmission. For example, meningococcal meningitis is a bacterial infection that is caused by the organism *Neisseria meningiditis,* which can be transmitted via the direct route through droplet contact. The infectious respiratory secretions can transmit a meningococcal infection if they come in contact with a susceptible host's mucous membrane. Control measures are focused on preventing this contact from occurring by requiring the health care worker to use a mask to cover the mouth and nose when coming in close contact with a patient who has untreated meningococcal meningitis.

Airborne organisms, such as *Mycobacterium tuberculosis* (TB), varicella (chicken pox), and rubeola (measles), which can be transmitted from person to person, require respiratory isolation to prevent transmission to individuals entering the patient's room. This type of isolation requires special ventilation to prevent the air in the room from drifting out into the hallway or being recirculated within the hospital. Special masks that filter very small particles are required to be worn by individuals entering the room.

Standard Precautions

Standard Precautions, sometimes referred to as Universal Precautions or Body Substance Isolation, refer to the basic precautions that are to be used on all patients, regardless of their diagnosis. The general premise of Standard Precautions is that all body fluids have the potential to transmit any number of infectious diseases, both bacterial and viral. Certain basic principles must be followed to prevent direct and indirect transmission of these organisms. Nonsterile exam gloves should be worn for touching any moist body fluid. This includes urine, stool, saliva, emesis, sputum, blood, and any type of drainage. A good rule of thumb to follow is "If it's wet and it's not yours—wear gloves!" Other personal protective equipment, such as face shields and protective gowns, should be worn whenever there is a risk of splashing body fluids into the face or onto clothing.

Portal of Entry

Infectious organisms must have a way to enter a susceptible host. The human body is designed to keep infectious agents out. Intact skin is the first line of defense against infectious disease transmission. Once the skin is compromised, through a cut, puncture, or abrasion, a portal of entry has been established and an infectious organism can enter the host. In health care, and especially in critical care, the skin of the patient is compromised in many ways, through the use of intravenous and central venous catheters, pressure ulcer development from prolonged bedrest, and surgical procedures.

The mucous membranes provide primary defense mechanisms to prevent organisms from entering the host. If the primary mechanisms of the respiratory, gastrointestinal, and genitourinary tracts are overcome, they can also become a portal of entry. These defense mechanisms, such as mucous production, acid production, mucociliary activity, and the presence of normal body flora, can be overcome in the critical care setting by endotracheal and nasogastric intubation, administration of gastric-acid–neutralizing medications, and antibiotics that reduce the normal body flora.

Susceptible Host

The final link in the chain of infection is that of the susceptible host. Without the susceptible host, there can be no disease transmission. Unfortunately, there are few sure ways to make a host unsusceptible. Vaccinations can make a host immune to certain bacterial and viral infections. This is a very easy way to break the last link in the chain. Other ways to make a host less susceptible include adequate nutrition, rest, and reduced stress. It is easy to see why the critical care patient is at higher risk of succumbing to infectious disease transmission.

Microorganisms

Normal Flora

Human beings are covered by microorganisms. They inhabit both the internal and external surfaces of the body. These microorganisms that live in harmony on and in our bodies are referred to as normal body flora (Table 11–6). These organisms rarely cause disease.

There are certain body sites which are normally void of all microorganisms and are considered sterile. These body sites are:

- Trachea, bronchi, sinuses
- Cerebrospinal fluid
- Blood
- Bladder
- Peritoneal fluid
- Synovial fluid

Pathogenic Organisms

Pathogenic organisms are those that can multiply in a host and cause damage. Some organisms that are considered normal flora, such as *Staphylococcus aureus,* can cause dis-

TABLE 11–6. COMMON NORMAL BODY FLORA

Skin
Staphylococcus aureus
Staphylococcus epidermidis
Diphtheroids
Streptococcus viridans
Enterobacter species
Yeasts

Upper Respiratory Tract
Klebsiella pneumoniae
Haemophilus influenzae
Staphylococcus aureus
Staphylococcus epidermidis
Streptococcus pneumoniae
Mycoplasma pneumoniae

Colon
Pseudomonas aeruginosa
Escherichia coli
Klebsiella pneumoniae
Enterobacter species
Proteus species
Streptococcus faecalis (enterococcus)
Clostridium perfringens
Yeasts

ease in certain circumstances. Many nosocomial infections are the result of normal flora becoming pathogenic or being introduced into normally sterile body sites. This type of infection is referred to as endogenous.

Colonization versus Infection

Colonization refers to the growth and multiplication of an organism or organisms in or on a host without tissue invasion or damage. It may be chronic, long-term colonization with the organism becoming part of the host's normal flora or transient carriage such as a health care worker's hands becoming colonized with bacteria for a period of time before they are finally eliminated through handwashing. It is likely that critical care patients are heavily colonized with hospital flora because their natural host defenses are diminished due to underlying illness and their increased exposure to microorganisms due to a large number of invasive devices.

Infection refers to the invasion and multiplication of the organism in the tissue. This invasion and multiplication elicits an immune response and may or may not result in clinical signs and symptoms of infection.

Trying to determine whether or not a positive culture represents a true infection or simply colonization is not always an easy task. Symptoms of infection include fever, redness, development of purulent (green) drainage, and pain. Laboratory findings indicative of infection include:

- The presence of many polymorphonuclear leukocytes (PMNs or polys)
- A large number of organisms seen on smear and culture

- Predominance of a single organism as opposed to many different species

The absence of these somatic signs and symptoms and laboratory findings points more toward colonization than infection. Patients who are colonized do not necessarily require antibiotic treatment to eradicate the microorganism since no tissue damage has occurred.

Asepsis

Basic asepsis is one of the cornerstones of good infection control practice in any health care setting. Unfortunately, it is one of the most frequently forgotten principles. Following the basic principles of asepsis is extremely important in the critical care unit, where patients become colonized with hospital organisms, many of which may be highly resistant to antibiotic treatment.

There are two types of asepsis. Practices that prevent or reduce the transmission of microorganisms from person to person are referred to as medical asepsis or clean technique. Surgical asepsis describes practices that are designed to keep areas and objects completely free from microorganisms. This is also known as sterile technique.

Handwashing

Basic handwashing is defined by the Centers for Disease Control and Prevention (CDC) as vigorous rubbing together of lathered hands for 10 seconds followed by a thorough rinsing under a stream of running water. Particular attention should be paid around rings and under fingernails. It is best to keep natural fingernails well trimmed and without polish. Cracked nail polish is a good place for microorganisms to hide. Artificial fingernails are not recommended for use in any health care setting because they are virtually impossible to clean without a nail brush and vigorous scrubbing. Handwashing should be performed prior to donning exam gloves to carry out patient care activities and after removing exam gloves. Washing should occur any time bare hands become contaminated with any wet body fluid and should be done before the body fluid dries. Once it dries, microorganisms begin to colonize the skin, making it more difficult to remove them. Plain soaps suspend microbial particles so they can be rinsed away, while antimicrobial soaps actually kill microorganisms on the skin. An antimicrobial soap, such as chlorhexidine gluconate, should be used in the critical care setting.

Dry, cracked skin, a long-standing problem associated with handwashing, has new significance with the emergence of bloodborne pathogens. Frequent handwashing, especially with antimicrobial soap, can lead to extremely dry skin. The frequent use of latex exam gloves has been associated with increased sensitivities and allergies, causing even more skin breakdown. All of this skin breakdown can put the health care provider at risk for bloodborne pathogen transmission, as well as for colonization or infection with bacteria. Attention to skin care is extremely important for the critical care practitioner who is using antimicrobial soap and latex gloves frequently. Lotions and emollients should be used to prevent skin breakdown. If skin breakdown does occur, the employee health nurse should be consulted for possible treatment or work restriction until the condition resolves.

Sterile Technique

Sterile technique should be followed for procedures whenever a patient's normal host defenses have been compromised, such as when inserting a Foley catheter or intravenous line, changing a surgical wound dressing, or tracheal suctioning. Because sterility cannot be visualized, certain principles must be adhered to in order to guarantee the sterility of an item or field. Once opened, a sterile field is considered contaminated if:

- A nonsterile item touches it.
- It becomes wet.
- It is covered.
- It is left unattended.

The sterile field should be observed at all times to ensure that contamination has not occurred. It is helpful to have one person observing the sterile procedure for breaks in the sterile field, such as leaning against the sterile field with nonsterile clothing.

Critical Items

Sterile means the absence of all microorganisms. Any item that is to be introduced into a sterile body cavity or tissue or that will allow blood to flow through it must be sterile. These are referred to as "critical items." Sterility can be achieved through a number of methods including gas sterilization (ethylene oxide), steam under pressure (autoclave), and chemical sterilization (paracetic acid). Prior to sterilization the items must be thoroughly cleaned to remove any biological material. Because sterility cannot be seen with the naked eye, items that have been sterilized are identified in some manner to let the user know that the product indeed has been sterilized. This may be a chemical tape or label on the package that has turned a specific color after sterilization has occurred.

Semicritical Items

Items that will come into contact with mucous membranes or nonintact skin are referred to as "semicritical." Items that fall into this category are laryngoscope blades, glass thermometers, endoscopes, and vaginal speculums. If any of these items is to be reused, it must be thoroughly cleaned with an instrument cleaner to remove any biological material and then receive high-level disinfection. This process eliminates all but the most resistant bacterial spores. Sterilization is not necessary for these items because the body areas they will be touching are not sterile. High-level disinfection can be achieved by soaking in a cold sterilant, such as a 2% glutaraldehyde, for a period of time. Once an item has been soaked in a glutaraldehyde, it should be rinsed in sterile water to prevent contamination with water pathogens. If the high-level disinfected item is rinsed in tap water, this should be followed by an alcohol rinse to remove any contamination from the tap water. This process can be labor intensive, so that many semicritical items have become disposable to eliminate this need for high-level disinfection.

Noncritical Items

Noncritical items are those items that come in contact with intact skin, such as a bedpan or blood pressure cuff. These items require low-level disinfection which can be achieved using a hospital-grade disinfectant. Phenolic, quaternary ammonium, and 70% to 90% isopropyl alcohol fall into this category.

It is important to remember that items are processed in certain ways because of what they do—not because of what body fluid is on them. A noncritical item never needs more than low-level disinfection even if it is contaminated with blood.

Nosocomial Infections in the Critically Ill Patient

In general, intensive care units have the highest incidence of nosocomial infections due to the high use of multiple invasive devices and the frequent presence of debilitating underlying diseases. Pulmonary infections are the most common nosocomial infections in the critical care setting. Other important infections include urinary tract, blood-stream, and surgical site infections.

Nosocomial Pneumonia

Rates of nosocomial pneumonia have been reported to be 10 to 20 times higher in the critical care patient and 7 to 21 times higher in the intubated patient. The added insult of a nosocomial pneumonia can significantly increase length of stay and cost between $10,000 and $30,000. Nosocomial pneumonias are also associated with a high mortality rate, varying anywhere from 20% to 60% depending on the acuity and underlying diseases of the patient, as well as the bacterial etiology of the infection. Mortality tends to be higher when infection is due to *Pseudomonas* organisms. Details of specific risk factors and control measures for the prevention of nosocomial pneumonia are presented in Chapter 13, Respiratory System.

Urinary Tract Infection

Urinary tract infections (UTIs) are other common nosocomial infections, usually occurring after urinary catheterization. Although UTIs are considered benign infections in many patients, their occurrence in the critically ill patient may lead to bacteremia and increased morbidity and mor-

tality. Host factors that increase the risk for UTI include advanced age, debilitation, and the postpartum state.

The most common pathogens identified in UTI are: *Escherichia coli, Klebsiella, Proteus, Enterococcus, Pseudomonas, Enterobacter, Serratia,* and *Candida.* It is not surprising to note that, with the exception of *Serratia,* these organisms normally colonize the colon. Infection with *Serratia* suggests exogenous contamination.

Microorganisms may be introduced into the bladder via the catheter after passing through the distal urethra and meatus. More commonly, microorganisms travel along the outside of the indwelling catheter or through the inside of the catheter if the drainage system has been opened.

Control Measures for UTI

The use of indwelling urinary catheters should be limited to the following circumstances:

- To relieve urinary tract obstruction
- To permit urinary drainage in patients with bladder dysfunction and retention
- To aid in surgery
- To accurately measure output in critically ill patients

Indwelling catheters should never be used for convenience with an incontinent patient.

Strict adherence to aseptic technique is essential in preventing UTI. All indwelling catheters should be inserted using aseptic technique and sterile equipment. Handwashing before and after any manipulation of the catheter or apparatus is essential. Nonsterile exam gloves should be worn during specimen collection, emptying of drainage bags, and manipulation of the catheter. This not only protects the health care provider from unwanted contact with urine, it also acts as a barrier protecting the patient from the normal skin flora of the health care provider.

A closed drainage system should be used and maintained. If breaks in the system cannot be avoided, the catheter-tubing junction should be disinfected with alcohol and care taken not to contaminate the exposed ends. Irrigation of indwelling catheters should be avoided unless obstruction is expected, and then continuous irrigation using a closed system is recommended. If intermittent irrigation is necessary, strict aseptic technique should be used. Sterile irrigant and irrigating equipment should be used for each irrigation.

When emptying urinary drainage bags it is necessary to use a separate collecting container for each patient. The drainage spout and the nonsterile collecting container should never come into contact with each other. If this does occur, the drainage spout should be disinfected with alcohol prior to reinserting it into the drainage bag.

Obtaining urine specimens for laboratory analysis should be done through the sampling port designed for this purpose in the closed drainage system. After disinfecting the sampling port, obtain the specimen using a sterile needle and syringe.

Bloodstream Infections

Nosocomial bloodstream infections (BSIs) have been reported to add 2 weeks to a patient's length of stay, with additional costs of $40,000 for those who survive. Crude mortality rates have been reported from 25% to 50%. These infections occur at a higher rate in critical care units than in the general hospital units, and have been correlated with the presence of invasive devices and increased lengths of stay in the critical care unit.

Control Measures for BSI

The portal of entry for primary bloodstream infections is usually through an invasive line, such as a central venous, intravenous, or arterial catheter. The main control measure for preventing nosocomial BSI is to limit the use of invasive devices. When such devices are necessary, strict aseptic technique should be observed during insertion, dressing changes, monitoring, and other interventions involving the devices.

The standard recommendation is that peripheral IV lines remain in place no longer than 48 to 72 hours, and arterial lines no longer than 96 hours. There is no standard recommendation for routine removal of central venous catheters when required for prolonged periods. If the patient begins to show signs of sepsis that could be catheter-related, these catheters should be removed. More important than the length of time the catheter is in place is how carefully the catheter was inserted and cared for while in place. All catheters that have been placed in an emergency situation should be replaced as soon as possible and at least within 24 hours of insertion. Dressings should be left in place until the catheter is removed, or the dressing becomes damp, loosened, or soiled. Intravenous tubing should be changed no more frequently than every 72 hours, with the exception of tubing for blood, blood products, or lipids (every 24 hours).

Secondary BSI is defined as a bloodstream infection that can be traced to a previous infection at another site, such as a wound infection or pneumonia. The prevention strategy for secondary BSI is to treat the underlying source of the infection.

Surgical Site Infections

The risk of surgical site infection following an operative procedure can be associated with a number of host risk factors, including prolonged hospitalization prior to surgery, underlying disease such as diabetes and malnutrition, obesity, and smoking. Underlying infections should be treated prior to surgery whenever possible. Exogenous risk factors include prolonged duration of operation, inappropriate use of prophylactic antibiotics, and surgical site preparation.

Preparation of the surgical site by shaving with a razor has been shown to increase the risk of surgical site infection in all classes of surgery. The rate of infection is higher in patients who were shaved the night before their surgical procedure compared to those who were shaved just prior to the operation. For this reason, if shaving is necessary, it is best done immediately prior to the procedure. The preferred method is to remove hair using an electric clipper or a depilatory.

After surgery, good attention to aseptic technique is essential for dressing changes. Sterile technique should be used until the incision site is primarily healed, at which time clean dressing technique may be used.

Risks To Health Care Workers

The term *hospital* tends to connote a place for healing, treatment, and getting well. It may be difficult for health care workers to imagine that this seemingly healthful environment could pose health risks to them. One of the costs of state-of-the-art technology and treatment is that the providers of this care are at increased risk of exposure to biological and chemical hazards.

Bloodborne Pathogens

Bloodborne pathogens are viruses that can be transmitted through contact with blood or certain body fluids. Most notable are the human immunodeficiency virus (HIV), hepatitis B virus, and hepatitis C virus. The body fluids that contain enough viral particles to transmit an infection include:

- Blood
- Semen
- Vaginal secretions
- Pericardial fluid
- Pleural fluid
- Peritoneal fluid
- Synovial fluid
- Cerebrospinal fluid
- Amniotic fluid
- Breast milk

Any other body fluid that contains visible blood or in which body fluids cannot be differentiated should be considered potentially infectious.

The route of transmission for bloodborne pathogens in the health care setting is directly through mucous membrane or nonintact skin contact, or indirectly through vehicle contact such as a sharp instrument. The portal of entry is percutaneous or mucous membranes.

The Occupational Safety and Health Administration (OSHA) mandates that certain safety measures be followed by health care workers to prevent transmission of bloodborne pathogens in the workplace. There are five basic areas of control: engineering controls, work practice controls, personal protective equipment, housekeeping measures, and hepatitis B vaccination.

Engineering Controls

Engineering controls are safety devices that remove the hazard from the workplace. Examples of engineering controls are sharps containers, needleless systems for administering intermittent IV therapy, and resheathable syringes. It has been difficult to entirely engineer out the risks that sharp instruments play in the health care setting. Manufacturers have struggled with developing safety devices that still provide the functionality required by the clinicians who use them. Health care employers are required to evaluate available products and to implement them if they will reduce exposures while at the same time performing the desired clinical function.

Work Practice Controls

Policies that direct how health care workers should perform are referred to as work practice controls. Universal Precautions are a work practice control that is required of all health care settings. The more stringent Body Substance Isolation may be used if it is preferred by the institution. Other work practice controls include:

- Minimize splashing, spraying, and generation of droplets of blood and body fluids.
- No bending, breaking, recapping, or manipulating of needles.
- No eating, drinking, smoking, or applying lip balm or contact lenses in areas where blood or body fluids are present.

Personal Protective Equipment

Personal protective equipment is worn to provide additional protection from bloodborne pathogens. This is worn in addition to the regular clothing or uniform and is to be worn in the work area only.

GLOVES

Nonsterile exam gloves are to be worn whenever performing venipuncture, handling the nonintact skin or mucous membranes of a patient, or handling specimens of blood or body fluid that are not in secondary containers. Latex exam gloves have been associated with skin sensitivities and allergies, and substitutions may need to be made if this condition occurs. Nonlatex exam gloves can offer adequate protection against bloodborne pathogens. Some vinyl exam gloves, however, are not form fitting and may pose a risk if dexterity is needed, as for phlebotomy.

Although gloves will not prevent exposure from needlesticks, there is some evidence that if a needle with HIV-infected blood is passed through a layer of latex it will reduce the viral load. This will reduce the likelihood of transmitting HIV via needlestick.

FACE PROTECTION

When performing procedures that may result in splashing, spraying, or generation of droplets, the health care worker must wear face protection. Adequate face protection will protect the eyes, nose, and mouth. This may be in the form of a full-face shield or a mask with eye protection. Attention should be paid to the fluid resistance of the face protection. Regular eyeglasses that leave gaps around the eyes do not offer enough protection from splashes of body fluid. Safety glasses are designed for solid projectiles, and may not offer enough protection against a big splash of body fluid. Face and eye shields should offer full protection against a spray or splash of body fluid to the face.

PROTECTIVE CLOTHING

Impervious gowns and/or lab coats are to be worn if there is a risk of blood or body fluid being splashed or sprayed onto clothing. This protective clothing should be worn over the general work clothes and should offer full protection against splashes and sprays. This means that lab coats must be buttoned, and protective gowns must be worn with the closures in the back. Protective clothing is not to be worn out of the work area and is to be removed immediately if it becomes soiled with blood or body fluid.

Housekeeping Measures

The environment should be maintained in a clean and sanitary condition. Blood and body fluid spills must be promptly cleaned up using a low-level disinfectant. Health care workers should exercise caution when cleaning blood spills, especially if there is broken glass or other sharp objects involved.

LINEN

Linen should be handled using Universal Precautions. All linen should be bagged at the point of origin and should not be sorted or rinsed or carried close to the body. Gloves should be worn for handling any wet linen.

LABELING

A biohazard symbol (Figure 11–2) is required to identify any area where blood or body fluids may be present. This is a universal symbol and must have a background of bright orange/red with lettering of a contrasting color.

INFECTIOUS WASTE

Each state defines infectious waste and regulates the disposal methods for infectious medical waste. It is important to know and understand your particular state regulation regarding approved disposal methods. All infectious waste must be labeled with a biohazard symbol.

Hepatitis B Vaccination

All health care employers are required to provide the hepatitis B vaccine to any employee at risk of having exposure to bloody or body fluids while at work. Vaccination

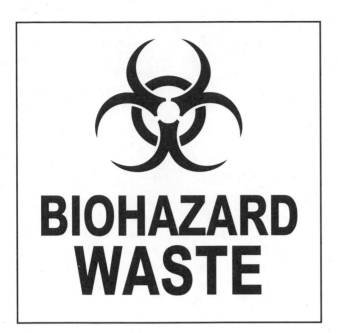

Figure 11–2. Biohazard symbol.

with the hepatitis B vaccine breaks the last link in the chain of infection, that of the susceptible host. The vaccine is very effective, giving full immunity to 9 out of 10 people vaccinated.

Postexposure Evaluation and Follow-up

Even if all the control measures are implemented to prevent exposure to bloodborne pathogens, occasionally an exposure does occur. Each exposure must be reported so that a full evaluation can be completed. Even if the exposed health care worker doesn't think the exposure is "high-risk," the exposure should be reported. By evaluating trends in exposure data additional control measures may be introduced to prevent future exposures from occurring.

Employers are required to provide the exposed employee with a medical evaluation following an exposure. This evaluation may include vaccination, lab tests, or other medical treatment. Testing should be done to determine the HIV and hepatitis B status of the source patient. State law may require informed consent prior to testing for HIV. In addition, some institutions are offering hepatitis C screening of the source patient.

Respiratory Pathogens

Respiratory pathogens are those pathogens that can be transmitted via the airborne route. These pathogens require specific isolation measures, as mentioned earlier in this chapter, to prevent transmission to health care workers. Additional measures may need to be taken if exposure occurs.

Tuberculosis

Exposure to tuberculosis can occur if a health care worker has unprotected contact with a patient with infectious *Mycobacterium tuberculosis*. To prevent these exposures, all patients with known or suspected tuberculosis should be placed in respiratory isolation and appropriate respiratory protection should be worn by all individuals entering the room. Early identification and treatment of patients with tuberculosis is the main control measure to prevent transmission.

Populations With Higher Prevalences of Tuberculosis

The incidence of tuberculosis is higher in the following groups of individuals:

- Contacts of persons with active TB
- Foreign-born persons from areas with high prevalence of TB (Asia, Africa, the Caribbean, Latin America)
- Medically underserved minority populations
- Homeless persons
- Correctional facility inmates (current or former)
- Alcoholics
- Injecting drug abusers
- Elderly

In general, persons who have been infected with TB have a 10% lifetime risk of developing active TB disease that can then be transmitted to others. This risk increases if the person has other underlying risk factors.

Populations With Higher Risk Of Progressing To Active TB Disease

- Persons who have recently been infected (within the previous 2 years)
- Children under 4 years old
- Persons with fibrotic lesions on chest x-ray
- Persons with certain medical conditions (HIV, silicosis, gastrectomy or jejunoileal bypass, being 10% below ideal body weight, chronic renal failure, diabetes mellitus, immunosuppression from chemotherapy, and some malignancies)

Prophylactic antituberculous medication may be prescribed to lower the risk of developing active TB disease. The recommended prophylactic medication is INH (isoniazid) for 6 to 9 months. Administration of this medication requires close medical follow-up to prevent toxicities. If the TB infection is a result of an exposure to a patient with drug-resistant TB, prophylaxis may be of no benefit.

All health care workers should have a TB skin test, known as purified protein derivative (PPD), placed at least annually. Skin testing may be indicated more frequently depending on the risk of transmission of TB in the individual facility.

Rubeola (Red Measles)

All health care workers should be immune to red measles. It is generally assumed that persons born before 1957 are immune due to having had the disease in childhood. All individuals born after 1957 should receive two measles vaccines to make them unsusceptible hosts.

Varicella (Chicken Pox)

Chicken pox is a common childhood disease characterized by upper respiratory symptoms and the development of large vesicles over the entire body. In childhood this disease is usually nothing more than a nuisance for parents who have to stay home from work to care for their sick child. In adults, however, chicken pox can lead to serious illness, including the development of pneumonia. In rare cases hospitalization is required. A small percentage of health care workers are not immune to the varicella virus. For these individuals, exposure to varicella will require work restriction during the incubation period (from day 10 through day 21 after exposure) and if they develop active disease. Use of the chicken pox vaccine should be considered for non-immune health care workers.

Shingles (Varicella Zoster)

Once a person has had chicken pox, the virus remains dormant in the body, along the nerve roots. If the body's normal immune function is weakened, as with chronic conditions such as HIV infection or in the normal aging process, the virus will reactivate as varicella zoster, more commonly known as shingles. The recurrence may be localized or disseminated. Transmission of varicella can occur from a person with active varicella zoster to individuals who are not immune to chicken pox.

Chemical Hazards

The requirements for sterilization, disinfection, and cleaning of patient care equipment and the environment expose the health care worker to a number of chemicals that may pose significant health risks. OSHA mandates that employers keep Material Safety Data Sheets (MSDSs) on each chemical used within the facility. These information sheets provide the user with all pertinent safety information regarding the chemical, including health risks and emergency medical treatment in the event of an exposure.

Antineoplastic agents may also contribute significantly to the health risks of health care workers. The U.S. Department of Health and Human Services makes recommendations for medical follow-up of employees handling antineoplastics. These recommendations suggest preplacement and periodic medical evaluations of workers handling these agents that include:

- complete work evaluation and history
- examination that includes the skin, liver, hematopoietic, and nervous systems

The Hazard Communication Standard mandates that each employee receive education and training in the safe handling of all chemicals that they will be exposed to during the performance of their job duties. All health care workers should familiarize themselves with their employer's hazard communication plan and follow all policies and procedures for the safe handling of chemicals.

SELECTED BIBLIOGRAPHY

What Heals: Humanizing Technology

Moore N: Planetree: Changing the way we think about patients. *Alternative Therapies in Health and Medicine.* 1995;1:14–15.

Planetree: The new industry standard for satisfying customers. *Hospital Entrepreneurs' Newsletter.* 1988;4(2).

Infection Control

Bennett JV, Brockmann PS (eds.): *Hospital infections,* 3rd ed. Boston: Little, Brown, 1994.

Soule BM (ed.): *The APIC curriculum for infection control practice,* vols. 1–3. Dubuque, IA: Kendall/Hunt, 1983.

Wenzel RP (ed.): *Prevention and control of nosocomial infections,* 2nd ed. Baltimore: Williams & Wilkins, 1993.

Transportation

American Association of Critical-Care Nurses: *Guidelines for the transfer of critically ill patients.* Aliso Viejo, CA: AACN, 1993.

Tice P: Intra hospital transport of critically ill adults: Potential physiologic changes and nursing implications. *Focus on Critical Care.* 1991;18(5):424–428.

Pathologic Conditions

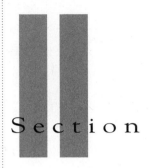

Section

Cardiovascular System

▶ Knowledge Competencies

1. Identify indications for, complications, and nursing management of patients undergoing coronary angiography and percutaneous transluminal coronary angioplasty.

2. Describe the etiology, pathophysiology, clinical presentation, patient needs, and principles of management of patients with acute ischemic heart disease.

3. Discuss the etiology, pathophysiology, clinical presentation, patient needs, and principles of management of patients in shock, heart failure, and hypertensive crisis.

■ *What Heals: Integrating Alternative Therapies*

It has been observed anecdotally for a long time that stressors are related to an increased incidence of myocardial infarction and sudden cardiac death. Scientific studies, however, are replacing such personal testimonials. These studies support the notion that a person's psychologic state can actually produce body illness. It has been shown, for example, that longevity is affected by events such as recent bereavement and grief, loss in job status, divorce, and financial distress. Impressive evidence also exists to document that emotions such as anxiety, fear, and social isolation are associated with coronary artery disease, hypertension, dysrhythmias, myocardial ischemia, and sudden cardiac death. What do these types of studies tell us? They provide conclusive evidence that the body and mind do communicate and that consciousness can play an important negative and villainous role in matters of illness.

Evidence also is rapidly accumulating to support the link between positive emotions and healing. Consider the results, for example, of several investigations evaluating the effects of music on cardiovascular patients. These studies document that acute cardiac patients who participate in music sessions report significant psychologic benefits, reduced anxiety and depression, lowered heart rates, increased peripheral temperatures, reduced cardiovascular complications, and lowered systolic blood pressures and mean arterial pressures. Alternative therapies such as progressive relaxation and Benson's relaxation technique also have been studied in cardiac rehabilitation patients and shown to have significant effects on diastolic blood pressure and lowered levels of anxiety and depression. Likewise, the use of progressive relaxation with patients undergoing coronary revascularization surgery has been found to significantly lower values related to anesthesia time, time on cardiopulmonary bypass, units of blood, and degree of postoperative hypothermia.

We know that medical science has focused on the anatomic, physiologic, cellular, genetic, and pharmacologic methods of accessing healing. This focus has concentrated solely on the body side of the body-mind equation. Data now are available to help us

239

understand how the mind and body are connected and how they communicate. We now know that alternative therapies also can be used to access healing. Perhaps this knowledge provides us with the missing link in bridging the mysterious gap between the body and mind. Perhaps it also provides the missing link in treating patients. What if we were to discover, after all these centuries, that the body approach to treating illness has missed its mark in terms of desired patient outcomes because it has not taken into account the profoundly devastating effects nor the enormously healing effects of the mind. What if treating body ailments with body-oriented therapies is only half of the answer? What might be the outcomes if we addressed both sides of the body-mind equation?

The answer to this question was dramatically exemplified in one study (Ornish D, et al., 1983). Experimental subjects who ate a low-fat diet, exercised, stopped smoking, and participated in stress management and group support were found to have a regression of their coronary artery lesions when com-

pared to a control group. Alternative therapies were used together with conventional therapies in this study and were able to achieve what has never been done before—the ability to reverse coronary artery disease.

Our role for the future is clear. We must learn to incorporate alternative therapies at the bedside to treat the psychologic sequelae inherent in all illness. In addition, however, we must learn to supplement the best of traditional medical therapy with the best of alternative therapy as a means of activating inner healing as well as augmenting the effects of drugs, surgery, and technologic therapies. The results could revolutionize the way we deliver care and might significantly improve outcomes such as morbidity, mortality, and quality-of-life issues.

CEG & BMD

Adapted from Guzzetta CE, Dossey BM: Cardiovascular nursing: Holistic practice. *St. Louis, MO: Mosby-Year Book, 1992, pp. 98–99, 300–301.*

SPECIAL ASSESSMENT TECHNIQUES, DIAGNOSTIC TESTS, AND MONITORING SYSTEMS

Assessment of Chest Pain

Obtaining an accurate assessment of chest pain history is an important aspect of differentiating cardiac chest pain from other sources of pain (e.g., musculoskeletal, respiratory, anxiety). Ischemic chest pain, caused by lack of oxygen to the myocardium, must be quickly identified for therapeutic

interventions to be effective. The most important descriptors of ischemic pain include: precursors of pain onset, quality of the pain, pain radiation, the severity of the pain, what relieves the pain, and timing of onset of the current episode of pain which brought the patient to the hospital. Each of these descriptors can be assessed using the "PQRST" nomogram (Table 12–1). This nomogram prompts the clinician to ask a series of questions which help clarify the characteristics of the cardiac pain.

TABLE 12–1. CHEST PAIN ASSESSMENT

	Ask the Question:	Examples:
P (Provoke)	What provokes the pain or what precipitates the pain?	Climbing the stairs, walking; or may be unpredictable—comes on at rest
Q (Quality)	What is the quality of the pain?	Pressure, tightness; may have associated symptoms such as nausea, vomiting, diaphoresis
R (Radiation)	Does the pain radiate to locations other than the chest?	Jaw, neck, scapular area, or left arm
S (Severity)	What is the severity of the pain (on a scale of 1 to 10)?	On a scale of 1 to 10, with 10 being the worst, how bad is your pain?
T (Timing)	What is the time of onset of this episode of pain that caused you to come to the hospital?	When did this episode of pain that brought you to the hospital start? Did this episode wax and wane or was it constant? For how many days, months, or years have you had similar pain?

TABLE 12–2. INDICATIONS FOR CARDIAC CATHETERIZATION

Right Heart
- Measurement of right-sided heart pressures:
  suspected cardiac tamponade
  suspected pulmonary hypertension
- Evaluation of valvular disease (tricuspid or pulmonic)
- Evaluation of atrial or ventricular septal defects
- Measurement of AVo_2 difference

Left Heart
- Diagnosis of obstructive coronary artery disease
- Identification of lesion location prior to CABG surgery
- Measurement of left-sided heart pressures
  suspected left heart failure or cardiomyopathy
- Evaluation of valvular disease (mitral or aortic)
- Evaluation of atrial or ventricular septal defects

Coronary Angiography

Coronary angiography is a common and effective method for visualizing the anatomy and patency of the coronary arteries. This procedure, also known as cardiac catheterization, is used to diagnose atherosclerotic lesions or thrombus in the coronary vessels. Coronary angiography is also used for evaluation of valvular disease, including stenosis or insufficiency, septal defects, congenital anomalies, and cardiac wall motion abnormalities (Table 12–2).

Procedure

Prior to cardiac catheterization the patient should be NPO for at least 8 to 12 hours, in the event that emergency intubation is required during the procedure. Benadryl and aspirin are typically administered prior to beginning the procedure as a precautionary measure against allergic reaction to the dye and to prevent catheter-induced platelet aggregation during the procedure. Typically, patients remain awake during the procedure, allowing them to facilitate the catheterization process by controlling respiratory patterns (e.g., breath holding during injection of radiopaque dye to improve the quality of the image). An anxiolytic agent, such as diazepam, is frequently administered during the procedure to decrease anxiety or restlessness.

An intracoronary catheter is inserted through a "sheath" or vascular introducer placed in a large artery, most commonly the femoral artery (Figure 12–1A). The catheter is then advanced into the ascending abdominal aorta, through the aortic arch, and into the coronary arterial orifice located at the base of the aorta (Figure 12–1B). Ionic dye, visible to the observer or operator under fluoroscopy (x-ray), is then injected into the coronary arterial tree via the catheter. If the cardiac valves, septa, or ventricular wall motion is being evaluated, the catheter is advanced directly into the left ventricle, followed by injection of dye (Figure 12–1C). In a right heart catheterization, the catheter is inserted into the venous system via the inferior vena cava, passed through the right ventricle, and advanced into the pulmonary artery.

Interpretation of Results

The coronary vascular tree consists of a left and a right system (Figure 12–2). The left system consists of two main branches, the left anterior descending (LAD) artery and the left circumflex (LCX) artery. The right system has one main branch, the right coronary artery (RCA). Both systems have a number of smaller vessels which branch off these three primary arterial vessels. A clinically significant stenosis is considered to be an obstruction of 75% or greater in a major coronary artery or one of its major branches. If there is significant disease of only one of the major arteries, the patient is said to have single-vessel disease. If two major vessels are affected, there is two-vessel disease, and if significant disease exists in all three major coronary arteries, then the patient has three-vessel disease. Frequently, the microvasculature, or smaller vessels branching off the major coronary artery, may also have blockages. It is common, however, to refer to these multiple lesions as single-vessel disease.

A ventriculogram is obtained by radiographic imaging during the injection of dye after advancing the catheter from the aorta, through the aortic valve, and into the left ventricle (Figure 12–1C). A cineventriculogram provides information on ventricular wall motion, ejection fraction, and the presence and severity of mitral regurgitation. Ejection fraction, or the percentage of blood volume ejected from the left ventricle with each contraction, is the gold standard for determining left ventricular function and is helpful in selecting treatment strategies. Ejection fractions > 55% to 60% are considered to be normal. The left ventricular ejection fraction is one of the most important predictors of long-term outcome following acute myocardial infarction. Patients with ejection fractions less than 20% have nearly a 50% 1-year mortality.

Complications

During the cardiac catheterization a number of complications may occur, including arrhythmia; coronary vasospasm; allergic reaction to the dye; atrial or ventricular perforation resulting in pericardial tamponade; embolus to an extremity, a lung, or, rarely, the brain; myocardial infarction; or death. Common management and prevention strategies for catheterization complications are summarized in Table 12–3.

Percutaneous Transluminal Coronary Angioplasty

Percutaneous transluminal coronary angioplasty (PTCA), also termed angioplasty or balloon angioplasty, is a cardiac catheterization with the addition of a balloon apparatus on

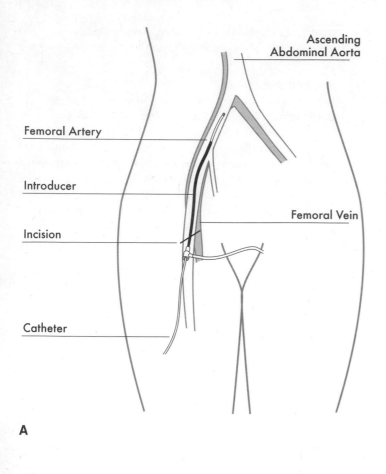

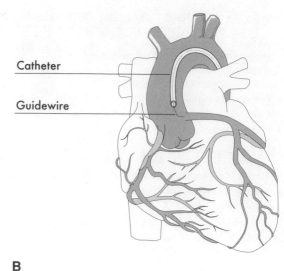

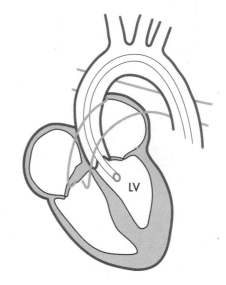

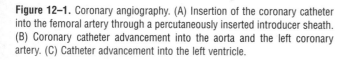

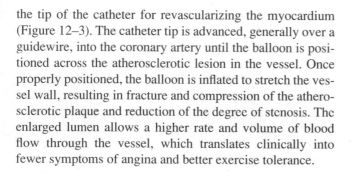

Figure 12–1. Coronary angiography. (A) Insertion of the coronary catheter into the femoral artery through a percutaneously inserted introducer sheath. (B) Coronary catheter advancement into the aorta and the left coronary artery. (C) Catheter advancement into the left ventricle.

the tip of the catheter for revascularizing the myocardium (Figure 12–3). The catheter tip is advanced, generally over a guidewire, into the coronary artery until the balloon is positioned across the atherosclerotic lesion in the vessel. Once properly positioned, the balloon is inflated to stretch the vessel wall, resulting in fracture and compression of the atherosclerotic plaque and reduction of the degree of stenosis. The enlarged lumen allows a higher rate and volume of blood flow through the vessel, which translates clinically into fewer symptoms of angina and better exercise tolerance.

Complications

Angioplasty is associated with the same complications found during cardiac catheterization. In addition, complications related to manipulation of the coronary artery itself

may also occur. The most common serious complications include a 2% to 10% incidence of complete occlusion of the vessel ("abrupt closure"), acute myocardial infarction (1% to 5% incidence), and the need for emergency coronary artery bypass surgery (1% to 2% incidence). The most important predictor of complications of myocardial infarction and abrupt vessel closure is reduced coronary flow through the lesion prior to the procedure. A universal scale, the TIMI Scale, is used to quantify this rate of coronary flow (Table 12–4).

Other Devices Used For Percutaneous Coronary Revascularization

In addition to routine balloon angioplasty, a number of other devices are now commonly used for percutaneous coronary

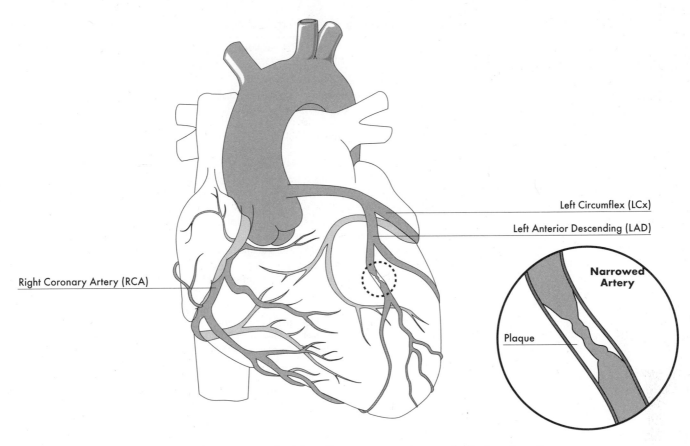

Figure 12–2. Coronary artery circulation with a coronary vessel narrowed with plaque formation.

AT THE BEDSIDE
▶ *Unstable Angina*

Mr. Smith, 62 years old, presented to the emergency department with complaints of pain in his chest and jaw. The pain, originally occurring only with exertion and resolving with rest, had become increasingly persistent over the past 2 to 3 days. On the evening of his arrival, Mr. Smith experienced a 15-minute episode of severe pain while watching television. This episode he characterized as a "tight, burning feeling in my chest, and an aching in my jaw" which did not vary with respiratory effort and was accompanied by diaphoresis, nausea, and shortness of breath.

On arrival to the ED Mr. Smith's pain and nausea had resolved, pulse oximetry showed oxygen saturation of 98% on room air, and his vital signs were:

B/P	148/86 mm Hg
HR	90 beats/minute
RR	18 breaths/minute
T	37.6°C orally

On physical examination heart sounds were normal, without S_3, S_4, or murmurs. Initial diagnostic tests revealed:

ECG	Normal sinus rhythm with nonspecific ST-T wave changes
Chest x-ray	Normal cardiac silhouette, clear lung

A more detailed assessment of Mr. Smith's history revealed increasing dyspnea on exertion and fatigue for the previous 6 months. Despite these symptoms, he had continued his daily 2 1/2-mile walking routine, sometimes experiencing shortness of breath several times during the walk. Mr. Smith reported smoking cigarettes in the past, one pack per day for 20 years, but quit 25 years ago. No ankle swelling, nocturnal dyspnea, or orthopnea were reported, nor was Mr. Smith aware of any family history of cardiac problems, coronary artery disease, diabetes, or hypertension.

Mr. Smith was started on aspirin based on his history and the likelihood of underlying coronary artery disease. He was then admitted for observation and evaluation of cardiac enzymes.

TABLE 12–3. CARDIAC CATHETERIZATION: COMMON COMPLICATIONS AND NURSING INTERVENTIONS

Complication	Intervention
Local bleeding due to catheter site artery damage (hematoma, hemorrhage, pseudoaneurysm)	Keep patient flat; head of bed (HOB) < 30°. Discontinue heparin infusion if present. Compress the artery just above the incision (pedal pulse should be faint). Monitor for hypotension, tachycardia, or dysrhythmia. Embolectomy or vascular repair may be deemed necessary following groin ultrasound.
Coronary artery dissection	Stent will typically be placed during procedure. Monitor for dysrhythmia or tamponade. Administer heparin.
Tamponade due to perforation of the heart	Typically this will be evident in the catheter lab at the time of perforation. Monitor patient for equalization of cardiac pressures. Emergency surgery may be required for repair.
Peripheral thromboembolism	Extremity will exhibit pain, pallor, pulselessness, paresthesias, and paralysis; may also be cool to touch. Heparin or other anticoagulant should be continued. Thrombolytic therapy may be administered directly to the clot using a tracking catheter. Surgical intervention may be necessary.
Thromboembolism: CVA due to embolus	Monitor for signs and symptoms of neurologic compromise including speech patterns, orientation, vision, equal grips and pedal pushes, and sensation.
Pulmonary embolism	Provide supplemental O_2. Monitor for adequate arterial oxygen saturation and respiratory rate. Continue administration of heparin or other anticoagulant IV. Direct thrombolytic therapy may be administered using a tracking catheter; direct extraction of the clot may also be attempted. Ventilation/perfusion scan or pulmonary arteriograms may be done to verify thrombus location.
Arrhythmia	Direct irritation of the ventricular wall by the catheter tip poses the greatest risk; postprocedure risk is extremely low. Monitor the patient in lead V_1.
Infection	Use aseptic technique for all dressing changes. Monitor catheter insertion sites for erythema, inflammation, heat, or exudate. Monitor patient temperature trends.
Pulmonary edema due to recumbent position, stress of angiographic contrast, or poor left ventricular function	Elevate HOB 30°. Administer diuretics as necessary. Consider use of flexible sheath or brachial access.
Acute tubular neurosis and renal failure	Hydrate patient well prior to and following procedure with continuous infusion of NS (typically 8 hours before and 8 hours after at 100 ml/hour). Monitor urine specific gravity trends and continue to infuse NS until specific gravity returns to within normal limits. Monitor for elevations in serum creatinine.
Vasovagal reaction	Administer pain medications prior to sheath removal. Monitor BP and heart rate before and after sheath removal, then every 15 minutes for four times after removal.

	CK Total	CK MB
ED	169 u/L	5 ng/ml
4 hours later	163 u/L	5 ng/ml

Six hours after presenting to the ED, Mr. Smith had recurrent tightness in his chest. An ECG showed T-wave inversion in the anterior leads. Sublingual nitroglycerin 0.4 mg was administered every 5 minutes with complete relief of the pressure following the second tablet. A heparin drip was started. Subsequent cardiac enzymes showed:

	CK Total	CK MB
8 hours	159 u/L	4 ng/ml
12 hours	152 u/L	4 ng/ml

Other laboratory results were normal with the exception of elevated cholesterol and triglycerides on the lipid panel. Following receipt of these results, Mr. Smith was scheduled for an exercise tolerance test.

The ECG recorded a heart rate of 118 beats/minute after 6 minutes of exercise. Onset of chest tightness during the last minute of exercise was described as similar to that which brought him to the hospital and correlated with 1.5-mm ST depression in leads V_4 to V_6. A cardiac catheterization was scheduled.

Coronary angiography showed a 75% obstruction of the left anterior descending artery and 90% obstruction of the diagonal branch of the same artery. Left ventricular ejection fraction (LVEF) was 55%. A coronary angioplasty (PTCA) was performed on both lesions.

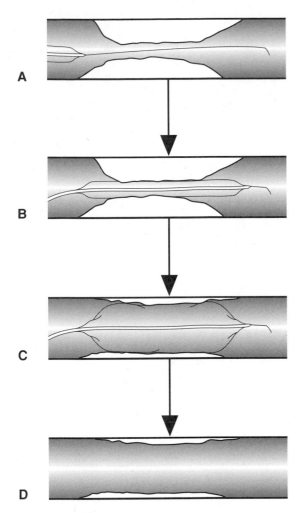

Figure 12–3. Percutaneous transluminal coronary angioplasty (PTCA). (A) PTCA catheter being advanced into the narrowed coronary artery over a guidewire. (B) Catheter position prior to balloon inflation. (C) Balloon inflation. (D) Coronary vessel following catheter removal.

TABLE 12–4. TIMI SCALE FOR QUANTIFYING CORONARY BLOOD FLOW

Grade		Definition
0	No perfusion	There is no antegrade flow beyond the point of occlusion.
1	Penetration without perfusion	Contrast material passes beyond area of obstruction but "hangs up" and fails to opacify entire coronary bed distal to obstruction for duration of cineangiographic filming sequence.
2	Partial perfusion	Contrast material passes across obstruction and opacifies coronary bed distal to obstruction at a slower rate than its entry into or clearance from comparable areas not perfused by previously occluded vessel, e.g., the opposite coronary artery or coronary bed proximal to obstruction.
3	Complete perfusion	Antegrade flow into bed distal to obstruction occurs as promptly as antegrade flow into bed proximal to obstruction, and clearance of contrast material from the involved bed is as rapid as clearance from an uninvolved bed in same vessel or opposite artery.

From: The TIMI Study Group: The thrombolysis in myocardial infarction (TIMI) trial: Phase I findings. New England Journal of Medicine. *1985;312:932.*

PATHOLOGIC CONDITIONS

Acute Ischemic Heart Disease

Myocardial ischemia is the lack of adequate blood supply to the heart, resulting in an insufficient supply of oxygen to meet the demands of the heart muscle. This supply-demand mismatch, known as ischemia, is most often due to thrombus formation at a site of atherosclerotic plaque rupture within a coronary artery. Decreased oxygen supply to myocardial tissue may cause a variety of symptoms such as chest discomfort (angina), shortness of breath, diaphoresis, and/or nausea. Unstable angina, defined as angina which is of new onset, increasing in frequency, or occurring at rest, and acute myocardial infarction (AMI) are referred to as the "acute coronary syndromes" which form the spectrum of acute ischemic heart disease.

Etiology and Pathophysiology

Intracoronary thrombus formation, and the resulting obstruction of coronary blood flow, is the pathophysiologic mechanism of acute ischemic heart disease. Preexisting atherosclerosis and spasm of the smooth muscle wall of the coronary arteries, termed fixed obstructions, may also contribute to reduced flow. In some situations coronary artery spasm may play a major role, unrelated to underlying atherosclerosis. These occurrences are rare and are sometimes associated with cocaine abuse seen in myocardial infarction in young patients.

revascularization. Intracoronary stents are small metallic mesh tubes placed across the stenotic area and expanded with an angioplasty balloon (Figure 12–4, A–E). Once expanded, the tube is permanently anchored in the vessel wall. Stents are effective in decreasing the rate of abrupt vessel closure seen with traditional PTCA. Atherectomy catheters and lasers are also used; however, patient outcomes are not significantly better than those achieved with traditional balloon catheters and may result in higher rates of complication, including acute myocardial infarction. Each of these devices may offer advantages over traditional balloon angioplasty catheters in situations involving specific vascular anatomy (e.g., ostial lesions) or lesion morphology (e.g., high degree of calcified plaque).

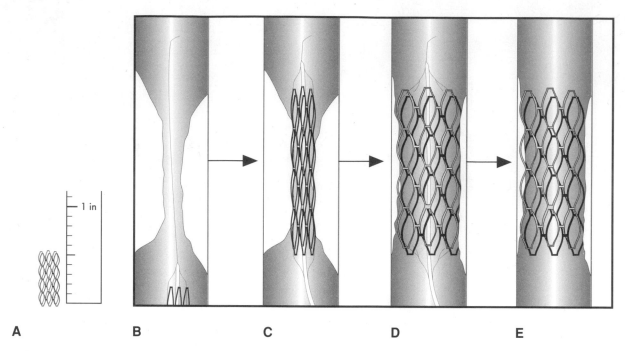

Figure 12–4. Intracoronary stent. (A) Size of stent device when fully deployed. (B) Insertion of stent into a narrowed area of a coronary artery on a balloon-inflatable catheter. (C) Inflation of the balloon catheter to expand the stent. (D) Inflation complete with stent fully expanded. (E) Stent following removal of balloon catheter.

The formation of a thrombus in coronary arteries is initiated by the fissuring and rupture of atherosclerotic plaque in the vessel wall of the coronary artery (Figure 12–5). A continuous, dynamic process occurs whereby plaque may become unstable, for example, during periods of active accumulation of more lipid into the core of the plaque. The plaque then ruptures, dispelling its contents into the lumen of the coronary artery and causing activation of clotting factors at the site of plaque rupture. The rupture of plaque and resultant thrombus formation may eventually occlude the coronary artery.

While most people have some degree of atherosclerotic plaque formation by age 30, the vast majority of these plaques are considered "stable." They are covered by smooth fibrous caps allowing adequate blood flow through the coronary arteries, and they are not prone to the events leading to unstable angina or myocardial infarction. In young growing plaques, the fibrous cap may thin and rupture, resulting in unstable angina, ischemia, and/or myocardial infarction.

A variety of factors predispose a plaque to fissure and rupture. Characteristics of plaque at increased risk for rupture include:

- *Location of the lesion in the vascular tree*. Areas of greater turbulence of flow and dynamic activity during the cardiac cycle are at higher risk.
- *Size of the lipid pool within the plaque*. A large amount of lipid inside the plaque core is more likely to be associated with plaque disruption.
- *Infiltration of the plaque with macrophages*. Macrophages are thought to weaken the integrity of the fibrous cap of the plaque, making it more susceptible to fissuring.

While these three characteristics determine the likelihood of plaque rupture, they are not easily identified by clinical assessment, stress testing, or cardiac catheterization.

A plaque may be caused to fissure and/or rupture by a number of environmental or hormonal factors, known as "triggers" (Table 12–5). These triggers may disrupt the

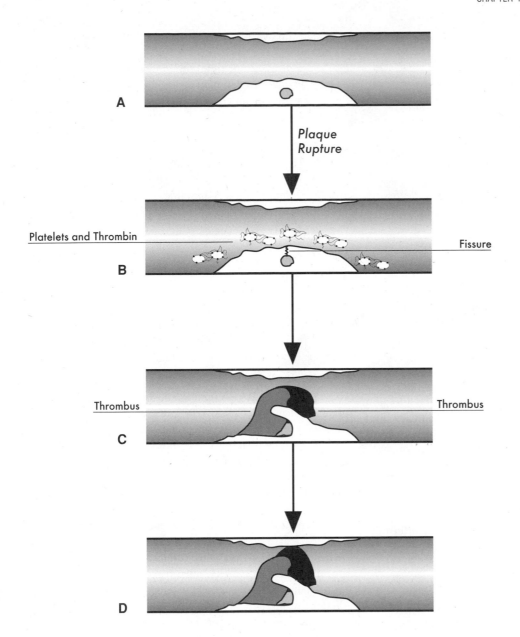

A

Plaque Rupture

Platelets and Thrombin

B

Fissure

Thrombus

C

Thrombus

D

Figure 12–5. Atherosclerotic plaque formation. (A) Stable plaque. (B) Plaque with cap disruption. (C) Moderate amount layered thrombus. (D) Occlusive thrombus.

plaque and precipitate an acute coronary event. Some of the triggers for atherosclerotic plaque rupture can be manipulated or controlled, such as blood pressure, blood glucose level, and stress. In the clinical setting, management of these variables may decrease the risk for acute myocardial infarction, reinfarction, and/or reocclusion, and should be closely monitored.

When these triggers combine to cause plaque rupture, the lipid pool is exposed and a rough surface on the intima of the vessel wall occurs, stimulating the local effects of hormonal and immune factors and initiating thrombus formation. At the same time, the fibrinolytic system is stimulated, creating a dynamic process of simultaneous attempts to form and dissolve the clot. Because of the dynamic nature of the clotting process, the thrombus may be completely or only partially obstructive, or may fluctuate inter-

mittently between the two stages. Regardless of the maturity of the clot, the process of thrombus formation may lead to obstruction of blood flow, diminishing oxygen delivery to distal myocardium and creating a mismatch between the supply of and demand for oxygen.

Because the underlying pathology of the ischemia-related diagnoses is the same (plaque rupture and thrombus formation), ischemic heart disease encompasses the entire spectrum of ischemic coronary events which are sometimes referred to as the acute coronary syndromes. A continuum of clinical events may result from the supply-demand mismatch including unstable angina, non-Q-wave myocardial infarction, or Q-wave myocardial infarction (Figure 12–6).

Following a decrease in oxygen supply to the myocardium, the cell membranes of "hypoxic" myocytes develop increased permeability. The cell is no longer able

TABLE 12–5. HORMONAL AND ENVIRONMENTAL TRIGGERS OF PLAQUE RUPTURE

Acute	Chronic
Hemodynamic Reactivity	**Basal Hemodynamic Forces**
• Morning increase in blood pressure	• Increased resting blood pressure
• Morning increase in heart rate	• Increased resting heart rate
• Physical exertion	**Basal Hemostatic Variables**
• Emotional stress	• Location of the plaque
• Exposure to cold	• Size of the lipid pool within the core plaque
Hemostatic Reactivity	• Degree of macrophage infiltration of the plaque
• Increased coronary blood flow velocity	**Chronic Risk Factors**
• Increased viscosity of blood	• Gender (male > female)
• Decreased tPA activity	• Increasing age
• Increased platelet aggregation	• Diabetes mellitus
Vasoreactivity	• Hypercholesterolemia
• Increased plasma epinephrine	• Cigarette smoking
• Increased plasma cortisol	

to regulate its internal and external environment, and the cell dies, releasing cytotoxic substances into the bloodstream. Cardiac myocytes release significant amounts of CK-MB (cardiac-specific creatine kinase) when they die, causing elevation in this laboratory value and confirming the MI diagnosis.

Clinical Presentation

Clinical presentation across the spectrum of acute coronary syndromes is similar, with clinical presentation differing slightly depending on the involved vessels (Table 12–6).

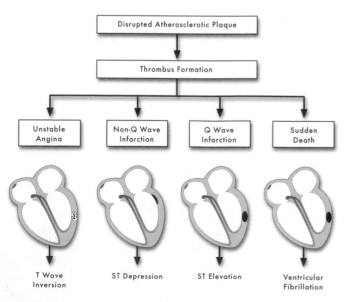

Figure 12–6. Pathophysiologic steps leading to acute coronary events.

1. Pain or discomfort, usually in the chest (Table 12–1)
   • Pressure or tightness in the chest
   • Jaw or neck pain
   • Left arm ache or pain
   • Epigastric discomfort
   • Scapular back pain
2. Nausea/vomiting
3. Hemodynamic instability
   • Hypotension (systolic BP < 90 mm Hg, or 20 mm Hg below baseline)
   • Cardiac index (< 2.0 L/minute/m^2)
   • Elevated PAD and/or PCWP
   • Skin cool, clammy, diaphoretic
4. Dyspnea
5. Arrhythmia
   • LBBB
   • Tachycardia/bradycardia
   • Frequent premature ventricular contractions
   • Ventricular fibrillation
6. Anxiety, sense of impending catastrophe
7. Denial

Some patient populations are predictably different in their description of chest pain, such as women and diabetics. Women may be prone to deny chest pain for longer periods of time than men, delaying their arrival to the emergency department and often rendering them ineligible for thrombolytic therapy. In addition, women are typically postmenopausal when signs and symptoms of atherosclerotic disease become apparent. This predominantly older patient population may pose problems of its own such as anxiety, fear of the inability to care for oneself following myocardial infarction, and other concerns to geriatric patient populations which must be considered.

Diabetics are another patient population with predictable differences in symptomatic presentation. Diabetics have atypical pain secondary to neuropathies, and early development of atherosclerotic disease. Coronary artery disease in this patient population is diffuse, and poor distal vascular anatomy is common. Lesion morphology in diabetic patients is also more difficult to revascularize, either using percutaneous or surgical methods.

Diagnostic Tests

Unstable Angina

1. *12-Lead ECG*. Transient changes may occur and resolve; most commonly T-wave inversion and/or ST-segment depression.
2. *Cardiac Enzymes (CK and CK-MB)*. Normal (Figure 12–7).
3. *Cardiac Catheterization*. Not recommended in the acute setting, except in the case of continued pain

TABLE 12–6. CLINICAL PRESENTATION OF MYOCARDIAL ISCHEMIA AND INFARCTION

Type MI	Arterial Involvement	Muscle Area Supplied	Assessment	ECG Changes	Likely Dysrhythmias	Possible Complications
Anteroseptal wall	LAD	Anterior LV wall Anterior LV septum Apex LV Bundle of His Bundle branches	↓ LV Function → ↓ CO, ↓ BP ↑ PAD, ↑ PCWP S_3 and S_4, with CHF Rales with pulmonary edema	**Indicative:** ST elevation with or without abnormal Q waves in $V_{1,2,3,4}$ Loss of R waves in precordial leads **Reciprocal:** ST depression in II, III, AVF.	RBBB, LBBB AV blocks Atrial fibrillation or flutter Ventricular tachycardia (VT) Tachycardia (septal)	Cardiogenic shock VSD Myocardial rupture Heart blocks may be permanent (LBBB) High mortality associated with this location of MI
Posterior septal lateral	RCA Circumflex branches (right and left)	Posterior surface of LV SA node 45% AV node 10% Left atrium Lateral wall of LV	Murmurs indicating VSD (septal) PA catheter to assess R to L shunt in VSD Signs/symptoms of LV aneurysm with lateral Displaced PMI leading to signs and symptoms of mitral regurgitation	**Lateral Indicative:** ST elevation I, AVL, $V_{5,6}$ Loss of R wave and ↑ ST in I, AVL, V_{5-6} **Posterior Indicative:** Tall, broad R waves (> 0.04 sec) in V_{1-3} ↑ ST V_4R (right sided 12 lead, V_4 position) **Posterior Reciprocal:** ST depression in $V_{1,2}$, upright T wave in $V_{1,2}$	Bradycardia Mobitz I (posterior)	RV involvement Aneurysm development Papillary muscle dysfunction Heart blocks frequently resolve
Inferior or "diaphragmatic"	RCA	RV, RA SA Node 50% AV Node 90% RA, RV Inferior LV Posterior IV Septum Posterior LBBB Posterior LV	Symptomatic bradycardia: ↓ BP LOC changes diaphoresis ↓ CO ↑ PAD ↑ PCWP Murmurs: associated with papillary muscle dysfunction mid/holosystolic rales, pulmonary edema, nausea	**Indicative:** ↑ ST segments in II, III, AVF Q waves in II, III, AVF **Reciprocal:** ST depression in I, AVL, V_{1234}	AV blocks; often progress to CHB which may be transient or permanent; Wenchebach; bradyarrhythmias	Hiccups Nausea/vomiting Papillary muscle dysfunction MR Septal rupture (0.5%–1%) RV involvement associated with atrial infarcts especially with atrial dysrhythmias
Right ventricular infarction	RCA	RA, RV, inferior LV SA Node AV Node Posterior IV Septum	Kussmaul's sign JVD Hypotension ↑ SVR, ↓ PCWP ↑ CVP S_3 with noncompliant RV Clear breath sounds initially Hepatomegaly, peripheral edema, cool clammy pale skin	**Indicative:** 1- to 2-mm ST segment elevation in V_4R ST- and T-wave elevation in II, III, AVF Q waves in II, III, AVF ST-elevation decreases in amplitude over V_{1-6}	First-degree AV block Second-degree AV block, type I Incomplete RBBB Transient CHB Atrial fibrillation VT/VF	Hypotension requiring large volumes initially to maintain systemic pressure. Once RV contractility improves fluids will mobilize, possibly requiring diuresis.

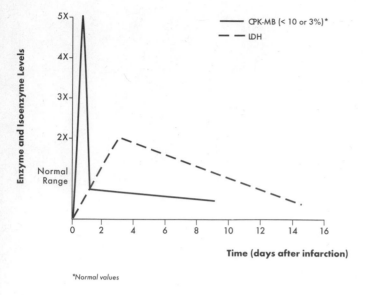

Figure 12–7. Peak cardiac enzyme changes with acute myocardial infarction (AMI).

without relief with NTG. Report is normal, or with visible atherosclerotic disease, but without complete occlusion or thrombus.

Myocardial Infarction

1. *12-Lead ECG.* Thirty-five percent of AMI have ST-segment elevation (see Chapter 21, Advanced ECG Concepts). Approximately 65% of AMI have no ECG changes or other diagnostic changes.
2. *Creatine Kinase (CK and CK-MB)* (Figure 12–7)
   • Total CK > 150 to 180 u/L
   • MB band > 10 ng/ml or > 3% of total
   • Peaks at 12 hours after symptom onset
3. *Troponin T.* > 0.1 ng/ml.
4. *Cardiac Catheterization.* Ventricular wall motion abnormalities (also may be seen by echocardiography); total occlusion of one or more coronary arteries.

Patient Needs and Principles of Management

Because most complications of acute ischemic heart disease directly result from reduced coronary flow, a primary objective in patient management is to optimize blood flow to the myocardium. Additional goals are to prevent complications of ischemia and infarction, alleviate angina, and reduce anxiety.

▶ Optimize Blood Flow to the Myocardium

Regardless of whether a patient presents with unstable angina or acute myocardial infarction, restoration and maintenance of coronary blood flow is important to improve patient outcomes. Interventions to optimize blood flow to the myocardium include pharmacologic measures, such as antiplatelet or antithrombin agents, and mechanical measures, such as percutaneous coronary revascularization (e.g., angioplasty, stent, or other) or coronary artery bypass grafting (CABG). The intervention selected and the optimal timing of the intervention will depend on whether the occlusion of the artery is total or partial. This determination must be made as accurately and as quickly as possible, as a totally occluded artery will soon result in tissue necrosis or myocardial infarction (Figure 12–8). All unstable arteries benefit from the following interventions which stabilize the artery and optimize coronary arterial flow.

Medical Management

1. Decrease activity of coagulation system with pharmacologic therapy (Figure 12–9):
   • *Antiplatelet agents:* ASA, IIa/IIIb receptor agents (e.g., Abciximab or Reopro and Integrilin)
   • *Antithrombin agents:* Indirect (e.g., heparin), direct (e.g., Hirudin)
2. Increase ventricular filling time (decrease heart rate):
   • Beta blockers
   • Bedrest for 24 hours
3. Decrease preload:
   • Nitrates
   • Diuretics
   • Morphine sulphate
4. Decrease afterload:
   • ACE inhibitors (angiotensin-converting enzyme inhibitors)
   • Hydralazine
5. Decrease myocardial oxygen consumption (MVo_2):
   • Beta blockers
   • Bedrest for 24 hours

Totally occluded arteries require, in addition to the above pharmacologic interventions, further reperfusion

Patient Needs and Principles of Management, Cont.

therapy, such as thrombolysis, angioplasty, or CABG in order to effectively restore blood flow to the coronary artery. In the event of left main coronary artery stenosis or three-vessel disease, acute CABG is usually considered. In the acute setting, thrombolytic therapy is often the fastest, most universally available method for reperfusion. The indications, contraindications, comparison of different agents, and common complications of thrombolytic therapy are listed in Tables 12–7 through 12–10.

Surgical Management

Coronary artery bypass grafting is one method of revascularization generally used in patients with atherosclerosis of three or more coronary vessels or in the case of significant left main coronary artery disease. CABG is performed both electively, as well as emergently, and may be performed either prior to or following a myocardial infarction. The CABG procedure requires "induction" with general anesthesia, initiation of cardiopulmonary

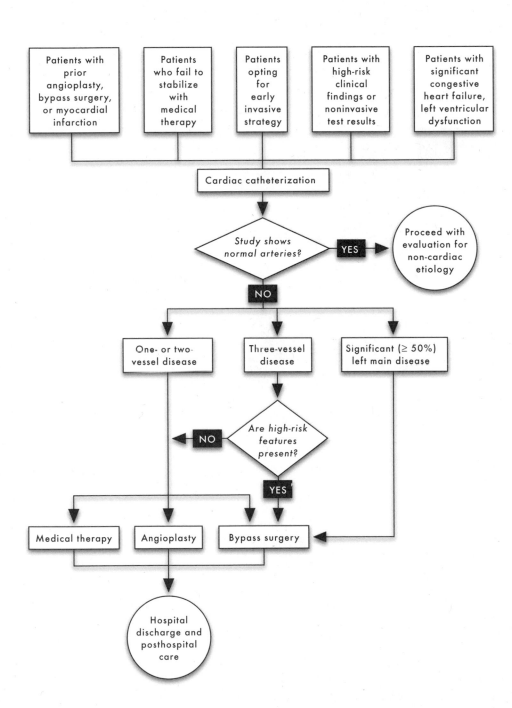

Figure 12–8. Treatment decision tree for coronary revascularization. (U.S. Department of Health and Human Services: *Unstable angina: Diagnosis and management.* AHCPR Publication number 94-0602. Clinical Practice Guideline number 10. May 1994.)

Patient Needs and Principles of Management, Cont.

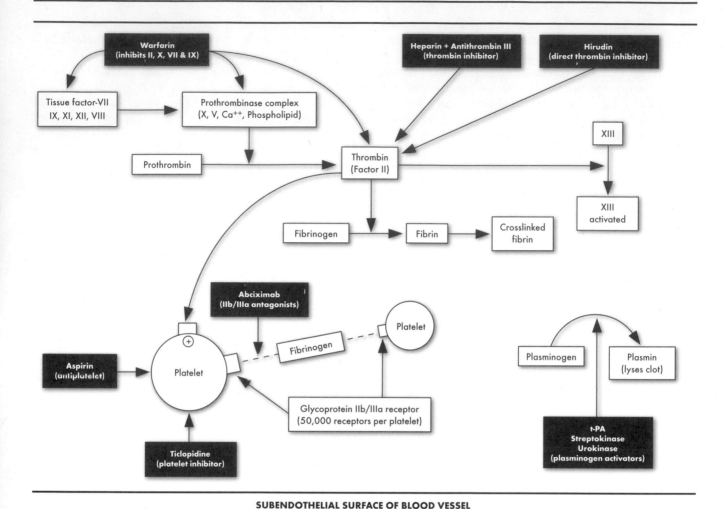

Figure 12–9. Coagulation sequence and site of antithrombotic/antiplatelet drug activity.

bypass (blood is diverted outside of the body to a pump which mechanically oxygenates the blood before returning it to the arterial circulation), and placement of a graft into the coronary arterial tree (Figure 12–10). The graft, generally a leg vein or left internal mammary artery (LIMA) graft, is inserted past the distal end of the blockage in the coronary artery and, in the case of a leg vein graft, anastomosed to the aorta. Multiple grafts may be inserted based on the number of blockages present and the availability of viable insertion sites in the patient's native coronary tree.

INDICATIONS FOR CORONARY ARTERY BYPASS GRAFTING

The indications for CABG and long-term patient outcome following this procedure have been intensively reviewed over the past decade. In general, patients with three-vessel disease, poor left ventricular ejection fraction (< 35%), or significant disease in the left main coronary artery have lower long-term morbidity and mortality with surgical

TABLE 12–7. INDICATIONS AND CONTRAINDICATIONS FOR THROMBOLYTIC THERAPY

Indications
- Chest pain > 20 minutes, but typically less than 12 hours
- ST elevation ≥ 1 mm in two contiguous leads
- LBBB
- High-risk patients with chest pain > 12 hours in duration may still be candidates if pain persists

Absolute Contraindications
- Active internal bleeding
- History of intracranial bleeding, cerebral neoplasm, or other intracranial pathology
- Stroke or head trauma within 6 months
- Known allergy to the drug chosen

Relative Contraindications
- Major surgery or GI bleeding within 2 months
- Traumatic puncture of noncompressible vessel
- Pregnancy or 1 month postpartum
- Uncontrolled hypertension (systolic > 200 or diastolic > 110)
- Trauma within 2 weeks, including CPR with rib fracture

Patient Needs and Principles of Management, Cont.

TABLE 12–8. COMPARISON OF COMMON THROMBOLYTIC AGENTS

	Streptokinase (SK)	Alteplase (tPA)	Eminase (APSAC)
Mechanism of action	Streptococci bacteria; binds free and fibrin-bound plasminogen and activates it to form plasmin; plasmin dissolves clots	Genetically made through recombinant DNA technology	Chemically inert plasminogen-streptokinase activator complex
Cost	$320	$2200	$1800
Dose	1.5 million units IV over 30–60 minutes	0.75 mg/kg (total dose ≤ 100 mg) IV bolus 10% of total dose, then administer remainder over 90 minutes	30-mg bolus over 3–5 minutes
Time to reperfuse	45–55 minutes	45–55 minutes	45–55 minutes
Chemical half-life	23 minutes	5 minutes	90–150 minutes
Clinical duration of action	18–20 hours	12 hours	24–30 hours
Antigen-producing	Yes	No	Yes
Specificity (clot vs. hemostatic plug)	None	None	None
Systemic fibrinogenolysis	4+*	2+	4+
Platelet activation	3+	3+	3+
Other		Must be refrigerated; good for 30 minutes after mixing	

Drug activity on a scale of 1 (minimal or no activity) to 4 (high activity).

revascularization (CABG) compared to medical therapy or percutaneous interventions such as angioplasty or stent. CABG may also be indicated as an emergent "rescue" procedure in patients whose coronary artery severely dissects or fractures during an attempted percutaneous procedure.

CONTRAINDICATIONS FOR CORONARY ARTERY BYPASS GRAFTING

Several populations of patients may be considered poor candidates for coronary bypass, including the very elderly, debilitated patients, patients with severely diseased distal coronary vasculature (e.g., some diabetics), and patients with extremely poor left ventricular ejection fractions (e.g., < 10% to 15%). Patients with low ejection fractions often have difficulty being weaned from cardiopulmonary bypass following the procedure. Other contraindications are those related to general anesthesia risk, including severe COPD, pulmonary edema, or pulmonary hypertension.

TABLE 12–9. COMPLICATIONS OF THROMBOLYTIC THERAPY

Complication	Percentage Occurrence
Groin bleeding, local (compressible external)	25%–45%
Intracerebral bleeding	1.45%
Retroperitoneal bleeding (noncompressible internal)	1%
Gastrointestinal bleeding	4%–10%
Genitourinary bleeding	1%–5%
Other bleeding	1%–5%

POSTOPERATIVE MANAGEMENT

The following is a general overview of the early postoperative management of CABG patients:

1. *Maintain hemodynamic stability.* A variety of cardiac drugs are administered to maintain hemodynamic stability in the first 24 hours postoperatively. The following hemodynamic values may serve as guides for vasopressor administration and intravascular fluid therapy. In general, values greater or lower than the following require intervention:

MAP	70 to 80 mm Hg
CI	2.0 to 3.5 L/minute/m^2
PAD/PCWP	10 to 12 mm Hg (used primarily to evaluate need for volume replacement)
CVP	5 to 10 mm Hg (used primarily to evaluate need for volume replacement)
HR	Intrinsic or paced rhythm in range of 80 to 100/minute to keep CI ≥ 2.0

2. *Maintain ventilation and oxygenation.* Ventilation and oxygenation are maximized in the early postoperative period with mechanical ventilation. Within 2 to 12 hours, most patients have recovered from the anesthesia effects and are sufficiently stable to allow weaning from mechanical ventilation. Individuals with preexisting pulmonary problems may require longer periods of intubation until weaning can be suc-

Patient Needs and Principles of Management, Cont.

TABLE 12–10. PHARMACOLOGIC INTERVENTIONS IN MYOCARDIAL INFARCTION

Drug	Management
Nitroglycerin (IV)	**Drug preparation** Standard concentration of IV nitroglycerin is 100 mg in 500 ml NS or D5W. V preparations of nitroglycerin should not be concentrated more than 400 mg in 500 ml. The effectiveness and necessity of special tubing to prevent absorption of drug into the administration set has recently been challenged. Follow your hospital policy or procedure. **Drug administration** Nitroglycerin has been shown to be useful in the management of ischemic pain. In most patients it can safely be increased at a rate of 10 to 20 µg every 10 minutes until pain relief is achieved. Hypotension is the most prevalent side effect and BP should be monitored prior to each incremental increase in dose. Onset of action is immediate, peak of action is immediate, duration of action is only 3 to 5 minutes, and metabolism is by the liver. Nitroglycerin may either be tapered at 10 to 20 µg every 15 minutes, with nitropaste being applied at the halfway point during the taper, or the full dose of paste can be applied 30 minutes prior to shutting the NTG off entirely with no taper.
Thrombolytic agents	See Table 12–8 for information on action, dosing, and infusion rates. tPA is most effective when administered via "front-loaded" technique, which is described in the package insert and Table 12–8. Reperfusion arrhythmias, such as frequent PVCs, may occur but should not trigger initiation of antiarrhythmic therapy unless repeated runs of VT, 5 beats or more, occur.

cessfully accomplished. Following weaning and extubation, supplemental O_2 therapy usually is required for 1 to 2 days to maintain PaO_2 or SaO_2 in normal ranges. Postoperative atelectasis is a common occurrence after cardiopulmonary bypass, usually requiring frequent pulmonary interventions (e.g., coughing and deep breathing, incentive spirometry, ambulation) to maintain ventilation and oxygenation.

3. *Prevention of postoperative complications.*
   A. Bleeding from vascular graft anastomosis sites: Frequent monitoring of mediastinal tube drainage, hematocrit, and coagulation status; avoidance of even brief periods of hypertension.
   B. Cardiac tamponade: Frequent assessment for signs/symptoms of tamponade (pulsus paradoxus; increased CVP and decreased mediasti-

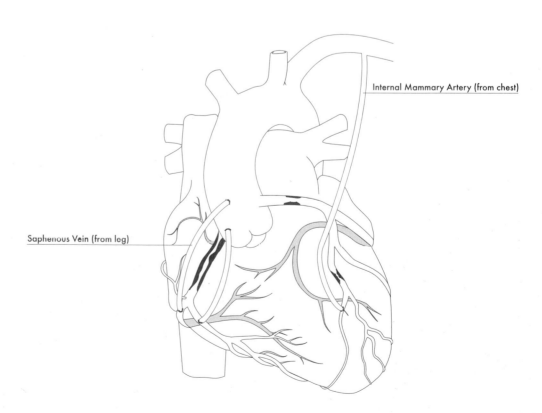

Internal Mammary Artery (from chest)

Saphenous Vein (from leg)

Figure 12–10. Coronary artery bypass grafting (CABG).

nal tube drainage; decreased heart sounds, BP, and cardiac output).

C. Infection: Antibiotics are used prophylactically for 24 hours; temperature spike within 24 hours postoperatively is not abnormal (usually related to pulmonary atelectasis).

D. Cardiac arrhythmias: ECG monitoring, treat unstable rhythms, maintain K^+ within normal limits with IV replacement.

E. Relief of postoperative pain and anxiety: Analgesic administration is typically required to ensure pain relief, especially to facilitate ambulation and coughing/deep breathing.

▶ Preventing Complications Associated with Coronary Obstruction

Complications associated with acute ischemic syndromes include: recurrent ischemia, infarction or reinfarction, onset of congestive heart failure, and arrhythmias.

1. *Prevent recurrent ischemia, infarction, or reinfarction.* Continue pharmacologic interventions to inhibit prothrombotic events, including ischemia and infarction (e.g., antiplatelet and antithrombin agents). Assess for recurrent angina with frequent chest pain assessment and serial 12-lead ECG and ST-segment ischemia monitoring.

2. *Continuously monitor for dysrhythmias.* Monitor, if possible, for 24 to 72 hours following an ischemic episode.

3. *Minimize potential for congestive heart failure (CHF).* Minimize myocardial oxygen consumption with the administration of beta blockers, limit physical activity (bedrest), and avoid increases in metabolic rate (e.g., fever). Decrease left ventricular afterload with the administration of ACE inhibitors.

▶ Alleviating Pain

Relief of pain improves coronary flow by decreasing the level of circulating catecholamines, thereby decreasing blood pressure (afterload) and heart rate (myocardial oxygen consumption). Nitrates typically relieve anginal pain by dilating coronary arteries and increasing flow, thereby improving myocardial oxygenation and directly treating the source of the pain. Another pharmacologic intervention commonly used to relieve pain in ischemia is morphine sulfate. While morphine is a potent narcotic which has been criticized for masking cardiac pain, it is also a potent vasodilator and effectively vasodilates coronary as well as peripheral arteries, resulting in mild afterload reduction. Severe pain, unable to be relieved with nitrates or a combination of nitrates and morphine, is typically an indication for immediate interventional PTCA if available, or transfer to a referring institution for emergency PTCA.

▶ Reducing Anxiety

The reduction of anxiety in ischemic heart disease is important for a number of reasons. The most important physiologically is the reduction of catecholamine secretion and decrease in sympathetic tone following relaxation in the anxious patient. This effect has been shown to decrease the incidence of arrhythmias and promote vasodilation and afterload reduction. Decreasing anxiety should also increase the patient's ability to process new information regarding his or her diagnosis, and to better understand instructions for tests or procedures that will be done.

Relief of pain typically is most effective in reducing patient anxiety. In the event that pain is not relieved with nitroglycerin, or thrombolytics in the initial treatment of ischemia, pain relievers such as morphine sulfate and/or anxiolytics such as Ativan (short-acting) are usually effective.

A number of interventions may be done at the bedside to promote relaxation, including specific relaxation and imagery techniques, meditation, music therapy, and/or the use of audiocassette relaxation tapes. Providing the patient and family with adequate information regarding unfamiliar surroundings, when the physician may be available to speak with them, possible "unknowns" such as tests or procedures, and important expectations such as visitation guidelines helps to provide a sense of security and facilitates relaxation by increasing the patient's level of comfort with the situation. Anxiety can also be decreased by offering the patient opportunities for control in the acute setting. Examples include the timing of simple activities such as visitor presence, bathing, and eating.

AT THE BEDSIDE
▶ *Cardiac Imagery*

Many cardiac patients surround themselves with negative thinking and negative images of their body, their heart, and their health. Patients describe images of their healing heart following an AMI as a black hole inside the heart (image of the infarct), a mussy, flabby sack (image of congestive heart failure), a big, hot, swollen inflamed bag (image of pericarditis), and even as biologically incorrect as blood being unable to circulate throughout the heart chambers because of the heart attack (they thought the coronary blockage was inside the heart). Yes, it seems that patients are very good at conjuring up demons, negative images, and negative thinking. We have done a good job in passing on to the patient the images and words that describe their malfunction and the pathophysiology. Could it be, however, that we have not done as well in transmitting to our patients the images they need to conjure up healing, health, and recovery?

We know that what we think and what we feel change our physiology. What if we made an effort to give the patient healing, healthy, and correct biologic images on which to focus during his or her recovery? Process imagery is a strategy for guiding patients in a step-by-step biologic healing process. For example, following an AMI, our teaching could include, early on, images of healthy, healing scar formation, images of a strong scar (maybe like superglue), new collateral circulation (maybe like a beautiful new lattice network), and strong pipes (coronaries) through which blood is flowing without tension. End-state imagery is another strategy for guiding patients to rehearse being in a final, healed state. An end-state image for an AMI patient would be visions of a strong, healed heart and successfully returning to family activities, exercise, a healthy diet, work, and sexual activity. Combining these strategies with relaxation, music, and guided imagery sessions can be a powerful technique. At the very least, dispelling misconceptions, suggesting visions of healing and recovery, and teaching biologically correct images, as well as acknowledging and supporting effective coping behaviors, are therapeutic interventions that we all need to incorporate into our practice.

Adapted from Guzzetta CE: *Capsules and Comments in Critical Care Nursing.* 1993;1:34.

AT THE BEDSIDE
▶ *Congestive Heart Failure*

Mr. Gaston, 75 years old, presented to the emergency department with diaphoresis and severe dyspnea. Initial assessment revealed the following:

RR	32/minute
BP	110/90
HR	110 beats/minute, irregular
JVD	Bilateral 7-mm elevation
Lungs	Bibasilar rales throughout the lower lobes
Cardiovascular	S_1, S_2 with an S_3

A pulse oximeter revealed 83% oxygen saturation. Labwork, including an arterial blood gas sample, was done with the following results:

PaO_2	60 mm Hg
$PaCO_2$	28 mm Hg
pH	7.51
SaO_2	93%

Oxygen was initiated at 40% by face mask. An ECG was done which showed left ventricular hypertrophy, left bundle and branch block, and Q waves. His chest x-ray showed an enlarged cardiac silhouette and bilateral infiltrates. A pulmonary artery (PA) catheter was placed and the following parameters were found:

RA	10 mm Hg
PA	41/35 mm Hg
PCWP	32 mm Hg
CO	3.8 L/minute
CI	1.9 L/minute/m^2

A dobutamine drip was started at 2.5 µg/kg/minute, and furosemide 40 mg IV was given. Cardiac catheterization was performed the next morning with the following findings:

LAD	95%
RCA	50%
LCX	75%
EF	28%
Severe asyneresis	

Congestive Heart Failure

Congestive heart failure (CHF) is a broad term referring to the inability of the heart to pump sufficient blood to meet the oxygen and nutrient requirements of the body. A number of underlying disease processes may contribute to this "weak pump" syndrome, with coronary atherosclerosis, valvular heart disease, hypertension, and cardiomyopathy as the most common causes. Although the underlying causes are diverse, the progressive process which occurs in response to one of these initiating events is the same.

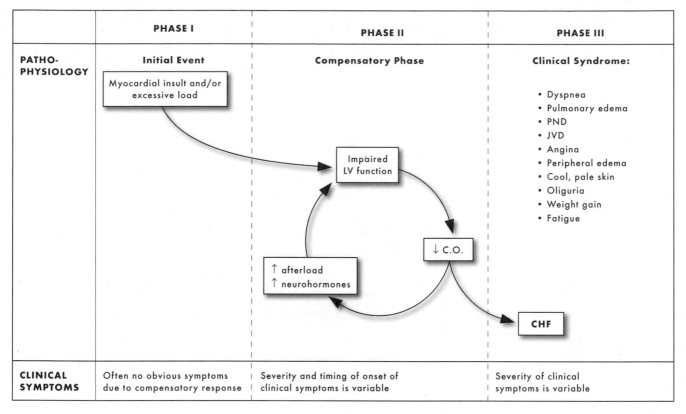

	PHASE I	**PHASE II**	**PHASE III**
PATHO-PHYSIOLOGY	**Initial Event** Myocardial insult and/or excessive load	**Compensatory Phase** Impaired LV function ↑ afterload ↑ neurohormones ↓ C.O. CHF	**Clinical Syndrome:** • Dyspnea • Pulmonary edema • PND • JVD • Angina • Peripheral edema • Cool, pale skin • Oliguria • Weight gain • Fatigue
CLINICAL SYMPTOMS	Often no obvious symptoms due to compensatory response	Severity and timing of onset of clinical symptoms is variable	Severity of clinical symptoms is variable

Figure 12–11. Pathophysiology of heart failure during phases I, II, and III.

Etiology, Risk Factors, and Pathophysiology

While CHF may result from a number of underlying etiologies, those causing left ventricular systolic dysfunction are the most common contributors. The pathophysiology of CHF is a three-stage process, beginning with an initial insult to the myocardium (phase I), followed by a response phase (phase II), and resulting in the clinical syndrome known as CHF, characterized by exhaustion of compensatory mechanisms (phase III) (Figure 12–11). Regardless of the precipitating event, the physiologic progression of the syndrome, once initiated, is the same.

Phase I

Phase I of CHF is characterized by an initiating event (e.g., myocardial infarction, viral infection, valvular heart disease, hypertension, idiopathic cardiomyopathy) which causes loss of myocytes. This cell loss or permanent damage to the myocytes can be either localized or diffuse, resulting in compromised ventricular function. To date, over 700 initiating factors such as acute ischemic damage, viruses, toxins, and others have been isolated as contributors to myocardial insult and heart failure.

- *Result of Phase I: Decreased stroke volume secondary to an initial insult to the myocardium.*

Phase II

A number of adaptive mechanisms occur in response to the initial insult in an effort to maintain adequate cardiac output to meet the body's needs. This phase is sometimes referred to as the "compensatory" phase (Figures 12–11 and 12–12). These compensatory mechanisms or responses include the Frank-Starling response, myocardial remodeling, and the neurohormonal response.

FRANK-STARLING RESPONSE

As cardiac output decreases and the sympathetic nervous system is activated, alpha-1 receptors are stimulated, resulting in arteriolar and venous vasoconstriction. This adaptive response initially results in increased venous return to the ventricle, increased ventricular end-diastolic volume, stretching of the ventricular myocytes, and improved stroke volume. Later, as overstretching of the ventricle occurs, this compensatory mechanism is lost, resulting in left ventricular decompensation and myocardial hypertrophy (Figure 12–13).

MYOCARDIAL HYPERTROPHY (REMODELING)

In response to increased vascular volume and decreased myocardial function (loss of the Frank-Starling response), the left ventricle dilates and hypertrophies. This distortion of the normal left ventricular anatomy causes mitral regurgitation and further left ventricular dilatation. Angiotensin II,

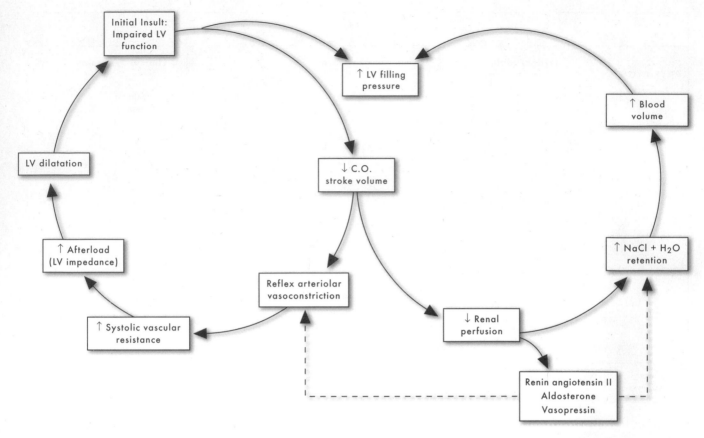

Figure 12–12. Compensatory mechanisms of heart failure.

produced in the renal medulla in response to low renal blood flow, directly induces myocyte hypertrophy as well. The result of these factors is decreased left ventricular reserve (stretch), increased preload (high residual volume in the ventricle following systole), and further mitral regurgitation.

NEUROHORMONAL RESPONSE

In response to decreased stroke volume and decreased renal perfusion, several neurohormonal systems are activated, each of which acts to compensate for the decrease in stroke volume. These include:

1. *Adrenergic nervous system.* Adrenergic nervous system activity is heightened in the setting of impaired ventricular function as a direct result of baroreceptor stimulation. These baroreceptors mediate the sympathetic nervous system, which in turn stimulates the beta-1 receptors. This results in an increase in heart rate and contractility.

2. *Renin-angiotensin-aldosterone system.* Decreased renal perfusion stimulates the release of renin, increasing the production of angiotensin I and II and the release of aldosterone. This causes arteriolar vasoconstriction, decreased cardiac output, increased arterial blood pressure and peripheral resistance, increased ventricular filling pressures, sodium and potassium retention (imbalance), increased volume

overload, increased left ventricular wall stress, increased ventricular dilation and hypertrophy, and increased sympathetic nervous system arousal.

3. *Arginine vasopressin system.* Arginine vasopressin (AVP) is a potent vasoconstrictor which is normally inhibited by stretch receptors in the atria during atrial distension. In heart failure, these receptors are less sensitive, causing a decrease in AVP inhibition. This results in systemic vasoconstriction, further increasing afterload (the pressure against which the ventricle must pump in order to get blood out of the ventricle). Increases in AVP availability also lead to an inability to excrete free water, hypoosmolarity, and, in general, inability to autoregulate further AVP production.

4. *Atrial natriuretic peptide.* Atrial natriuretic peptide (ANP) is a counterregulatory hormone that opposes all three of the above systems, resulting in vasodilation and sodium excretion. ANP is produced in response to atrial distension and results in decreased formation of renin, decreased effects of angiotensin II, decreased release of aldosterone and vasopressin, and enhanced renal excretion of sodium and water. In chronic heart failure the levels of ANP remain elevated, but are less so than in the acute phase (phase II).

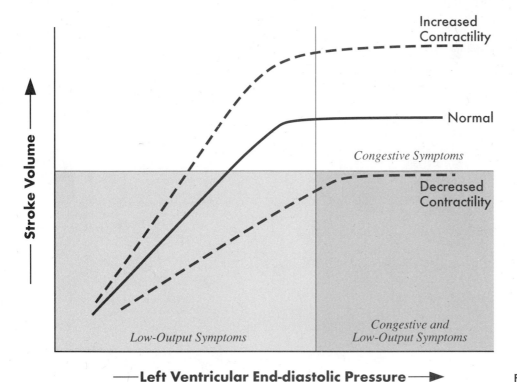

Figure 12–13. Frank-Starling curve.

The effects of the compensatory mechanisms in phase II lead to an increase in circulating volume and perfusion to vital organs. Eventually, these mechanisms are self-limiting and a vicious cycle of increased afterload and volume overload results. The neurohormonal response is no longer beneficial in the chronic state but, as seen in phase III, becomes detrimental.

- *Result of Phase II: Ventricular hypertrophy, weakened myocytes, increased arteriolar resistance, increased vascular volume, and increased ventricular wall stress occur in an effort to maintain adequate cardiac output.*

Phase III

When the adaptive mechanisms of phase II fail, the clinical syndrome of heart failure follows. This third phase of heart failure is extremely variable in onset and presentation. The clinical expression and course of the disease is determined by the extent of the initial insult and myocyte damage, the severity of hemodynamic burden (volume overload), and the patient's individual neurohormonal response to these changes. Phase III is characterized by a progressive deterioration of cardiovascular functioning due to the relationship between compromised LV function and excessive cardiac afterload (Figure 12–14).

- *Result of Phase III: Clinical signs and symptoms of heart failure are evident, resulting in decreased functional status and activity intolerance for the patient.*

Clinical Presentation

Regardless of the underlying cause of the weak pump, patients with heart failure present with clinical signs and symptoms of intravascular and interstitial volume overload, as well as manifestations of inadequate tissue perfusion. Common findings in CHF include:

- Dyspnea (especially with exertion, commonly severe in the acute setting)
- Postural nocturnal dyspnea (PND)
- Pulmonary edema (pronounced crackles)
- Jugular venous distension (JVD)
- Chest discomfort or tightness
- Peripheral edema
- Cool, pale, cyanotic skin
- Oliguria
- Reported weight gain
- Fatigue

More specific physical signs and symptoms may vary in individuals depending on the ventricle which is primarily involved. A summary of clinical findings specific to left and right ventricular failure is presented in Table 12–11.

Because subjective assessment of symptoms and their severity may vary from clinician to clinician, a classification system is commonly used to standardize symptom severity in CHF. One system, the Killip Classification, is used primarily at initial evaluation to predict severity of illness. A second system, known as the New York Heart

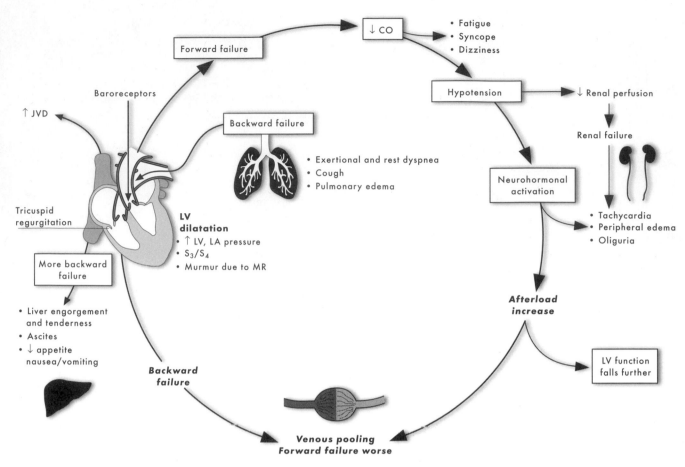

Figure 12–14. Clinical features of heart failure.

Association Functional Classification System, is used to provide systematic assessment of patient status and to benchmark improvement or deterioration from initial evaluation (Table 12–12).

A number of conditions, both cardiac and noncardiac, are similar to heart failure in their clinical presentation and should be ruled out as possible diagnoses in the initial assessment. These conditions include myocardial infarction (MI), pulmonary disease, arrhythmias, anemia, renal failure, nephrotic syndrome, and thyroid disease.

TABLE 12–11. CLINICAL SIGNS AND SYMPTOMS SPECIFIC TO RIGHT- AND LEFT-SIDED HEART FAILURE

Right Heart Failure	Left Heart Failure
Signs and Symptoms of Hepatic Congestion	**Signs and Symptoms of Pulmonary Congestion**
JVD	JVD
Liver enlargement and tenderness	Pulmonary edema
Positive hepatojugular reflex (pressure on liver increases JVD)	Rales
Dependent edema	Atrial fibrillation or other atrial arrhythmias secondary to atrial distension
Ascites	Pulsus alternans (every other beat diminished)
Decreased appetite, nausea, vomiting	Dyspnea
Cardiac Pressures	Cough
Increased RV pressure	Hyperventilation
Increased RA pressure	Dizziness, syncope, fatigue
Heart Sounds	**Cardiac Pressures**
S_3 (early sign)	Increased LV and LA pressure
S_4 (may also present)	Increased pulmonary artery pressures
Wide split S_2	**Heart Sounds**
Pansystolic murmur at lower left sternal border secondary to stretching of tricuspid ring	S_3 and (occasionally) S_4
	Pansystolic murmur at apex secondary to mitral regurgitation

TABLE 12–12. CLASSIFICATION OF CARDIOVASCULAR DISABILITY

Killip Classification

Class
I   Asymptomatic
II Basilar rales, S_3
III Pulmonary edema
IV Shock

New York Heart Association Functional Classification

Class
I   Patients with cardiac disease but without resulting limitations of physical activity. Ordinary physical activity does not cause undue fatigue, palpitation, dyspnea, or anginal pain.
II Patients with cardiac disease resulting in slight limitation of physical activity. They are comfortable at rest. Ordinary physical activity results in fatigue, palpitation, dyspnea, or anginal pain.
III Patients with cardiac disease resulting in marked limitation of physical activity. They are comfortable at rest. Less than ordinary physical activity causes fatigue, palpitation, dyspnea, or anginal pain.
IV Patient with cardiac disease resulting in inability to carry on any physical activity without discomfort. Symptoms of cardiac insufficiency or of the anginal syndrome may be present even at rest. If any physical activity is undertaken, discomfort is increased.

Diagnostic Tests

- *12-Lead ECG:* Acute ST-T wave changes, low voltage, left ventricular hypertrophy, atrial fibrillation or other tachyarrhythmias, bradyarrhythmias, Q waves from previous myocardial infarction.
- *Chest x-ray:* Cardiomegaly, cardiothoracic ratio greater than 0.5.
- *CBC:* Low red cell count (anemia).
- *UA:* Proteinuria, red blood cells, or casts.
- *Creatinine:* Elevated.
- *Albumin:* Decreased.
- *Serum sodium and potassium:* Decreased.
- *Pulmonary artery pressures:* Elevated.
- *Cardiac index:* < 2.0 L/minute/m^2.
- *Echocardiography:* Dilated left ventricle, right ventricle, or right atria; hypertrophied left ventricle; valve incompetence; diffuse or segmental hypocontractility; atrial thrombus; pericardial effusion; left ventricular ejection fraction $< 40\%$.
- *Radionuclide ventriculography:* More precise measure of right ventricular dysfunction and LVEF.

Patient Needs and Principles of Management

Acute management of CHF has changed dramatically over the past decade, from an emphasis on the micromanagement of hemodynamic parameters, primarily using positive inotropes, to an emphasis on functional capacity and long-term survival with the use of neurohormonal blocking agents. This shift is due to a better understanding of the neurohormonal response and the dependence of the body on these mechanisms for compensation in low output states. Goals of patient management in CHF revolve around four general principles: (1) treatment of the underlying cause (e.g., ischemia, valvular dysfunction), (2) management of fluid volume overload, (3) improvement of ventricular function, and (4) patient and family education.

▶ Limiting the Initial Insult and Treating the Underlying Cause

The most effective, but often the most difficult, management strategy for CHF is to limit the damage done by the initial insult. This limitation of myocardial damage and cell loss maximizes the amount of viable ventricular muscle, myocardial contractility, and overall ventricular function.

1. Administer thrombolytic therapy as soon as possible for eligible patients in the setting of acute myocardial infarction (see the previous section on acute ischemic heart disease).

2. Revascularization may be warranted in patients with persistent ischemia as a preventive measure against eventual tissue necrosis.
3. Valve replacement or other surgical corrections should be undertaken as soon as possible to prevent prolonged overstretching of the ventricular myocardium.

▶ Management of Fluid Volume Overload

Decrease preload by the use of diuretic therapy, limitation of dietary sodium, and restriction of free water.

1. Diuretics should be initiated according to the severity of the patient's signs and symptoms. More severe symptoms require intravenous therapy and loop diuretics, while less severe symptoms may be managed adequately on thiazide diuretics.
2. Sodium and fluid restriction should be monitored carefully, with sodium intake not exceeding 2 g per day and free water not exceeding 1500 ml in a 24-hour period.
3. Serum sodium and potassium should be monitored on a regular basis to prevent inadvertent electrolyte imbalances (each day or two in the acute setting, depending on the aggressiveness of therapy).

Patient Needs and Principles of Management, Cont.

▶ Improvement of Left Ventricular Function

Improvement in left ventricular function is accomplished by decreasing the workload on the heart with preload and afterload reduction and by augmenting ventricular contractility. Ventricular function is often measured directly in the acute setting by monitoring cardiac index. As has been demonstrated by a number of large clinical trials, traditional micromanagement of hemodynamic variables, such as cardiac index with inotropic drugs, may be detrimental to long-term patient outcome. Current recommendations do not advocate this as an initial management strategy.

1. Decrease preload (see above).
2. Decrease afterload by administration of pharmacologic therapy, including ACE inhibitors and vasodilators. ACE inhibitors are recommended in all heart failure patients unless otherwise contraindicated. Contraindications to ACE therapy include: previous intolerance, potassium greater than 5.5 mEq/L, hypotension with systolic blood pressure less than 90 mm Hg, and serum creatinine greater than 3.0 mg/dl. Cautious initiation of low-dose therapy in patients with contraindications may still be considered. Vasodilators may also be used in conjunction with diuretics and ACE inhibitors if further afterload reduction is necessary. Especially in the case of underlying atherosclerotic disease, still the largest single contributor to heart failure, nitrates are often used concomitantly with ACE inhibitors and diuretics to augment afterload reduction.
3. Increase myocardial contractility, ACE inhibitors should be considered as the first-line drug, with digoxin recommended for severe heart failure due to left ventricular systolic dysfunction and in mild to moderate cases of failure when optimal doses of ACE inhibitors and diuretics have failed to relieve patient symptoms.
4. A relatively new recommendation is the use of low-dose beta blockage. Caution should still be taken when initiating this therapy in patients with significant respiratory compromise. Anticoagulation therapy is also recommended for prevention of pulmonary embolism in patients with atrial or ventricular septal stasis, a history of atrial fibrillation, or prior pulmonary embolism.
5. Cardiac assist devices can provide temporary maintenance or preservation of ventricular function, especially as a bridge to cardiac transplantation. These devices are inserted percutaneously or surgically using the medial sternotomy or thoracotomy approach (Chapter 22, Advanced Cardiovascular Concepts). Risks related to insertion of these devices include infection and long-term weaning difficulties in the event that an organ donor is not available.
   A. *Intraaortic Balloon Pump (IABP).* Femoral or brachial artery cannulation with the IABP allows for ventricular support, but restricts the patient to bedrest (femoral primarily) and compromises arterial flow to the cannulated limb.
   B. *Left Ventricular Assist Device (LVAD).* Left ventricular apical cannulation allows ambulation and physical rehabilitation while awaiting heart transplant. A large external pump circulates the blood.
   C. *Myoplasty.* The insertion of autologous skeletal muscle (generally latissimus dorsi) into the ventricular wall via removal of the third rib. This procedure requires a 2-month "muscle training" process once the transplant is in place and therefore requires a relatively stable heart failure candidate.

▶ Patient Education

Patients who present with CHF to the critical care unit have high acuity levels, require more intensive interventions, and have an increased need for emotional support surrounding the serious nature of the hospital admission. Previous admissions for CHF make patients more aware of the serious nature of acute episodes. Patient education which is appropriately addressed in the acute care setting includes:

1. Crisis intervention is necessary, both with the patient and the family. Include encouragement to verbalize fears related to role adaptations or changes in family responsibility, lifestyle alterations and limitations, and death and dying. The completion of advanced directives and living wills should be initiated if not previously addressed.
2. Family involvement in the critical care phase should be strongly encouraged, including assistance with activities of daily living such as bathing, and "patterning" of daily activities to allow for frequent periods of rest and spacing of exertional activity. In addition, family involvement in reading or other leisure activity with the patient is often restful and relaxing, and may be useful as a diversional activity. If possible, the family should also be present for reinforcement of patient teaching regarding the medical regimen, the importance of fluid and sodium restriction, and the need for daily weights.

Shock

Shock is the inability of the circulatory system to deliver enough blood to meet the oxygen and nutrient requirements of body tissues. This clinical syndrome may result from ineffective pumping of the heart (cardiogenic shock), insufficient volume of circulating blood (hypovolemic shock), or massive vasodilation of the vascular bed causing maldistribution of blood (vasogenic shock). Although the specific definition of shock and strategies for patient management vary according to the underlying pathophysiology, the principle of ineffective or insufficient oxygen delivery to meet the needs of body tissues remains consistent.

AT THE BEDSIDE
▶ *Shock Following Acute Myocardial Infarction*

Mr. Simpson, 49 years old, was found slumped in his living room chair, cool and clammy but still breathing. His wife phoned emergency medical services, which arranged air transportation to the local emergency room. On arrival Mr. Simpson's vital signs were as follows:

BP	68/44
HR	122 beats/minute
RR	33 breaths/minute
T	36.1°C, orally
Sa0$_2$	91%

Oxygen at 60% by face mask had been initiated in flight, as well as intravenous normal saline running wide open, 450 ml having already infused. Dopamine was started at a rate of 5 μg/kg/minute. A stat ECG showed "tombstone" ST elevation in the anterior leads, with reciprocal changes in leads II, III, and a VF. Mr. Simpson was taken for immediate PTCA. In the lab, cardiac catheterization findings were as follows:

LAD	99% proximal lesion
RCA	70% mid lesion
LCX	Normal
LVEF	13%
Wall motion	Left ventricular akinesis

On return to the ICU, Mr. Simpson's nurse obtained hemodynamic parameters as follows:

PA	45/25 mm Hg
RA	15 mm Hg
PCWP	22 mm Hg
CO	4.0 L/minute
CI	1.5 L/minute/m^2

Etiology, Risk Factors, and Pathophysiology

The ineffective delivery of oxygen to the tissues leads to cellular dysfunction, rapidly progressing to organ failure and finally to total body system failure. The cause of the initial onset of the shock syndrome may be from any number of underlying problems, including heart problems, fluid loss, and trauma. Because the body responds in the same way, differences between cardiogenic, hypovolemic, and vasogenic shock are obvious to the clinician only after the initial assessment has provided key information about the patient's acute illness. Given the history, the clinician can classify shock into one of three major pathological groups and proceed to further determine the patient's needs with the help of diagnostic testing. Since interventions for patient management will be directed at the cause, it is essential for the underlying pathophysiology to be clearly understood.

Cardiogenic Shock

In cardiogenic shock, the heart is unable to pump enough blood to meet the oxygen and nutrient needs of the body. Pump failure is caused by a variety of factors, the most common being left ventricular failure. A number of other factors may cause pump failure, however, and are typically categorized as coronary or noncoronary causes (Table 12–13).

In all cardiogenic shock cases, the heart ceases to function normally as a pump, resulting in decreases in stroke volume and cardiac output. This leads to a decrease in blood pressure and tissue perfusion. The inability of the ventricles, particularly the left ventricle, to empty adequately and maintain adequate forward flow is sometimes referred to as "forward failure" (Figure 12–15). The inadequate emptying of the ventricle increases left atrial pressure, which then increases pulmonary venous pressure. As a result, pulmonary capillary pressure increases, resulting in pulmonary edema. This retrograde congestion is sometimes referred to as "backward failure."

TABLE 12–13. CAUSES OF CARDIOGENIC SHOCK

Coronary Causes
- Myocardial infarction with resultant cell death in a significant portion of the ventricle
- Rupture of ventricle or papillary muscle secondary to myocardial infarction
- Dysfunctional ischemic tissue—"shock ventricle"—which occurs as a result of myocardial ischemia, not involving cell death, and is therefore transient

Noncoronary Causes
- Myocardial contusion
- Pericardial tamponade
- Ventricular rupture
- Arrhythmia (PEA—pulseless electrical activity—new name)
- Valvular dysfunction resulting in ventricular congestion
- Cardiomyopathies
- End-stage congestive heart failure

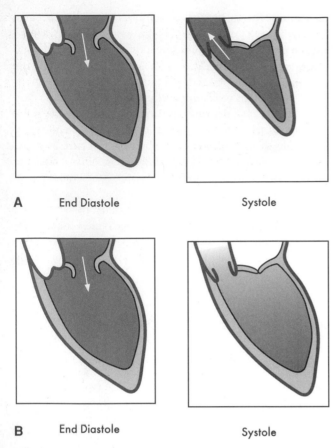

A End Diastole   Systole

B End Diastole   Systole

Figure 12–15. Cardiogenic Shock. (A) Normal cardiac filling. (B) Cardiac filling during cardiogenic shock.

Hypovolemic Shock

Hypovolemic shock occurs when there is inadequate volume in the vascular space. This volume depletion may be caused by blood loss, either internal or external, or by the vascular fluid volume shifting out of the vascular space into other body fluid spaces (Table 12–14). The loss of vascular volume results in insufficient circulating blood to maintain tissue perfusion.

The pathophysiology of hypovolemic shock is related directly to decreased circulating blood volume. When an insufficient amount of blood is circulating, the venous blood returning to the heart is insufficient. As a result, right

TABLE 12–14. CAUSES OF HYPOVOLEMIC SHOCK

Sources of External Loss of Body Fluid
- Hemorrhage (loss of whole blood)
- Gastrointestinal tract (vomiting, diarrhea, ostomies, fistulas, nasogastric suctioning)
- Renal (diuretic administration, diabetes insipidus, Addison's disease, hyperglycemic osmotic diuresis)

Sources of Internal Loss of Body Fluid
- Internal hemorrhage
- Movement of body fluid into interstitial spaces ("third spacing," often the result of bacterial toxin, thermal injury, or allergic reaction)

and left ventricular filling pressures are insufficient, decreasing stroke volume and cardiac output. As in cardiogenic shock, when cardiac output is decreased, blood pressure is low and tissue perfusion is poor.

Vasogenic Shock

Vasogenic shock is characterized by an abnormal placement or distribution of vascular volume, occurring in three situations: (1) sepsis, (2) neurologic damage, and (3) anaphylaxis. In each of these situations, the pumping function of the heart and the total blood volume are normal, but the blood is not appropriately distributed throughout the vascular bed. Massive vasodilation occurs in each of these situations for various reasons, causing the vascular bed to be much larger than normal. In this enlarged vascular bed, the usual volume of circulating blood (approximately 5 L) is no longer sufficient to fill the vascular space, causing a decrease in blood pressure and inadequate tissue perfusion. For this reason vasogenic shock is also referred to as "relative hypovolemic" shock.

Of the vasogenic or "distributive" shock syndromes, septic shock is most commonly seen in the critical care setting. In the field or emergency room setting, anaphylaxis and neurogenic shock are also common and typically result from allergic reactions and trauma related spinal cord injury.

Stages of Shock

Regardless of underlying etiology, all three types of shock (cardiogenic, hypovolemic, vasogenic) activate the sympathetic nervous system, which in turn initiates neural, hormonal, and chemical compensatory mechanisms in an attempt to improve tissue perfusion (Figure 12–16). Cellular changes that occur as a result of these compensatory mechanisms are similar in all types of shock. Progression of these cellular changes follows a predictable, four-stage course.

Initial Stage

The initial stage of shock represents the first cellular changes resulting from the decrease in oxygen delivery to the tissue. These changes include decreased aerobic and increased anaerobic metabolism, leading to increases in serum lactic acid. No obvious clinical signs and symptoms are apparent during this stage of shock.

Compensatory Stage

The compensatory stage is comprised of a number of physiologic events which attempt to compensate for decreases in cardiac output and restore adequate oxygen and nutrient delivery to the tissues (Figure 12–17). These events can be organized into neural, hormonal, and chemical responses. Neural responses include pressoreceptors in the aorta and carotid arteries which detect changes in arterial blood pressure and respond by activating the vasomotor center of the

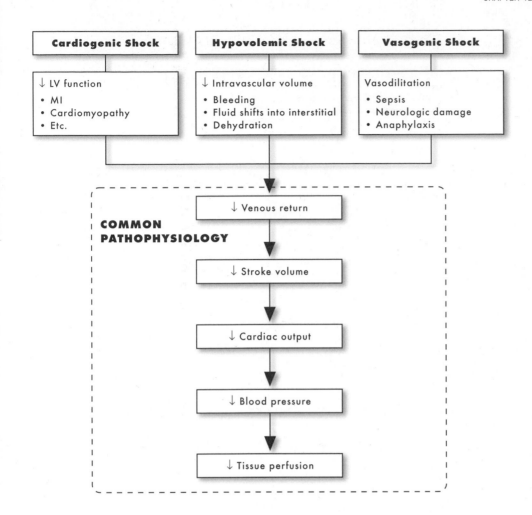

Figure 12–16. Pathophysiology of Shock.

medulla. Hypovolemia and resultant hypotension lead to activation of the sympathetic nervous system. The sympathetic nervous system initiates neural, hormonal, and chemical compensatory mechanisms in an attempt to decrease the vascular space and elevate the blood pressure. The sympathetic nervous system then vasoconstricts peripheral circulation, shunting blood to vital organs. As blood is shunted to vital organs, renal blood flow is decreased, stimulating the hormonal response.

Hormonal responses include increased production of catecholamines and adrenocorticotropic hormone (ACTH) and activation of the renin-angiotensin-aldosterone system. As a direct result of decreased renal blood flow, renin is released from the juxtaglomerular cells, activating angiotensinogen and producing angiotensin I. Angiotensin I, circulating in the blood, is converted to angiotensin II and III in the lungs. As was discussed in more detail in the CHF section, this hormonal response results in direct vasoconstriction, as well as release of aldosterone from the renal cortex and antidiuretic hormone (ADH) from the pituitary gland. Sodium and potassium retention, in conjunction with increased ADH, ACTH, and circulating catecholamines, effectively increases intravascular volume, heart rate, and blood pressure, and decreases urine output.

Chemical responses during the compensatory stage are related to the respiratory ventilation-perfusion imbalance which occurs as a result of sympathetic stimulation, redistribution of blood, and resultant decreased pulmonary perfusion. A respiratory alkalosis ensues, adversely affecting the patient's level of consciousness, restlessness, and agitation.

These compensatory mechanisms are effective for finite periods of time which may vary depending on the individual and presence of comorbidities. The younger and healthier the patients prior to the shock episode, the more likely they are to survive a prolonged episode of shock. In the absence of vascular volume replacement, these intrinsic vasopressors eventually fail as a compensatory mechanism, and the patient enters the progressive, and finally refractory, stages of shock, usually resulting in death.

Progressive Stage

The progressive stage is characterized by end organ failure due to cellular damage from prolonged compensatory changes. The compensatory changes, which were effective in supporting blood pressure and therefore tissue perfusion, are no longer effective and severe hypoperfusion ensues. Lack of oxygen and nutrients results in organ failure, typi-

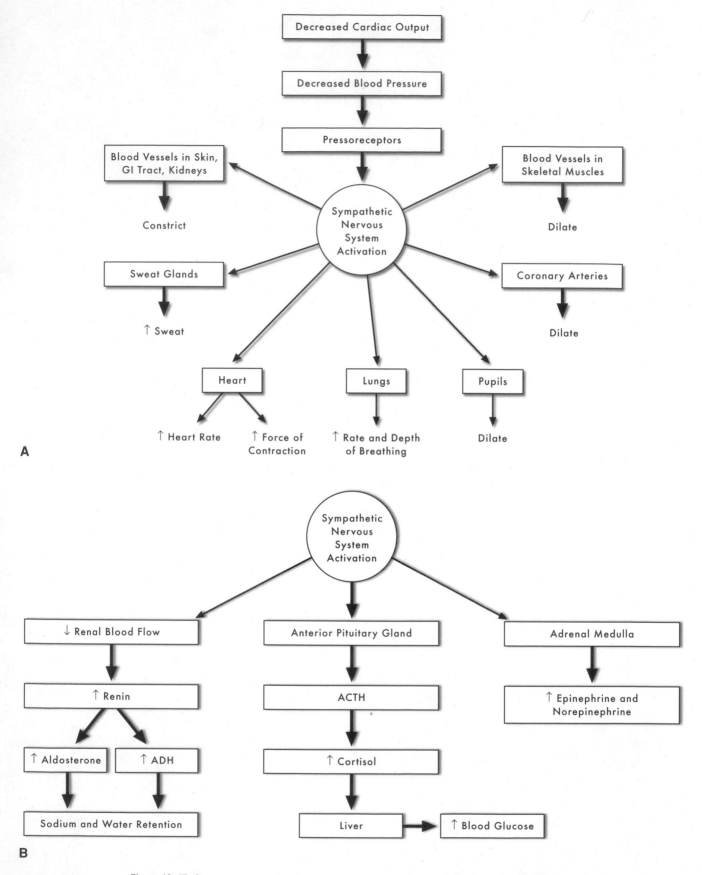

Figure 12–17. Compensatory response to shock. (A) Neural compensation. (B) Hormonal compensation.

cally beginning with gastrointestinal and renal failure, followed by cardiac failure and loss of liver and cerebral function.

Refractory Stage

The refractory stage, as its name implies, is the irreversible stage of shock. At this stage cell death has progressed to such a point as to be irreparable, and death is imminent.

Clinical Presentation

Clinical signs and symptoms vary depending on the underlying cause of shock and the stage of shock in which the patient presents.

Initial Stage

No visible signs and symptoms are evident from ongoing cellular changes in this stage.

Compensatory Stage

Consciousness	Restless, agitated, confused
Blood pressure	Normal or slightly low
Heart rate	Increased
Respiratory rate	Increased (> 20 breaths/minute)
Skin	Cool, clammy, may be cyanotic
Peripheral pulses	Weak and thready
Urine output	Concentrated and scant (< 30 ml/hour)
Bowel sounds	Hypoactive, possible abdominal distension
Labs:	
Glucose	Increased
Sodium	Increased
Pao_2	Decreased
$Paco_2$	Decreased
pH	Increased

Progressive Stage

Consciousness	Unresponsive to verbal stimuli
Blood pressure	Inadequate (< 90 mm Hg)
Heart rate	Increased
Respiratory rate	Increased, shallow
Skin	Cold, cyanotic, mottled

Peripheral pulses	Weak and thready, may be absent
Urine output	Scant (< 20 ml/hour)
Bowel sounds	Absent
Labs:	
Amylase	Increased
Lipase	Increased
SGPT/SGOT	Increased
LDH	Increased
CPK	Increased
Creatinine	Increased
BUN	Increased
Pao_2	Increased
$Paco_2$	Increased
pH	Decreased
HCO_3	Decreased

Diagnostic Tests

Cardiogenic

ECG	Tachycardia
Pulmonary arterial pressure	PAD/PCWP high (> 12 mm Hg), RA high (> 8 mm Hg)
Echocardiogram	Ventricular wall motion abnormalities, cardiac tamponade, ventricular rupture

Hypovolemic

Pulmonary arterial catheter	PAD/PCWP low (< 8 mm Hg), RA low (< 5 mm Hg)
Ultrasound	Groin or retroperitoneal hemorrhage

Vasogenic

Septic	Positive blood cultures
Anaphylactic	Arterial blood gas shows inadequate oxygenation
Neurogenic	Computed tomography scan and magnetic resonance imaging shows spinal cord damage

Patient Needs and Principles of Management

Differences in the underlying cause of shock lead to some variation in the principles of management. The basic goals of therapy for all forms of shock, however, include the need to correct the underlying cause of shock, improvement of oxygenation, and restoration of adequate tissue perfusion.

► Correction of the Underlying Cause of Shock

Cardiogenic: Remove coronary obstruction, if present, and restore blood flow.

Hypovolemic: Identify source and stop bleeding if possible; correct fluid shunting or third spacing with electrolyte management.

Vasogenic:

- Anaphylactic: Intubate for oxygenation and treat the underlying allergic reaction using antidote or steroid therapy.
- Septic: Antibiotic therapy and removal of infected tissue (e.g., bowel) or device (e.g., central arterial or venous line).

- Neurogenic: Severing of the cord may be irreversible; however, intubation will provide respiratory support while the underlying cause is identified.

► Improve Oxygenation

1. Assess for patent airway and intubate if necessary.
2. Administer oxygen at 100% or as necessary until Pao_2 is adequate (> 60 to 70 mm Hg).

► Restore Adequate Tissue Perfusion

1. Administer fluid volume expanders (normal saline, lactated Ringer's solution, or plasmanate) in large rapid boluses. Type and cross-match for blood type and administer blood as necessary for hypovolemic shock.
2. Initiate vasoactive drug therapy.

Hypertension

Hypertension is typically a chronic disease of blood pressure elevation which is often masked, especially in the early years of onset, by lack of warning signs or symptoms. *Hypertensive crisis* is an acute episode or exacerbation, occurring infrequently in a small percentage of hypertensive patients and characterized by the pivotal effect the particular episode and its treatment may have on the patient's long-term outcome. In most cases, the numerical or absolute value of the arterial blood pressure is less important than its impact on the individual's underlying risk of target organ damage, specifically cerebrovascular, coronary, and renal disease.

Etiology, Risk Factors, and Pathophysiology

Although a number of clinical syndromes commonly are associated with hypertension and many underlying etiologies may contribute to the progression of hypertensive disease, the pathophysiology of hypertension is similar regardless of the underlying disease entity.

An acute hypertensive crisis begins with elevation of the systolic or diastolic blood pressure causing a threat, direct or indirect, to an organ or body system. Acute, severe increases in pressure may cause serious, life-threatening cerebrovascular and cardiovascular compromise. Prolonged hypoperfusion of an organ system leads to ischemia, necrosis, and organ system failure.

Classification of Hypertension

Due to the increased risk of such events in all hypertensive patients, morbidity and mortality directly related to hypertension is high, and long-term, consistent therapy in all stages of hypertension is necessary.

Benign Hypertension

Benign hypertension is characterized by slightly elevated blood pressure (140 to 150 systolic/90 diastolic, in adults) for long periods of time, with little if any end organ damage. Benign hypertension does not tend to cause acute problems or complications, unless other comorbid conditions, such as atherosclerotic disease, are present. The pressure does not typically exacerbate or precipitate an acute emergent event (generally not greater than 140 to 150 systolic/90 diastolic, in adults).

Accelerated Hypertension

Often used interchangeably with malignant hypertension, the stage known as "accelerated hypertension" is generally considered a precursor to malignant hypertension, and is characterized by an increase in the basal blood pressure.

Malignant Hypertension

Hypertension typically is a chronic disease in which elevation in blood pressure occurs slowly, over a period of several years. Because of its gradual onset, the body adapts to increased pressures in the vascular bed and the patient frequently is asymptomatic for years, eventually able to tolerate pressures of up to 200/120 mm Hg without experiencing significant symptoms or clinical events. This type of presentation often is identified "accidentally," secondary to hospitalization for another problem. Generally patients with malignant hypertension are at risk for significant end organ damage due to the severity of high pressure in the vascular bed and inability of the circulatory system to further adapt or compensate in the event of additional stressors.

Hypertensive Crisis

Hypertensive crisis is characterized by a severe elevation in blood pressure, relative to the individual's baseline blood pressure, which causes risk of end organ damage and poor long-term outcome due to permanent organ system damage if the immediate episode is not treated quickly and aggressively.

Special Populations

In pregnant women and children a less severe elevation in blood pressure may result in significant end organ damage and is therefore considered to be a "hypertensive crisis" at values much lower than would be expected to be problematic in the average adult. The absolute value of the blood pressure will vary significantly depending on the situation and the individual involved. For example, preeclampsia, considered to be a hypertensive crisis in pregnancy, may occur at pressures as low as 130 to 160/100 mm Hg.

Clinical Presentation

Diagnosis of hypertensive crisis is not based on the absolute value of the blood pressure, but rather on the following combined criteria:

- Rapidity of the rise of the blood pressure
- Duration of prior hypertension
- Clinical determination of the immediate threat to vital organ function
- Headache
- Blurred vision
- Nosebleed
- Dizziness or vertigo
- TIA
- Diminished peripheral pulses or bruits
- Carotid or abdominal bruit
- Heart sounds with S_3 and/or S_4
- Systolic and/or diastolic murmurs
- GI bleeding
- Pulmonary edema
- Shortness of breath
- Fatigue
- Malaise
- Weakness
- Nausea and vomiting
- Hematuria
- Dysuria
- Funduscopic findings: arteriovenous thickening, arteriolar narrowing, hemorrhage, papilledema, or exudates

Diagnostic Tests

- *Chest x-ray:* Myocardial hypertrophy, pulmonary infiltrates
- *Computed tomography:* Arteriolar narrowing and arteriovenous thickening
- *Specific tests to target organ damage:*
  - Renal angiography
  - Coronary angiography
  - Carotid/cerebral angiography
- *Magnetic resonance imaging:* Cerebral vascular malperfusion

Patient Needs and Principles of Management

Management of the patient with acute exacerbation of hypertension, or hypertensive crisis, revolves around three primary objectives: reduction of arterial pressure, evaluation and treatment of target organ damage, and preparation/planning for continuous and consistent outpatient follow-up.

▶ Reduction of Arterial Pressure

1. *Ascertain correct arterial blood pressure.* Verify arterial blood pressure, being sure to ascertain bilateral measurements with the correct cuff size if using sphygmomanometry, as well as orthostatic pressures if possible (lying and sitting up, if standing is not possible). Each measurement should be 2 minutes apart and both right and left measurements should be documented. If bilateral measurements are greater than 10 mm Hg different, the higher reading should be used to gauge therapy. In most acute situations, priority should be given to establishing a stable arterial access site for direct, invasive monitoring of blood pressure.

2. *Initiate pharmacologic intervention.*
   - *Acute.* Pharmacologic intervention is the fastest, most effective means of reducing arterial blood pressure. A number of agents are used in the acute setting for management of hypertensive crisis (Table 12–15). Aggressiveness of pharmacologic intervention should be based on the severity of blood pressure elevation (immediate risk of stroke), the immediate risk of irreversible target organ damage (renal and hepatic function related to drug metabolism and clearance also should be considered), and any confounding conditions or risk factors which are present (for example, the fetus in preeclampsia). In general, acute severe (accelerated malignant/stage 3 and 4) hypertension should be treated as quickly and aggressively as can be tolerated by the patient in order to prevent the immediate risk of hypertensive encephalopathy, dissecting aortic aneurysm, myocardial infarction, or intracranial hemorrhage. Maintenance of cerebral perfusion pressure is imperative during treatment, and overly aggressive pharmacologic management poses the threat of cerebrovascular compromise due to a sudden drop in arterial pressure and inability of the autoregulatory mechanism to adjust. Other organ systems dependent on higher pressure for perfusion include the renal and coronary systems. A sudden, severe drop in systemic arterial pressure may result in ischemic episodes or acute renal failure.

   - *Nonacute.* Dietary alteration and relaxation or biofeedback techniques may be used in addition to pharmacologic measures to reduce the morbidity and mortality of hypertension. Although these measures are most effective when employed long term as part of a cohesive outpatient follow-up program, initiating these strategies in the acute setting may help to emphasize their importance.

▶ Evaluation and Treatment of Target Organ Disease

Concomitant to initiation of pharmacologic intervention, the assessment and prevention of target organ disease is important to avoid irreversible damage. Target organs typically at risk include the brain, heart, kidneys, and eyes. Strategies to prevent damage to these organ systems during hypertensive crisis include:

1. *Brain.* Reduce diastolic pressure by one-third (not to go below 95 mm Hg) using aggressive pharmacologic measures (see Table 12–15).

TABLE 12–15. COMMON DRUGS USED TO MANAGE ACUTE HYPERTENSIVE EPISODES

Nitroprusside	• Dilates arterioles and veins.
	• Administer IV at 0.5 to 10.0 mg/kg/minute (mix in normal saline only; 100 mg in 500 ml). Cover bottle with foil to avoid light exposure.
	• Titrate up to desired blood pressure, recognizing that the effect will be evident within 1 minute of change in dose.
Trimethaphaur	• Ganglionic blocker; also dilates arterioles/veins.
	• May be preferable in patients with aortic dissection.
	• Administer IV at 0.5 to 5 mg/minute.
	• Patient should be in sitting position if possible.
Nitroglycerin	• Dilates veins more than arterioles.
	• Administer IV at a rate of 5 to 100 µg/minute. Mix 100 mg in 500 ml NS or D_5 IV.
Diazoxide	• Dilates arteriolar tone only.
	• No individual titration necessary.
	• Administer dose of 50 to 150 mg rapidly. Effect noted in 1 to 5 minutes. Repeat same dose in 10 minutes if no effect; total dose not to exceed 600 mg/day.
	• Do NOT use if MI or aortic dissection suspected (diazoxide is a positive inotrope).
Enalapril	• An angiotensin-converting enzyme (ACE) inhibitor.
	• Administer IV at a rate of 5 mg/minute.
Labetalol	• Beta-receptor agonist (beta blocker).
	• Particularly indicated in patients with suspected MI or angina.
	• Administer 5 mg bolus over 5 minutes and repeat three times. IV drip may then be started.

2. *Heart.* Reduce diastolic and systolic pressure by one-third; administer combination therapy if possible (vasodilator and beta blocker) or ACE inhibitor for afterload reduction; monitor for ischemic changes on ECG.

3. *Kidneys.* Reduce systolic and diastolic blood pressure using pharmacologic measures; monitor serum creatinine and urine specific gravity as well as proteinuria and hematuria; for patients with severe existing renal impairment, use of ACE inhibitors may exacerbate their renal compromise and is therefore contraindicated in patients with bilateral renal artery stenosis; administer diuretics to maintain serum sodium and adequate diuresis.

4. *Eyes.* Reduce systolic and diastolic blood pressure; observe retina for evidence of hemorrhage, exudate, or papilledema; instruct the patient with blurring of vision regarding his or her environment, especially location of the call bell.

▶ Patient Education on Lifestyle Modification and Follow-Up

Following control of hypertension in the acute phase, patient education should be initiated regarding the serious and chronic nature of the disease. Often, the clinician may have an opportunity in the acute stage to make an impact regarding the seriousness of uncontrolled hypertension and its potentially debilitating effects. Prior to beginning the educational process, assessment should include:

1. Family history of hypertension, cardiovascular disease, coronary artery disease, stroke, diabetes mellitus, and hyperlipidemia.
2. Lifestyle history including weight gain, exercise, and smoking habits.
3. Dietary patterns including high sodium, alcohol, and dietary fat intake or low potassium intake.
4. Knowledge of hypertension and impact of previous medical therapy for hypertension (compliance/side effects/results or efficacy).

AT THE BEDSIDE
▶ *Thinking Critically*

You are taking care of a patient, 4 days post anterior MI, who just transferred into the ICU from an intermediate floor with severe shortness of breath. Your initial assessment reveals the following:

HR	128 beats/minute
BP	110/82
RR	36 breaths/minute
T	37.6°C, orally
Lung sounds	Coarse, bilateral rales in lower lobes, poor respiratory effort
Heart sounds	S_1, S_2, S_3
Skin	Flushed, diaphoretic, +2 pedal edema (Doppler pulses)
ECG	NSR, with prolonged ventricular repolarization (tall QRS complex)

What is your initial intervention? The underlying cause for this patient's respiratory compromise is most likely what? Management of this condition would most likely include what interventions?

SELECTED BIBLIOGRAPHY

What Heals: Integrating Alternative Therapies

Aiken LH, Henrichs TF: Systematic relaxation as a nursing intervention technique with open heart surgery patients. *Nursing Research.* 1971;20:212.

Barry J, Selwyn AP, Nabel EG, et al.: Frequency of ST-segment depression produced by mental stress in stable angina pectoris from coronary artery disease. *American Journal of Cardiology.* 1988;61:989.

Bohachick P: Progressive relaxation training in cardiac rehabilitation: Effects on psychologic variables. *Nursing Research.* 1984; 33:283.

Bolwerk CA: Effects of relaxing music on state anxiety in myocardial infarction patients. *Critical Care Nursing.* 1990;13:63.

Davis C, Cunningham SG: The physiologic responses of patients in the coronary care unit to selected music. *Heart and Lung.* 1985;14:291.

Deanfield JE, Shea M, Kensett M, et al.: Silent myocardial ischaemia due to mental stress. *Lancet.* 1984; November: 1001.

Eliot R, Buell J: Role of emotions and stress in the genesis of sudden death. *Journal of the American College of Cardiology.* 1985;5:95B.

Freeman LJ, Nixon PGF, Sallabank P, et al.: Psychological stress and silent myocardial ischemia. *American Heart Journal.* 1987; 114:477.

Guzzetta CE: *Effects of relaxation and music therapy on coronary care unit patients admitted with presumptive acute myocardial infarction.* Rockville, MD: U.S. Department of Health and Human Services, Division of Nursing, Grant NU 00824, August 1987.

Guzzetta CE: Effects of relaxation and music therapy on coronary care unit patients with presumptive acute myocardial infarction. *Heart and Lung.* 1989;18:609.

Hyman RB, Feldman HR, Harris RB, et al.: The effects of relaxation training on clinical symptoms: A meta-analysis. *Nursing Research.* 1989;38:216.

Lown B, Temte JV, Reich P, et al.: Basis for recurring ventricular fibrillation in the absence of coronary heart disease and its management. *New England Journal of Medicine.* 1976;294:623.

Munro BH, Creamer AH, Haggerty MR, et al.: Effect of relaxation therapy on post-myocardial infarction patients' rehabilitation. *Nursing Research.* 1988;37:231.

Ornish D, Brown SE, Scherwitz LW, et al.: Can lifestyle changes reverse coronary heart disease? The lifestyle heart trial. *Lancet.* 1990;336:129.

Ornish D, Scherwitz LW, Doody RS, et al.: Effects of stress management training and dietary change in treating ischemic heart disease. *Journal of the American Medical Association.* 1983;249:54.

Rahe RH, et al.: Recent life changes, myocardial infarction and abrupt coronary death: Studies in Helsinki. *Archives of Internal Medicine.* 1974;133:221.

Reich P, DeSilva RA, Lown B, et al.: Acute psychological disturbance preceding life-threatening arrhythmias. *Journal of the American Medical Association.* 1981;246:233.

Rosenman RH, Brand RJ, Jenkins CD, et al.: Coronary heart disease in the Western Collaborative Group Study: Final follow-up experience of $8\frac{1}{2}$ years. *Journal of the American Medical Association.* 1975;233:872.

Rossi EL: *The psychobiology of mind-body healing: New concepts of therapeutic hypnosis.* New York: WW Norton, 1986.

Rozanski A, Bairey N, Krantz DS, et al.: Mental stress and the induction of silent myocardial ischemia in patients with coronary artery disease. *New England Journal of Medicine.* 1988;318:1005.

Ruberman W, Weinblatt E, Goldberg JD, et al.: Psychosocial influences on mortality after myocardial infarction. *New England Journal of Medicine.* 1984;311:552.

Selwyn AP, Ganz P: Myocardial ischemia in coronary disease. *New England Journal of Medicine.* 1988;318:1058.

Updike P: Music therapy results for ICU patients. *Dimensions in Critical Care Nursing.* 1990;9:39.

Wolff HG: *Stress and disease.* Springfield, IL: C Thomas, 1953.

Cardiac Imagery

Dossey BM: Imagery: Awakening the inner healer. In Dossey BM, Keegan L, Guzzetta CE, Kolkmeier L: *Holistic nursing: A handbook for practice.* Gaithersburg, MD: Aspen, 1988.

Lowery BJ: Psychological stress, denial, and myocardial infarction. *Capsules and Comments in Critical Care Nursing* (abstract and comment 1-11). 1993;1:15–16.

General Cardiovascular

Andreoli KG, Zipes DP, Wallace AG, Kinney MR, Fowkes VK: *Comprehensive cardiac care,* 6th ed. St. Louis, MO: CV Mosby, 1987.

Baas LS: *Essentials of cardiovascular nursing.* Gaithersburg, MD: Aspen, 1991.

Guzzetta CE, Dossey BM: *Cardiovascular nursing: Bodymind tapestry.* St. Louis, MO: CV Mosby, 1984.

Wingate S. *Cardiac nursing: A clinical management and patient care resource.* Gaithersburg, MD: Aspen, 1991.

Coronary Angiography

Tilkian AG, Daily EK: *Cardiovascular procedures: Diagnostic techniques and therapeutic procedures.* St. Louis, MO: CV Mosby, 1986.

Zorb SL: *Cardiovascular diagnostic testing: A nursing guide.* Gaithersburg, MD: Aspen, 1991.

Coronary Revascularization

Osguthorpe SG, Tidwell SL, Ryan WJ, Paull DL, Smith TL: Evaluation of the patient having cardiac surgery in the post operative rewarming period. *Heart and Lung.* 1990; 19(2): 570–574.

Seifert, PC: *Cardiac surgery.* St. Louis, MO: Mosby-Year Book, 1994.

Acute Ischemic Heart Disease

Braunwald E, Mark D, Jones R, et al.: *Unstable angina: Diagnosis and management.* Clinical Practice Guideline No. 10. AHCPR Publication number 94-0602. Rockville, MD: Agency for Health Care Policy and Research, Public Health Service, U.S. Department of Health and Human Services, May 1994.

Califf RM, Mark DB, Wagner GS (eds.): *Acute coronary care,* 2nd ed. Chicago: Mosby-Year Book, 1995; pp. 525–541.

Fuster V, Dyken ML, Vokonas PS, Hennekens C: Aspirin as a therapeutic agent in cardiovascular disease. *Circulation.* 1993; 87(2):659–675.

Kirklin JW, Akins CW, Blackstone EH, Booth DC, Califf RM, Cohen LS, et al.: ACC/AHA guidelines and indications for coronary artery bypass graft surgery. A report of the American College of Cardiology/American Heart Association Task Force on Assessment of Diagnostic and Therapeutic Cardiovascular Procedures (Subcommittee on Coronary Artery Bypass Graft Surgery). *Circulation.* 1991;83(3):1125–1173.

Pasternak R, Braunwald E, Sobel B: Acute myocardial infarction. In Braunwald E: *Heart disease. A textbook of cardiovascular medicine.* Philadelphia: WB Saunders, 1992; pp. 1200–1291.

Congestive Heart Failure

Konstam M, Dracup K, Baker D, et al.: *Heart failure: Evaluation and care of patients with left-ventricular systolic dysfunction.* Clinical Practice Guideline No. 11. AHCPR Publication number 94-0612. Rockville, MD: Agency for Health Care Policy and

Research, Public Health Service, U.S. Department of Health and Human Services, June 1994.

Lindpainter K, Ganten D: The cardiac renin-angiotensin system: An appraisal of present experimental and clinical evidence. *Circulation*. 1991;68:905–921.

Packer M: The neurohormonal hypothesis: A theory to explain the mechanism of disease progression in heart failure. *Journal of the American College of Cardiology*. 1992;20(1): 248–254.

Smith T, Braunwald E, Kelly R: The management of heart failure. In Braunwald E: *Heart disease. A textbook of cardiovascular medicine*. Philadelphia: WB Saunders, 1992, pp. 464–519.

Whitman G (ed.): Management of chronic heart failure. *Critical Care Nursing Clinics of North America*. 1993;5(4).

Shock

Rice V: Shock, a clinical syndrome: An update. Parts 1–4. *Critical Care Nurse*. 1991;11(4):20–27.

Hypertension

Johannsen JM: Update: Guidelines for treating hypertension. *American Journal of Nursing*. 1993; March: 42–49.

National Institutes Of Health: *The fifth report of the Joint National Committee on Detection, Evaluation, and Treatment of High Blood Pressure*. Bethesda, MD: NIH Publication No. 93-1088. January 1993.

Nolan C, Linas S: Accelerated and malignant hypertension. In Schrier R, Gottschalk CW (eds.): *Diseases of the kidney*, 4th ed. Boston: Little, Brown, 1988, pp. 1703–1781.

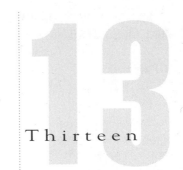

Respiratory System

Thirteen

▶ **Knowledge Competencies**

1. Identify indications for, complications of, and nursing management of patients receiving pulse oximetry, end-tidal CO_2 monitoring, and selected radiographic tests.

2. Describe the etiology, pathophysiology, clinical presentation, patient needs, and principles of management of acute respiratory failure (ARF).

3. Compare and contrast the pathophysiology, clinical presentation, patient needs, and manage-

ment approaches for common diseases leading to ARF:
- Adult respiratory distress syndrome (ARDS)
- Acute respiratory infections
- ARF in the chronic obstructive pulmonary disease patient (asthma, emphysema, bronchitis)
- Pulmonary embolism
- Pneumonia

■ *What Heals: The Art of Guiding*

A nurse healer is a guide who uses the art of guiding to help others uncover and recognize healing behaviors, make choices, and discover insights about how to cope more effectively. A guide also helps a person explore purpose and meaning in life as well as illness. Guiding is a special art and a healing intervention that can be used all the time.

We must remember that although patients may be critically ill, they still bring with them their own inner healing. In the midst of crisis, patients often forget their innate healing resources and need to be guided to get in touch with them.

Nurse: *"I'd like to spend a few minutes to talk to you about your illness. Most patients tell us that being in the intensive care unit is a pretty scary experience. (pause) They have many questions, concerns, and worries about*

being ill and being here. Talking about these concerns and finding ways to deal with them often make patients feel better and get better. Can you share with me some of your questions and thoughts about being here?"

Such an introduction establishes caring and the willingness to explore problems and methods of coping. As questions, concerns, and fears surface, the patient and nurse can work together to uncover the appropriate coping techniques and supportive interventions. Although the nurse healer guides the patient in the inner journey of self-discovery and coping by offering insights, options, and choices, we can never assume that we know the best course for a person. Patients must make their own choices and only they will know what each experience holds for them.

CED & BMD

SPECIAL ASSESSMENT TECHNIQUES, DIAGNOSTIC TESTS, AND MONITORING SYSTEMS

Chest X-Rays

Chest radiography provides visualization of heart and lungs and is an important tool in respiratory assessment. Chest x-rays should complement the bedside assessment. Critical care nurses need to know basic radiographic concepts and how to optimize portable chest x-ray technique, and need to learn a systematic way for viewing a chest x-ray film.

Chest x-rays are taken as part of routine screening procedures, when respiratory disease is suspected, to evaluate the status of respiratory abnormalities (e.g., pneumothorax, pleural effusion, tumors), to confirm proper invasive tube placement (i.e., endotracheal, tracheostomy, or chest tubes, or pulmonary artery catheters), or following traumatic chest injury.

Basic Concepts

An x-ray is a form of radiant energy, and a radiographic image is made by x-ray machines. Only a few rays are absorbed by air as beams pass through the atmosphere, whereas all rays are absorbed by metal as the beams attempt to pass through a sheet of metal. When nothing but air lies between the film cassette and the x-ray source, the radiographic image will be blackness or radiolucency. If density increases, more beams will be absorbed between the film cassette and the x-ray source, and the radiographic image will be whiteness or radiopacity. As the x-ray beam passes through the patient, the denser tissues absorb more of the beam, and the less dense tissues absorb less of the beam.

The lungs are primarily sacs of air or gas, so normal lungs look black on chest films. Conversely, the skeletal thorax will appear white, since bone is very dense and absorbs the most x-rays (Table 13–1). The heart and mediastinum appear gray because those structures are made up of mostly water. Breast tissue is made up of mostly fat and it will appear whitish-gray.

TABLE 13–1. BASIC X-RAY DENSITIES

Radiolucent (black)
Gas, air (dark or black)
• Lungs, trachea, bronchi, alveoli
Water (dark or gray)
• Heart, muscle, blood, blood vessels, diaphragm, spleen, liver
Fat (lighter or whitish-gray)
• Breasts, marrow, hilar streaking
Radiopaque (white)
Metal, bone (lightest or white)
• Ribs, scapulae, vertebrae
• Bullets, coins, teeth, ECG electrodes

Basic Views of the Chest

The most common method of obtaining a chest x-ray is the posterior-anterior (PA) view. PA chest x-rays are typically done in the radiology department with the machine about 6 feet away from the x-ray film cassette and the patient standing with the anterior chest wall against the x-ray plate and the back toward the x-ray machine. The patient is told to take a deep breath and hold it as the x-ray beam is delivered through the posterior chest wall to the x-ray film cassette. The PA view results in a very accurate, sharp picture of the chest.

Critically ill patients are rarely able to tolerate the positioning requirements of a PA chest x-ray. Most chest x-rays in critical care are obtained with an anterior-posterior (AP) view with the patient supine in bed, with or without back rest elevation. With portable AP chest films, the film cassette is placed behind the patient and the x-ray beam is delivered through the anterior chest to the x-ray film. The x-ray machine is only 3 feet away from the patient, which results in greater distortion of chest images, making the AP chest x-ray less accurate than the PA method. Of particular concern is that the heart size is enlarged on an AP film. When viewing chest x-rays, it is important to know whether a PA or AP view was used to avoid misinterpretation of heart size as cardiomegaly.

Distortions can be minimized by placing the patient in a high Fowler's position, or as erect as possible, with the thorax symmetrically placed on the x-ray film cassette. Explain the procedure to the patient and the need to avoid movement. All unnecessary objects lying on the anterior chest (such as ventilator tubing, safety pins, jewelry, ECG wires, nasogastric tubes) should be removed. If the patient is unconscious, taping the forehead in a neutral position may be necessary, especially in the high Fowler's position. All caregivers assisting with the chest x-ray need to protect themselves from radiation exposure by positioning themselves behind the x-ray machine or by using lead aprons covering the neck, chest, and abdomen.

Other chest x-ray views include: (1) lateral views to identify normal and abnormal structures behind the heart, along the spine, and at the base of the lung; (2) oblique views to localize lesions without interference from the bony thorax or to get a better picture of the trachea, carina, heart, and great vessels; (3) lordotic views to better visualize the apical and middle regions of the lung and to differentiate anterior from posterior lesions; and (4) lateral decubitus (cross-table) views, done with the patient supine or side-lying, to assess for air/fluid levels or free-flowing pleural fluid.

Systematic Approach to Chest X-Ray Interpretation

A systematic approach should be used when analyzing a chest x-ray film. It is important to first make sure that the film has been properly labeled (correct name and medical record number) and to identify the right and wrong sides

TABLE 13–2. STEPS FOR INTERPRETATION OF A CHEST X-RAY FILM

Step 1
Look at the different densities (black, gray, and white), and answer the question, *"What is air, fluid, tissue, and bone?"*

Step 2
Look at the shape or form of each density, and answer the question, *"What normal anatomic structure is this?"*

Step 3
Look at both right and left sides, and answer the question, *"Are the findings the same on both sides or are there differences (both physiologic and pathophysiologic)?"*

Step 4
Look at all the structures (bones, mediastinum, diaphragm, pleural space, and lung tissue), and answer the question, *"Are there any abnormalities present?"*

Step 5
Look for all tubes, wires, and lines, and answer the question, *"Are the tubes, wires, and lines in the proper place?"*

From: Thelan L, Davie J, Urden L, Lough M: Critical care nursing: Diagnosis and management, *2nd ed. St. Louis, MO:* Mosby-Year Book, 1994.

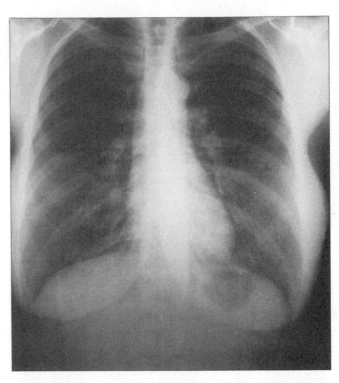

Figure 13–2. Normal chest x-ray. *(From: Sanchez F: Fundamentals of chest x-ray interpretation.* Critical Care Nurse. *1986; 6(5):42..)*

before placing the film on the viewbox. If previous films are available, place them next to the new films for comparison. View the chest x-ray from the lateral borders, moving to the medial aspects of the thorax and asking a series of questions found in Table 13–2.

Begin the chest x-ray analysis by comparing the right side to the left side using the following sequence (Figures 13–1 and 13–2): (1) soft tissues—neck, shoulders, breasts, and subcutaneous fat; (2) trachea—the column of radiolucency readily visible above the clavicles; (3) bony thorax—note size, shape, and symmetry; (4) intercostal spaces—note width and angle; (5) diaphragm—dome-shaped with distinct margins, right dome 1 to 3 cm higher than left dome; (6) pleural surfaces—visceral and parietal pleura appear like a thin hairlike line along the apices and lateral chest; (7) mediastinum—size varies with age, sex, and size; (8) hila—large pulmonary arteries and veins; and (9) lung fields—largest area of the chest and most radiolucent (Figure 13–3).

Normal Variants and Common Abnormalities

When the soft tissues are examined, the two sides of the lateral chest should be symmetric. A mastectomy will make one lung look more radiolucent than the other due to the absence of fatty tissue. The trachea should be midline, with the carina visible at the level of the aortic knob or second intercostal space (Figure 13–2). The most common cause of tracheal deviation is a pneumothorax which causes a tracheal and mediastinal shift to the area away from the pneumothorax (Table 13–3).

Bony thorax inspection reveals general body build. Clavicles should be symmetric and may have an irregular notch or indentation in the inferior medial aspect of the

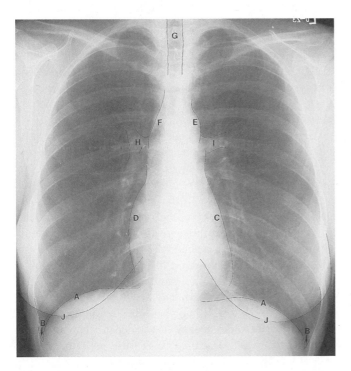

Figure 13–1. Normal chest x-ray. Normal chest x-ray film taken of a 28-year-old female from a posteroanterior (PA) view. The backward L in the upper right corner is placed on the film to indicate the left side of the chest. Some anatomic structures can be seen on the x-ray: (A) diaphragm; (B) costophrenic angle; (C) left ventricle; (D) right atrium; (E) aortic arch (referred to as aortic knob); (F) superior vena cava; (G) trachea; (H) right bronchus (right hilum); (I) left bronchus (left hilum); and (J) breast shadows.

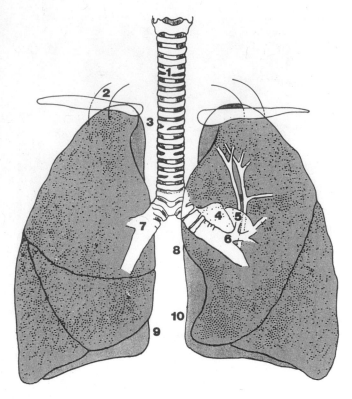

Figure 13–3. Mediastinal structures visible on a chest x-ray. (1) Trachea, (2) first rib, (3) superior vena cava, (4) aortic knob, (5) pulmonary artery, (6) left main bronchus, (7) right main bronchus, (8) left atrium, (9) right atrium, and (10) left ventricle. *(From: Sanchez F: Fundamentals of chest x-ray interpretation.* Critical Care Nurse. *1986;6(5):53.)*

clavicle called a rhomboid fossa, a normal variant. Deformities of the thorax can be detected, such as scoliosis, funnel chest, or pigeon chest. Decreases in the density (less white) of the spine, ribs, and other bones may indicate loss of calcium from the bones due to osteoporosis or long-term steroid dependency. Careful examination of the intercostal spaces (ICS) and rib angles may indicate pathology. Chronic obstructive pulmonary disease (COPD) patients will have widened ICS and the angle of the ribs to the spine increases to 90° instead of the normal 45° angle due to severe hyperinflation. Conversely, narrowed ICS may be visible in cystic fibrosis patients with severe interstitial fibrosis. Rib fractures, if present, are commonly visible along the lateral borders of the rib cage.

Elevation of the diaphragm can be a result of abdominal distention, phrenic nerve paralysis, or lung collapse. Depression or flattening of the diaphragm can occur when 11 or 12 ribs show on a chest x-ray as a result of COPD. Normal costophrenic angles can be seen where the tapered edges of the diaphragm and the chest wall meet. Since breast tissue can obscure the angles in females, these angles are more distinct in males. Obliteration or "blunting" of the costophrenic angle can occur with pleural effusion or atelectasis.

Identification of a pleural space on a chest x-ray is an abnormal finding. The pleural space is not visible unless air (pneumothorax) or fluid (pleural effusion) enters it. These findings commonly are seen in the ICU population.

Two terms often heard regarding the mediastinum are "shifting" and "widening." Mediastinal structures, usually the trachea, bronchi, and heart, can shift with atelectasis, with the shift directed toward the alveolar collapse. Pneumothorax also can shift the mediastinum away from the area of involvement. A widening of the mediastinum can indicate several pathologic conditions, such as cardiomegaly, aneurysms, or aortic disruption. Bleeding into the mediastinum, following chest trauma or cardiac surgery, also may cause widening of the mediastinum.

Heart size can be estimated easily by measuring the cardiothoracic ratio on a PA film. The heart diameter normally is 50% or less of the thoracic diameter to the inside of the ribs on full inspiration. This method for determining normal heart size cannot be used when viewing AP chest x-rays, the most common type taken of the critically ill.

The lung fields should be assessed for any areas of increased density (whiteness) or increased radiolucency (blackness) which can indicate an abnormality. Density increases when water, pus, or blood accumulates in the lung. Increased radiolucency is caused by increased air in the lungs, as may occur with COPD. A fine line present on the right side of the lung at the sixth rib level (midlung) is a normal finding, representing the horizontal fissure separating the right upper and middle lobes.

Invasive Lines

Chest x-rays are frequently obtained in critical care to confirm proper placement of invasive equipment (endotracheal tubes, central venous and pulmonary artery catheters, intraaortic balloons, nasogastric tubes, chest tubes). All invasive tubes have radiopaque lines running the length of the tube which are visible on the x-ray (Figure 13–4). When in the proper position, an endotracheal tube should be 2 to 4 cm above the carina. Look for a thin white line in the trachea and follow it down to the level of the clavicles and measure the space between the end of the tube and the carina. In some patients the tip of the endotracheal tube will be slightly less that 2 cm above the carina to ensure that the inflated balloon is below the vocal cords.

Identify all white lines and follow their paths. The nasogastric tube should run the length of the esophagus with the tip of the tube in the stomach. The stomach can be identified by the radiolucency just under the diaphragm on the left side, which is called the gastric air bubble. Pulmonary artery catheters should be viewed running through the right atrium and right ventricle into the pulmonary artery. These can be difficult to identify at first, but be sure and look at both sides of the hila (right and left pulmonary arteries found on either side of the mediastinum).

Identify all items in the chest, such as temporary or permanent pacing wires, pacing generators, automatic

TABLE 13–3. CHEST X-RAY FINDINGS

Assessed Area	Usual Adult Findings	Remarks
Trachea	Midline, translucent, tubelike structure found in the anterior mediastinal cavity	Deviation from the midline suggests tension, pneumothorax, atelectasis, pleural effusion, mass, or collapsed lung
Clavicles	Present in upper thorax and are equally distant from sternum	Malalignment or break indicates fracture
Ribs	Thoracic cavity encasement	Widening of intercostal spaces indicates emphysema; malalignment or break indicates fractured sternum or ribs
Mediastinum	Shadowy-appearing space between the lungs that widens at the hilum	Deviation to either side may indicate pleural effusion, fibrosis, or collapsed lung
Heart	Solid-appearing structure with clear edges visible in the left anterior mediastinal cavity; heart should be less than one-half the width of the chest wall on a posteroanterior film	Shift may indicate atelectasis or tension pneumothorax; if heart is greater than one-half the chest wall width, congestive heart failure or pericardial fluid may be present
Carina	The lowest tracheal cartilage at which the bronchi bifurcate	If the end of the endotracheal tube is seen 3 cm above the carina, it is in the correct position
Main-stem bronchus	The translucent, tubelike structure visible to approximately 2.5 cm from hilum	Densities may indicate bronchogenic cyst
Hilum	Small, white, bilateral densities present where the bronchi join the lungs; left hilum should be 2 to 3 cm higher than the right hilum	A shift to either side indicates atelectasis; accentuated shadows may indicate emphysema or pulmonary abscess
Bronchi (other than main stem)	Not usually visible	If visible, may indicate bronchial pneumonia
Lung fields	Usually not completely visible except as fine white areas from hilum; fields should be clear as normal lung tissue is radiolucent; normal "lung markings" should be present to the periphery	If visible, may indicate atelectasis; patchy densities may be signs of resolving pneumonia, silicosis, or fibrosis; nasogastric tubes, pulmonary artery catheters, and chest tubes will appear as shadows and their positions should be noted
Diaphragm	Rounded structures visible at the bottom of the lung fields; right side is 1 to 2 cm higher than the left; the costophrenic angles should be clear and sharp	An elevated diaphragm may indicate pneumonia, pleurisy, acute bronchitis, or atelectasis; a flattened diaphragm suggests chronic obstructive pulmonary disease; unilateral elevation indicates a pneumothorax or pulmonary infection; the presence of scarring or fluid causes blunting of costophrenic angles; 300 to 500 ml of pleural fluid must be present before blunting is seen

From: Talbot I, Meyers-Marquardt M: Pocket guide to critical assessment. *St. Louis, MO: CV Mosby, 1990.*

implantable defibrillators, chest tubes, and surgical wires or clips.

Helpful Hints

Chest x-rays should be taken after every attempt to insert central venous catheters to detect the presence of an accidental pneumothorax. A common error is to mistake the scapulae for a pneumothorax, especially on AP views.

Two common abnormal x-ray signs frequently discussed are the silhouette sign and the air bronchogram. In order for any structure to be visible, the density of its edge must contrast with the surrounding density. The loss of contrast is called the silhouette sign. It means that two structures of the same density have come in contact with each other and the borders are lost. For example, the heart is a water density, so if the alveoli near the left heart border fill with fluid, the two densities are the same and there will be a loss of contrast and no left heart border. An air bronchogram is air showing through a greater density, such as

water. Normally, the bronchi are not seen on a normal chest x-ray, except for the main-stem bronchi, because they have thin walls, contain air, and are surrounded by air in the alveoli (two structures of the same density). If water surrounds the bronchi, as in pneumonia and pulmonary edema, then the bronchi filled with air will be in contrast to the water density and will be visible.

Computed Tomography and Magnetic Resonance Imaging

Computed tomography (CT) and magnetic resonance imaging (MRI) allow for the three-dimensional examination of the chest in situations where two-dimensional chest x-rays are insufficient. CT and MRI are particularly advantageous over chest x-rays to evaluate mediastinal and pleural abnormalities, particularly those with fluid collections. Pleural effusions or empyemas, malpositioned or occluded chest tubes, mediastinal hematomas, and mediastinitis are problems for which CT and MRI are more sensitive than chest x-rays.

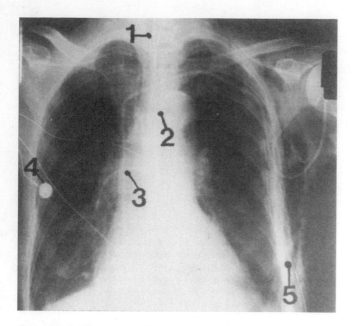

Figure 13–4. Chest x-ray with markers identifying invasive devices. (1) Endotracheal tube, (2) nasogastric tube, (3) pulmonary artery catheter in right pulmonary artery, (4) ECG electrode, and (5) chest tube. *(From: Sanchez F: Fundamentals of chest x-ray interpretation.* Critical Care Nurse. *1986; 6(5):60.)*

The need for transportation to the radiology department and positioning restrictions within the scanning devices pose certain risks to critically ill patients. Of particular concern is the automatic movement of patients during the procedure into and out of the scanning device. Accidental disconnection of invasive devices can easily occur if additional tubing lengths and potential obstructions are not considered. Decreased visualization of patients during the procedures requires vigilant monitoring of cardiovascular and respiratory parameters and devices, as well as establishing a method for conscious patients to alert nearby clinicians in case of difficulties. The strong magnetic field of MRI units may interfere with ventilator performance and necessitate manual ventilation, leading to potential alterations in arterial blood gas values.

MRI testing can be a frightening experience for the patient. Anxiety-related reactions, occurring in up to almost one-third of patients, range from mild apprehension to severe anxiety. These reactions can result in cancellation of the test or interference with its results. It is suggested that all patients receive basic information regarding the MRI procedure, including details of the small chamber they will be placed in, the noise and temperature they will experience, and the duration of the procedure. If possible, use of the prone position, some form of relaxation or music tape, and the presence of a family member or friend should be considered. In addition, short-acting anxiolytics should be used for patients who need them.

Pulmonary Angiograms

Pulmonary angiograms are one of the most sensitive tools for diagnosis of pulmonary emboli. Through a catheter advanced into the pulmonary artery, contrast material is injected during rapid filming. Emboli appear as filling defects, or dark circumscribed areas, within the white vascular images of the artery.

The invasive nature of this diagnostic test, coupled with potential reactions to the contrast material, restricts its use to situations where other less invasive tests (e.g., clinical signs or symptoms, ventilation-perfusion scans) are ambiguous.

End-Tidal CO$_2$ Monitoring

Measurement of the carbon dioxide level of exhaled gases provides a reasonable estimate of arterial carbon dioxide (PaCO_2) levels. This is accomplished by capnometry, in which a special sensor, connected into the ventilatory circuit close to the endotracheal tube, sends infrared light through the exhaled gas to a photodetector on the other side of the tube (Figure 13–5). CO$_2$ levels are then continuously displayed by the microprocessing unit in a graphic pattern, or capnogram.

Capnography is useful especially as a visual trending tool, alerting clinicians to potential changes in PaCO_2 levels. Changes in metabolic rates and alveolar ventilation, gas leaks, and ventilator equipment problems are clinical situations in which capnography can provide an early indication of PaCO_2 changes. End-tidal CO$_2$ monitoring does not accurately reflect PaCO_2 levels, so it should be used as an adjunct to arterial blood gas (ABG) analysis, not as a replacement. A variety of clinical situations may lead to distortions of the readings this noninvasive monitoring device (e.g., airway secretions), limiting its use to primarily that of a trend-monitoring tool.

PATHOLOGIC CONDITIONS

Acute Respiratory Failure

Each of the case studies below represents a common situation in a critical care unit—respiratory dysfunction. This rapid onset of respiratory impairment (that is, severe enough to cause potential or actual morbidity or mortality if untreated) is termed *acute respiratory failure* (ARF). Although the origin of the respiratory failure may be a medical or surgical problem, the management approaches share similar features.

Acute respiratory failure is a change in respiratory gas exchange (CO$_2$ and O$_2$) such that normal cellular function is jeopardized. Acute respiratory failure is defined as a PaO_2 < 60 mm Hg and PaCO_2 > 50 mm Hg. Actual PaO_2 and PaCO_2 values which define acute respiratory failure

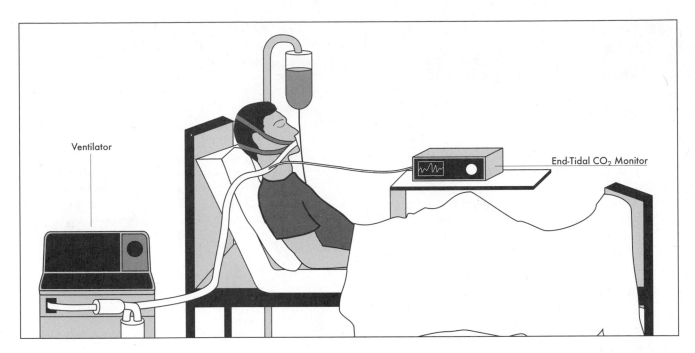

Figure 13–5. End-tidal CO_2 monitor.

vary, depending on a variety of factors that influence the patient's normal (or baseline) arterial blood gas values. Factors such as age, altitude, chronic cardiopulmonary disease, or metabolic disturbances may alter the "normal" blood gas values for an individual, requiring an adjustment

to the classic definition of acute respiratory failure. For example, if PaO_2 levels in a 75-year-old male living in Denver are normally 56 mm Hg, acute respiratory failure would not be diagnosed until PaO_2 levels have decreased to 50 mm Hg or less.

AT THE BEDSIDE
▶ *Motor Vehicle Accident (MVA)*

Gary B., 22 years old, was admitted to the surgical ICU following a motor vehicle accident in which he suffered blunt chest trauma, bilateral fractured femurs, and a concussion. During his second day in the unit, his arterial blood gases began deteriorating (decreases in PaO_2, increases in $PaCO_2$), and he required increasing amounts of supplemental oxygen to maintain PaO_2 levels > 60 mm Hg. Gary was dyspneic, restless, and somewhat agitated. He verbalized a fear of impending death.

	Admission	Day 2
Respiration rate	24/minute	34/minute
Chest x-ray	clear	infiltrates
ABGs	40% FM	100% FM
PaO_2	120 mm Hg	58 mm Hg
$PaCO_2$	33 mm Hg	30 mm Hg
pH	7.42	7.51
HCO_3	24 mEq/L	21 mEq/L

AT THE BEDSIDE
▶ *Postanesthesia*

Mrs. A. was admitted to the surgical ICU following thoracic surgery for the removal of a malignant tumor of the right upper lobe. She was intubated and was being manually ventilated by the anesthesiologist with a manual resuscitation bag (MRB) with 10 L/minute of O_2 inflow. A right pleural chest tube was draining minimal amounts of blood, with no evidence of air leaks or obstructions.

Mrs. A. was unresponsive to verbal and pain stimulation on admission. No spontaneous respirations were noted after a brief period of disconnection from the MRB. Fifteen minutes after initiation of mechanical ventilation (SIMV of 10 breaths/minute, TV of 10 ml/kg, PEEP of 5 cm H_2O, 0.40 FIO_2), ABGs were:

PaO_2	145 mm Hg
$PaCO_2$	41 mm Hg
pH	7.38
HCO_3	24 mEq/L

Etiology, Risk Factors, and Pathophysiology

Many abnormalities can lead to acute respiratory failure (Table 13–4). Regardless of the specific underlying cause, the pathophysiology of acute respiratory failure can be organized into four main components: impaired ventilation, impaired gas exchange, airway obstruction, and ventilation-perfusion abnormalities.

Impaired Ventilation

Conditions that disrupt the muscles of respiration or their neurologic control can impair ventilation and lead to acute respiratory failure (Table 13–4). Decreased or absent respiratory muscle movement may be due to fatigue from excessive use, atrophy from disuse, inflammation of nerves, nerve damage (e.g., surgical damage to the vagus nerve during cardiac surgery), or CNS depression, or following administration of neuromuscular blocking agents. Impaired respiratory muscle movement decreases movement of gas into the lungs, resulting in alveolar hypoventilation. Inadequate alveolar ventilation causes retention of CO_2 and hypoxemia.

Impaired Gas Exchange

Conditions that damage the alveolar-capillary membrane impair gas exchange. Direct damage to the cells lining the alveoli may be caused by inhalation of toxic substances (gases or gastric contents), leading to two detrimental alveolar changes. The first is an increase in alveolar permeability, increasing the potential for interstitial fluid to leak into

the alveoli and cause noncardiac pulmonary edema (Figure 13–6A). The second alveolar change is a decrease in surfactant production by alveolar type II cells, increasing alveolar surface tension, which leads to alveolar collapse (Figure 13–6B).

Another cause of impaired gas exchange occurs when fluid leaks from the intravascular space into the pulmonary interstitial space (Figure 13–6C). The excess fluid increases the distance between the alveolus and the capillary, decreasing the efficiency of the gas exchange process. The interstitial edema also compresses the bronchial airways, which are surrounded by interstitial tissue, causing bronchoconstriction. Capillary leakage may occur when pressures within the cardiovascular system are excessively

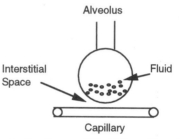

A. Leakage of Fluid into Alveolus

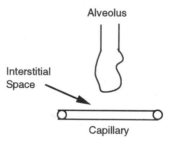

B. Atelectasis

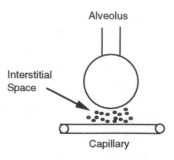

C. Interstitial Edema

Figure 13–6. Pathophysiologic processes in acute respiratory failure due to impaired gas exchange. (A) Increased alveolar membrane permeability. (B) Alveolar collapse from decreased surfactant production. (C) Increased capillary membrane permeability and interstitial edema.

TABLE 13–4. CAUSES OF ACUTE RESPIRATORY FAILURE IN ADULTS

Impaired Ventilation
Spinal cord injury (C-4 or higher)
Phrenic nerve damage
Neuromuscular blockade
Guillain-Barré syndrome
CNS depression
   Drug overdoses (narcotics, sedatives, illicit drugs)
   Increased intracranial pressure
   Anesthetic agents
Respiratory muscle fatigue

Impaired Gas Exchange
Pulmonary edema
Adult respiratory distress syndrome (ARDS)
Aspiration pneumonia

Airway Obstruction
Aspiration of foreign body
Thoracic tumors
Asthma
Bronchitis
Pneumonia

Ventilation-Perfusion Abnormalities
Pulmonary embolism
Emphysema

high (e.g., in heart failure) or when pathologic conditions elsewhere in the body release biochemical substances (e.g., serotonin, endotoxin) which increase capillary permeability.

Airway Obstruction

Conditions that obstruct airways increase resistance to airflow into the lungs, causing alveolar hypoventilation and decreased gas exchange (Figure 13–7). Airway obstructions can be due to conditions that: (1) block the inner airway lumen (e.g., excessive secretions or fluid in the airways, inhaled foreign bodies), (2) increase airway wall thickness (e.g., edema or fibrosis) or decrease airway circumference (e.g., bronchoconstriction) as occurs in asthma, or (3) increase peribronchial compression of the airway (e.g., enlarged lymph nodes, interstitial edema, tumors).

Ventilation-Perfusion Abnormalities

Conditions disrupting alveolar ventilation or capillary perfusion lead to an imbalance in ventilation and perfusion. This decreases the efficiency of the respiratory gas exchange process. In an effort to keep the ventilation and perfusion ratios balanced, two compensatory changes occur: (1) to avoid wasted alveolar ventilation when capillary perfusion is decreased (e.g., with pulmonary embolism), bronchiolar constriction occurs to limit ventilation to alveoli with poor or absent capillary perfusion (Figure 13–8B); (2) to avoid capillary perfusion of alveoli that are not adequately ventilated (e.g., with atelectasis), arteriole constriction occurs and shunts blood away from hypoventilated alveoli to normally ventilated alveoli (Figure 13–8C). As the number of alveolar-capillary units affected by these compensatory changes increases, gas exchange eventually is affected negatively.

Each of these pathophysiologic changes results in inadequate CO_2 removal and/or O_2 absorption. The severity of acute respiratory failure can be further increased when anxiety and fear of impending death develop, a common consequence of severe dyspnea and hypoxemia. These symptoms increase oxygen demands and the work of breathing, further compromising O_2 availability for crucial organ function and depleting respiratory muscle strength.

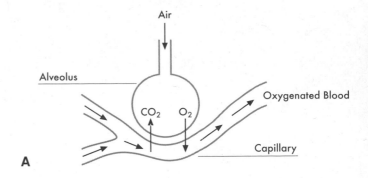

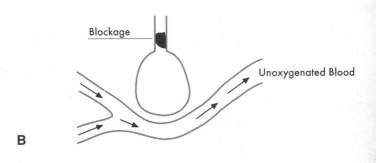

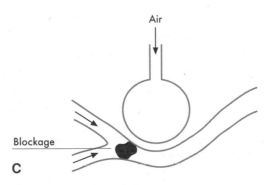

Figure 13–8. Pathophysiologic processes in acute respiratory failure from ventilation-perfusion abnormalities. (A) Normal ventilation and perfusion relationship. (B) Decreased ventilation and normal perfusion. (C) Normal ventilation and decreased perfusion.

Clinical Presentation

Signs and Symptoms

Hypoxemia (PaO_2 < 60 mm Hg)

- Restlessness
- Dyspnea
- Confusion
- Anxiety
- Tachypnea
- Tachycardia
- Diaphoresis

Hypercarbia ($PaCO_2$ > 50 mm Hg)

- Hypertension
- Irritability
- Somnolence (late)
- Cyanosis (late)
- Loss of consciousness (late)

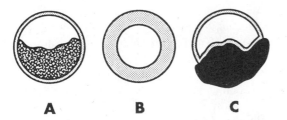

Figure 13–7. Mechanism of airway obstruction. (A) Fluid secretions present within airway. (B) Intraluminal edema narrowing airway diameter. (C) Peribronchial compression of airway.

Pallor or cyanosis of skin
Use of accessory muscles of respiration
Abnormal breath sounds (rales, rhonchi, wheezes)
Manifestations of primary disease (see description of individual diseases below)

Diagnostic Tests

- Arterial blood gases—PaO_2 < 60 mm Hg and $PaCO_2$ > 50 mm Hg; or PaO_2 and $PaCO_2$ in abnormal range for that individual.
- Tests specific to underlying cause (see description of individual diseases below).

AT THE BEDSIDE

Gary: "I remember feeling panicky, couldn't catch my breath, feeling all closed in. The room was too hot. That mask on my face was suffocating me. All I wanted to do was get outside so I could breathe easier."

Patient Needs and Principles of Management

The management of the patient in acute respiratory failure revolves around four primary areas: improvement of oxygenation and ventilation, treatment of the underlying disease state, reduction of anxiety, and prevention and management of complications.

▶ Improvement of Oxygenation and Ventilation

Most causes of acute respiratory failure are treatable, with a return of normal respiratory function following resolution of the pathophysiologic condition. Aggressive support of respiratory function is required, however, until there is resolution of the underlying condition.

1. Provide supplemental O_2 to maintain PaO_2 > 60 mm Hg. The use of noninvasive methods for O_2 administration (nasal cannula or face masks) is preferable if acceptable PaO_2 levels can be achieved. Continued hypoxemia despite noninvasive O_2 delivery methods necessitates intubation and mechanical ventilation.
2. Improve ventilation with the administration of bronchodilators, mucolytic agents, and other airway management modalities (chest physiotherapy, suctioning, positioning) as indicated.
3. Intubate and initiate mechanical ventilation if noninvasive methods fail to correct hypoxemia and hypercarbia or if cardiovascular instability develops. The mode of mechanical ventilation, rate, and tidal volume vary depending on the underlying cause of respiratory failure and a variety of clinical factors. Modes of ventilation which decrease the work of breathing (control, assist/control, synchro-

nized intermittent ventilation [SIMV] with high minute ventilation [MV] rates, pressure support [PS]) will typically be used for the first 24 hours since respiratory muscle fatigue is common. Positive end expiratory pressure (PEEP) levels > 5 cm H_2O may be required if FIO_2 levels > 0.6 are needed to eliminate hypoxemia. Closely monitor the cardiovascular status during increases of PEEP, which may decrease venous return and cardiac output. Neuromuscular blockade may be needed initially to prevent ineffective respiratory efforts by the patient and to maximize gas exchange.
4. During suctioning, closely observe for signs and symptoms of hypoxemia (decreases in SaO_2; increases in heart rate, respiratory rate, restlessness, diaphoresis, and arrhythmias). Use of a PEEP valve on the manual resuscitation bag (MRB) when ventilator PEEP levels are > 5 cm H_2O, and use of an MRB which delivers 100% O_2 may be necessary to prevent cardiopulmonary changes during suctioning. If changes still occur despite these interventions, it may be necessary to keep the patient on the ventilator during hyperoxygenation and suction through a special endotracheal tube adaptor. Suctioning should only be performed when clinically indicated, and never on a routine schedule.
5. Prior to intrahospital transport, verify adequacy of ventilatory support equipment to maintain cardiopulmonary stability. Verify that PEEP on the transport equipment is maintained. Some ventilators used for transport do not have the capability to provide more advanced ventilatory modes (e.g., PS, reverse I:E ratio).

▶ Treatment of Underlying Disease State

Correction of the underlying cause of the acute respiratory failure should be done as soon as possible. See the specific management approaches for each disease state later in the chapter.

▶ Reduction of Anxiety

1. Maintain a calm, supportive environment to avoid unnecessary escalation of anxiety. Give brief explanations of activities and approaches being done to relieve ARF. Vigilance and presence of health care providers during anxiety periods is crucial to avoid panic by patients and visiting family members.
2. Teach diaphragmatic breathing to slow the rate and increase the depth of respirations. Place one hand on the patient's abdomen. Instruct the patient to inhale deeply, causing the hand on the abdomen to rise. During exhalation, have the patient feel the hand on the belly sink down toward the spine. Explain that the chest should not be moving at all. After a minute or two, ask the patient to place his or her hands on the belly to continue the exercise. Guide the patient in a relaxation breathing script (Table 13–5) to control the rate and depth of respirations and reduce anxiety. This exercise may be followed by listening to soothing music of the patient's choice to deepen the level of relaxation.

AT THE BEDSIDE

Primary Nurse: "I could see that Gary's anxiety and fear were increasing his respiratory difficulties. He seemed panicked by his lack of control over his breathing. As we waited for the medical management modalities to relieve his pulmonary abnormalities, I knew it would be critical to decrease Gary's anxiety and fear. Using simple, brief directions, I guided him in some diaphragmatic breathing and relaxation exercises to slow his inspirations and reduce his anxiety. I also made sure that someone was always in the room with him until we got his hypoxemia corrected. Having his mom or dad there was a great support for Gary, and for me when I had to briefly leave the room to get supplies or such. I even taught his parents how to do relaxation exercises with Gary."

3. Administer mild doses of anxiolytics (i.e., lorazepam or diazepam) which do not depress respiration. To enhance the placebo response of the anxiolytic, explain the purpose of the medication and have the patient imagine the medication flowing through the bloodstream to relax each muscle in the body. Diaphragmatic breathing exercises should also be continued.

▶ Prevention and Management of Complications

1. *Ventilator and neuromuscular blockade related:* See Chapter 6, Airway and Ventilatory Management, for detailed management strategies.
2. *Pulmonary aspiration:* Provide continuous gastric aspiration, and ensure proper inflation of ET cuff at all times. Refer to additional prevention strategies for nosocomial pneumonia on page 290.
3. *Gastrointestinal bleeding:* Check gastric aspirate for presence of occult blood every 8 to 12 hours. Protect gastric mucosa in high-risk patients with nonalkalinizing gastric protective agents (e.g., sucralfate).
4. *Barotrauma:* Avoid unnecessary increases in airway pressures (e.g., "bucking" the ventilator, excessive coughing) and assess for signs and symptoms of pneumothorax, pneumomediastinum, and other barotrauma complications. See Chapter 6, Airway and Ventilatory Management, for additional strategies.

TABLE 13–5. RELAXATION BREATHING SCRIPT

Purpose: To slow respiratory rate and increase depth of breathing.
Time: 3 to 5 minutes

Begin with diaphragmatic breathing and continue with a short head-to-toe relaxation script (see Chapter 8, Alternative Therapies).

Relaxation Breathing Script

". . . now return your concentration to your breathing. Slow diaphragmatic breathing . . . letting your belly blow up like a balloon as you inhale and letting it sink back to your spine as you exhale. This is the kind of relaxed breathing we do each night before we fall asleep. Feel the relaxation . . . As you feel the air moving in your nose, down the back of your throat, and into your lungs, hear yourself saying way in the back of your mind . . . 'One . . . feel the air moving slowly back out as your belly sinks back to your spine.' As your next breath fills your lungs, hear yourself saying deep inside of you . . . 'Two . . . Feel the air moving slowly back out.' As you take the next breath deep into your lungs, hear yourself saying deep inside of you . . . 'Three . . . And feel the air moving back out.' As you inhale your next breath, hear yourself saying deep inside of you . . . 'Four. Start this cycle over.' Repeat this cycle as often as you wish . . . counting one to four . . . and then start over again."

Acute Respiratory Distress Syndrome (ARDS)

The case study of Gary B., presented at the beginning of the section on pathologic conditions, is typical of a patient who develops acute respiratory distress syndrome (ARDS). ARDS is an acute physiologic syndrome characterized by noncardiac pulmonary edema caused by increased alveolar capillary membrane permeability. ARDS is one of the most lethal of the diseases or syndromes that lead to respiratory failure.

Etiology, Risk Factors, and Pathophysiology

The risk factors for the development of ARDS can be categorized into conditions that lead to direct damage to the alveolar-capillary membrane (primary causes) and those that are thought to be mediated by cellular or humoral injury to the capillary endothelial wall (secondary causes) (Table 13–6). Whether primary or secondary causes, the pathological processes involved in ARDS are characterized by excessive alveolar-capillary membrane permeability, interstitial edema, and diffuse alveolar injury (Figure 13–6). Direct damage to the alveolar membrane can easily occur when toxic substances are inhaled, such as during fires or chemical spills.

TABLE 13–6. PRIMARY AND SECONDARY CAUSES OF ARDS

Primary Causes (Direct Damage to the Alveolar Membrane)
Aspiration of gastric contents
Pulmonary contusion
Near drowning
Inhalation of smoke or toxic substances
Diffuse pneumonias (viral and bacterial)

Secondary Causes (Mediated by Cellular or Humoral Injury to the Capillary Endothelium)
Systemic sepsis
Hypovolemic shock associated with chest trauma or sepsis
Acute pancreatitis
Fat emboli
Trauma
DIC
Massive blood transfusions

Alveolar and interstitial edema, microatelectasis, and ventilation-perfusion mismatching in ARDS lead to severe hypoxemia and poor lung compliance ("stiff lungs"). In the setting of trauma and sepsis, this abnormality in microvascular permeability occurs in capillary beds throughout the body. Typically, this multiorgan disorder is not clinically apparent, with clinical manifestations isolated to the respiratory system. When multisystem organ failure (MSOF) does occur, it is seen in ARDS patients who develop bacterial infections and sepsis (see Chapter 14, Multisystem Problems).

The development of a gram-negative pulmonary infection is a frequent sequela of ARDS. The ARDS process disrupts normal macrophage function and increases the risk of infection.

Mortality from ARDS is high, frequently occurring several days to weeks after the onset of the syndrome.

Clinical Presentation

Signs and Symptoms

- Dyspnea
- Tachypnea (rates often > 40/min)
- Intercostal retractions
- Copious secretions
- Panic, fear of impending death
- Rales and/or rhonchi

Diagnostic Tests

- Chest x-ray shows diffuse, bilateral pulmonary infiltrates without increased cardiac size
- $PaO_2/PAO_2 < 0.2$
- PCWP < 18 mm Hg
- Static compliance (TV/[inspiratory plateau pressure − PEEP]) < 40 ml/cm H_2O

Patient Needs and Principles of Management

Much of the management of ARDS relies on supportive care and the prevention of complications. To date, interventions to limit the disease progression or reverse the underlying structural defects are not known.

▶ Improvement of Oxygenation and Ventilation

Interventions specific to ARDS to improve oxygenation and ventilation include the following:

1. Administer high FIO_2 levels with a high-flow system or rebreathing mask. A constant positive airway pressure (CPAP) mask may be tolerated in alert, cooperative patients. Continuous, vigilant monitoring for contraindications of noninvasive CPAP (decreased LOC, nausea/vomiting, increased dyspnea, or panic) is imperative.
2. Intubation and mechanical ventilation are necessary if CV instability is present, severe hypoxemia persists, or fatigue develops.

- Begin oxygen support at an F_{IO_2} of 1.0 with PEEP at a level to achieve an acceptable Pa_{O_2} (> 50 mm Hg) without hemodynamic compromise. Decrease F_{IO_2} levels to < 0.6 once Pa_{O_2} is > 50 mm Hg, and then decrease PEEP support.
- Decrease the work of breathing by using assist-control or SIMV modes with initially high rates.
- Adjust TV, inspiratory flow rates, and PEEP levels to keep peak airway pressures < 45 cm H_2O, if possible.

3. Muscle relaxation and/or sedation may be required for intubation and for the first 24 to 48 hours after intubation to maximize gas exchange. "Fighting the ventilator" is a common complication of ventilatory support in the severely dyspneic, hypoxemic patient.

4. Decrease oxygen consumption by minimizing fever, activity level, and respiratory effort.

5. Improve oxygen-carrying capacity with transfusions for hemoglobin levels below normal.

6. Minimize suctioning the airway to avoid oxygen desaturation and risk of nosocomial pneumonia. Use of closed system suctioning may be necessary if desaturation is severe during suctioning, particularly in patients on high levels of PEEP and F_{IO_2}.

▶ Reduction of Anxiety

These measures are the same as those previously described for ARF management.

▶ Achievement of Effective Communications

Refer to Chapter 6, Airway and Ventilatory Management, for a detailed discussion of communication techniques for intubated patients.

▶ Maintain Hemodynamic Stability and Adequate Perfusion

1. Minimize CV instability by careful monitoring during PEEP therapy and administration of fluids to correct hypovolemia.

2. Vasoactive drugs may be required to maintain adequate perfusion.

▶ Prevention of Complications

In addition to complications listed for ARF:

1. ARDS patients are at higher risk for development of nosocomial pneumonias. Follow the prevention strategies delineated for nosocomial pneumonias below. Prophylactic antibiotics have not been shown to decrease nosocomial pneumonia rates in ARDS patients. Meticulous attention to hand washing and removal of invasive devices as soon as possible are key prevention strategies.

2. The incidence of barotrauma, pulmonary embolism, GI bleeding, and electrolyte disorders is particularly high in ARDS.

Pneumonia

Respiratory infection is a common cause of acute respiratory failure. Infections developed before hospitalization (community-acquired) and those acquired during hospitalization (nosocomial) can lead to significant morbidity and mortality, and require critical care management. The mortality rate exceeds 50% for severe, community-acquired pneumonias, and ranges from 30% to 60% for critically ill patients who develop a nosocomial pneumonia.

A variety of respiratory infections occur in critically ill patients, including bronchitis, asthma, and pneumonia. This section focuses on pneumonia, the most common respiratory infection and the most common cause of respiratory failure in critically ill patients.

Etiology, Risk Factors, and Pathophysiology

At high risk for the development of pneumonia are the young, the elderly, those with chronic cardiopulmonary disease, and immunocompromised individuals. In addition, immobility, decreased level of consciousness, and intubation place hospitalized patients at high risk for development of nosocomial pneumonias.

The major routes of entry of causative organisms are aspiration of oropharyngeal or gastric contents into the lung, inhalation of aerosols or particles containing the organisms, and hematogenous spread of the organism into the lung from another site in the body (Figure 13–9). Most pneumonias are due to aspiration of bacteria colonizing the oropharynx or upper GI tract. Pneumonia develops when the normal bronchomucociliary clearance mechanism or phagocytic cells are overwhelmed by the number or virulence of organisms aspirated or inhaled into the airways. The proliferation of organisms in the pulmonary parenchyma elicits an inflammatory response, with large influxes of phagocytic cells into the alveoli and airways and production of protein-rich exudates. This inflammatory response impairs the distribution of ventilation and decreases lung compliance, resulting in increased work of breathing and the sensation of dyspnea. Hypoxemia results from the shunting of blood through poorly ventilated areas of pulmonary consolidation. The inflammatory response leads to fever and leukocytosis.

Pneumonia also can develop through hematogenous spread, when organisms remote from the lungs gain access to the blood, become lodged in the pulmonary vasculature, and proliferate. Pneumonias with a hematogenous origin usually are distributed diffusely in both lung fields, rather than localized to a single lung or lobe.

Several factors present in critically ill patients increase the risk for the development of nosocomial pneumonia. Aspiration of oropharyngeal and gastric secretions is increased in the presence of endotracheal tubes, nasogastric tubes, poor GI motility, gastric distention, and immobility; all of these are common situations in critically ill patients.

Treatments that neutralize the normally acidic gastric contents, such as antacids, H_2 blockers, or tube feeding, allow increased growth of gram-negative bacteria in gastric contents. This increases the potential for aspiration of gram-negative bacteria and hematogenous spread.

The high frequency of gastric and pulmonary intubation further increases the risk for pneumonia. Within 24 hours of admission to a critical care unit, there is colonization of the pharynx with gram-negative bacteria. Approximately 25% of colonized patients develop a clinical infection (tracheobronchitis or pneumonia). Critically ill patients at high risk for nosocomial pneumonias are those immunocompromised from malignancy, AIDS, and chronic cardiac or respiratory disease; the elderly; or those with depressed alveolar macrophage function (oxygen, corticosteroids). Frequent changes in ventilatory equipment also increase the risk for nosocomial pneumonias in patients on ventilators.

While a variety of similar organisms cause community- and hospital-acquired pneumonias, their frequency distribution is different (Table 13–7). Of particular concern in hospital-acquired infections is the polymicrobial origin of the pneumonia and the potential for causative organisms to be resistant to antimicrobial therapy.

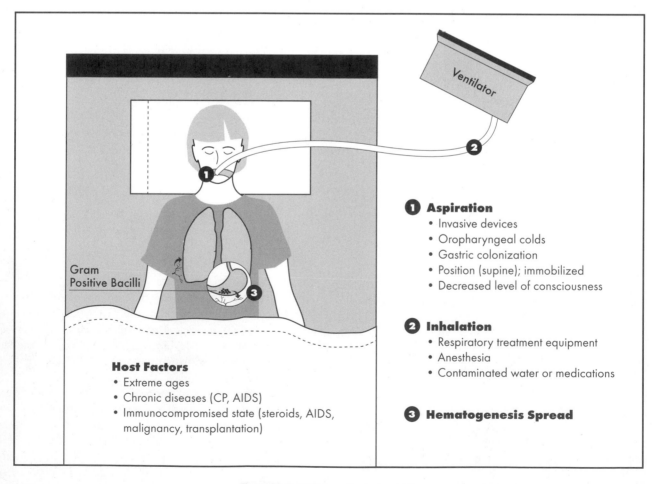

Figure 13–9. Pathogenesis of pneumonia.

TABLE 13–7. INFECTIOUS ETIOLOGIC AGENTS IMPLICATED IN SEVERE COMMUNITY-ACQUIRED PNEUMONIA REQUIRING ICU SUPPORT AND BACTERIAL CAUSES OF NOSOCOMIAL PNEUMONIA IN ICU PATIENTS

Etiologic Agent	Frequency, %	Antibiotic
Community-Acquired Pneumonias		
Streptococcus pneumoniae	40	Penicillin G
Haemophilus influenzae	5	Ampicillin or cefuroxime
Staphylococcus aureus	10	Nafcillin or vancomycin for resistant strains
Enterobacteriaceae	10	Cefotaximine and gentamicin
Legionella pneumophila	10	Erythromycin and rifampin
Mycoplasma pneumoniae	5	Erythromycin
Viral	2	
Lung abscess	10	Penicillin and metronidazole
Nosocomial Pneumonias		
Enterobacteriaceae	30–50	Cefotaximine and gentamicin
Staphylococcus aureus	10–30	Nafcillin or vancomycin for resistant strains
Pseudomonas aeruginosa	10–20	Piperacillin
Streptococci	10–15	Penicillin
Legionella spp.	5–15	Erythromycin and rifampin
Haemophilus influenzae	2–10	Ampicillin or cefuroxime
Anerobes	2–5	Penicillin and metronidazole

Adapted from: Hall JB, Schmidt GA, Woods LD (eds.): Principles of critical care. New York: McGraw-Hill, 1992, pp. 1250, 1260, 1261. With permission.

Clinical Presentation

Signs and Symptoms

- Fever
- Cough, typically productive
- Purulent sputum or hemoptysis
- Dyspnea
- Pleuritic chest pain
- Tachypnea
- Rales
- Abnormal breath sounds (rales, bronchial breath sounds)

Diagnostic Tests

- Gram stain and culture of sputum for causative organisms. May require fiberoptic bronchoscopy with brush specimen or bronchoalveolar lavage specimen retrieval in situations where pneumonia responds poorly to treatment.
- Infiltrates on chest x-ray. Infiltrates may be either localized or diffuse in nature.
- Elevated WBC
- Abnormal arterial blood gases (hypoxemia, hypocapnia)

Patient Needs and Principles of Management

▶ Treatment of Underlying Disease

Appropriate antimicrobial therapy should be initiated based on likely causative organisms until definitive culture results are obtained (Table 13–7). Fluid should be administered to correct hypovolemia and hypotension, if present. Hypotension that is unresponsive to fluid therapy should alert the clinician to the potential for septic shock.

▶ Improvement of Oxygenation and Ventilation

Similar to ARF management, with the following additions:

1. PEEP and CPAP are unlikely to improve oxygenation in the presence of pneumonia, and may exacerbate the ventilation-perfusion abnormalities associated with pneumonia. These techniques should be used with caution in pneumonia.
2. Voluminous, tenacious repository secretions may require endotracheal intubation to assist with clearance. Chest physiotherapy may be helpful to increase secretion clearance, particularly when lobar atelectasis is present. Fiberoptic bronchoscopy may also be required to assist with secretion management.

▶ Prevention of Nosocomial Pneumonias

In addition to the high morbidity and mortality associated with pneumonia in critically ill patients, high priority must be given to strategies to prevent the development of noso-comial pneumonias. The development of a nosocomial pneumonia in a critically ill patient increases requirements for ventilatory support (MV, oxygen, time). It is estimated that a nosocomial pneumonia increases hospitalization 4 to 10 days, and increases costs by $20,000 to $40,000 per episode. Prevention strategies include the following:

- Decrease the risk of cross-contamination or coloniza-tion via the hands of hospitalized personnel. Hand washing is the most effective strategy. Hospital staff should be vaccinated each year for influenza.
- Minimize tracheal trauma. Suction only when nec-essary to clear secretions from large airways.
- Maintain a closed system on ventilator/humidifier circuits, and avoid pooling of tubing, condensation, or movement into ET tubes. Disinfect and sterilize respiratory equipment and change routine equip-ment according to guidelines. Ventilator circuits should be routinely changed no more frequently than every 48 hours.
- Avoid neutralization of gastric contents with antacids and H_2 blockers. Use nonalkalinizing gas-

tric protective agents (e.g., sucralfate) for patients at high risk for GI bleeding. Since tube feedings also neutralize the gastric contents, duodenal feeding may have some advantage over gastric feedings. Intermittent gastric feeding may be better than con-tinuous to allow gastric acidity to return and decrease gram-negative bacterial overgrowth.
- Systemic or topical application of prophylactic agents to decrease gram-negative bacterial growth has been advocated. However, the benefit has not been clearly established, and costs can be significant.
- Decrease the risk of aspiration. Avoid supine posi-tioning, if possible. Use small-bore gastric/duodenal tubes when possible. Good mouth care is important (particularly in intubated patients), and the orophar-ynx should be suctioned prior to cuff deflation. Early detection and correction of gastric reflux problems and ambulation as soon as possible are important.
- Use sterile technique for endotracheal suctioning.
- Provide nutritional support to improve host defenses.
- Eliminate invasive devices and equipment as soon as possible.

Pulmonary Embolism (PE)

Etiology, Risk Factors, and Pathophysiology

Pulmonary embolism is a complication of deep vein throm-bosis (DVT), long bone fracture, or air entering the circula-tory system. There are many risk factors for pulmonary embolism (Table 13–8), with critically ill patients being especially prone due to the presence of central venous and PA catheters, immobility, use of muscle relaxants, and con-gestive heart failure.

Thromboemboli

Venous thrombi form at the site of vascular injuries or where venous stasis occurs, primarily in the leg or pelvic veins. Thrombi that dislodge travel through the venous cir-culation until they become wedged in a branch of the pul-monary circulation. Depending on the size of the thrombi, and the location of the occlusion, mild to severe obstruction of blood flow occurs beyond the thrombi.

The primary sequela, and major contributor to mortal-ity, of the pulmonary obstruction is circulatory impairment. The physical obstruction of the pulmonary capillary bed increases right ventricular afterload, dilates the right ventri-cle, and impedes coronary perfusion. This predisposes the right ventricle to ischemia and right ventricular failure (cor pulmonale).

A secondary consequence of thromboemboli is a mis-matching of ventilation to perfusion in gas exchange units beyond the obstruction (Figure 13–8C), resulting in arterial hypoxemia. This hypoxemia further compromises oxygen delivery to the ischemic right ventricle.

Air Emboli

Air or other nonabsorbable gases entering the venous system also travel to the right heart, pulmonary circulation, arteri-oles, and capillaries. A variety of surgical and nonsurgical sit-uations predispose patients to the development of air embolization (Table 13–8). Damage to the pulmonary endothelium occurs from the abnormal air-blood interface, leading to increased capillary permeability and alveolar flooding. Bronchoconstriction also occurs with air emboliza-tion. In addition to hypoxemia, P_{CO_2} removal is also impaired.

Arterial embolization may occur if air passes to the left heart through a patent foramen ovale, present in approximately 30% of the population. Peripheral emboliza-tion to the brain, extremities, and coronary perfusion leads to ischemic manifestations in these organs.

Fat Emboli

Fat enters the pulmonary circulation most commonly when released from the bone marrow following long bone frac-tures (Table 13–8). Nontraumatic origins of fat emboliza-

TABLE 13–8. RISK FACTORS FOR DEVELOPMENT OF PULMONARY EMBOLISM

Thromboemboli
Obesity
Prior history of thromboembolism
Advanced age
Malignancy
Estrogen
Immobility
Paralysis
Congestive heart failure
Postpartum
Postsurgical
Posttrauma
Hypercoagulability states
Central venous and PA catheters

Air Emboli
Neurosurgery
Liver transplant
Harrington rod insertion
Open-heart surgery
Arthroscopy
Pacemaker insertion
Cardiopulmonary resuscitation
Gastroscopy
Positive pressure ventilation
Scuba diving
Intravenous infusion
Central venous catheter insertion or removal

Fat Emboli
Long bone fracture
Blunt trauma to liver
Pancreatitis
Lipid infusions
Sickle cell crisis
Burns
Cardiopulmonary bypass
Cyclosporine administration

---

tion also occur and are thought to be due to the agglutination of low-density lipoproteins or liposomes from nutritional fat emulsions. The presence of fat in the pulmonary circulation injures the endothelial lining of the capillary, increasing permeability and alveolar flooding.

Clinical Presentation

The diagnosis of PE is based primarily on clinical signs and symptoms. Since many of the signs and symptoms are nonspecific, PE frequently is difficult to diagnosis. In critically ill patients, diagnosis is especially difficult due to alterations in communication and level of consciousness, and the nonspecific nature of other cardiopulmonary alterations.

Signs and Symptoms

- Dyspnea
- Pleuritic pain
- Apprehension
- Diaphoresis
- Evidence of DVT
- Hemoptysis
- Tachypnea
- Fever
- Tachycardia
- Shock symptoms with large PE

Diagnostic Tests

- Chest x-ray: Evaluate for basilar atelectasis, elevation of the diaphragm, and pleural effusion, although most patients have nonspecific findings on chest x-ray; diffuse alveolar filling in air embolism.
- Arterial blood gas analysis: Hypoxemia with or without hypercarbia.
- ECG: Signs of right ventricular strain (right axis deviation, right bundle branch block) or precordial strain; sinus tachycardia.
- PA pressures: Elevated with a decreased cardiac output.
- Ventilation-perfusion scan: Decreased perfusion to areas with emboli. Scan sensitivity is decreased in intubated patients and in the presence of COPD.
- Pulmonary angiography: Slightly higher risk of complications with this procedure, but sensitivity and specificity are high.

Patient Needs and Principles of Management

The key to preventing morbidity and mortality from pulmonary embolism is early diagnosis and treatment to prevent reembolization. Objectives include the improvement of oxygenation and ventilation, improvement of cardiovascular function, prevention of reembolization, and prevention of pulmonary embolus.

▶ Improvement of Oxygenation and Ventilation

Oxygen therapy is usually very effective in relieving hypoxemia associated with PE. When cardiopulmonary compromise is severe, mechanical ventilation with neuromuscular blockade may be required to achieve optimal oxygenation.

► Improvement of Cardiovascular Function

Controversy exists as to the benefit of vasoactive drug administration (such as norepinephrine and/or inotropic agents) to improve myocardial perfusion of the right ventricle. In severe embolic events, where cardiac failure is profound, additional therapy to hasten clot resolution may be warranted. Surgical removal of a massive pulmonary embolus may be performed when cardiovascular compromise is severe and unresponsive to other modalities, and there are contraindications to thrombolytic therapy.

► Prevention of Reembolization

Several strategies are employed to prevent the likelihood of future embolization and cardiopulmonary compromise:

1. Limiting activity to prevent dislodgement of additional clots.
2. Use of anticoagulation therapy with heparin to maintain a PTT 1.5 to 2.5 times the control when no contraindication exists.
3. Insertion of vena cava filters to prevent emboli from legs, pelvis, and inferior vena cava from migrating to pulmonary circulation. Filters are placed percutaneously in the inferior vena cava (Figure 13–10).

► Prevention of Pulmonary Embolus

- Subcutaneous, low-dose heparin administration in high-risk patients. Routine use of this prevention strategy in critically ill patients who have no contraindications for heparin therapy is thought to decrease PE.
- Sequential compression devices (SCDs) (Table 13–9; Figure 13–11) to prevent venous stasis for high-risk patients (Table 13–8). In high-risk surgical patients, intraoperative application may improve effectiveness.
- Placement of prophylactic vena cava filters in high-risk patients.
- Early fixation of long bone fractures to prevent fat emboli.
- Early mobilization. As soon as hemodynamic stability is achieved, and there are no other contraindications to mobilization, activity level should begin increasing to include sitting in a chair several times/day and short periods of ambulation.

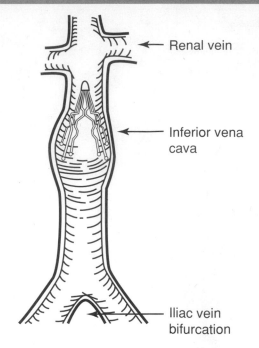

Figure 13–10. Percutaneous introduction of an inferior vena cava filter (Greenfield filter) for pulmonary embolism. *(From: Sticklin LA, Walkenstein M: Vena cava filters: A nursing perspective.* Oncology Nursing Forum *1993;20:509. With permission.)*

TABLE 13–9. TIPS FOR SAFE AND EFFECTIVE USE OF SEQUENTIAL COMPRESSION DEVICES

Contraindications for sequential compression device use:
- Massive leg edema
- Extreme leg deformities
- Arterial ischemia, severe arteriosclerosis
- Inflammation
- Severe phlebitis
- Trauma
- Pulmonary edema
- Skin disorders in legs (rash, ulcers, new skin grafts)

Follow manufacturer's directions carefully to ensure proper sizing of SCD stockings.

Assess frequently for signs of excessive compression:
- Tingling
- Leg pain
- Foot or leg discoloration
- Cool leg extremities
- Change in pulse strength

Patient Needs and Principles of Management, Cont.

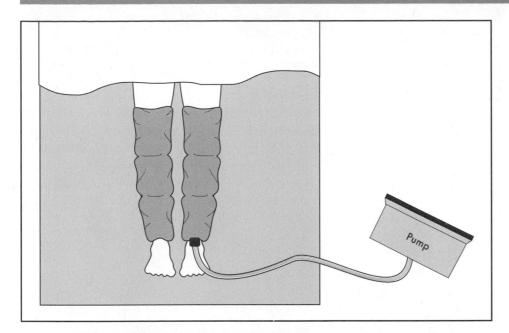

Figure 13–11. Sequential compression device (SCD) for prevention of deep vein thrombosis and pulmonary embolism.

ARF in the Patient with Chronic Obstructive Pulmonary Disease (COPD)

Individuals with chronic obstructive pulmonary disease (bronchitis, asthma, emphysema) are at high risk for the development of acute respiratory failure. Altered host defenses, increased secretion volume and viscosity, impaired secretion clearance and airway changes, and common pathophysiologic changes predispose the COPD patient to frequent episodes of acute respiratory failure. The etiology, clinical presentation, and management of ARF in the COPD patient varies somewhat from ARF without chronic underlying pulmonary dysfunction. This section of the chapter highlights differences in ARF management in the patient with underlying COPD.

Etiology, Risk Factors, and Pathophysiology

Any systemic or pulmonary illness can precipitate ARF in patients with COPD. In addition to the etiologies of ARF listed in Table 13–4, diseases or situations which decrease ventilatory drive, muscle strength, chest wall elasticity, or gas exchange capacity, or increase airway resistance or metabolic oxygen requirements can easily lead to ARF in patients with COPD (Table 13–10). The most common precipitating events include:

- *Airway infection* (pneumonia, bronchitis). Frequent antibiotic administration, hospitalization, and impaired cough and host defenses in COPD increase acute airway infections. Infections are commonly caused by gram-negative enteric bacteria or *Legion-*

TABLE 13–10. PRECIPITATING EVENTS OF ACUTE RESPIRATORY FAILURE IN COPD

Decreased ventilatory drive
Oversedation
Hypothyroidism
Brain stem lesions

Decreased muscle strength
Malnutrition
Shock
Myopathies
Hypophosphatemia
Hypomagnesemia
Hypocalcemia

Decreased chest wall elasticity
Rib fractures
Pleural effusions
Ileus
Ascites

Decreased lung capacity for gas exchange
Atelectasis
Pulmonary edema
Pneumonia
Pulmonary embolus
Congestive heart failure

Increased airway resistance
Bronchospasm
Increased secretions
Upper airway obstructions
Airway edema

Increased metabolic oxygen requirements
Systemic infection
Hyperthyroidism
Fever

ella, with *Haemophilus influenzae* and *Streptococcus pneumoniae* causing acute bronchitis.

- *Pulmonary embolus.* The high incidence of right ventricular failure in COPD increases the risk of pulmonary embolus from right ventricular mural thrombi.
- *Congestive heart failure.* In the presence of cor pulmonale, treatment of left-sided, congestive heart failure is often delayed due to difficulties in early diagnosis.
- *Noncompliance with medication regime.* The complicated treatment regime for management of COPD, which includes frequent administration of both oral and inhaled agents, frequently leads to underuse of medications.

The development of ARF in COPD patients places a tremendous burden on the pulmonary system. The chronic disease process leads to impairment of ventilation, poor gas exchange, and airway obstruction. The additional burden of an acute disease process, even a relatively minor one, further impairs ventilation and gas exchange and/or increases airway obstruction. Compensatory mechanisms can easily be overwhelmed, with lethal consequences.

Clinical Presentation

Signs and symptoms are similar to ARF, but usually more pronounced.

Diagnostic Tests

- Chest x-ray: Evidence of COPD (flat diaphragms, hyperinflation of air fields), in addition to x-ray findings specific to the cause of the ARF.
- ABG: $Pa_{CO_2} > 45$ mm Hg and higher than baseline levels during stable, chronic disease periods.

Patient Needs and Principles of Management

The presence of chronic respiratory dysfunction and an acute respiratory problem leads to some changes in the typical management of acute respiratory failure.

▶ Treatment of Underlying Disease State

Treatment is directed at both the acute precipitating event and the chronic airflow obstruction problems associated with COPD.

1. Increase airway diameter with bronchodilators and reduce airway edema with corticosteroids. Beta-adrenergic or anticholinergic agents are more effective bronchodilators than theophylline (Table 13–11). Higher than usual doses may be necessary until the precipitating event is resolved. Bronchospasm that is refractory to bronchodilators in severe asthma cases, also called status asthmaticus, may require subcutaneous epinephrine administration. Epinephrine is only given to young patients with no evidence of cardiac disease.
2. Treat pulmonary infections with appropriate antibiotics.
3. Improve secretion removal. Strategies to improve secretion removal include adequate hydration, corticosteroids, coughing, heated moist aerosolization, and chest physiotherapy. Secretions are particularly thick and tenacious in asthma patients. Monitor response to these therapies and discontinue them if no additional benefits are observed.

▶ Improvement of Oxygenation and Ventilation

1. Correction of hypoxemia is done by small increases in FiO_2 levels, preferably with a controlled O_2 delivery device such as a Venturi mask. Frequent monitoring of arterial blood gases is essential to ensure adequate arterial oxygenation (Pa_{O_2} of 55 to 60 mm Hg or baseline values during nonacute situations) without significantly increasing Pa_{CO_2} levels. Higher than necessary FiO_2 levels may increase Pa_{CO_2} by suppressing the hypoxic ventilatory drive of some COPD patients and/or increasing the ventilation-perfusion ratio.
2. Position the patient to maximize ventilatory efforts and relaxation/rest during spontaneous breathing. A high Fowler's position and leaning on an overbed table is often the position of greatest comfort prior to intubation and mechanical ventilation.
3. Relaxation techniques and diaphragmatic, pursed lip breathing are especially helpful to decrease anxiety and improve ventilatory patterns. Anxiolytics and other sedatives should be used cautiously to avoid decreasing minute ventilation.
4. The decision to intubate and mechanically ventilate the patient is based primarily on the deterioration of mental status, coupled with knowledge of the patient's baseline pulmonary function and functional status, and the reversibility of the underlying

cause. Somnolence and inability to cooperate with treatments are other strong indicators for intubation and ventilation. Weaning from mechanical ventilation is frequently more difficult, and in some cases not possible, in the presence of COPD. Informed discussions with the patient and family regarding intubation options should be undertaken. The presence of an advanced directive can help guide clinician's actions when patients are unable to make treatment decisions themselves.

5. Ventilatory management of COPD patients differs little from ARF alone. Slow correction of hypercarbia should be done to avoid life-threatening alkalemia from preexisting metabolic compensation. Following intubation, respiratory muscle recovery from fatigue typically requires 48 to 72 hours. During this phase efforts to "wean" the patient are best avoided unless dramatic progress was made in removing the underlying cause of the respiratory failure. Respiratory muscle rest should be ensured by providing a mode of ventilation that decreases respiratory effort. Following the 48- to 72-hour rest period, respiratory muscle conditioning (intermittent mandatory ventilation [IMV], increasing the triggering sensitivity, etc.) should begin gradually by decreasing IMV support or increasing the triggering sensitivity. Periods of rest should continue to be provided to prevent fatigue. The development of auto-PEEP and barotrauma is increased in patients with COPD, necessitating smaller tidal volumes (7 to 10 ml/kg), higher respiratory rates (15 to 18/minute), and short inspiratory and long expiratory times.

TABLE 13–11. BRONCHODILATOR CATEGORIES USED IN STATUS ASTHMATICUS

Category	Examples
Beta agonists (goal is β_2 specificity)	Albuterol, β_2 specific (often given as a continuous aerosol treatment)
	Epinephrine (β_1 and β_2)
Anticholinergics	Ipratropium bromide
	Glycopyrrolate
Methyxanthines	Aminophylline

▶ Nutritional Support

Typically, patients with COPD have protein-calorie malnutrition, as well as low levels of phosphate, magnesium, and calcium. These chronic nutritional deficits lead to muscle weakness and may interfere with the weaning process. Early enteral or parenteral feeding of these patients is essential to avoid further deterioration in their nutritional status during acute illness. Parenteral feeding may be best initially since dyspnea in the nonintubated patient makes oral feeding difficult and aerophagia leads to decreased GI motility. Large carbohydrate loads increase CO_2 production during nutritional support, requiring higher minute ventilation rates to avoid hypercapnic acidosis. The administration of lipid calories should account for 50% of the nutritional support during mechanical ventilation. Higher amounts may be needed during weaning attempts to minimize minute ventilation requirements related to nutritional CO_2 production.

▶ Prevention and Management of Complications

In addition to the complications associated with ARF, the following complications commonly are observed in COPD patients with ARF:

1. *Arrhythmia:* High incidence of both atrial and ventricular arrhythmia in patients with COPD due to hypoxemia, acidosis, heart disease, medications, and electrolyte abnormalities. Cardiac monitoring and correction of the underlying cause is the goal, with pharmacologic treatment of arrhythmia only for life-threatening situations.

2. *Pulmonary embolus:* High incidence. Observe for signs and symptoms and follow the usual treatment/prevention guidelines.

3. *GI distention and ileus:* Aerophagia is common in dyspneic patients, increasing the incidence of this complication.

4. *Auto-PEEP and barotrauma:* High incidence, especially in the elderly and in individuals with high ventilation needs.

AT THE BEDSIDE
■ *Thinking Critically*

You are caring for a patient in acute respiratory failure with the following interventions:

- Mechanical ventilatory support (assist-control rate 10/minute TV 800 ml, PEEP 15 cmH$_2$O, F$_{IO_2}$ 0.85)
- Pa$_{O_2}$ 63 mm Hg
- MAP 68 mm Hg on vasoactive drug support (dopamine 7 µg/kg/minute)
- Neuromuscular blockade (vecuronium)
- Sedation (Ativan)

How might the level of PEEP this patient is receiving affect his response to suctioning? What precautions could you take to avoid or respond to potential complications?

SELECTED BIBLIOGRAPHY

Critical Care Management of Respiratory Problems

Civetta J, Taylor R, Kirby R (eds.): *Critical care,* 2nd ed. Philadelphia: JB Lippincott, 1992.

Conn RB (ed.). *Current diagnosis,* 8th ed. Philadelphia: WB Saunders, 1991.

Curtis JR, Hudson LD: Acute respiratory failure in chronic obstructive pulmonary disease. In Carlson R, Gohab M (eds.): *Principles and practice of medical intensive care.* Philadelphia: WB Saunders, 1993, pp. 793–805.

Hall JB, Schmidt GA, Wood LDH (eds.): *Principles of critical care.* New York: McGraw-Hill, 1992.

Ventilator Management

Luce J, Pierson D, Tyler M: *Intensive respiratory care,* 2nd ed. Philadelphia: WB Saunders, 1993.

DuPuis YG: *Ventilators: Theory and clinical application,* 2nd ed. St. Louis, MO: CV Mosby, 1992.

McPherson S: *Respiratory therapy equipment,* 4th ed. St. Louis, MO: CV Mosby, 1990.

Techniques to Reduce Anxiety

Clark S, Fontaine D, Simpson T: Recognition, assessment and treatment of anxiety in the critical care setting. *Critical Care Nurse.* 1994; August suppl: 2–16.

Melendez J, McCrank E: Anxiety-related reactions associated with magnetic resonance imaging. *Journal of the American Medical Association.* 1993;270:745–747.

Chest X-ray Interpretation

Detternmeier P: *Pulmonary nursing care.* St. Louis, MO: Mosby-Year Book, 1992.

Hall J, Schmidt G, Wood L: *Principles of critical care: companion handbook.* New York: McGraw-Hill, 1993.

Holloway N: *Nursing the critically ill adult,* 4th ed. Menlo Park, CA: Addison-Wesley, 1993.

Kersten L: *Comprehensive respiratory nursing.* Philadelphia: WB Saunders, 1989.

Sanchez F: Fundamentals of chest x-ray interpretation. *Critical Care Nurse.* 1986;6:41–52.

Stillwell S: *Critical care nursing reference.* St. Louis, MO: Mosby-Year Book, 1992.

Thelan L, Davie J, Urden L, Lough M: *Critical care nursing: Diagnosis and management,* 2nd ed. St. Louis, MO: Mosby-Year Book, 1994.

Miscellaneous

Boggs R, Wooldridge-King M: *AACN procedure manual for critical care,* 3rd ed. Philadelphia: WB Saunders, 1993.

Craven D, Steger K: Nosocomial pneumonia in the intubated patient. New concepts on the pathogenesis and prevention. *Infectious Disease Clinics of North America.* 1993;3(4):843–866.

Sticklin LA, Walkenstein M: Vena cava filters: A nursing perspective. *Oncology Nursing Forum.* 1993;20:509.

Tablan OC, Anderson LJ, Arden NH, Breiman RF, et al.: Guideline for prevention of nosocomial pneumonia. Parts I & II. *American Journal of Infection Control.* 1994;22:247–292.

Multisystem Problems

■ *What Heals: Enhancing the Placebo Response*

The placebo response (see What Heals: The Powerful
Placebo, Chapter 9) probably is present, more or less,
in each one of us. If it is true that a placebo healing
response can occur naturally in all clinical situations,
what would happen if *we tried* consciously to
enhance its effects in our patients? It is known that
how a drug is given or how a procedure is performed
and by whom can influence the outcome of the
placebo response. The placebo response, therefore, is
influenced greatly by the faith that the patient has in
the caregiver and in the patient's expectation that the
drug or therapy will work. Likewise, it is influenced
by the faith that the caregiver conveys to the patient
regarding the drug or therapy, as well as the trust and
rapport established between the two.

To enhance the placebo response when administering medications, for example, we can discuss with
patients what is known about the medication's
potency and effectiveness. When patients receive
intravenous morphine for pain, we can ask them to
visualize the powerful painkilling medicine being
injected into their veins and to see the molecules traveling to the source of the pain to relieve it. We can
suggest that they work with the medication to
enhance its effectiveness by allowing the relaxed,
warm, and comfortable feeling associated with the
morphine to flow throughout their body.

The essence of the placebo response is associated with positive attitudes and emotions. Many of
the self-regulation modalities such as imagery, music
therapy, and relaxation, as well as exercise, increase
endorphin production. When patients believe they are
receiving a highly effective medication or therapy
and when they believe that they are doing something
to enhance healing, endorphin levels can rise.
Patients, therefore, actually can influence the course
of their own illness as well as their response to therapy through the impact of their own consciousness.
Because basic nursing interventions such as touching,
giving back rubs, preoperative teaching, positioning,

and distraction all have the potential to increase endorphin levels, it is critical that we discuss the possible therapeutic benefits of each therapy. When we realize that what we say to patients can actually influence the placebo response, then we will develop a variety of new communication skills to enhance the healing response in our patients and maximize the benefits of all the nursing care we give.

CEG & BMD

Adapted from: Guzzetta CE: Placebo response. In Guzzetta CE, Dossey BM: Cardiovascular nursing: Holistic practice. *St. Louis, MO: Mosby-Year Book, 1992, pp. 392–393.*

PATHOLOGICAL CONDITIONS

Systemic Inflammatory Response Syndrome (SIRS), Sepsis, and Multiple Organ Dysfunction Syndrome (MODS)

The case studies presented below represent two distinct clinical situations, both of which caused the systemic inflammatory response syndrome (SIRS). SIRS is the systemic inflammatory response to a clinical insult, such as an infection or burn (Table 14–1). The stimulus for SIRS can be singular or multifactorial. Examples of situations which can precipitate SIRS are burns, trauma, transfusions, pancreatitis, or infection. Following the insult, an inflammatory response is initiated as a normal physiologic response. The inflammatory response consists of vasodilatation, increased microvascular permeability, cellular activation and release of mediators, and coagulation (Figure 14–1). In SIRS, however, there is an excessive release of these mediators, which leads to severe tissue damage, with hypoperfusion of major body systems.

AT THE BEDSIDE
▶ *Sepsis*

Mary Jean W., a 70-year-old Caucasian female, was transferred from the emergency department (ED) of a rural community hospital, and admitted to the medical intensive care unit (MICU) complaining of acute onset of diffuse abdominal pain, coffee-ground emesis, and bright red blood via the rectum. She had experienced a syncopal episode while in the bathroom at home, and had sustained facial bruises. In the ED, an IV of 0.9% NS was infused at 125 ml/hour; an NG was placed and set to low intermittent suction yielding coffee-grounds material; and a #16 Fr Foley was inserted with cloudy amber urine returned.

Review of Systems in ED

Skin:	2 cm ecchymosis above R eye, and inner canthus R eye
Lymph:	1 cm R axillary node
HEENT:	Sclera anicteric; no petechiae
Cardiac:	No bruits; no JVD; Gr III/VI systolic murmur at apex
	EKG: Sinus rhythm, ST depression II, III, AVF, V_4–V_6, T-wave inversion AVL
Lungs:	Diffusely decreased breath sounds; fine crackles at bases
Abd:	slightly distended, + high-pitched BS; soft, diffusely tender, no rebound tenderness, + voluntary guarding
Extrem:	1 + pretibial pitting edema of lower extremities; no tenderness
Neuro:	Cranial nerves 2-12 intact, awake and alert
VS:	BP 76/35 HR 108 RR 24 Temp 39.4 C
Labs:	WBC 43K, 87(s) 5(l) 8(m)
	LFTs increased
	ABG 7.33/28/116/96% on 2 L/minute O_2

The patient was taken to surgery very early the following morning for an exploratory laparotomy.

Post-Op Day #1

Patient returned from OR hyperdynamic, was unable to manifest a hyperthermic response, and required maximum ventilatory and inotropic support. Patient arrested and was resuscitated.

Post-Op Day #2

Patient arrested and expired.

TABLE 14–1. DEFINITIONS

Infection
Microbial phenomenon characterized by an inflammatory response to the presence of microorganisms or the invasion of normally sterile host tissue by those organisms.

Bacteremia
The presence of viable bacteria in the blood.

Systemic Inflammatory Response Syndrome
The systemic inflammatory response to a variety of severe clinical insults. The response is manifested by two or more of the following conditions:
  Temperature > 38.0°C
  Heart rate > 90/minute
  Respiratory rate > 20 breaths/minute or $Paco_2$ < 32 mm Hg
  WBC > 12,000 cells/mm^3, < 4000 cells/mm^3, or > 10% immature (band) forms

Sepsis
The systemic response to infection. This systemic response is manifested by two or more of the following conditions as a result of infection:
  Temperature > 38.0°C
  Heart rate > 90/minute
  Respiratory rate > 20 breaths/minute or $Paco_2$ < 32 mm Hg
  WBC > 12,000 cells/mm^3, < 4000 cells/mm^3, or > 10% immature (band) forms

Severe Sepsis
Sepsis associated with organ dysfunction, hypoperfusion, or hypotension. Hypoperfusion and perfusion abnormalities may include, but are not limited to, lactic acidosis, oliguria, or an acute alteration in mental status.

Septic Shock
Sepsis with hypotension, despite adequate fluid resuscitation, along with the presence of perfusion abnormalities that may include, but are not limited to, lactic acidosis, oliguria, or an acute alteration in mental status. Patients who are on inotropic or vasopressor agents may not be hypotensive at the time that perfusion abnormalities are measured.

Hypotension
A systolic BP of < 90 mm Hg or a reduction of > 40 mm Hg from baseline in the absence of other causes for hypotension.

Multiple Organ Dysfunction Syndrome
Presence of altered organ function in an acutely ill patient such that homeostasis cannot be maintained without intervention.

From: ACCP/SCCM Consensus Committee: Critical Care Medicine. *1992;20:866.*

SIRS is manifested in a variety of ways: fever, tachycardia, tachypnea, altered level of consciousness, and decreased urine output. These findings may or may not be the result of an infection. If not the result of an infection, an infection may develop subsequent to the insult. If the response is allowed to progress unchecked, the result may be the development of sepsis and/or dysfunction of one or more organ systems, or multiple organ dysfunction syndrome (MODS). The systemic inflammatory response syndrome, sepsis, and multiple organ dysfunction syndrome can be thought of as a progression of illness. The key is early identification of signs and symptoms of the SIRS, and prompt development of a treatment plan to avoid progression to sepsis or MODS. Early intervention is paramount to successful outcomes in these patients.

The systemic inflammatory response is a natural defense against an insult. The initial signs exhibited by both patients in the case studies occur as a result of the body's desire to maintain homeostasis at a time when there are increased demands. In order to maintain adequate perfusion and preservation of organ function, the body adopts a defense strategy, the systemic inflammatory response (Figure 14–2). This response is generated by the release of mediators from different cells in the body. These mediators are the foundation of the systemic inflammatory response, causing most of the signs and symptoms observed in SIRS. For example, a very important mediator is tumor necrosis factor (TNF). TNF is secreted by white blood cells (macrophages) in response to stimulation. TNF has been shown to cause tachycardia, tachypnea, and fever, all of

AT THE BEDSIDE
▶ *SIRS*

The patient is a 65-year-old male who was admitted to the burn unit with diffuse partial and full-thickness burns following a propane tank explosion. The initial assessment upon arrival to the unit was:

VS: BP 80/50 HR 144 RR ventilated rate of 14 Temp 38.6

Patient is responsive to verbal stimuli but very lethargic. His urine output has dropped dramatically in the last hour.

Labs: WBC 13.2

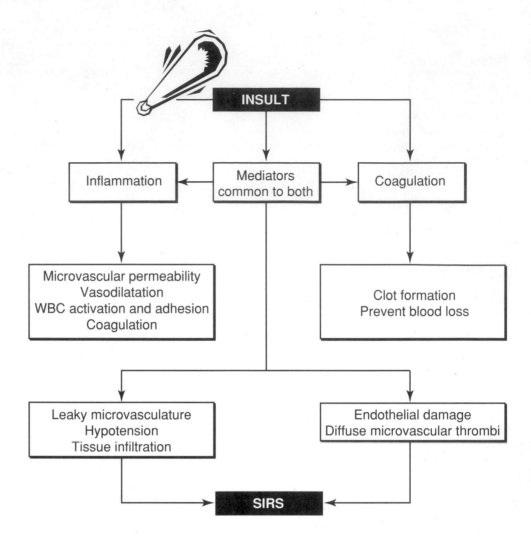

Figure 14–1. Interactive cascade of inflammation and coagulation leading to SIRS. (*Secor V: The inflammatory response.* Critical Care Nursing Clinics of North America. *1994;6(2):255.)*

which were manifestations in the two case studies. Other mediators will cause different clinical signs and symptoms.

Etiology, Risk Factors, and Pathophysiology

SIRS

SIRS is a series of systemic events that are manifested in many different ways in response to an insult to the body. This response is a cellular reaction that initiates a number of mediator-induced reactions, and is both inflammatory and immune in nature (Figure 14–2).

There are essentially four different types of cells that are activated as part of the response to an insult or stimulus: polymorphonuclear cells (neutrophils), macrophages, platelets, and endothelial cells. These cells are activated to become either directly involved in the reaction (i.e., platelets aggregation) or are stimulated to produce and release certain chemical mediators into the circulation, such as cytokines or plasma enzymes. Once activated, "a checks and balances system" is normally in place to control the inflammatory response. In some situations, however, when the response is large or the injury diffuse, local control of the response is lost, leading to excessive mediator release with consequent organ damage.

The common cold, or viral syndrome, is an example of a normal systemic inflammatory response that is contained. Some of the manifestations are the same as those experienced by critically ill patients, such as fever, malaise, increased white blood cell count, or arthralgia. The difference is that the inflammatory immune response with a viral cold is contained and not allowed to develop unregulated. The mediators for the response to the common cold are very similar to the mediators for the response to burns or pancreatitis. The difference is that the insult is not as severe, and the body has the ability to "shut off," or down-regulate, the response as needed. In fact, healthy volunteers have been administered low dosages of mediators such as endotoxin or tumor necrosis factor, and have developed "flulike" symptoms in response.

A general understanding of the various mediators responsible for the SIRS is important (Table 14–2). Mediators can be divided into five groups: cytokines, plasma

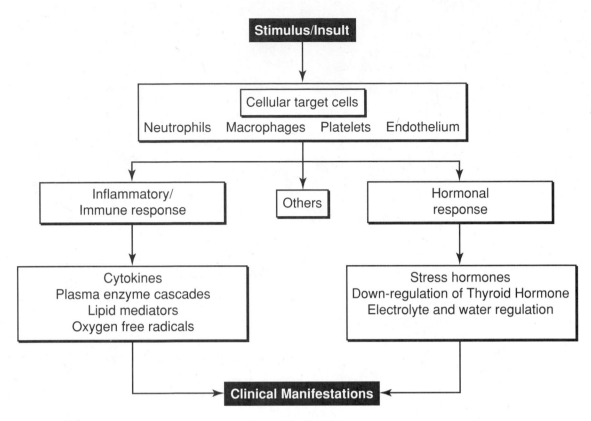

Figure 14–2. Diagram of cascade of events from the stimulus of the systemic inflammatory response to clinical manifestations.

enzyme cascades, lipid mediators, toxic oxygen-derived metabolites, and unclassified mediators such as nitric oxide and proteases. These mediators are stimulated after cellular activation in response to a certain stimulus (e.g., infection, trauma, pancreatitis). Cytokines are active chemical substances which are secreted by cells in response to some stimulus. If secreted by lymphocytes, they are called lymphokines, and if secreted by monocytes or macrophages, they are called monokines. Examples of cytokines include tumor necrosis factor (TNF), interleukin (IL), interferon (IFN), and colony-stimulating factors such as granulocyte colony-stimulating factor (G-CSF).

In addition to cytokines, there also is activation of different enzymatic plasma cascades. Examples of these include the complement cascade and the various coagulation cascades. There also are various lipid mediators which are either stimulated or produced as part of a cellular destructive process. These lipid mediators include arachidonic acid metabolites, leukotrienes, prostaglandins, and platelet activating factor. Oxygen-derived free radicals are another group of mediators which exert a negative effect as part of the SIR. Examples of these include hydrogen peroxide and hydroxyl radical. Nitric oxide and proteases are other mediators that are not grouped into any of the previ-

ous categories, but are mediators of various responses to an insult.

In addition to the mediators which are stimulated as part of the inflammatory and immune responses, there also are mediators related to hormonal stimulation and regulation. The hormonal response component of the SIR is characterized by the release of stress hormones (catecholamines, glucagon, cortisol, and growth hormone), suppression of thyroid hormone, and hormonal regulation of fluid and electrolyte balance.

Sepsis

Sepsis is the manifestation of the SIR in response to an infectious process (Table 14–1). The source of infection may be bacterial, viral, fungal, or on rare occasions, rickettsial or protozoal. Specific mediators may vary depending on the specific microbial invaders. For example, two of the main mediators in sepsis are endotoxin and exotoxin. Both of these mediators can be responsible for the enhanced response of the inflammatory, immune, and hormonal systems.

The risk factors for development of sepsis are many and include malnutrition, immunosuppression, prolonged antibiotic use, and the presence of invasive devices (Table

TABLE 14-2. MANIFESTATIONS AND MEDIATORS OF THE SYSTEMIC INFLAMMATORY RESPONSE SYNDROME*

Manifestations	Cause	Possible Mediators
Neurological		
↓ Mental status	↓ CO	TNF
↓ CPP	Hypotension	
	↑ HR	
	↓ Arterial pressure	IL-2
	↓ SVR	
	↓ EF	
	Negative inotropic effect	PAF
	Myocardial depression	MDF
	Ventricular dilation	
	↓ EF	
Agitation	Hypoxemia	TNF, IL-2, PAF, MDF
		Leukotrienes
		Lactate
Cardiovascular		
Changes in CO		TNF, IL-1, IL-2, PAF, MDF
	↑ CO	Prostaglandins
	Vasodilation	NO, Prostacyclin, PGE$_2$
	↓ SVR	Complement, NO
	Hypotension	Endorphins, NO
	Massive vasodilation	Bradykinin, NO
	Vasoconstriction	Thromboxane
		Prostacyclin
	Loss of vascular integrity, leakage of intravascular fluid into interstitium, edema	Endotoxin
Tachycardia	↑ HR	Catecholamines
		TNF
New extra heart sounds or murmurs		Any of the above
Bounding pulse		Any of the above
Pulmonary		which ↑ CO
Tachypnea		TNF
↑ Vascular markings on x-ray		TNF
		O$_2$ free radicals
↑ Crackles on auscultation		TNF
↑ A-a gradient	Pulmonary vasoconstriction	Thromboxane A$_2$
	↑ PVR, bronchoconstriction	
	Bronchoconstriction	Bradykinin, PAF
	Pulmonary vasoconstriction	Leukotrienes
	Damages endothelial cell in lung capillary causing ↑ capillary permeability and microvascular leak	O$_2$ free radicals
	↑ Adherence of neutrophils in pulmonary vasculature	IL-1
	Bronchoconstriction; causes bronchospasm	Complement
	↑ Microvascular permeability	Bradykinin
	Procoagulant activity	TNF
	Vasoconstriction, platelet aggregation	Arachidonic acid metabolites (prostaglandins, thromboxane, leukotrienes)
	Excessive coagulation	PAF
Peripheral Vascular		
↑ Third-space edema		TNF
Warm extremities, bounding pulses, mottled skin		TNF
Hemostasis	↑ Intravascular coagulation leading to vascular obstruction, endothelial damage, and tissue ischemia	Coagulation cascade
Vascular and tissue damage		Proteases
Gastrointestinal		
↓ BS	Anything causing low flow to the gut	
	Vasoconstriction of mesentery	Leukotrienes
	Abdominal distension	Leukotrienes
	GI ulceration, particularly in duodenum and jejunum	PAF
↑ Residuals	Anything causing low flow to the gut	
Abdominal distension	↑ Gut permeability	Leukotrienes
Heme + NG drainage or stool	Low flow	TNF
↑ LFTs	Anything causing low flow to the gut	
Renal		
↓ Urine output	Low flow	TNF
	↑ GFR, may cause renal hypoperfusion and hypofiltration	Endothelin I
↑ Creatinine/BUN	Low flow	TNF
Skin		
↑ or ↓ Temp		TNF, IL-1, prostaglandins
Edema		TNF
Fever	Enhanced immune cell activity	TNF
Hemopoietic		
↑ or ↓ WBC		
Bandemia		
Thrombocytopenia		Thromboxane A
		Arachidonic acid metabolites
		PAF
		Complement

*Legend: TNF = tumor necrosis factor; IL-1 = interleukin 1; IL-2 = interleukin 2; PAF = platelet-activating factor; MDF = myocardial depressant factor; NO = nitric oxide; PGE$_2$ = prostaglandin E$_2$.

TABLE 14–3. RISK FACTORS FOR DEVELOPMENT OF SEPSIS

Host-Related Factors
Malnutrition
Immune deficiency disorders
Immunosuppression
Skin breakdown
Fragile skin/mucous membranes
Traumatic injuries
Burns
Pressure sores
IV drug abuse
ETOH abuse
Chronic illness
Diabetes mellitus
Neoplastic disease
Cirrhosis
Renal failure
Cardiac disease
Pulmonary disease
Pregnancy associated with prolonged rupture of membranes
Immune senescence (elderly)
Poor mobility
Bedridden status
BPH
Decreased mucociliary transport mechanisms
Decreased cough and clearance function
Increased response to influenza vaccine
UTI
Vaginal colonization with GBS
Perineal colonization with *Escherchia coli*
Premature rupture of membranes

Treatment-Related Factors
Invasive diagnostic devices
Invasive therapeutic devices
Surgical procedures
Prolonged hospitalization
Therapeutic immunosuppression
Chemotherapy
Radiation therapy
Splenectomy
Urinary catheters
Use of H_2 receptor antagonists (leading to gastric bacterial overgrowth and aspiration pneumonia)
Aggressive resuscitation
Prolonged TPN
Extensive antibiotic therapy
Pain/stress

Adapted with permission from: Klein DM, Witek-Janusek L: Advances in immunotherapy of sepsis. Dimensions of Critical Care Nursing. *1992; 11(2):75–81.*

14–3). It is important to remember that a large number of infections in critically ill patients are nosocomial and can lead to sepsis. Many of these nosocomial infections can be prevented with simple measures (Chapter 11, Safety Issues). Hand washing is the single most effective method for preventing nosocomial infections.

MODS

Multiple organ dysfunction is the worsening progression of the systemic inflammatory response. If SIRS is allowed to persist unchecked, or becomes too overwhelming, the patient will develop clinical manifestations of organ dysfunction. Previously termed organ failure, the syndrome has been more appropriately called organ dysfunction because, in actuality, organs show manifestations of dysfunction before they fail. Very few organs fail entirely. The mortality rates for MODS vary depending on the underlying cause, with mortality rates ranging from 50% to 100% as the number of involved organs increases.

MODS can be classified as either primary or secondary. In primary MODS, organ dysfunction is a direct effect of an insult to an organ that has been compromised. For example, aspiration causes lung dysfunction, or acetaminophen overdose causes liver dysfunction. With primary MODS, the onset occurs relatively soon after the insult. In secondary MODS, the organ dysfunction occurs as the result of persistent and prolonged mediator release following an insult such as a thermal burn or pancreatitis. Generally the time frame for secondary MODS is 7 to 10 days; however, this onset is variable.

Clinical Presentation

SIRS

The clinical manifestations of SIRS vary depending on the host, as well as the type and extent of the injury. Table 14–2 summarizes the common manifestations of SIRS as well as possible causes and responsible mediators. Close monitoring and assessment are essential for the detection of early signs of SIRS. Early recognition and treatment are extremely important for positive patient outcomes.

MODS

The clinical manifestations of primary and secondary MODS are the same as in SIRS and depend on which organs are affected. The reader is referred to the clinical manifestations of SIRS presented previously in this chapter, as well as the other chapters on individual organ systems, for manifestations and treatment of disruptions in organ systems.

Diagnostic Tests

- Complete blood cell count: White blood cell count > 12,000 cells/mm^3, or < 4000 cells/mm^3, or > 10% immature bands.
- Arterial blood gas: Paco_2 < 32 mm Hg.
- Chest x-ray: May be normal or show signs of infiltrates.
- Culture and sensitivity: Generally will be positive from a normally sterile source.
- CAT scan: May be negative or show abscess collection.

Patient Needs and Principles of Management

The treatment of a patient with SIRS or sepsis consists of several objectives: treatment of the underlying cause, maximizing oxygen delivery, and providing support for nutritional status, dysfunctional organ systems, and the patient and family's psychological well-being.

► Treatment of the Underlying Cause

The management plan begins with recognition and treatment of the source or stimulus of the response. Until this is done, no other therapy can be successfully applied. This may mean drainage of an abscess or removal of an infected invasive line, vascular graft, or orthopedic device. Once the source has been identified, appropriate antibiotic therapy needs to be initiated.

► Maximizing Oxygen Delivery

Parallel to the administration of antibiotics are measures to maximize oxygen delivery.

1. *Assess oxygen delivery.* The components of oxygen delivery which need to be assessed and optimized include cardiac output (CO), oxygen saturation (SaO_2), hemoglobin (Hgb), and to a lesser extent, partial pressure of oxygen (PaO_2).
2. *Maximize cardiac output.* A significant number of patients with SIRS will increase their cardiac output as a compensatory response to meet increased cellular oxygen demands. However, a major pathological problem of SIRS is the increase in the permeability of the capillary bed. As a result, intravascular volume is difficult to maintain. This necessitates the administration of fluids. Typically, a patient will require a combination of both crystalloid and colloid fluid replacement. The exact type of fluid and amount is usually dependent upon the preference of the institution and the patient's needs. Pharmacologic support also may be required to maximize cardiac output. The choice of drugs also is dependent upon individual institutional preferences and the patient's needs. Refer to Chapter 9, Pharmacology, for more detailed information.
3. *Maximize oxygenation.* Along with maximizing cardiac output, oxygenation needs to be addressed. Maintaining SaO_2 above 92% to 94% and PaO_2 above 60 mm Hg are acceptable goals. This will allow adequately oxygen availability and maximization of delivery. Concurrent is the need for sufficient hemoglobin to ensure adequate oxygen-carrying capacity. There is some disagreement on what are the appropriate hemoglobin and hematocrit levels for this type

of patient; however, as a general rule, 10 g of hemoglobin and 30% for the hematocrit are acceptable.
4. *Decrease oxygen demand.* Decreasing oxygen demand is an important aspect of maximizing oxygen delivery. Methods to reduce oxygen demand include:

- Reducing tachycardia and tachypnea
- Reducing hyperthermia
- Alleviating pain
- Alleviating shivering
- Providing comfort measures
- Consolidating activities

In taking action in these areas, unnecessary oxygen consumption can be minimized, thus improving the supply to other tissues in greater need of oxygen.

Notice there has been no mention of maintaining an optimal blood pressure. The reason for this is that although maintenance of blood pressure is critical, adequate blood pressure does not imply adequate perfusion. For this reason, measurements of oxygen delivery and consumption are used to assess adequacy of perfusion, and not blood pressure alone. There is great variability in perfusion among patients with similar mean arterial pressures. A patient with a mean arterial pressure of 100 mm Hg may not have adequate tissue perfusion. In contrast, a patient with a mean arterial pressure of 50 may have sufficient tissue perfusion. The point is that an evaluation of perfusion is not based on pressure assessment alone.

► Providing Support for Dysfunctional Systems

An important objective in the management of SIRS and MODS is to provide support to dysfunctional organ systems. Renal dysfunction, a common sequela of SIRS, should be aggressively managed to prevent fluid and electrolyte imbalances which may increase mortality. Refer to the chapter in this book specific to each organ system for approaches commonly used to support failing organs.

► Providing Nutritional Support

Nutritional support may be provided by the enteral or parenteral route, although the former is the preferred route. Most critically ill patients can tolerate a standard type of tube feeding or parenteral formula, with rare situations that require feeding modifications (e.g., volume overload, organ dysfunction, or gastrointestinal abnormalities). General guidelines for nutritional support include 25 to 35 kcal/kg/day for total caloric intake and 1.5 to 2.0 g protein/kg/day. It is helpful to have a nutrition specialist assist with nutritional planning.

Patient Needs and Principles of Management, Cont.

▶ Providing Psychological Support

The care of the patient with SIRS or sepsis is physically and mentally demanding. There are many interventions that are essential just to maintain life. Adequate pain control and sedation are vital. It is easy to lose sight of the patient and family's psychological needs. These needs must not be overlooked. Specific information regarding pharmacologic and nonpharmacologic pain and sedation management are covered in Chapter 7, Pain Management, and Chapter 8, Alternative Therapies. Meeting patients' psychosocial needs is addressed in Chapter 3, Planning Care for Critically Ill Patients and Families, as well as in Chapter 8.

In addition to pain and sedation management, information management is very important. Including the patient and family in critical decisions helps to maintain patient-focused care. Collaborative decisions among the patient, family, and health care team should be promoted. Allowing for the influence of different cultural values in the decision-making process is also important.

AT THE BEDSIDE
▶ *Sensory Teaching*

During critical illness, nurses need to seize opportunities to explain to patients what has occurred as well as what things will occur in the near future. Many critically ill patients are not interested, however, in an intellectual discussion of the indications or need associated with a particular test or procedure—that is, they really are not interested in the "whys." They are much more interested in the sensory experience—that is, learning the details of the personal experience they will encounter. When facing a diagnostic test, procedure, treatment, or surgery, patients want to know what the experience is going to feel like, whether it will be painful or uncomfortable, and what they will experience in terms of touch, smell, sound, or taste. Patients undergoing MRI, for example, may not be interested in the full details of why the test was ordered. Explaining that the test will help to evaluate the extent of injuries may be all the information that a patient desires to know. Most will want to know, however, that the MRI will not be painful, but involves some muscle discomfort from laying on a small table in a long narrow tunnel for about an hour and is associated with very loud noises while the test is being performed. This kind of education, called *sensory teaching*, has been shown to be highly effective in helping patients prepare for and cope with the stress of new situations, therapies, and surgery.

Overdoses

Drug and/or alcohol overdoses, as well as poisonings, can result in multiple organ dysfunction. Overdoses can be deliberate or accidental. Accidental overdose may involve one substance or multiple substances, and can be acute (inaccurate dosing of pediatric medications) or chronic (inadvertent, unnecessary dosing of asthma medication or over-the-counter medications). The level of intoxication or overdose varies with the element and amount ingested, the time until the patient is treated, and the underlying physical and emotional condition of the patient. The priority of care, as in all emergency situations, is maintenance of the patient's airway, breathing, and circulation.

Etiology, Risk Factors, and Pathophysiology

Alcohol Overdose

Alcohol overdose is most often seen in alcoholics, in young persons who have not yet reached "legal" drinking age, or in combination with other drugs as a suicidal gesture. There are four types of alcohol seen in alcohol intoxication:

- Ethanol (ethyl or grain alcohol)
- Methanol (wood alcohol)
- Ethylene glycol (antifreeze)
- Isopropyl alcohol (rubbing alcohol)

Alcohol dissolves readily in the lipid components of the plasma membranes of the body, and thus enters the brain quickly, resulting in a rapid effect on the central nervous system.

In ethanol intoxication, serum levels range from 200 mg/dl (mild intoxication) to > 500 mg/dl (coma). A serum

AT THE BEDSIDE
▶ *Alcohol Overdose*

R. F., a 19-year-old male, is brought to the ED by his roommates who state that he fell from a third-floor balcony of their campus residence. Your initial assessment reveals a depressed level of consciousness, with decreased response to stimuli, facial contusions and lacerations, and apparent dislocations of the right shoulder and right knee. While reviewing his initial serum chemistry results, you note that the serum alcohol level is 430 mg/dl.

alcohol level of 100 mg/dl is the legal upper limit for driving a car in most of the United States.

In the case of methanol intoxication, serum levels range from 50 mg/dl (mild intoxication to 100 mg/dl (severe intoxication). Metabolic acidosis is manifested as decreased bicarbonate levels on arterial blood gas, and indicates that the generation of hydrogen ions by the liver exceeds the ability of the kidney to excrete hydrogen ions. This excess of systemic hydrogen ions will result in pulmonary compensation via hyperventilation, as the body makes an effort to decrease its level of CO_2. Refer to Chapter 6, Airway and Ventilatory Management, for further information on acid-base imbalance.

Ethylene glycol intoxication is characterized by CNS depression, cardiopulmonary complications, pulmonary edema, and renal tubular degeneration. Serum chemistry reveals metabolic acidosis, as described above, and renal toxicity. An aggregation of hydrogen ions can result in increased production and accumulation of lactic acid, which tends to impair renal function. Renal toxicity should be suspected when the serum pH < 7.35, serum creatinine > 2.0 mg/dl, and BUN > 100 mg/dl.

AT THE BEDSIDE
▶ *Drug Overdose*

A. G., a 36-year-old male, is brought by his spouse to the ED complaining of "palpitations and shortness of breath, and feeling overheated." Your initial assessment reveals sinus tachycardia at a rate of 170, BP 210/110, circumoral cyanosis, and a small amount of bright red blood oozing from his right nares. Oral temperature is 39.8°C (103.6°F). As you continue your assessment, the patient begins to experience tonic-clonic movements of the extremities, which progress to generalized motor seizures and loss of consciousness.

Isopropyl alcohol intoxication is distinguished from other types of alcohol intoxication by the presence of ketoacids in both the urine and serum. Metabolic acidosis is a reflection of excess ketoacids, requiring buffering by the bicarbonate ions.

Drug Overdose

Drug overdose may involve any type of medication. The majority of overdoses involve analgesics, antidepressants, sedatives, cough and cold drugs, and street drugs (cocaine, crack cocaine, PCP, LSD). Street drugs are used to elevate mood, or to produce unusual states of consciousness. Psychoactive drugs often are chemically similar to neurotransmitters such as serotonin, dopamine, and norepinephrine, and act by either directly or indirectly altering neurotransmitter-receptor interactions. Medullary inspiratory neurons are highly sensitive to depression by drugs, especially barbiturates and morphine, and death from an overdose of these agents is often secondary to respiratory arrest. Refer to Table 14–4 for presenting signs and symptoms of common agents of drug overdose.

Clinical Presentation

Alcohol Overdose

Excess ingestion of any type of alcohol may cause central nervous system symptoms such as sluggish reflexes, emotional instability, or out-of-character behavior. Amnesia may result for events that occurred during the period of intoxication. Unconsciousness usually occurs before a person can drink enough for fatal consequences to occur, but the rapid consumption of alcohol can cause death by either respiratory depression or aspiration during vomiting. There are signs and symptoms that are specific to each type of alcohol ingested:

- *Acute ethanol intoxication:* Muscular incoordination, slurred speech, stupor, hypoglycemia, flushing, seizures, coma, depressed respirations, and hyporeflexia
- *Methanol intoxication:* CNS depression, metabolic acidosis, and visual disturbances
- *Ethylene glycol intoxication:* CNS depression, cardiopulmonary complications, pulmonary edema, and renal tubular degeneration
- *Isopropyl intoxication:* CNS depression, areflexia, respiratory depression, hypothermia, hypotension, and GI distress

Drug Overdose

The specific signs and symptoms of drug overdose are dependent upon the substance ingested. However, there are several signs and symptoms that are commonly seen in most patients. These include changes in mental status (typically, decreased level of consciousness), behavioral

TABLE 14–4. SIGNS AND SYMPTOMS OF OVERDOSE

Opioids
Change in LOC
Respiratory depression, aspiration
Hypotension
Miosis
↓ Gastric motility

Barbiturates
↓ LOC
Hypothermia

Sedatives
Respiratory depression

Hypnotics
Shock
Cardiac dysrhythmias
Pulmonary edema

Cocaine
Hyperexcitability
Headache
Hypertension
Tachycardia
Nausea/vomiting, abdominal pain
Fever
Delirium, convulsions, coma

PCP (Phenylcyclidine)
Violent behavior
Hallucinations
Seizures
Rhabdomyolysis
Hypertensive crisis

LSD
Severe agitation
Dilated pupils
Hallucinations

Tricyclics
Seizures
Coma
Dysrhythmias, ECG changes
Heart failure
Shock

Salicylates
Tinnitus
Vertigo
Vomiting
Hyperthermia
Altered mental status

Acetaminophen
GI distress
Hepatotoxicity
Hepatic necrosis

changes, and respiratory depression. The signs and symptoms of drug overdose for particular drugs are summarized in Table 14–4.

Diagnostic Tests

Alcohol Overdose

A differential diagnosis to rule out other medical conditions, such as hypoglycemia or hyperglycemia, which may mimic overdose or intoxication, is an important component of the initial assessment. Since alcohol ingestion interferes with the liver's ability to produce glucose, alcohol-induced hypoglycemia in the intoxicated patient is a fairly common scenario.

Prior to any diagnostic test, it is extremely important to obtain a history either from the patient, family member or friend, or the person who found the patient to determine the probable substance that was ingested. Once the substance is potentially identified there are diagnostic tests which are helpful in aiding the treatment of patients following alcohol intoxication. These include:

- Ethanol and methanol serum levels will be elevated if these were ingested. Most labs can run these tests. Isopropyl serum levels are not run as commonly as ethanol and methanol levels.
- Serum creatinine and BUN levels may be elevated due to renal dysfunction.
- Liver functions may be elevated due to hepatotoxic effects of certain types of alcohol.
- Serum glucose and electrolytes may be abnormal.

Drug Overdose

Diagnostic studies for patients following drug overdose include:

- Toxicology screen, which can be either broad-spectrum tests, including testing for the presence of such substances as amphetamines, barbiturates, benzodiazepines, and narcotics, or specific screens, if the substance is known.
- Arterial blood gas, which will indicate respiratory or metabolic disturbances.
- Serum glucose and electrolytes, which can be abnormal.

Patient Needs and Principles of Management

The principles of management of patients following alcohol intoxication or drug overdose are similar. These principles are maintenance of a patent airway, prevention of complications, elimination of ingested substances or toxic metabolites, and maintenance of hemodynamic stability.

▶ Maintenance of Patent Airway

1. Maintain adequate minute ventilation. Stimulate the patient to breathe. If the patient cannot spontaneously maintain minute ventilation, then intubation and mechanical ventilation may be required.
2. Monitor pulse oximetry and blood gas values.
3. Position the patient with the head of the bed slightly elevated.
4. Suction the patient's airway as needed.

▶ Prevention of Complications

1. Orient the patient to surroundings.
2. Insert a nasogastric tube for stomach decompression/decontamination.
3. Keep the head of the bed elevated to prevent aspiration.
4. Pad bed side rails, and restrain the patient as necessary to prevent self-injury.
5. Provide constant reassurance to the patient and family.
6. Provide pharmacologic interventions, as indicated:

   - IV naloxone: Counteraction of CNS and respiratory depression; differentiates alcohol intoxication from narcotic overdose.
   - IV diazepam: Termination of seizure activity (drug overdose).
   - IV phenytoin: Termination of seizure activity refractory to diazepam (drug overdose).

   - IV phenobarbital: Termination of seizure activity refractory to both diazepam and phenytoin (drug overdose).
   - Dextrose 50% IV: Prevention of Wernicke's encephalopathy; counteracts alcohol-induced hypoglycemia (alcohol overdose).
   - 100 mg thiamine IM: prevention of Wernicke's encephalopathy; given concurrently with dextrose 50% (alcohol overdose).

▶ Elimination of Ingested Substances of Toxic Metabolites

1. Gastric lavage to remove stomach contents and flush GI tract.
2. Osmotic diuresis with mannitol and glucose (alcohol overdose).
3. Induced emesis if the patient is awake and able to protect the airway.
4. Gastric decontamination and catharsis with activated charcoal, polyethylene glycol, and magnesium citrate (drug overdose).
5. Hemodialysis and hemoperfusion for severe drug intoxication for selected substances.

▶ Maintenance of Hemodynamic Stability

1. Administration of fluid to maintain intravascular fluid volume.
2. Pharmacologic interventions for drug overdose:

   - IV propranolol: Slowing of tachycardia.
   - Lidocaine: Termination of ventricular tachycardia, and return to normal sinus rhythm.
   - Nitroprusside: Management of preexisting hypertension exacerbated by or refractory to propranolol.

3. Treatment for shock: Refer to Chapter 12, Cardiovascular System, for a discussion of shock.

SELECTED BIBLIOGRAPHY

What Heals: Enhancing the Placebo Response

Dossey L: *Space, time, and medicine.* Boston: Shambhala Publications, 1982.

Rossi EL: *The psychobiology of mind-body healing: New concepts of therapeutic hypnosis.* New York: WW Norton, 1986.

SIRS, Sepsis, MODS

Abraham E (guest ed.): Sepsis: Cellular and physiologic mechanisms. *New Horizons: The Science and Practice of Acute Medicine.* 1993;1(1).

Ackerman MH (ed.): Sepsis. *Critical Care Nursing Clinics of North America.* 1994;6(2).

Bone RC: The pathogenesis of sepsis. *Annals of Internal Medicine.* 1991;115:457–469.

Hazinski MF: Mediator-specific therapies for the systemic inflammatory response syndrome, sepsis, severe sepsis, and septic shock: Present and future approaches. *Critical Care Nursing Clinics of North America.* 1994;6(2):309–319.

Klein DM, Witek-Janusek L: Advances in immunotherapy of sepsis. *Dimensions of Critical Care Nursing.* 1992;11(2):75–89.

Secor VH: The inflammatory/immune response in critical illness: Role of the systemic inflammatory response syndrome. *Critical Care Nursing Clinics of North America.* 1994;6(2):251–264.

Stengle J, Dries D: Sepsis in the elderly. *Critical Care Nursing Clinics of North America.* 1994;6(2):421–427.

Witek-Janusek L, Cusack C: Neonatal sepsis: Confronting the challenge. *Critical Care Nursing Clinics of North America.* 1994;6(20):405–419.

Overdose

Dean BS, Verdile VP, Krenzelok EP: Coma reversal with cerebral dysfunction recovery after repetitive hyperbaric oxygen therapy for severe carbon monoxide poisoning. *American Journal of Emergency Medicine.* 1993;11(6):616–618.

Deglin JH, Vallerand AH: *Davis's drug guide for nurses,* 3rd ed. Philadelphia: FA Davis, 1993.

Delaney K: Handling an opioid overdose. *Emergency Medicine.* 1993;25(1):127, 130, 136.

Eliastam M, Sternbach GL, Bresler MJ (eds.): *Manual of emergency medicine,* 5th ed. St. Louis, MO: CV Mosby, 1989.

Nikas DL: The neurologic system. In Alspach JG (ed.): *Core curriculum for critical care nursing,* 4th ed. Philadelphia: WB Saunders, pp. 315–471.

Parsons PE: Respiratory failure as a result of drugs, overdoses, and poisonings. *Clinics in Chest Medicine.* 1994;15(1):93–102.

Rudolph JP: Automated gastric lavage and a comparison of 0.9% normal saline solution to tap water irrigation. *Annals of Emergency Medicine.* 1985;14:1156–1159.

Seger D: The science (or lack thereof) in the treatment of carbon monoxide poisoning. *American Journal of Emergency Medicine.* 1994;12(3):389–390.

Sheehy SB: *Emergency nursing: Principles and practice,* 3rd ed. St. Louis, MO: CV Mosby, 1992.

Soloway RAG: Street-smart advice on treating drug overdoses. *American Journal of Nursing.* 1993;93(4):65–71.

Sue YJ, Shannon M: Pharmacokinetics of drugs in overdose. *Clinical Pharmacokinetics.* 1992;23(2):93–105.

Tibbles PM, Perrotta PL: Treatment of carbon monoxide poisoning: A critical review of human outcome studies comparing normobaric oxygen with hyperbaric oxygen. *Annals of Emergency Medicine.* 1994;24(2):269–276.

Tintinalli JE, Krome RL, Ruiz E: *Emergency medicine: A comprehensive study guide,* 3rd ed. New York: McGraw-Hill, 1992.

Vander AJ, Sherman JH, Luciano DS: *Human physiology: The mechanisms of body function,* 6th ed. New York: McGraw-Hill, 1994.

Verdile VP, Dean BS, Krenzelok EP: Hyperbaric therapy for carbon monoxide poisoning. *American Journal of Emergency Medicine.* 1994;12(3):389–390.

Weinman SA: Emergency management of drug overdose. *Critical Care Nurse.* 1993;13(6):45–51.

Wright JE, Shelton BK: *Desk reference for critical care nursing.* Boston: Jones & Bartlett, 1993.

Neurologic System

■ *What Heals: Multisensory Stimulation*

Patients who experience a cerebrovascular event and are unable to communicate are in need of meaningful outside stimulation to help them relate to their surroundings. A multisensory stimulation program can be developed by the nurse in collaboration with the family. Because it is generally believed that hearing is the last sense to leave and the first one to return, the program should incorporate verbal and auditory stimulation. For example, call the patient by name, explain all care being administered, and reorient the patient to date, time, place, circumstance, and person. Talk to the family to determine the patient's interests and recommend that conversations focus on these areas. Encourage family and friends to relate and share what is happening within the family unit and social circle. Ask the family to tape the patient's favorite musical selections, which can be played at the patient's bedside (preferably with headphones) for 15 minutes several times a day. Encourage relatives and friends to send taped messages instead of cards.

Visual stimulation also needs to be a part of the program. Family photographs and familiar pictures or objects can be placed in an area that the patient will see when the patient opens his or her eyes. That could mean climbing a ladder to tape a picture on the ceiling. Likewise, stimulating taste should not be overlooked. If the patient is unable to eat, the patient's familiar mouthwash and toothpaste can be used. Finally, tactile stimulation might include both procedural and intentional touch, soft touch, pressure, and exposure to various textures such as a washcloth.

Because it is not known how much these patients are able to perceive, all caregivers and visitors must presume that these patients will hear what is said to them and will be aware of what is being done to them.

CEG & BMD

SPECIAL ASSESSMENT TECHNIQUES, DIAGNOSTIC TESTS, AND MONITORING SYSTEMS

Neurologic Assessment

Observation is the key to rapid detection of neurologic problems. Good observation skills include knowing what to observe, how to elicit the response to observe, and what to do when the response is not as expected. Skilled serial observation, coupled with accurate documentation, allows for detection of subtle changes in neurologic status.

There is no set way of performing a neurologic evaluation, although learning a simple routine and sticking to it seems to offer the best results. Each patient must have an individualized assessment based on his or her presenting signs and symptoms. By essentially "picking and choosing" from a menu of assessment tools, the nurse can save time by not having to perform inappropriate procedures.

Level of Consciousness

Identifying the patient's level of consciousness (LOC) is the easiest way to assess the patient's ability to interact with the environment. A variety of terms often are used to describe the level of consciousness, such as alert, lethargic, obtunded, or comatose (Table 15–1). It is easier to say that the patient opens his or her eyes only to a sternal rub than it is to describe that behavior as obtunded and hope that everyone else understands that term as the evaluator intended. Rather than using one of these terms, however, it is preferable to use what the patient says or does as descriptors of LOC. For example, when nailbed pressure is given, the patient has no movement in any limbs, but the eyes flicker open and the head deviates to the right. Another reaction might be that the patient states that he or she is at the zoo and that there are bugs on the wall. Monitor the patient frequently for slow, subtle changes or rapid changes in LOC. LOC is one of the easiest assessment parameters to monitor and one of the earliest indicators of

changes in neurologic status. Detecting changes in LOC can be crucial to the patient's survival and a positive outcome.

Glasgow Coma Scale

The one "standard" tool used to monitor neurologic status in critical care is the Glasgow Coma Scale (Table 15–2). This tool is based on the responsiveness of the patient and ability to follow commands. The best response in each category is selected and the patient is given a score for that response. Then scores are totaled for the three categories to determine the Glasgow coma score. The best score, representing no LOC impairment, would be 15. Scores less than 8 generally represent coma. It is important to note that this tool is an assessment guide and must be individualized to the patient. Rating motor response can be one of the most confusing categories of this scale (Figure 15–1). Different movements of the patient may be interpreted differently by different individuals. All four extremities should be assessed independently for response. For example, delivering a noxious stimuli (sternal rub, trapezius squeeze) to a patient may elicit a response in which the arms move upward towards the chest. If the patient attempts to push the examiner away with the hands, that is localization; if the patient extends the legs and curls the arms inwards, that is decorticate posturing or flexion. An easy way to remember decorticate and decerebrate posturing is that decorticate is "into the core," or flexion, and decerebrate is "away" from the body, or extension. Decorticate posturing signifies that there is damage in the cerebral hemispheres, but that below this level the structures are intact. Decerebrate posturing signifies damage to the midbrain, pons, and/or

TABLE 15–1. DEFINITIONS FOR COMMON TERMS USED TO DESCRIBE LEVEL OF CONSCIOUSNESS

Term	Definition
Alert	Awake and fully conscious; able to demonstrate reliable and responsive behavior.
Confused	Disoriented to time, place, or person; agitation, restlessness, or irritability may be present.
Lethargic	Oriented to time, place, and person, but has a sluggish response time for speech, motor, or cognitive activities.
Obtunded	Arousable with stimulation; responds verbally or follows simple commands with stimulation; else appears sleepy.
Stuporous	Minimal interaction with environment except when maximally stimulated with repeated noxious stimuli; responds with grunts or incomprehensible sounds.
Comatose	Appears to be sleeping; generally has no appropriate interactions with the environment, even with repeated noxious stimuli.

TABLE 15–2. GLASGOW COMA SCALE

Behavior	Score*
Eye Opening (E)	
Spontaneous	4
To speech	3
To pain	2
None	1
Motor Response (M)	
Obeys commands	6
Localizes pain	5
Withdraws to pain	4
Abnormal flexion	3
Extensor response	2
None	1
Verbal Response (V)	
Oriented	5
Confused	4
Inappropriate words	3
Incomprehensible sounds	2
None	1

*Coma score = E + M + V (Scores range from 3 to 15)

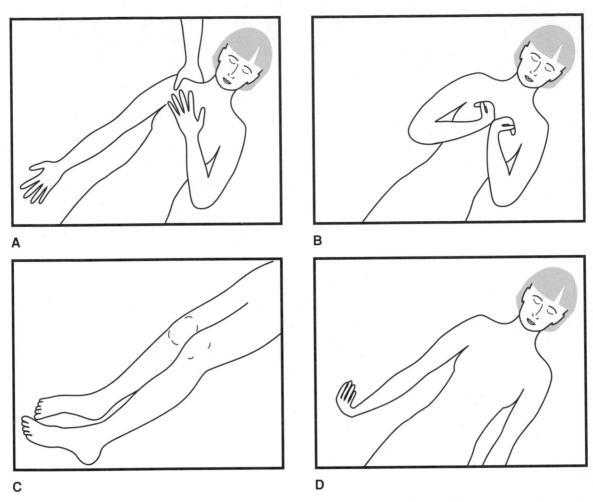

Figure 15–1. Motor movement to noxious stimuli rating on Glasgow Coma Scale. (A) Localization movement toward the site of noxious stimuli (trapezius squeeze) in a quick motion. (B) Decorticate posturing (into the core) is abnormal flexion with internal rotation of the upper extremities at the wrist. (C) Lower extremity posturing is plantar flexion with internal rotation, seen with both decorticate and decerebrate posturing. (D) Decerebrate posturing is abnormal extension with external rotation of the upper extremities at the wrist.

medulla oblongata. A mixture of posturing means that the level of injury in the brain is not symmetrical. For example, one side may have more damage than the other. Of the two, decerebrate posturing is considered to be worse than decorticate posturing as an indicator of clinical outcome. The presence of either posturing or a change from decorticate to decerebrate posturing should be brought to the attention of the physician immediately. These are ominous signs of extension of the lesion into the upper brain stem.

Pupillary Response
Pupillary changes usually are seen late in the course of neurologic difficulty. Careful observation of pupillary size, shape, reactivity, and equality is important to assist the clinician in predicting events and potential outcome. Pupils should be measured in millimeters, not quantified by words like "large," "small," "pinpoint," or "blown." Serial measurement of the pupil also enables the clinician to monitor

progression of potentially life-threatening problems such as herniation. Pupillary changes are not always a good predictor of outcome and should not be relied on as a primary clinical indicator. Don't forget that certain medications can affect pupil size and reactivity. For example, atropine can dilate pupils and narcotics can cause them to become very constricted.

Vital Signs
Vital signs are an extremely important part of any critical patient's assessment. In the neurologic patient, the systemic blood pressure (BP) and the respiratory rate are key concerns. Identification and regulation of the BP are important to maintain homeostasis in the brain. Uncontrolled BP can precipitate catastrophic events such as stroke, hemorrhage, shock, herniation, or even death. The Cushing response is one of impending disaster. The classic triad involves a rise in BP with a widened pulse pressure, a slowing of the heart

rate, and an increase in intracranial pressure. This is a very late response exhibited in neurologic deterioration and is of minimal value in identifying early, significant changes in the patient's condition.

Respiratory Patterns

Respiratory patterns also are of great importance in assisting the clinician with recognition of pathological processes within the brain. Respiratory failure can occur when the medulla is compressed. Respiratory changes also are seen with certain diseases which cause coma states and decreases in level of consciousness. Some of the more common respiratory patterns are discussed below (Figure 15–2).

Cheyne-Stokes Respiration

This pattern of respiration can be identified by the classic periods of apnea followed by a rhythmic progression of hyperpnea. Usually the periods of hyperpnea are longer than the periods of apnea. This type of pattern can be seen in some healthy individuals during sleep with no pathologic disease process, but often the pattern suggests the beginning of a neurologic problem. It most often is seen in patients who exhibit bilateral hemispheric injury, such as stroke, or in expanding lesions of the posterior fossa, such as cerebellar hemorrhage.

Ataxic (Biot's) Respiration

This pattern of respiration is easily identified by the random, irregular pattern of deep and shallow breathing. The often slow rate of this pattern can progress to complete apnea, requiring ventilatory support. Regular sleep patterns or sedative usage can promote this type of pattern; therefore, the use of sedatives, hypnotics, or tranquilizers is discouraged unless apnea monitoring or mechanical ventilation is available. This pattern is often seen in patients with medullary, cerebellar, or brain stem lesions.

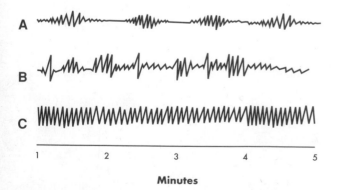

Figure 15–2. Respiratory patterns associated with neurologic impairment. (A) Cheyne-Stokes respiration—periods of apnea followed by increasing hyperpnea, seen in stroke and cerebellar hemorrhage. (B) Ataxic (Biot's) respiration—random irregular pattern of deep, shallow breathing, seen in medullary, cerebellar, or brain stem lesions. (C) Central neurogenic hyperventilation—sustained, rapid, regular, deep hyperpnea, which is rare but can be seen in pons and low midbrain lesions.

Central Neurogenic Hyperventilation

This pattern of respiration is characterized by sustained rapid, regular, and deep hyperpnea. This type of breathing pattern is seen in unconscious, severely head-injured patients without brain stem injury and more often in hypoxic patients with large pulmonary shunts with hypoxemia. Arterial blood gas analysis reveals a low $PaCO_2$, a high PaO_2, and an elevated pH. Lesions can usually be found in the pons and low midbrain regions of the brain.

Brain Stem Assessment

Brain stem evaluations are performed when there is significant loss of consciousness. Cranial nerve (CN) assessment evaluates the integrity of the brain stem and the cranial nerves that exit from it. Corneal reflexes evaluate the adequacy of function of CNs V and VII, the trigeminal and facial nerves. This test is performed with either a wisp of cotton from a cotton ball or the stretched-out end of a cotton swab lightly drawn across the cornea; a normal response is a blink. Absence of this response does not indicate irreversible brain damage; however, when seen with abnormal eye movements, it can mean significant brain stem damage. If there is no blink, the eye should be taped closed *without* an eye patch and artificial tears should be instilled. Eye patches can cause corneal abrasion or ulceration to the eye if the lids are not completely closed. A single strip of hypoallergenic tape should be used from the top of the orbital arch over the closed eyelid to the top of the zygoma.

Extraocular eye movements are controlled by three CNs: III, IV, and VI. These abnormal eye movements include:

1. *Nystagmus:* a jerking, rhythmical movement of one or both of the eyes
2. *Dysconjugate gaze:* each eye moving independently of the other
3. *Extraocular palsies:* individual nerve involvements in one or both of the eyes that inhibit eye movement in a certain direction

Dysconjugate gaze almost always is predictive of brain stem injury. Extraocular palsies are less predictive of brain stem injury because they may be related to increases in intracranial pressure or individual damage to that nerve. Nystagmus and dysconjugate gaze are easily assessed by lifting the eyelids and observing the movement of the eyes. Extraocular palsies require a cooperative patient who is able to follow commands for assessment purposes. The patient should be able to follow the examiner's finger in eight fields of movement: laterally left and right; upward to the left, right, and center; and downward to the left, right, and center. Gaze disorders can signal numerous types of deficits, from cranial nerve damage to muscle damage to brain stem damage.

The oculocephalic reflex, or doll's eye response, is commonly evaluated when determining brain death. It is one of the most confusing signs to evaluate. The oculocephalic reflex is only evaluated in unconscious patients because it is not present in awake patients. This reflex should never be evaluated in patients with suspected cervical spine injuries. The eyelids are held open by the examiner and the head is quickly rotated side to side. A normal response is for the eyes to deviate opposite to the direction the head is turned; e.g., they should remain looking at the examiner in both directions. If the eyes do not deviate or are noted to be "roving," this is an abnormal response. Do not use "positive" or "negative" to describe your findings. If you are unsure of what is normal or abnormal, describe what you see.

Evaluation of the oculovestibular reflex (or the cold calorics examination) is another possibly confusing examination. It also is used when determining brain death or brain stem integrity. The instillation of about 10 to 20 ml of iced water into the ear against an intact tympanic membrane causes conjugate deviation of the eyes towards the irrigated side in the patient with an intact brain stem. Patients who have interrupted brain stem function will either have no response or dysconjugate eye movement. This test should only be performed on patients with intact tympanic membranes. Again, when identifying the patient's response, refrain from using "positive" or "negative" to describe your findings. Describe what you see as a response to the iced water instillation.

Lumbar and Cisternal Punctures

Lumbar and cisternal punctures can be used for therapeutic as well as diagnostic purposes. They can be performed to sample cerebrospinal fluid (CSF) from the spinal canal and to instill medication or spinal anesthesia into the subarachnoid space. The most common area in which to do this is the lumbar area; however, cisternal puncture can be performed when the lumbar area is inaccessible due to structural abnormalities or there is a blockage preventing free flow of CSF. Lumbar and cisternal punctures are performed to sample CSF when there is a question of an infectious process (meningitis, syphilis), multiple sclerosis, or Guillain-Barré syndrome. They are contraindicated in patients who have increased intracranial pressure due to herniation or coagulopathies.

Both of these tests involve the insertion of a hollow needle by the physician into the spinal canal. Lumbar punctures are performed at the L3-L4 or L4-L5 space to prevent damage to the conus. Cisternal punctures are performed at the base of the skull into the cisterna magna (Figure 15–3). Both of these tests can be performed at the bedside and require little preparation. Patients may require some sedation if they are uncooperative, and assistance will be required to help position the patient. Lumbar punctures require the patient to lie on the left side in a fetal position. The patient also can be sitting on the side of the bed with

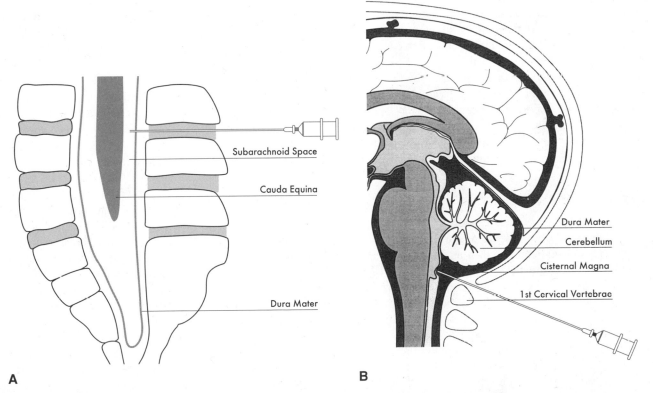

A   B

Figure 15–3. Lumbar and cisternal punctures. (A) Lumbar puncture performed at L3-4 or L4-5 space with hollow needle. (B) Cisternal puncture performed at base of the skull into the cisterna magna with hollow needle.

the chin tucked and hands under the knees or sitting at the edge of the bed over a bedside table. However, this position often is less than desirable or optimal in the critically ill patient. The fetal position widens the intervertebral space, allowing the needle to pass through easily. For cisternal punctures the patient sits on the edge of the bed, with the chin tucked and someone in front bracing the patient's shoulders. A local anesthetic is injected, and then the hollow needle is inserted into the subarachnoid space. Pressures are measured upon opening up the spinal column. Opening pressures in a horizontal position range from 6 to 13 mm Hg, or 80 to 180 mm H_2O. Pressures greater than 200 mm H_2O are considered abnormal. CSF samples are obtained for analysis, usually cell counts with differentials, chemistries, and culture with sensitivities. Once the needle is removed, a small self-adhesive bandage is placed over the insertion site and the patient is returned to a supine position.

During lumbar punctures, the physician may perform a Queckenstedt procedure to assess for the free flow of CSF in the spinal column. This is done by manually compressing the jugular vein for 10 seconds. A blood pressure cuff around the neck can also be used, although this can be quite upsetting to the patient. If there is no compression on the spinal column, the pressure measurement in the manometer should rise to approximately 250 to 300 mm H_2O, and then drop back to normal when the pressure is released. Any blockages, such as tumors, clots, bone fragments, or scar tissue, will prevent or slow down the rise in the manometer.

Postprocedure care involves maintaining the patient on bedrest for 4 to 6 hours, encouraging fluids, and monitoring the insertion site for any signs of bleeding, weeping of fluid, or development of hematoma. Patients often complain of headaches which are related to the loss of CSF, local pain at the insertion site, or pain radiating to the thigh if a nerve root was hit during the procedure. Pain medications may be given for site pain if indicated. Headaches should be treated with forced fluids, maintaining the head of the bed flat or less than 30 degrees, maintaining a dark quiet room with dim lights, or with administration of analgesics.

Computerized Tomography (CT Scan)

Computerized tomography, better known as CT scanning, is a common diagnostic tool in neurological patients. It consists of two parts—computerized data analysis and x-rays. A single x-ray beam is directed toward the head in a scanning motion to give a series of views resembling horizontal slices of the brain. The machine scans the head in a 180-degree arc and collects the x-ray beams in the computer. The density of the brain structures allows the computer to translate the collected x-ray beams into a three-dimensional picture of the brain and other structures in the head. The result is a series of finely cut pictures as small as 2 mm in thickness showing fine detail of bony structures, CSF, and brain tissue. Bone is visualized as white on film because it

is most dense, and CSF is visualized as black because of its low density. Brain tissue is seen in varying shades of white and gray, making it easier to distinguish between tumor, infarction, or tissue. A CT scan can be performed with an iodinated contrast medium to allow for better visualization of large vessels or vascular lesions. CT scans are indicated for suspected space-occupying lesions, edema, hydrocephalus, head trauma, or infarctions. They can help to determine the cause of dementia, seizures, headaches, or even visual changes with suspected cerebral origin. Although CT scans are quick, easy to perform, and painless, the patient must be cooperative for the scan to be accurate. Movement at any time during the scan can cause blurry films. Sedation may be required when patients are restless, uncooperative, or claustrophobic. Essentially the only risk related to CT scans is that of an allergic reaction to the contrast agent. The amount of radiation delivered to the patient is equivalent to that of a plain skull film.

During CT scans, no additional monitoring is required. Education is vital prior to the study to ensure that the patient is aware of the importance of lying still. Care must be taken prior to and during the procedure to position the patient correctly and prevent falls from the table, as there are no side rails. Often, the scanners will have protective padding or Velcro holding strips to assist with this. There are no postprocedural interventions associated with this test.

Magnetic Resonance Imaging and Angiography

Magnetic resonance imaging (MRI) is a more sophisticated test that offers greater anatomic detail and better resolution than a CT scan without using ionized radiation. The system consists of a magnet, a spectrometer, and an image display. Controlled bursts of radio pulse waves are delivered inside a magnetic tube causing resonance inside certain atomic nuclei. The energy which is emitted is sent into the computer, where three-dimensional images are constructed. These images are displayed on a view screen and can then be copied onto film for future viewing. The viewing of the MRI is the reverse of the CT scan. In the MRI, the bone is seen as black, and the CSF is seen as white.

MRI scans are most useful in diagnosing disorders of the brain stem, posterior fossa, and spinal cord. MRI scans also offer an advantage over CT scans in the discovery of demyelinating disorders such as multiple sclerosis, acoustic neuromas, and cerebellar atrophy. MRI can also be used to detect suspected lesions that are not able to be seen on CT, such as early cerebral infarction and intramedullary tumors. The time requirement for MRI scans is much longer than that of CT scans, which can be a disadvantage when needing to make treatment decisions based on diagnostic results.

Contraindications for MRI are listed in Table 15–3. Implanted metallic objects may become dislodged or slip inside the large magnetic tube and can cause severe patient injury. The magnet can also damage internally magnetized units, such as cardiac pacemakers, causing them to mal-

TABLE 15–3. CONTRAINDICATIONS FOR MRI

Implanted Ferromagnetic Devices
Vascular clips (aneurysm clips)
Metal heart valves
Eye prostheses with metal shards
Middle or inner ear prostheses

Electromechanical Devices
Implantable TENS units
Permanent pacemakers
AICD units
Insulin pumps
Metal life support equipment

Patient History
Lodged bullets or shrapnel
Metal shards in eyes from steel factory
Metal joint replacements

function or become demagnetized. External metallic equipment, such as IV pumps and ventilators, can make MRI studies difficult. The use of long tubing and portable monitoring equipment can help in some instances. Metal joint replacements are not an absolute contraindication to MRI, but they can cause significant artifacts on the films.

Patient education is important prior to scanning. Patients must be screened closely for any of the listed contraindications. In addition, they must remove all metal objects, such as jewelry, nonpermanent dentures, prostheses, hairpins, or clothing with snaps or zippers. They must be advised of the loud "booming" noise of the scanner. Offer patients ear plugs or place towel rolls next to their ears. Patients who are claustrophobic also may experience some anxiety or feelings of isolation; therefore, premedication with a sedative may be needed (see the MRI section in Chapter 13, Respiratory System). Inform the patients that the nurse or technician is in full view of them in the scanner and that they can talk to them if they feel uncomfortable on the table. Ensure the safety and comfort of the patients with safety belts and blankets for positioning. Offer the patients prism glasses so that they can see their feet and the room outside the scanner. There are no postprocedure interventions associated with this test.

Magnetic resonance angiography (MRA) is a specialized computer MRI program that has the ability to highlight specific cerebral vasculature in a three-dimensional image. With the use of contrast-enhancing media, more complex views are obtained of the vasculature of the brain. MRA is useful especially in suspected arteriovenous malformations, aneurysms, and cavernous angiomas, a rare vascular problem. The disadvantage of this procedure is, again, the time constraint and metal contraindications.

Electroencephalography

The electroencephalogram (EEG) is simply a measurement of the brain's activity. This is done by attaching a varying number of electrodes to standard locations on the scalp.

These electrodes are attached to a recorder which amplifies the activity and records it on paper. Different areas of the brain have patterned waveforms that can be measured against "normals" that have been established for age group and brain location.

Usually, the EEG is not used solely for diagnostic purposes, but as an adjunct to clinical evaluation. As a primary diagnostic tool, an EEG is useful in determining seizure focus for epileptics, identifying burst suppression during neurosurgical operative procedures, and identifying level of brain wave activity in brain death protocols. As an adjunctive tool, an EEG is useful in differentiating mass lesions from epilepsy, evaluating causes of coma (structural versus metabolic), and even differentiating seizure disorders from psychogenic states (catatonia, hysteria).

The EEG usually lasts 40 to 60 minutes with a portable machine for bedside use. The patient is instructed to lie still with the eyes closed. A mild sedative may be prescribed for restless or uncooperative patients, but the interpreter of the EEG must be aware of this as medications may cause changes in the recording. Documentation during the study will be done by the technician and may include changes in blood pressure, changes in level of consciousness, medications the patient is currently taking or has taken within 48 hours, movement or posturing of the patient, and any noxious stimuli introduced to the patient. It is best to plan nursing care around the time of the test so that no interventions will be done during this exam. Ideally, the patient should not have caffeine products, sedatives, tranquilizers, or anticonvulsants prior to the tests as these may skew the results. Fasting should also be avoided; hypoglycemia may change the EEG pattern.

EEG testing can be done utilizing many different techniques. An EEG can be done during sleep to assist with the diagnosis of temporal lobe epilepsy. Photic stimulation can be used to precipitate seizures in photosensitive patients. Hyperventilation is also a technique used to increase the chance of seizure activity.

When the EEG is complete, the removal of the electrode paste is done with acetone or witch hazel. Medications that were held prior to the study should be resumed. If the patient had a sleep EEG performed, 2 to 3 hours of undisturbed rest may be of benefit.

PATHOLOGIC CONDITIONS

Encephalopathy

Etiology, Risk Factors, and Pathophysiology

Encephalopathy is a global term used to describe any dysfunction of the brain. There are many different causes of encephalopathy, some known and some unknown. Some causes of encephalopathy include viruses (the most common cause), bacteria, parasites, toxic substances, and even

AT THE BEDSIDE
▶ *Anoxic Encephalopathy*

Barry M., a 26-year-old male, was drinking while driving and was involved in a motorcycle accident. He was found beside a tree and his helmet was found about 25 feet away from him cracked into two pieces. He was unresponsive at the scene and was intubated by the paramedics. Upon arrival at the local hospital emergency department the endotracheal tube was found to be in the esophagus. An emergent CT scan showed several linear skull fractures, a small hematoma and generalized edema. His Glasgow Coma Scale (GCS) score was 4 on arrival (1-E, 2-M, 1-V). Two days later, a serial CT demonstrated severe edema with obliteration of the ventricles and initial signs of herniation. His GCS has dropped to a score of 3 and he was made a "No Code Blue" by his family. He continued to maintain a stable blood pressure and a manageable intracranial pressure. One week later with a GCS of 4, a cerebral arteriogram showed adequate blood flow to both hemispheres of his cerebral cortex. Barry continues to survive in a long-term care facility in a comatose state.

some vaccines. Two common words associated with this term are "anoxic" and "metabolic." Again, they identify general types of problems and are considered to be nonspecific diagnoses unless the exact cause of the encephalopathy is known.

Etiology and Pathophysiology of Anoxic Encephalopathy

Cerebral anoxia is the lack of oxygen to the brain's tissues from little or no blood supply to the brain. The effects of oxygen starvation can be devastating within 4 to 6 minutes and irreversible after 10 minutes. Anoxia can be caused by a variety of events, such as cardiac arrest, respiratory arrest, stroke, bleeding, carbon monoxide poisoning, atherosclerosis, or incorrect intubation. Those who survive these injuries have varying degrees of focal neurologic deficits relative to the area of damaged brain.

Certain areas of the brain are at a higher risk of incurring anoxic injuries than others and include the cortical and parenchymal gray matter. The arteries supplying blood to these areas are the most distal, and in times of low perfusion, as in cardiac arrest, these areas will be the first to shut down. The effects of anoxia can include massive cerebral ischemia, edema, necrosis, and brain death. Anoxia can lead to a poor quality of life and little, if any, functional ability. Cerebral anoxia, however, is not the same as brain dead. By definition, patients with brain death are comatose, unaware of their surroundings and unable to respond to any external stimuli. Not all comatose patients are brain dead if they can maintain cerebral blood flow. Lack of higher cortical function is common in comatose patients because cerebral blood flow and brain stem function are independent of hemispheric functioning.

Etiology and Pathophysiology of Metabolic Encephalopathy

Various medical conditions can cause brain dysfunction and changes in responsiveness because of their effects on brain metabolism. Metabolic encephalopathy can be due to meningitis, hepatic coma, hypoglycemia, liver failure, alcohol toxicity, delirium tremens, or hypoxia related to lung disease. The etiology of metabolic encephalopathy is speculated to be related to diminished blood flow, brain hypoxia, and/or changes in glucose metabolism.

Metabolic cerebral activity adjusts the cerebral blood flow to meet energy demands of the brain. Cerebral activity in a certain area can stimulate increased flow to that area. It is estimated that even while we sleep, our brains maintain 60% to 80% normal blood flow. Coma states and anesthetics significantly reduce the metabolic rate. Interruptions in energy production or utilization can cause problems which lead to neurologic changes.

Clinical Presentation

Anoxic Encephalopathy

- Memory problems (hallmark of anoxia)
- Loss of function (weakness, paralysis)
- Seizures
- Paresthesias
- Behavior changes
- Motor speech difficulties (dysphasia, dysphagia)
- Persistent vegetative states
- Coma

Metabolic Encephalopathy

Clinical presentation of metabolic encephalopathy is related to the underlying pathologic condition. Generally, the signs and symptoms are as follows:

- Change in level of consciousness (confusion, attention deficits, cognitive changes)
- Seizures
- Respiratory disorders
- Motor changes (generalized weakness, posturing)
- Cranial nerve dysfunction
- Delirium tremens (extreme diaphoresis, tachycardia, hypertension, hallucinations, profound agitation or physical activity)

Diagnostic Tests

Anoxic Encephalopathy

- *CT scan:* May show areas of cerebral edema, ischemia, or infarction related to the area of injury, seen as a darker gray area on films.

- *MRI:* May be used if CT scan is negative; will show early cerebral infarction.
- *EEG:* Usually done 24 hours after insult; can offer prognostic information. Adequate rhythm in all fields indicates good recovery; irregular and slow rhythm in one or all areas lasting longer than 24 hours predicts functional impairment; no activity alternating with bursts of spikes and slow wave activity is predictive of short-term survival; and no activity for more than 6 hours indicates no recovery.

Metabolic Encephalopathy

- *Lumbar or cisternal puncture:* May assist in diagnosis of underlying causes of encephalopathy; contraindicated in patients with increased intracranial pressure.
- *CT scan:* Useful in identification of cerebral edema; may assist in diagnosis of underlying causes of the encephalopathy.
- *MRI:* May be used if CT scan is nonpredictive.
- *EEG:* Adjunctive diagnostic tool; see anoxic encephalopathy.

Patient Needs and Principles of Management

The major focus of care for patients with encephalopathies is the treatment of the underlying cause, if known, and limiting functional losses. For those who require continuous management by the health care team, routine serial exams by the critical care nurse can assist the multidisciplinary team in managing contractures, skin breakdown, nutrition, and medication effectiveness.

▶ Postinsult Care to Limit Functional Loses

1. *Respiratory support.* Temporary support of oxygenation with mechanical ventilation is common. The goal of mechanical ventilation is to maintain normal acid-base parameters. Oxygen consumption rises to two to three times normal to meet the increase in metabolic needs, so the need to maintain PaO_2 at greater than 100 mm Hg is essential. It also is important to keep $PaCO_2$ between 25 to 35 mm Hg because increases in carbon dioxide can cause vasodilation, which may increase intracranial pressure. It is important to monitor the taping of endotracheal tubes; if the tape is too tight around the patient's neck, internal jugular compression can occur, causing a rise in the intracranial pressure.
2. *Cardiovascular support.* Further damage to the brain can be caused by hypotension after an anoxic brain injury. Vasopressors may be needed to maintain systolic pressures higher than 110 mm Hg. Control of dysrhythmias is important to maintain adequate cardiac output to the brain.
3. *Nutritional support.* Gastric or feeding tubes are common for nutritional supplementation, especially in the presence of decreased LOC. Increased metabolic demands from the injury, coupled with febrile states, lead to higher caloric needs than usual. Albumin and prealbumin levels should be monitored every few days for signs of catabolism.
4. *Neurological support.* Medications are used to reduce brain swelling or to assist with reopening of blocked blood vessels. Phenytoin is known to cause stabilization of the cell membrane, which may slow the damage to the brain as well as prevent seizure activity. Heparinization may be necessary to avoid complications of immobility, such as deep vein thrombosis (DVT), as well as to enhance microcirculatory flow. Calcium channel blockers have proven useful in treating vasospasm. Maintaining the head of the bed ≥ 30 degrees assists in gravity drainage of cerebrospinal fluid. Neutral positioning prevents internal jugular compression and rises in intracranial pressure. Using towel rolls or sandbags to aid in positioning is acceptable, as are flat pillows to prevent forward extension of the head and neck. Agitation should be managed with sedatives such as lorazepam or diazepam in scheduled doses around the clock until the patient is calm and demonstrating manageable behavior. However, oversedation should be avoided so level of consciousness can be more carefully monitored.
5. *Discharge planning.* Family support is of utmost importance because the circumstances surrounding this diagnosis are often sudden, unexpected, and very overwhelming. Discharge planning may be difficult depending on the level of care that the patient requires. Mechanically ventilated patients requiring intense, skilled nursing care will be best suited for long-term care facilities equipped to handle them. Some families may prefer to care for the

Patient Needs and Principles of Management, Cont.

family member at home with considerable home health care involvement.

▶ Prevention

Monitoring of cardiopulmonary function, with rapid intervention for situations of low blood pressure, perfusion, and/or tissue oxygenation is critical to prevent anoxic encephalitis. Following intubations, initial and ongoing assessments of airway patency and oxygenation status are important.

Cerebrovascular Accident (Stroke)

Cerebrovascular accident (CVA), or stroke as it is more commonly known, accounts for the largest proportion of neurologic illnesses in the United States today. Hypertension and arteriosclerosis are the major underlying causes of stroke. In order to understand the destruction that is caused by stroke, one must be familiar with the brain's need for survival. Although the brain's weight is only 2% of the total body weight, it requires 20% of the total cardiac output, 20% of the total oxygen consumption, and approximately 75% of the total glucose consumption. All of this is supplied through the bloodstream. When there is an interruption in this process for more than 4 minutes, ischemia begins to develop. If this process is not reversed, cellular death begins to occur, leading to necrosis of brain tissue. Strokes can range from mild with very small deficits to massive, as evidenced by complete functional and neurological shutdown.

Etiology, Risk Factors, and Pathophysiology

There is a vast system of blood vessel architecture in the brain. One of the more significant areas of the brain to be aware of is the middle cerebral artery (MCA). It is one of the first branches of the internal carotid artery and supplies the lateral portion of the entire cerebral hemisphere, as well as most of the basal ganglia. The other branch of the internal carotid is the anterior cerebral artery (ACA), which supplies the anterior portion of the cerebral hemisphere. Occlusion of these arteries is caused most often by an embolus from the heart or proximal vessels. Occasionally, atherosclerosis narrows the lumen of these arteries, leading to thrombosis and occlusion. Atherosclerotic plaques of these areas are more common in individuals of Afro-American

AT THE BEDSIDE

Mother: "I wish they had never done anything to him when he wrecked. Then he'd be with the good Lord now. Instead, he has to lay here and suffer like an old dog."
Sister: "This isn't my brother. It's just his body laying there, all connected up to the tubes. You all are keeping him alive, and for what? He'll never come back to us like he was."

AT THE BEDSIDE
▶ *Cerebrovascular Accident (CVA)*

James T., a 71-year-old retired teacher, was admitted to the neurologic ICU after his family noticed slurred speech, difficulty in naming objects, and inappropriate use of certain objects (he would use a comb to attempt to brush his teeth). The patient denies having any difficulty and thinks his family is "off their rocker. I've never been sick a day in my world."

He has a significant family history of hypertension (two brothers), and both of his parents died of "blood clots in the brain." On physical exam, the patient has right-sided neglect, eye deviation to the right, dysnomia (called a flashlight a hatchet, was unable to identify a pen), notable weakness in the right upper extremity, a flat affect, and dysarthria. His blood pressure is 210/115, and he claims to take an aspirin a day "to keep my blood thin." A CT without contrast demonstrated a left temporoparietal intracranial hemorrhage.

With acute blood pressure management with nitroprusside changing to Procardia XL (for long-term management), James' blood pressure has been under control for 7 days. He transferred to the rehabilitation unit where he is currently undergoing intensive therapy for his hemiplegia, neglect, and dysarthria. His children are extremely supportive and desire to take him home with them after discharge.

or Japanese origin. The extent of an infarction following occlusion of the MCA or ACA is extremely variable and depends on the location and rapidity of the occlusive process, the patient's anatomy and past history, and other systemic factors.

The blood supply to the brain can be altered through several different processes. These include embolism, thrombosis, hemorrhage, and compression or spasm of the vessels.

Embolism

Embolism refers to the occlusion of a cerebral vessel by a foreign substance such as a fragment of fat, a tumor, a blood clot, or air. Typically, embolism is linked with heart disease that features bacterial vegetations or blood clots that are easily detached from the wall or valves of the heart. The incidence of cerebral emboli is increased in chronic atrial fibrillation, with prosthetic valves, and in atrial myxomas, coagulopathies, or chronic subacute bacterial endocarditis. The fragmented substance easily lodges at the bifurcation of the middle cerebral artery, sometimes breaking apart and traveling further into the cerebral vascular system. The onset of an embolic occlusion is rapid, with symptoms developing without warning. The extent of the damage is less severe than that caused by thrombosis or hemorrhage, with a more rapid recovery. Sometimes pieces of embolic plaque break apart and can move into smaller vessels, causing less damage than occlusion of the larger vessel.

Thrombosis

Thrombosis is the most common cause of cerebral infarction and is most often due to arteriosclerosis and the formation of plaque within an artery, decreasing blood flow to the brain. The main site of thrombosis is the carotid artery. Decreased blood flow causes brain tissue ischemia along the course of the affected vessel, leading to cerebral edema. This secondary edema often causes the greater damage rather than the infarct itself. The edema subsides within hours to days followed by neurological improvement.

Patients with a history of atherosclerosis or arteritis are at highest risk for thrombotic strokes. The symptoms of thrombosis are variable, depending on the site and size of the occluded vessel. Thrombotic strokes tend to develop while the patient is asleep or within an hour after rising. This differs from intracerebral hemorrhages, which often occur during active waking hours of the day, or from embolic strokes, which occur at any time during the day.

Hemorrhage

Hemorrhage can occur anywhere within the layers of the brain—above the dura (epidural), below the dura (subdural), in the subarachnoid space (subarachnoid), or within the brain tissue itself (parenchymal or intracerebral). Although the first three types of hemorrhage can lead to ischemia and stroke, the one most commonly identified with CVA is the intracerebral hemorrhage.

Intracerebral hemorrhage results from the rupture of a vessel within the brain. Hemorrhage due to hypertension and arteriosclerosis are common after age 50. Of all stroke types, hemorrhages cause the most devastating functional deficits and have the slowest recovery. Identified functional deficits depend on the area injured and the extent of the hemorrhage. Although thrombosis does occur more commonly, it does not cause death unless the thrombus is massive. Smaller hemorrhage sometimes can have more damaging effects. Although improvement is possible after hypertensive hemorrhage, it is less likely and rarely is there a full recovery to prestroke states. In addition, there is a high mortality rate associated with intracerebral hemorrhage.

Compression or Spasm of Vessels

Compression and arterial spasm generally cause infarction of the brain if left untreated. Compression results from tumors, large blood clots, or swollen brain tissue. The area of circulation that is compressed has little or no blood supply, causing ischemia and eventual necrosis of the brain tissue affected. Arterial spasm, which is due to irritation of the arterial wall, usually by blood, decreases blood supply to the area of the brain that is supplied by the constricted vessel. Short-term vasospasm does not always mean permanent damage to the area. If vasospasm can be detected early and treated properly, ischemia and infarction of the brain tissue can be avoided. Identification and treatment of vasospasm are discussed in Chapter 24, Advanced Neurologic Concepts.

Clinical Presentation

Strokes of vascular origin have an abruptly clinical presentation, followed by stabilization and varying degrees of clinical improvement. Strokes of nonvascular origin present with a gradual onset, followed by progressive neurological deterioration. Once tissue necrosis has developed, no known treatment is available to restore that area of the brain to its original state. General and focal signs of neurologic dysfunction are usually seen at their most intense period upon presentation of the patient. However, on occasion, focal signs can worsen and the depth of the coma can increase following presentation. This is called a "stroke in evolution."

Transient Ischemic Attacks (TIAs)

- Reversible periods of temporary focal ischemia
- Sudden loss of speech
- Hemiplegia
- Paresthesia
- Last a few minutes to a few hours
- First warning signs of stroke

Global Symptoms

- Headaches
- Vomiting
- Seizures

- Coma
- Hypertension
- Memory impairment
- Confusion and disorientation

Focal Symptoms (based on the area of ischemia or hemorrhage)

- Motor dysfunction (paralysis, weakness)
- Speech and language difficulties
- Visual changes
- Sensory loss
- Reflex changes

Right Hemispheric Strokes (nondominant side)

- Left hemiparesis or hemiplegia
- Left homonymous hemianopsia (loss of vision in half of the visual field on the named side)
- Deviation of the head/eyes to the right
- Astereognosis (inability to identify the environment using the senses)
- Tactile inattention
- Constructional and dressing apraxia (inability to perform movements necessary to perform the task, even though the name and purpose of the act are known)

Left Hemispheric Strokes (dominant side)

- Right hemiparesis or hemiplegia
- Right homonymous hemianopsia
- Right/left disorientation
- Expressive or receptive dysphasia (or mixed)
- Deviation of the head/eyes to the left

Posterior Circulation Strokes (arising from the vertebral/basilar arteries)

- Dysarthria
- Disorientation
- Dizziness and disequilibrium
- Dysphagia
- Diplopia or other visual deficits

Anterior Circulation Strokes (arising from carotid arteries)

- Hemiparesis (MCA involvement: hemiparesis greater in the arm than in the leg; ACA involvement: hemiparesis greater in the leg than in the arm)
- Hemiparesthesia
- Hemiapraxia
- Hemianopsia

Diagnostic Tests

Differential diagnosis of stroke can be made via CT scan or angiography, as well as clinical examination and presentation. Other tests include EEG, MRI, or even echoencephalograms to confirm the diagnosis of stroke. Laboratory data that are helpful include CBC, especially WBC; BUN; and glucose level.

Large cerebral lesions can produce conjugate deviation of the eyes. A quick way to assess where the lesion might be is to look at the direction of the eyes. Eyes will deviate toward the site of injury and in some cases, the head and eyes have limited movement in the opposite direction. Pupillary changes vary depending on the site of the stroke. Typically, the larger pupil will be on the opposite side from the lesion.

Neglect, simply stated, is a condition where the patient completely ignores a part of his body, usually the hemiplegic side. This is a frequent occurrence in the stroke population and is quite simple to assess. If the patient is alert and able to follow commands, ask him or her to draw a clock face. The patient will be unable to draw the clock face on the side of the neglect. If the patient is unable to draw or cannot follow commands, offer a familiar object to use (comb, toothbrush). Offer the object by placing it in different places in front of him or her—to the far right, to the far left, and directly in the center. The patient will not pick up the item on the side of neglect. The assessment may be as simple as calling the patient's name while standing to one side of the bed and observing whether the patient is able to find you in that field. Interventions to assist patients with neglect include changing their bed position so that they are always approached from the unaffected side, teaching them visual scanning of the area, placing needed personal items on the unaffected side, and offering them a mirror if possible. Always encourage patients to identify the side of neglect and make them aware of their limbs and limb position.

Motor assessment is very important in patients who present with subarachnoid hemorrhages as well as focal deficits from space-occupying lesions. A drift assessment is a sensorimotor assessment that is quite easy to perform as long as the patient is able to follow directions and participate. Instruct the patient to close his or her eyes and raise the arms with the palms facing the ceiling. A normal response is for the patient to maintain this position until told to stop. Patients with focal motor weakness will demonstrate varying degrees of pronator drift. This is seen when the weakened side will have a slow drift of the arm in a downward direction or even just a turn of the palm to the floor. Patients who have parietal injury may even show a drift upward as a compensatory mechanism. It is important to remember to have patients' eyes remain closed during the exam. With their eyes open, patients see what is happening and tend to want to compensate for their weakness with shoulder lifts, bending at the elbows, or simply just striving to elevate their arms. Identify drifts as right or left, positive or negative in your documentation. If it is a new finding, as always, notify the physician as it may signify a worsening of the patient's condition.

Patient Needs and Principles of Management

Management of stroke varies depending on the etiology. The goals of treatment are to restore circulation to the brain, stop the ischemic process, restore function when possible through rehabilitative measures, and facilitate coping. General management principles are as follows.

▶ Serial Neurologic Evaluations

Monitoring for stroke progression should include level or side of paralysis or paresis, further functional deficits, and changes in level of consciousness. Any change or progressive worsening of the deficit should be reported to the physician immediately.

▶ Restore Circulation to Brain and Stop Ischemic Process

1. *Maintain adequate cerebral blood flow.* Blood pressure should be kept within a range so as to maintain cerebral blood flow at premorbid states, yet not at a level which will lead to further hemorrhage or cerebral damage. Vasopressors may be needed to accomplish this, such as nitroprusside or dopamine. Aggressive fluid administration may be required to increase vascular volume and cardiac output to maintain cerebral blood flow.
2. *Airway maintenance.* Maintaining adequate oxygenation in situations where oxygen supply is compromised is vital. Artificial airways are helpful in patients with airway obstruction or snoring respirations. Avoid sedatives and opiates if at all possible because they tend to depress the respiratory center.

▶ Restore Function and Prevent Complications

1. *Activity progression.* Bedrest is initiated early, with progressive activity ordered as the patient has functional return. Physical therapy, occupational therapy, and speech therapy should be consulted as indicated by the neurological dysfunction.
2. *Prevent complications of immobility.* To reduce pooling of blood in the lower extremities, it is common to use compression devices or elastic stockings on the extremities. These devices work to compress the veins that allow pooling of blood behind valves in the lower legs. They force the blood upward into the vascular system and don't allow it to form clots that are easily dislodged and the source of many potentially fatal problems.

▶ Management of the Underlying Cause of the Stroke

1. *Anticoagulation.* Once vascular hemorrhage can be ruled out as a cause of stroke, anticoagulation therapy can be initiated. There are differing opinions on dosing and frequency of heparin administration. Subcutaneous and intravenous administration are the two methods of heparin administration employed most frequently, barring any contraindications. Contraindications would include severe hypertension, vascular hemorrhage, or active ulceration of the GI tract. Heparin therapy can be initiated prior to oral coumarin derivatives if indicated.
2. *Blood pressure management.* This includes identifying and correcting any factors that would lead to a reduced cardiac output, including prevention of shock and circulatory collapse. Hypertension management can be the most difficult aspect of care to manage.
3. *Surgery.* The most common surgical procedure for embolic or thrombotic stroke is carotid endarterectomy. The near or complete occlusion of the carotids can be demonstrated through Doppler flow studies or arteriograms. Intraoperative clamping and stripping of the carotids is completed to restore or improve cerebral blood flow. A significant problem associated with carotid clamping is called "shower emboli," a term used when small pieces of atherosclerotic plaque break off of the vessel near the area of clamping and float up toward the brain causing further damage to the cerebrum. This can be a significant risk to patients having this procedure. Other surgical procedures include artery reconstruction or arterial bypass of the occlusion. These procedures carry with them similar risks and outcomes. The most common surgical procedure for compression

AT THE BEDSIDE

Daughter: "Daddy probably won't like living with us at first—he is so independent. But the doctors say he won't be safe living alone after he is discharged."

Son: "I think it's killing Dad to know he's like this. He never wanted to be a burden to anyone, and now, he can't even tie his shoe without help. Heck, he doesn't even know what a shoe is. This is pitiful. I hope they can get him back to normal soon."

strokes due to tumors is a craniotomy and tumor removal (see Chapter 24, Advanced Neurologic Concepts, for a detailed discussion).

▶ Facilitate Coping

Stroke is a devastating illness to patients, families, and the community. It is unexpected, unwanted, and often carries a negative impact for the patient and family. Chronic, long-term care may be needed if neurological deficits are severe. Support groups, both national and community-based, are helpful not only for the patients, but also for their caregivers. Pet therapy, music therapy, and other alternative therapies have proven useful in assisting patients and families through this highly emotional time.

Seizures

Seizures are sudden bursts of electrical activity within the brain, either unilateral or bilateral. A seizure is a phenomenon or symptom, not a disease. Seizures can be a frequent event in the management of critically ill patients. It is estimated that 50% of open head traumas and 5% of closed head traumas will have seizures during their hospital course.

Etiology, Risk Factors, and Pathophysiology

The etiology of seizures is not always clear. In fact, over 80% of the patients who have them never really receive a specific diagnosis for them. The few known causes of seizures include congenital defects of the nervous system, infectious disease, head injury, brain tumors, strokes, drug and alcohol withdrawal, brain abscesses, metabolic problems, and degenerative neurological diseases (e.g., Alzheimer's disease, phenylketonuria). Epilepsy, sometimes confused with the term seizures, is recurrent or chronic seizures uncontrolled by medications. Status epilepticus is uncontrolled generalized seizures in rapid succession (see Chapter 24, Advanced Neurologic Concepts).

The characteristics of seizures help to determine their location in the brain. In 1985, a simple classification system was developed to assist health care professionals in identifying seizure types. Two broad categories exist with several subcategories: (1) generalized seizures (once known as grand mal seizures) and (2) partial seizures (once known as petit mal seizures).

Generalized seizures are convulsive actions that affect the entire body. Partial seizures occur when there is a focal electrical discharge in one specific area of the brain. These seizures are subdivided into two categories—simple and complex. Simple partial seizures are also known as focal motor or focal sensory seizures. Complex partial seizures account for about one-third the total number of seizures

AT THE BEDSIDE
▶ Seizures

Susan D., 28 years old and a clerk in the county courthouse, was brought to the emergency department by EMS personnel after her husband called to say she had fallen in the bathroom and had not gotten up. On arrival to the ED, her vital signs were stable: BP 118/76, HR 78, RR 22 and snoring. She was noted to be incontinent of bowel and bladder, eyes deviated to the right, and difficult to arouse with nailbed pressure. Her past medical history according to her husband included a motor vehicle accident 3 years ago with a closed head injury, two normal vaginal deliveries, and an appendectomy when the patient was 14 years old. On further discussion with her husband, he stated that he heard her go into the bathroom, then "a lot of noise went on in there like something fell." When her husband called to her, she did not respond. On his arrival to the bathroom, the patient was noted to be unresponsive, on her back with her arms drawn up to her chest, her head turned to the right, with a glassy stare on her face. This is when he called the EMS. With an unwitnessed seizure, the doctors could only postulate that this was a generalized tonic-clonic seizure. A loading dose of phenytoin was given with orders for round-the-clock dosing. Susan woke up about 6 hours later with no knowledge of the incident, other than to complain of muscle soreness and a terrific headache. Susan was discharged after 6 days, and returned to work after 2 months. She continued to have seizures until her medication was under control. She is unable to drive and relies on her husband for assistance.

seen. They also are known as psychomotor or temporal lobe seizures. When people think of seizures, this is the type they generally associate with.

Clinical Presentation

Simple Partial Seizures

- Stiffening or jerking in one extremity or one side of the body
- Tingling sensation in the same area
- No loss of consciousness
- Time frame of 5 to 15 seconds

Complex Partial Seizures

- Variable from person to person
- Purposeless activity
- Aura (warning sign that is usually sensory in nature and related to the seizure focus)
- Staring
- Confusion or no response
- Automatisms (smacking the lips, chewing motions, or fidgeting)
- Nonviolent, but will struggle or fight if restrained
- Amnesia (temporary)
- Time frame of 1 to 3 minutes
- May evolve to generalized seizures

Generalized Seizures

- No aura
- Loud cry (not from pain, but from air rushing past the vocal cords)
- Tonic phase: Body tightens (similar to decorticate posturing), becomes unconscious
- Clonic phase: Muscles alternate between spasms and relaxation, jerking spastic movements
- Biting of tongue
- Foaming at the mouth
- Loss of bowel and bladder control
- Apnea
- Time frame of 1 to 3 minutes
- Postseizure (most are temporary): Regains consciousness, is confused and fatigued, has headache, may have some speech difficulties, may have a weakness of the arm or leg, and may sleep for hours

Diagnostic Testing

- *MRI:* Used to determine site of seizure focus; not always reliable (depends on cause of seizures; e.g., tumors show as grey areas)
- *Continuous Video Monitoring:* Used in conjunction with continuous EEG recordings, this is the most helpful tool in diagnosing seizure disorders. This can also help to recognize different types of seizures and differentiate between seizures and other clinical disorders (e.g., TIAs, hysterical episodes).
- *Lumbar Puncture:* Used when an infectious process (e.g., meningitis) is the suspected source of seizure activity.

Patient Needs and Principles of Management

The treatment of seizures focuses first on the correction of the problem, whether it is metabolic, alcohol-related, or even stress-induced. General patient care for patients having seizures includes maintaining safety, maintaining an airway, monitoring and treating seizure activity, and preventing complications.

▶ Correction of the Underlying Causes

1. *Assess contributing factors.* Assess for hypoglycemia, electrolyte imbalances, drugs or alcohol, or infections. Consider seizure prophylaxis in the following populations: open and closed head injuries, brain abscesses, meningiomas, acoustic neuromas, or any cerebral hematoma.
2. *Surgical options.* For approximately 5% of patients with seizures uncontrolled by medications, temporal lobe surgery may be helpful. This surgery carries with it hope, risks, complications, and positive outcomes for some. Selection criteria include 3 to 5 years of chronic seizures without evidence of remission; intractable seizures uncontrolled by any medication; identified unilateral focus of seizure activity determined by sodium amytal testing, neuropsychological testing, and continuous EEG monitoring; and seizure focus in an area where removal will cause no major neurological deficit.

   The mortality risk is less than 1%, and morbidity is at 2% due to a potential for hemorrhage or infection. Once the area is removed (approximately a 1 cm by 1 cm area), the patient is returned to the intensive care unit for continuous EEG monitoring and progression of care. Length of stay in the ICU is variable, but generally lasts 1 to 2 days. The patients are kept on their seizure medications for the postoperative period, and then continuously monitored during the next year. If after 1 year the patient is seizure free, the medications are slowly

Patient Needs and Principles of Management, Cont.

weaned. If a seizure does occur during this year, the medications are restarted at the preoperative dose. About one-half the patients who have this surgery and are seizure free for the first year can eventually stop taking medication. Success of this surgery is determined by seizure control.

▶ Safety Maintenance

Patients should not be restrained during seizure activity; rather, gently guide their extremities to a safe position or use pillows or padding to ensure a safe environment. *Do not place tongue blades, padded spoons, or your fingers in the patient's mouth.* Artificial airways or bite blocks are acceptable if they are placed before the patient begins to bite down. Do not attempt to place anything in the patient's mouth after seizure activity begins, even if he or she is biting the tongue.

▶ Airway Maintenance

When patients have seizures, position them on their sides in the rescue position. Offer supplementary oxygen, such as a blow by or nasal cannula if they are apneic for a short period of time. Longer periods of apnea may necessitate an artificial airway or intubation. Monitor the patient for vomiting and potential aspiration as well as any acute signs of hypoxia (circumoral cyanosis, low oxygen saturations, etc.).

▶ Monitoring Seizure Activity

1. *Monitoring seizures.* There are three phases of seizures that are important to monitor. The prodromal phase is not always visible to the human eye, but has to do with any auras that may occur. It may even be a slight change in the person's mood. The ictal phase is when the seizure is actually occurring. Safety of the person is the number one priority at this time. Note how long the seizure lasts, what the progression is, if the person is incontinent, and if any eye deviation occurs (it usually goes to the side of the seizure focus and any injury). The postictal phase can last two to three times as long as the seizure. The person may be amnestic and have some sensory or motor deficits that are temporary.

2. *Medication treatment.* Some medications may be needed to keep the seizure activity under control. General principles of medication treatment are to start with one drug and increase until seizures are controlled; if an additional drug is needed, then weaning from one to the other is indicated. Some common medications used for seizure control include phenytoin (Dilantin), phenobarbital (Luminal), carbamazepine (Tegretol), clonazepam (Clonopin), felbamate (Felbatol), and gabapentin (Neurontin). Seventy-five percent of patients treated with medication are able to maintain seizure control and live productive lives.

SELECTED BIBLIOGRAPHY

What Heals: Multisensory Stimulation

Mirr M: Meaningful communication with unresponsive individuals: Is it possible? *Capsules and Comments in Critical Care Nursing.* 1994;2:1–4.

Mitchell SK, Yates RR: Cerebrovascular disease. In Dossey BM, Guzzetta CE, Kenner CV: *Critical care nursing: Body-mind-spirit,* 3rd ed. Philadelphia: JB Lippincott, 1992, pp. 588–589.

Encephalopathy

Alspach G (ed.): *AACN core curriculum for critical care nursing,* 4th ed. Philadelphia: WB Saunders, 1991.

American Nurses' Association: *Neuroscience nursing practice:*

Process and outcome criteria for selected diagnoses. Washington, D.C.: ANA, 1985.

Boss BJ: Cognitive systems: Nursing assessment and management in the critical care environment. *AACN Clinical Issues in Critical Care Nursing.* 1991;2(4):685–698.

Guin PR, Freudenberger K: The elderly neuroscience patient: Implications for the critical care nurse. *AACN Clinical Issues in Critical Care Nursing.* 1992;3(2):98–105.

Hickey JV: *The clinical practice of neurological and neurosurgical nursing,* 3rd ed. Philadelphia: JB Lippincott, 1992.

Krause MV, Mahan LK: *Food, nutrition and diet therapy,* 6th ed. Philadelphia: WB Saunders, 1979.

Luce JM, Pierson DJ: *Critical care medicine.* Philadelphia: WB Saunders, 1988.

Lundgren J: *Acute neuroscience nursing: Concepts and care.* Boston: Jones & Bartlett, 1986.

Marshall SB, Marshall LF, Vos HR, Chesnut RM: *Neuroscience critical care: Pathophysiology and patient management.* Philadelphia: WB Saunders, 1990.

Snyder M (ed.): *A guide to neurological and neurosurgical nursing,* 2nd ed. Albany, NY: Delmar, 1991.

Stewart-Amidei C: Assessing the comatose patient in the intensive care unit. *AACN Clinical Issues in Critical Care Nursing.* 1991; 2(4):613–622.

Thelan LA, Davie JK, Urden LD: *Textbook of critical care nursing diagnosis and management.* St. Louis, MO: CV Mosby, 1990.

Walleck C: Preventing secondary brain injury. *AACN Clinical Issues in Critical Care Nursing.* 1992;3(2):19–30.

Wright JE, Shelton BK (eds.): *Desk reference for critical care nursing.* Boston: Jones & Bartlett, 1993.

Cerebrovascular Accidents

Alspach G (ed.): *AACN core curriculum for critical care nursing,* 4th ed. Philadelphia: WB Saunders, 1991.

American Heart Association: *Stroke: Why do they behave that way?* Dallas: AHA, 1992.

American Nurses' Association: *Neuroscience nursing practice: Process and outcome criteria for selected diagnoses.* Washington, D.C.: ANA, 1985.

Hickey JV: *The clinical practice of neurological and neurosurgical nursing,* 3rd ed. Philadelphia: JB Lippincott, 1992.

Luce JM, Pierson DJ: *Critical care medicine.* Philadelphia: WB Saunders, 1988.

Lundgren J: *Acute neuroscience nursing: Concepts and care.* Boston: Jones & Bartlett, 1986.

Marshall SB, Marshall LF, Vos HR, Chesnut RM: *Neuroscience critical care: Pathophysiology and patient management.* Philadelphia: WB Saunders, 1990.

National Stroke Association: *What is a stroke?* Englewood, CO: NSA, 1990.

Snyder M (ed.): *A guide to neurological and neurosurgical nursing,* 2nd ed. Albany, NY: Delmar, 1991.

Thelan LA, Davie JK, Urden LD: *Textbook of critical care nursing diagnosis and management.* St. Louis, MO: CV Mosby, 1990.

Wright JE, Shelton BK (eds.): *Desk reference for critical care nursing.* Boston: Jones & Bartlett, 1993.

Seizures

Alspach G (ed.): *AACN core curriculum for critical care nursing,* 4th ed. Philadelphia: WB Saunders, 1991.

American Nurses' Association: *Neuroscience nursing practice: Process and outcome criteria for selected diagnoses.* Washington, D.C.: ANA, 1985.

Dupuis RE, Miranda-Massari J: Anticonvulsants: Pharmacotherapeutic issues in the critically ill patients. *AACN Clinical Issues in Critical Care Nursing.* 1991;2(4):639–656.

Hickey JV: *The clinical practice of neurological and neurosurgical nursing,* 3rd ed. Philadelphia: JB Lippincott, 1992.

Hodges K, Root L: Surgical management of intractable seizure disorders. *Journal of Neuroscience Nursing.* 1991;23(2): 93–100.

Luce JM, Pierson DJ: *Critical care medicine.* Philadelphia: WB Saunders, 1988.

Lundgren J: *Acute neuroscience nursing: Concepts and care.* Boston: Jones & Bartlett, 1986.

Marshall SB, Marshall LF, Vos HR, Chesnut RM: *Neuroscience critical care: Pathophysiology and patient management.* Philadelphia: WB Saunders, 1990.

O'Brien K: Managing the seizure patient. *Nursing 91.* 1991;January:63–65.

Snyder M (ed.): *A guide to neurological and neurosurgical nursing,* 2nd ed. Albany, NY: Delmar, 1991.

Thelan LA, Davie JK, Urden LD: *Textbook of critical care nursing diagnosis and management.* St. Louis, MO: CV Mosby, 1990.

Wright JE, Shelton BK (eds.): *Desk reference for critical care nursing.* Boston: Jones & Bartlett, 1993.

Sixteen

Hematology and Immunology Systems

▶ **Knowledge Competencies**

1. Analyze basic laboratory test results used to assess the status of the hematologic and immunologic systems for abnormalities:

   - Complete blood count
   - White blood cell differential
   - Erythrocyte sedimentation rate
   - Prothrombin time/international normalization ratio
   - Partial thromboplastin time
   - Fibrinogen
   - Fibrin split products/d-dimer

2. Describe the etiology, pathophysiology, clinical presentation, patient needs, and management approaches for common hematologic problems in critically ill patients:

   - Anemia
   - Disseminated intravascular coagulation (DIC)

3. Contrast the clinical presentation, patient needs, and principles of management of the neutropenic patient with that of a critically ill patient with an intact immune response.

■ *What Heals: Psychoneuroimmunology*

Each of us has experienced physiologic increases in heart rate and respirations when we become angry or scared. We also have experienced the physiologic response of relaxation when we are feeling rested, balanced, and at peace with ourselves. How then can our emotions change our physiology? Is it just a physiologic, autonomic event—or is it something more?

Psychoneuroimmunology (PNI) is a new field that examines the bidirectional impact of the psychologic mind state on immune function as moderated by the nervous and endocrine systems. The field of PNI has generated conclusive evidence that what we think and feel (our thoughts and emotions) can affect our neurologic, endocrine, and immune systems (either in positive or negative ways) at the cellular and subcellular levels. These findings help to explain the critical link between the mind and the body.

The discovery of the neuropeptide system has advanced the field of PNI and transformed our understanding of how the body and the mind communicate. Neuropeptides are amino acids that open the lock to receptor sites to facilitate or block specific cellular responses. The first neuropeptides discovered were endorphins (meaning the morphine within). Endorphins are called neuropeptides because they were first discovered in the brain and are composed of peptides.

Since the discovery of endorphins, dozens of other neuropeptides have been identified. Brain function can be regulated by these neuropeptides, which can alter behavior, mood states, and cellular function. Neuropeptides also have been found to be located not only in the brain but also in the brain stem, spinal cord, and gastrointestinal system and are capable of circulating throughout the body to communicate with all body parts.

Neuropeptides (called messenger molecules) and their receptors explain how emotions are experienced throughout the body. Because the autonomic, endocrine, and immune systems all make and use these messenger molecules, these systems are able to "talk" to each other. The autonomic, immune, and endocrine systems are all integrated by the neuropeptides which are responsible for connecting the body and emotions.

As nurses, we need to understand that we can help our patients to facilitate the process of body-mind communication in more intentional and deliberate ways. Research has found that body-mind inter-ventions such as relaxation therapies and imagery can produce positive emotions and feelings. Immunocompetence, for example, may be increased by such positive emotions, attitudes, thoughts, and feelings. By implementing such therapies we help patients not only to cope with the anxiety and stress of a critical illness but also to transform their negative emotions into desired thoughts and feelings to activate inner psychophysiologic healing.

CEG & BMD

Adapted from: The critical link between body and mind. In Guzzetta CE, Dossey BM: Cardiovascular nursing: Holistic practice. St. Louis, MO: Mosby-Year Book, 1992, pp. 78–79.

SPECIAL ASSESSMENT TECHNIQUES, DIAGNOSTIC TESTS, AND MONITORING SYSTEMS

A complete patient assessment will guide the selection of screening tests for hematologic and immunologic problems. Historical data are particularly important and should include family history, occupational exposures, lifestyle behaviors, diet, allergies, past medical problems, surgeries, transfusion of blood or blood products, and current medications. Abnormal physical assessment data from each body system collectively identify risk factors or acute abnormalities pertinent to hematologic and immunologic function. In addition, a variety of laboratory tests assist the clinician to evaluate problems in these systems (Table 16–1).

Complete Blood Count

The complete blood count (CBC) is the primary assessment tool for evaluation of the hematologic and immunologic status. The red blood cell (RBC) count and RBC indices, along with the hemoglobin (Hgb) and hematocrit (Hct) levels, provide valuable information regarding the oxygen-carrying capability of the blood. The total white blood cell (WBC) count and the WBC differential reveal the body's ability to muster an immunological response against foreign substances and to participate in the normal inflammatory process required for tissue restoration. Partial information concerning hemostasis is obtained from the platelet count, with additional studies required to fully evaluate the coagulation process.

RBC Count

The RBC count is based on the number of erythrocytes per cubic millimeter of blood. Normal values for males are higher than for females. A decrease in normal RBC count by 10% indicates anemia. Anemia may be caused by decreased production or increased destruction of RBC or loss of RBC by hemorrhage. An increase in the total number of RBC occurs as a compensatory mechanism in persons with chronic hypoxia or as an adaptation to high altitudes. Further assessment of the ability of the bone marrow to produce RBC is obtained by a reticulocyte count.

Hemoglobin

Hemoglobin is the primary carrier of oxygen to body tissues and returns carbon dioxide to the lungs for elimination. As the number of RBC changes, so does the Hgb content. The Hgb can be estimated by multiplying the total RBC count by 3. A decrease in Hgb to a level as low as 7 g/dl can be well tolerated, if the decrease occurs gradually. Patients with underlying cardiac or pulmonary disorders may become symptomatic with even small changes in the Hgb content of the blood.

Hematocrit

Hematocrit measures the RBC mass in relationship to a volume of blood. It is usually expressed as the percentage of cells per 100 ml of blood. Multiplying the Hgb value by 3 gives an estimate of Hct. The Hct is particularly sensitive to changes in the volume status of the patient, increasing with fluid losses and decreasing with increased plasma volume.

TABLE 16–1. NORMAL VALUES FOR HEMATOLOGIC AND IMMUNOLOGIC SCREENING TESTS*

Laboratory Test	Normal Value
RBC	Males: 4.6–6.2 million/mm^3
	Females: 4.2–5.4 million/mm^3
Hgb	Males: 13–18 g/dl
	Females: 12–16 g/dl
Hct	Males: 45%–54%
	Females: 36%–46%
RBC indices	
MCV	81–98 um^3
MCH	27–32 pg/cell
MCHC	32%–36%
Total WBC	5000–10,000 mm^3
WBC differential (% of total)	
Neutrophils	60%–70%
Segmented	56%
Bands	3%–6%
Eosinophils	1%–4%
Basophils	0.5%–1.0%
Monocytes	2%–6%
Lymphocytes	20%–40%
Platelet count	150,000–400,000 mm^3
Erythrocyte sedimentation rate	
Westergren method	Males: 0–15 mm/hour
	Females: 0–20 mm/hour
PT	11–15 seconds
Therapeutic anticoagulation	1.5 times normal
INR, therapeutic anticoagulation	2.0–3.0
PTT	30–45 seconds
APTT	15–25 seconds
Therapeutic anticoagulation	1.5–2.5 times normal
Fibrinogen	200–400 mg/dl
FSP	2–10 ug/ml
d-dimer	25 mg/dl

*Normals vary between laboratories. Refer to local laboratory standard values when interpreting test results.

Interpretation of Hgb and Hct results must also take into account the time the values were obtained in relationship to blood volume loss or fluid administration. For example, values obtained immediately after an acute hemorrhage may appear normal, as compensatory mechanisms have not had time to restore plasma volume. Restoration of plasma volume by compensation or crystalloid resuscitation will lower the Hgb and Hct.

RBC Indices

The RBC indices are mathematical calculations based on the RBC, Hgb, and Hct which describe the size, weight, and Hgb concentration of the individual erythrocyte. These indices are useful in determining the etiology of anemia.

Total WBC Count

Leukocytes, or WBC circulating in the blood, are measured as an indicator of the total amount of WBC in the body. Most WBC are not sampled in a CBC as they are marginated along capillary walls, circulating in the lymphatic system, or sequestered in lymph nodes and other body tissues.

Increased WBC, or leukocytosis, usually is caused by an elevation in one type of WBC line. It is most often associated with a normal immune system response to an infection, but is also a normal result of the inflammatory process. Overproduction of abnormal leukocytes in the bone marrow occurs during leukemia.

Leukopenia refers to a decrease in the total WBC number. This occurs when bone marrow production is inhibited or during infection when rapid consumption of WBC takes place. The life span of a circulating WBC is only hours to days; therefore, a constant replacement process is necessary to prevent leukopenia.

WBC Differential

Five different categories of leukocytes are measured in the differential and reported as a percentage of the total WBC count. The absolute count is calculated by multiplying the percentage of each type of cell by the total WBC count. Increases or decreases in one cell line help determine normal immune response or predict impaired immunity.

Neutrophils are the primary responders to infection and inflammation in the body. This type of WBC is released from the bone marrow in an immature form called a band. Bands quickly mature into segmented neutrophils with greater phagocytic properties to respond to infection. Most often leukocytosis is caused by an increased number of segmented neutrophils (neutrophilia). The term *left shift* generally is used to refer to leukocytosis with an increased percentage of bands. Neutropenia, or a decreased number of circulating neutrophils, places the body at increased risk for infection. An absolute neutrophil count of less than 1000/mm^3 severely compromises immune system function, particularly to bacterial infections.

Monocytes are phagocytic cells that circulate briefly in the blood before leaving the cardiovascular system to mature into macrophages in other body tissues. The circulating monocyte is an important scavenger WBC. As it performs phagocytosis, it sends out chemicals called cytokines which activate the lymphocytes of the blood.

Lymphocytes are WBC responsible for the body's specific immune response to infection. Subsets of these lymphocytes exist and are assessed by other laboratory tests. Lack of proper functioning lymphocytes or adequate numbers of these cells places the body at particular risk for viral and fungal infections. The CD4 cell is a subset of lymphocytes. It is the target of HIV infection leading to the development of acquired immunodeficiency syndrome (AIDS).

Eosinophils are thought to perform phagocytosis of immune complexes generated during allergic reactions. Therefore, increased percentages of these cells are seen during an allergic response. Basophils are another WBC associated with allergy. They are thought to break down during an allergic reaction, releasing their intracellular contents of heparin and histamine. This destruction causes a lower percentage of basophils following an allergic response.

Platelet Count

Platelets are disc-shaped fragments of megakaryocytes and are not true cells. They are called thrombocytes because of their role in the initiation of blood coagulation at the site of damaged blood vessel walls. Two-thirds of the body's platelets are circulating in the blood, with the remaining third sequestered within the spleen. Thrombocytopenia (decreased number of platelets) is associated with increased risk of spontaneous bleeding and is caused by decreased production, increased consumption, increased destruction, or increased sequestration of platelets. Hypercoagulability of the blood can result from increased circulating platelets caused by proliferative disorders and inflammation. Qualitative assessment of platelet function is determined by the bleeding time.

Erythrocyte Sedimentation Rate (ESR)

A nonspecific but useful test in monitoring inflammation and infection in the body is the ESR. It measures the rate RBC settle out of unclotted blood. Females normally have a higher rate than males. Different laboratory techniques have different normal values. Elevated ESR is seen in pregnancy, infection, inflammatory diseases, and cancer. Decreased ESR is seen in sickle cell anemia, polycythemia, or hypofibrinogenemia.

Coagulation Studies

Prothrombin Time (PT) and International Normalization Ratio (INR)

The PT evaluates the extrinsic pathway of fibrin clot formation stimulated by tissue trauma. Prolonged PT may be caused by abnormalities in coagulation factors V, VII, and X, prothrombin, fibrinogen, and vitamin K, and by liver disease or DIC. It is a test used to evaluate therapeutic anticoagulation with coumadin. PT results are reported in seconds.

Because of different reagents used in testing, PT values from different facilities are not standardized, so comparing results may lead to discrepancies. The INR is a calculation developed to standardize interpretation of PT results. The PT and INR are reported together, but the INR is now the recommended system for establishing the therapeutic range for oral anticoagulant therapy.

Partial Thromboplastin Time (PTT) and Activated Partial Thromboplastin Time (APTT)

The PTT and APTT are reported in seconds and are used to evaluate fibrin clot formation stimulated by the intrinsic pathway of coagulation. The APTT is a more sensitive test than the PTT. These tests are used to screen for congenital coagulation disorders and for monitoring anticoagulation with heparin therapy. Liver disease, vitamin K deficiency, and DIC prolong the PTT/APTT.

Fibrinogen

Fibrinogen, also known as coagulation factor I, is measured in the plasma. It may be increased during inflammatory response, pregnancy, or acute infection. Decreased levels are present with liver disease and DIC. If the fibrinogen level has been elevated, a downward trend, even though within normal range, can indicate a consumptive coagulopathy. Other specific clotting factor assays may be performed if a hereditary bleeding tendency is suspected.

Fibrin Split Products (FSP) and Fibrin Degradation Products (FDP)

The normal breakdown of a fibrin clot releases fragments with mildly anticoagulant properties called FSP or FDP. Excessive clot breakdown results in elevated amounts of FSP, contributing to a tendency for bleeding. Increased FSP are observed in DIC, obstetrical complications involving hemorrhage, and pulmonary embolism. Fibrinolytic drugs such as streptokinase, urokinase, or t-PA, used therapeutically in treating myocardial infarction, cause levels of FSP to rise.

d-dimer

Individual fragments of FSP can be identified. One fragment, the d-dimer, is a more specific indicator of fibrinolysis. Testing for d-dimer is used as a confirmation of DIC, but it will also be elevated when using fibrinolytic agents.

Additional Tests and Procedures

After obtaining basic laboratory screening tests, additional laboratory and diagnostic testing will be necessary to identify specific etiologies for hematologic and immunologic function.

For patients with hematologic disorders, a peripheral blood smear, a bone marrow aspiration, or further studies of specific clotting factors may be performed. Further immunologic testing may include complement levels, protein electrophoresis, serological testing for antibody responses, or phagocyte function studies.

Microbiological specimens for Gram's stain and culture help to identify sources of infection. Noninvasive studies such as ultrasound may determine liver, spleen, or lymph node abnormalities. Radiologic procedures (x-rays, CT scans, arteriograms) may be needed to identify areas of infection or hemorrhage.

PATHOLOGIC CONDITIONS

Critically ill patients often have combined abnormalities involving the hematologic and immunologic systems. The patient with sepsis and subsequent disseminated intravascular coagulation (DIC), as in this case study, typifies this situation. Anemia, immunocompromise, and coagulopathy are three distinct problems faced in the management of this patient. Each of these problems will be explored separately.

AT THE BEDSIDE
▶ *Sepsis and Disseminated Intravascular Coagulation*

Mr. Johnson, a 63-year-old Caucasian male, was admitted to the MICU with hypotension, alteration in mental status, and a fever of 102° rectally. He has a history of rheumatoid arthritis, right total hip replacement, and gastric ulcers. He is disoriented to place and time. Hemodynamic data revealed values consistent with septic shock. Dressings covering his intravascular lines show evidence of oozing from insertion sites. Nasogastric aspirate is coffee ground in appearance. His initial laboratory data show:

RBC	3.3 million/mm^3
Hgb	10.8 g/dl
Hct	31%
WBC	13,000/mm^3, with 79% neutrophils and 20% bands
Platelets	120,000/mm^3
Fibrinogen	325 mg/dl
Protime	16 seconds
PTT	60 seconds
FSP	40 µg/ml
d-dimer	>250 mg/ml

Anemia

Etiology, Risk Factors, and Pathophysiology

Anemia is the most common condition resulting from hematologic disease. Its etiology may be classified into disorders of RBC production, increased destruction of RBC, or acute blood loss.

A patient history gives important clues to the etiology of anemia. Decreased production may result from nutritional deficiencies in substrates for RBC production—iron, folic acid, or vitamin B$_{12}$. Those at high risk for iron deficiency anemia include children, adolescents, and pregnant women, or patients with malabsorption syndromes. Chronic blood loss from the GI tract or from heavy menstruation is the most important cause. Folic acid deficiency may be seen in alcoholics. Vitamin B$_{12}$ deficiency from the diet may occur in strict vegetarians and from lack of intrinsic factor (postgastrectomy or with pernicious anemia) or Crohn's disease.

Anemia may be associated with chronic illness, such as chronic inflammation, infection, cancer, liver disease, or renal failure. The life span of RBC is decreased in these chronic disease states, and the bone marrow does not compensate adequately with increased production. Cancer specifically involving the bone marrow will replace normal bone marrow and decrease new RBC generation. Anemia associated with chronic renal failure is more severe and involves a decrease in production of erythropoietin, resulting in decreased stimulation of bone marrow production of RBC.

Aplastic anemia represents a failure of the bone marrow to produce RBC (or any other cellular components of blood). A thorough medication history may reveal use of drugs with potential for bone marrow suppressive side effects. Cancer chemotherapeutic agents represent one such category of drugs. Other causes of aplastic anemia include exposure to toxins such as insecticides, congenital abnormality, and idiopathic (e.g., autoimmune) disorders.

Thalassemia represents a group of genetically inherited syndromes of abnormal hemoglobin synthesis. The abnormal RBC has a short life span as the cells are hemolyzed prematurely. Thalassemia can be considered an anemia resulting from both abnormal production and accelerated destruction.

Premature destruction of RBC leads to hemolytic anemia. This can occur episodically or chronically. Abnormalities intrinsic to the RBC are usually hereditary causes of hemolytic anemia, such as sickle cell disease or G6PD deficiency. Extrinsic sources of hemolysis include immune destruction as in a transfusion reaction, damage by artificial heart valves, cardiopulmonary bypass, or intraaortic balloon pumping.

Acute hemorrhage also will lead to anemia. Trauma, surgical blood loss, DIC, gastrointestinal bleeding, and bleeding from excessive anticoagulation frequently are encountered as causes of anemia in the critical care patient population. With acute hemorrhage, both cellular components and plasma are lost simultaneously. Until volume replacement from fluid resuscitation or mobilization of fluids from extracellular sources occurs, a drop in Hct will not be appreciated.

Regardless of the etiology of anemia, the critical effect of decreased RBC is a decrease in the oxygen-carrying capacity of the blood. Effects may be well tolerated if anemia develops slowly, but may be life-threatening if sudden blood loss occurs. Rapid loss of blood volume results in hypovolemic shock and cardiovascular instability, further reducing delivery of oxygen to body tissues.

Clinical Signs and Symptoms

Clinical manifestations are related to the body's compensatory mechanisms attempting to maintain perfusion of oxygen to vital tissues. As compensatory mechanisms are overwhelmed, more serious signs and symptoms occur. Patients with underlying pathology involving the pulmonary and cardiovascular system will not tolerate effects of anemia and become symptomatic more quickly.

Cardiovascular

- Tachycardia, palpitations
- Widened pulse pressure
- Increased cardiac output
- Decreased capillary refill

- New systolic flow murmur
- Orthostatic hypotension
- Chest pain
- ECG abnormalities (dysrhythmias, ischemic changes)
- Hypovolemic shock (hypotension, tachycardia, decreased cardiac output, increased systemic vascular resistance)

Respiratory

- Increased respiratory rate
- Dyspnea on exertion, progressing to at rest

Skin/Musculoskeletal

- Pallor of skin and mucous membranes
- Dusky nailbeds

- Intermittent claudication
- Muscle cramps
- Decreased skin temperature
- Clubbing of nails in chronic anemia

Neurologic

- Headache
- Light-headedness
- Faintness
- Roaring in the ears
- Irritability
- Restlessness
- Fatigue

Abdominal

- Enlarged liver and/or spleen

Patient Needs and Principles of Management

The management of the anemic patient must be guided by the severity of symptoms. The level of concern for Hgb and Hct decreases is determined by the patient's symptoms and if bleeding is suspected. Restoration of adequate oxygen delivery to tissues is a priority in the critically ill patient. Identification of the etiology of anemia and resolution of the underlying cause, if possible, also should be attempted.

▶ Improvement of Oxygen Delivery

Oxygen delivery is a product of the amount of Hgb in the blood, the saturation of the Hgb with oxygen, and the cardiac output. Management strategies focus on optimizing each of those components.

1. Administration of supplemental oxygen can enhance oxygen saturation. Use of oxygen, particularly during activity, may assist with dyspnea on exertion.
2. Adequate Hgb can be replaced in acute situations only by transfusion of packed RBC. Transfusion of one unit of packed RBC should increase the Hgb by 1 g/dl and Hct by 2% to 3%.
3. Cardiac output can be optimized with volume replacement, including packed RBC, in situations of bleeding and hypovolemia. Other manipulations of cardiac output must be guided by hemodynamic monitoring and calculations to assess oxygen delivery and oxygen consumption.
4. Monitoring vital signs, oxygen saturation, and sub-

jective patient data before, during, and after a change in therapy or activity will identify the patient's ability to tolerate anemia.
5. Use of cell savers and autotransfusion in surgical patients may help to reduce blood losses and anemia.
6. Minimizing activity and planning periods of rest are important nursing interventions for the anemic patient.

▶ Identification and Treatment of Underlying Disease State

Further diagnostic testing is indicated to determine the etiology of anemia. Radiological studies to locate sites of bleeding, particularly in the GI tract, may be necessary. Treatment of the underlying cause of anemia may vary from supportive care to the following:

1. Administer recombinant human erythropoietin to restore bone marrow production in chronic anemia. The response may take several weeks so it is not appropriate in situations in which acute correction of anemia is necessary. Chronic renal failure patients and patients receiving chemotherapy are two groups that may benefit from this treatment.
2. Supplemental oral ferrous sulfate may be indicated if iron deficiency anemia is present.
3. Dietary consultation may be needed prior to discharge to help patients and families plan meals with foods high in iron.

Immunocompromise

Etiology, Risk Factors, and Pathophysiology

All critically ill patients may be considered compromised hosts because their defense mechanisms are inadequate due to a combination of factors, such as age, nutritional status, underlying disease, medical therapy, or stress. Patients in the critical care unit are much more likely to develop a nosocomial infection than other hospitalized patients. The term *immunocompromised* is applied to patients whose immunological defense mechanisms are defective. Immunocompromised patients are prone to nosocomial infection, but may also develop opportunistic infection. Once infection develops in a critically ill patient, it may quickly progress to a systemic response to infection or sepsis.

Immune system protection from infection is categorized into three levels: natural defenses, nonspecific responses, and specific responses. Natural defenses include having intact epithelial surfaces (skin and mucous membranes) with normal chemical barriers (pH, secretions) present and all protective reflexes (blink, swallow, cough, gag, sneeze) intact. The nonspecific response to infection is activation of the phagocytic WBC (neutrophils and monocytes) to attack the foreign microorganisms (antigens) that have entered the body by passing or overwhelming the natural defenses. The monocytes play a key role in processing the invading antigen and presenting it to the WBC involved in the specific immune response.

Lymphocytes (B cells and T cells) are responsible for the orchestration of an immune response specific to the antigen. B lymphocytes create antigen-specific antibodies or immunoglobulins to aid in the destruction of the antigen and to protect the body from future encounters with the antigen. This is called *humoral immunity*. T lymphocytes have different subsets of cells created to modulate the immune system response (the T4 or CD4 cells) or cells which have cytotoxic properties (the T8 or CD8 cells) against the antigen. The immune response of the T lymphocytes is called *cell-mediated immunity*. Both types of lymphocytes work closely together in a specific immune response. However, humoral immunity is the primary protection against bacterial invasion and cell-mediated immunity is primarily targeted against intracellular infection by viral and fungal organisms.

Deficiencies in immune system function can be categorized into primary, or congenital, immune system defects and secondary, or acquired, immune system dysfunction. Immune deficiencies may be pinpointed to a specific cell type or may involve abnormalities in multiple components of the immune system. Secondary or acquired immunodeficiencies are the most likely type encountered in the critically ill patient population. Acquired immunodeficiency may be secondary to age, malnutrition, stress, chronic disease states, malignancy, drugs with immunosuppressive effects, or HIV infection.

Today, increased numbers of patients are undergoing organ transplantation and receiving immunosuppressive agents. More aggressive chemotherapeutic treatment of cancer is producing higher numbers of patients with bone marrow suppression. The dramatic growth in the number of people infected with HIV has also increased the number of immunosuppressed patients. All of these patients are at high risk for the development of neutropenia.

Neutropenia, an absolute neutrophil count below $500/mm^3$, generally increases susceptibility to infection. The cause and duration of neutropenia, the functional capability of the neutrophils, the state of the patient's natural barriers, and the endogenous and exogenous flora also contribute to the susceptibility of the individual patient to infection. The earlier infection can be detected, the more likely therapy is to be effective.

Detection of infection in the neutropenic patient may be more difficult. Due to lack of neutrophils, the patient may not be able to mount a vigorous inflammatory response; therefore, classic signs and symptoms of infection may be diminished or absent. For instance, purulent drainage is largely the result of dying neutrophils at the site of infection. The neutropenic patient may have an infection without evidence of purulent drainage. Pain may be the patient's only complaint. Any complaint of pain in this patient population must be fully investigated.

Clinical Signs and Symptoms

Local Evidence of Inflammation and Infection

- Redness
- Edema
- Warmth
- Pain
- Purulent drainage

General Evidence of Infection

- Fever or hypothermia
- Rigors or shaking chills
- Malaise
- Changes in level of consciousness
- Lymphadenopathy
- Tachycardia
- Tachypnea

System-specific

NEUROLOGICAL
- Headache
- Nuchal rigidity

RESPIRATORY
- Cough
- Change in color, amount of sputum

GENITOURINARY

- Dysuria
- Urgency
- Frequency
- Flank pain
- Abdominal pain
- Cloudy and/or bloody urine

GASTROINTESTINAL

- Nausea
- Vomiting
- Diarrhea
- Cramping abdominal pain
- Enlarged liver

Patient Needs and Principles of Management

Those patients with high risk for the development of infection must be identified upon admission to the critical care unit. Measures to protect and strengthen immune system function should be included in the plan of care. All health care team members must utilize measures to prevent the development of nosocomial infection. Close monitoring for signs and symptoms of a local or systemic inflammatory response to infection is especially important to detect infection early. Identification of the source and likely organisms causing infection will allow for initiation of broad-spectrum, empiric antimicrobial coverage. Culture and sensitivity reports will guide the choice of drug(s) specific to the organisms isolated from the patient.

▶ Identification of Patients with High Risk of Infection

Risk factors for immunocompromise are as follows:

1. Neonates and the elderly
2. Malnutrition
3. Medications with known immunosuppressive effects such as steroids, cancer chemotherapeutic agents, cyclosporin, or azathioprine
4. History of recent radiation therapy
5. Chronic systemic diseases such as renal or hepatic failure or diabetes mellitus
6. Known diseases involving the immune system such as HIV infection
7. Loss of protective epithelial barriers through:

   - Oral or nasogastric intubation
   - Presence of decubitus ulcers
   - Burns
   - Surgical wounds
   - Skin and soft tissue trauma

8. Invasive catheters or prosthetic devices in place such as:

   - Intravascular catheters
   - Indwelling bladder catheters
   - Heart valve replacements

   - Orthopedic hardware such as artificial joints, pins, plates, or screws
   - Cardiovascular devices such as pacemakers or implantable defibrillators
   - Synthetic vascular grafts
   - Ventricular shunts

▶ Implementing Measures to Protect and Strengthen Immune System Function

1. Take meticulous care of the skin and mucous membranes to prevent loss of barrier protection.
2. Use the enteral route for feeding when possible to maintain caloric intake and normal gut function.
3. Avoid the use of urinary bladder catheters.
4. Minimize patient stress and the release of endogenous glucocorticoids by relieving pain or using alternative methods such as guided imagery or music for relaxation, and other comfort measures (positioning, massage).
5. Administer colony stimulating factors (G-CSF or GM-CSF) to stimulate bone marrow production of neutrophils and monocytes.

▶ Implementing Measures to Prevent Nosocomial Infection

1. All personnel and visitors should wash their hands before and after contact with the patient. Hand washing remains the number one method to prevent nosocomial infection.
2. Institute universal blood and body fluid precautions with all patients and appropriate isolation for known or suspected patient infection.
3. Adhere to strict aseptic technique for all care of intravascular catheters and any invasive procedures performed at the patient's bedside.
4. Eliminate environmental sources of infection (e.g., fresh flowers, leftover fluids used for irrigations).
5. Track the time fluids, tubings, and catheters are used in administering IV fluids to the patient and change them at the prescribed intervals.

▶ Early Detection of Local or System Inflammatory Response to Infection

1. Monitor the patient closely for signs and symptoms consistent with infection and communicate abnormal findings to the physician.

2. Collect specimens for culture and sensitivity from potential sources of nosocomial infection (e.g., urine, sputum, blood, stool, wound drainage).

Coagulopathies

Etiology, Risk Factors, and Pathophysiology

Critically ill patients with coagulopathy may have a problem involving platelets, the coagulation cascade, fibrinolysis, or a combination of these three abnormalities. Inherited coagulation disorders occur less frequently than acquired disorders.

Platelets are the first to activate the coagulation process at the site of blood vessel injury. Quantitative platelet disorders can cause traumatic bleeding when the platelet count drops to between 50,000 and 100,000/mm^3. Spontaneous bleeding is possible at counts of 10,000 to 50,000/mm^3. Counts that reach 5,000 to 10,000/mm^3 are at high risk for spontaneous hemorrhage. Four general mechanisms are responsible for thrombocytopenia: decreased production, shortened survival, splenic sequestration, and intravascular dilution.

Patients may have adequate numbers of platelets but still have a bleeding tendency due to qualitative platelet disorders. Drug-induced suppression of platelet function commonly is associated with use of aspirin, nonsteroidal antiinflammatory agents, and beta-lactam antibiotics. Critically ill patients may be receiving multiple drugs with potential for impairment of platelet function. Patients with renal failure and uremia also may suffer from platelet dysfunction.

Coagulation cascade disorders are caused by both hereditary or acquired abnormalities in coagulation factors. Hemophilia types A and B are congenital deficiencies in factor VIII and factor IX. Von Willebrand's disease represents a deficiency or dysfunction of the plasma protein of the same name. Replacement of the deficient factor keeps these chronic diseases under control. Patients with these disorders may be monitored in critical care units when undergoing routine surgical procedures or when hospitalized for other medical problems.

Acquired coagulation cascade defects are associated with deficient coagulation factor production. This may be caused by a decreased amount of vitamin K, the vitamin essential to the formation of clotting factors II, VII, IX, and X. Critically ill patients are more susceptible to deficiency in vitamin K as a result of dietary deficiency, intestinal malabsorption, liver disease, use of coumadin, or antibiotic therapy. Vitamin K deficiency prolongs the PT.

Therapeutic anticoagulation using heparin or coumadin interferes with the clotting cascade. The intrinsic pathway and the final common pathway are affected by the administration of heparin. If bleeding from heparin in minimal, it can be controlled by decreasing the dose or temporarily stopping its administration. If bleeding is severe, the antidote to reverse heparin, protamine sulfate, may be administered intravenously. Heparin may also cause bleeding by inducing an immune-mediated thrombocytopenia.

Coumadin acts by inhibiting the production of vitamin K–dependent clotting factors. Effects from coumadin take several days to be observed after initiation of the drug. If significant bleeding occurs while on the coumadin, replacement of vitamin K–dependent factors by use of fresh frozen plasma may be necessary. Giving replacement vitamin K may also be helpful, but its effectiveness is dependent on the time taken by the liver to synthesize new clotting factors.

Use of thrombolytic agents (streptokinase, urokinase, t-PA, APSAC) to dissolve pathologic fibrin clots may result in patient bleeding from sites where a protective clot has formed. These agents are used in combination with heparin and antiplatelet drug therapy, which contribute to bleeding from the mechanisms previously described. This is a complex acquired coagulopathy involving patients in critical care units.

Another example of a complex acquired coagulopathy is DIC, a secondary problem which develops in patients already critically ill from a wide variety of disorders (Table 16–2). The many etiologies of DIC share the ability to activate the clotting cascade to form excessive amounts of circulating thrombin, which catalyzes fibrinogen to form fibrin. Fibrin forms microthrombi in the microcirculation

TABLE 16–2. ETIOLOGIES OF DISSEMINATED INTRAVASCULAR COAGULATION

Cardiovascular
Shock
Arterial aneurysm

Tissue Trauma
Burns
Crush injury
Head injury
Extracorporeal circulation
Malignant hyperthermia
Snake venom

Infections
Bacterial
Viral
Fungal

Obstetrical
Eclampsia
Amniotic fluid embolism
Abruptio placentae
Placenta previa
Abortion
Retained dead fetus

Neoplastic Disease
Acute leukemia
Adenocarcinoma

Immunological Reaction
Incompatible transfusion

TABLE 16–3. LABORATORY RESULTS SUGGESTING DIC

Test	Abnormality
Platelet count	Decreased
PT	Prolonged
PTT/APTT	Prolonged
Fibrinogen	Decreased
FSP/FDP	Increased
d-dimer	Increased

throughout the body. This fibrin deposition triggers the normal fibrinolytic process to break down clot formation.

Stimulation of the clotting cascade rapidly depletes existing platelets and coagulation factors, consuming them at rates faster than the body can replace them. Depletion of substrates of the coagulation process leaves the body at risk for spontaneous bleeding or hemorrhage from invasive procedures or trauma.

Microcirculation thrombosis can lead to tissue ischemia, infarction, and organ dysfunction. Single or multisystem organ dysfunction may occur.

Simultaneous activation of fibrinolysis releases the enzyme plasmin. Plasmin degrades fibrinogen to produce FDP. These end products of fibrin breakdown have weak anticoagulant properties. The FDP are normally cleared from the body by the reticuloendothelial system. Overproduction of FDP overwhelms the body's ability to clear them from the circulation, resulting in an increased level of circulating anticoagulants. Clots at new sites of injury are unable to form and existing clots are dissolved, leading to bleeding from both old and new sites.

DIC is an inappropriate, accelerated, systemic activation of the coagulation process, leading to a paradoxical clinical presentation of thrombosis and bleeding. This is superimposed over the underlying condition of the patient. Laboratory diagnosis requires careful interpretation of results (Table 16–3). In many cases absolute certainty regarding a diagnosis of DIC may not be possible. This does not impair the clinical management of the patient, because the primary goal of therapy is to treat the underlying condition. Management of DIC is usually conservative, managing significant bleeding with blood component therapy. Heparinization, although controversial, may be used in a subset of patients with organ dysfunction secondary to thrombosis.

Clinical Signs and Symptoms

Coagulopathy may be a subtle, occult process or a massive, obvious emergency. Assessment must encompass each body system, looking for evidence of abnormality in single or multiple components of the coagulation cascade.

Abnormal Platelet Numbers or Function

- Petechiae of skin or mucous membranes
- Spontaneous bleeding from gums or nose
- Thrombocytopenia
- Prolonged bleeding time

Abnormal Coagulation Factors

- Deeper hemorrhage into joints, subcutaneous tissue, or muscle
- Ecchymosis, purpura
- Bleeding responds slowly to local pressure
- Prolonged PT, APTT
- Decreased fibrinogen
- Decrease in level of specific coagulation factor

General Assessment for Bleeding and or Decreased Organ Perfusion as a Result of Microthrombosis

Skin/Musculoskeletal

- Petechiae
- Ecchymosis
- Purpura
- Oozing of blood from incisions, intravascular catheters
- Acral cyanosis of toes, fingers, nose, lips, ears
- Pain, swelling, and limited joint mobility
- Increased size of body part, increased girth

Neurologic

- Any change in level of consciousness, pupils, movement or sensation may indicate intracranial bleeding

- Impaired vision with retinal hemorrhage

GASTROINTESTINAL

- Guaiac positive gastric fluids
- Coffee ground emesis or gastric aspirate
- Melena or frank bloody stool
- Abdominal pain
- Enlarged liver or spleen

GENITOURINARY

- Vaginal bleeding
- Smoky to bright red urine
- Decreased urinary output

CARDIOVASCULAR

- Pericardial friction rub
- Muffled heart tones
- Hypovolemia and/or shock (with rapid loss of large volume of blood)

Patient Needs and Principles of Management

The management of coagulopathy varies with the type and severity of the disorder. The overall goal of therapy is to restore normal hemostasis. Supportive care focuses on the control and prevention of further bleeding associated with activities of daily living and therapeutic interventions.

▶ Restoration of Normal Hemostasis

1. Treatment of quantitative platelet disorders may involve transfusion of platelets. One unit of platelets may be expected to increase the platelet count by 5000 to 10,000/mm^3. Transfusion is recommended for levels less than 5000/mm^3, and prophylactically between 5000 and 33,000/mm^3. Increasing platelet count to higher levels may be necessary for invasive procedures or surgery.
2. Destruction of platelets by immune mechanisms may be treated with steroids or IV immunoglobulin infusion. If related to use of heparin, then heparin should be discontinued. Splenectomy may be a last resort.
3. Dysfunctional platelets may be treated by stopping the offending agent, such as aspirin or NSAIDs. If caused by uremia, short-term improvement may be achieved by administering IV desmopressin (DDAVP). Dialysis will also improve platelet function.
4. Acute replacement of all coagulation factors can be accomplished with transfusion of fresh frozen plasma. Cryoprecipitate will replace fibrinogen, factor VIII, and von Willebrand's factor. For hemophiliac patients, factor VIII or factor IX concentrates are used to replace the specific factor deficiency.

5. IV vitamin K may be used to treat coumadin-related bleeding or vitamin K deficiency.
6. Heparin therapy may be stopped, or the dosage decreased or reversed with IV protamine sulfate.

▶ Control and Prevention of Bleeding

1. Modify nursing care measures to minimize trauma and prevent skin and mucous breakdown:

   - Use sponge sticks for oral care.
   - Use electric razor or no shaving.
   - Avoid use of suppositories, tampons, or catheters.
   - Minimize use of automatic BP cuffs.
   - Minimize peripheral blood sampling.
   - Avoid IM injections.
   - Pad side rails; avoid restraint use.
   - Handle patients gently when turning or moving.
   - Gently remove adhesive dressings.
   - Avoid nasotracheal suctioning; do not extend suction catheters past end of artificial airways.

2. Modify nursing care procedures to control bleeding:

   - Apply direct pressure after invasive procedures for at least 5 to 10 minutes or until bleeding has stopped.
   - *After* removal of intravascular line, elevate arm above level of heart or for central line elevate the head to decrease venous pressure.
   - Use cold saline mouth rinses for oral bleeding.
   - Use ice packs on hematomas or hemarthrosis.
   - Do not dislodge or attempt to remove blood clots.

AT THE BEDSIDE
■ *Thinking Critically*

You are caring for a 63-year-old white male admitted from an assisted living center with acute alteration in mental status and fever. He has a history of rheumatoid arthritis, right total hip replacement, and gastric ulcers. His medications include:

- Prednisone
- Methotrexate
- Trilisate
- Carafate
- Tagamet
- Ferrous sulfate
- Folic acid

What are this patient's risk factors for potential hematologic and immunologic problems while hospitalized?

SELECTED BIBLIOGRAPHY

Anemia

Hematologic problems. Springhouse, PA: Springhouse Corp., 1990.

Blood Product Administration

Higgins MJ, Klein HG: Blood products in the intensive care unit. In Parrillo JE, Bone RC (eds.): *Critical care medicine: Principles of diagnosis and management.* St. Louis, MO: CV Mosby, 1995.

Immunocompromised Patients

Workman ML, Ellerhorst-Ryan J, Hargrave-Koertge V: *Nursing care of the immunocompromised patient.* Philadelphia: WB Saunders, 1993.

DIC

Snyder P: Disseminated intravascular coagulation. In Urban NA, Greenlee KK, Krumberger JM, Winkelman C (eds.): *Guidelines for critical care nursing.* St. Louis, MO: CV Mosby, 1995.

Gastrointestinal System

■ *What Heals: Gut Feelings and Intuition*

Have you ever had a gut feeling that something bad was about to happen to one of your patients? Did you ever just know that your patient was soon going to have a cardiac arrest even though you had no hard data to support it? This gut feeling, called *intuition,* occurs commonly for some nurses. Actually, intuitive thinking occurs for each one of us. Some of us ignore it, some try to hide it, and some try to cultivate it each day.

Intuition is a process by which we know more than we can explain. Likewise, clinical intuition has been described as a process by which the nurse knows something about the patient which cannot be verbalized or for which the source cannot be determined.

Most nurses recognize the importance of the rational, analytic, and verbal (or left-brain) way of thinking that directs our daily nursing practice. Many are unaware, however, of the significance of a nonverbal and intuitive (right-brain) way of thinking. Traditionally, in critical care we have placed value on only the facts—the hard data—with little room for gut feelings, intuition, or soft data. The idea that only hard data are important in critical care practice limits our potential as nurses. Our practice involves not only

analytic thinking, but also a qualitative, yet undefinable, intuitive process used to organize fragmented findings into meaningful wholes. When analytic and intuitive thinking are used together, whole-brain thinking emerges.

Some exciting "hard data" have been published to support the notion that intuitive processes are important in nursing practice. From these studies, we know that intuitive thinking generally is found to occur in the more experienced and technically proficient nurse, particularly when a caring relationship is developed with the patient and day-to-day ongoing care is provided. Intuition is fostered when the nurse is emotionally receptive and open to subtle cues and feelings and has a desire to "tune in" to the situation. Likewise, intuitive thinking is diminished when the nurse's physical and emotional energy levels are low as in situations of personal stress or illness. Self-confidence is another facilitating factor that enables nurses to believe in their intuitive experience and act on this knowledge without any discomfort about a lack of objective data.

It is clear that we need to find ways to cultivate intuitive thinking in nursing. Although intuitive thinking cannot be taught directly, it is possible to teach the skills necessary to recognize subjective data and to verbalize feelings, cues, and decisions surrounding intuitive experiences. We can encourage nurses to use their intuition in combination with analytic, objective thinking when assessing patients and clinical situations. We can support nurses who have experienced intuitive events and invite them to share, review, and analyze the process with others. Novice nurses can be provided with subtle, repeated, clinical cue patterns that will assist them in recognizing intuitive information, thereby increasing their confidence about inter-

preting the cues and acting on their decisions. Ultimately, we can systematically evaluate the usefulness of intuition in making correct decisions in the treatment and care of patients. But perhaps most important, we can encourage nurses to trust their intuition.

CEG & BMD

Adapted from: Guzzetta CE: Nursing process and standards of care. In Dossey BM, Keegan L, Guzzetta CE, Kolkmeier L: Holistic nursing: A handbook for practice. Gaithersburg, MD: Aspen, 1995; and Guzzetta CE: Research in critical care nursing. In Guzzetta CE, Dossey BM: Cardiovascular nursing: Holistic practice. St. Louis, MO: Mosby-Year Book, 1992.

PATHOLOGIC CONDITIONS

Acute Upper Gastrointestinal Bleeding

Life-threatening gastrointestinal (GI) bleeding originates most commonly in the upper GI tract and requires immediate therapy to prevent complications. Patients presenting with sudden blood loss are at risk for decreased tissue perfusion and oxygen-carrying capability, which can affect every organ system in the body.

Etiology, Risk Factors, and Pathophysiology

A variety of abnormalities within the GI tract can be the source of upper GI bleeding (Table 17–1). The most common cause of upper GI bleeding is peptic ulcer disease. Its pathogenesis is related to hypersecretion of gastric acid, coupled with impaired GI tract mucus secretion. Normally, mucus protects the gastric wall from erosive effects of acid. Peptic ulcers occur in the stomach and the duodenum, and are characterized by a break in the mucosal layer which penetrates the muscularis mucosa (innermost muscular layer), resulting in bleeding. Infection of the mucosa by *Helicobacter pylori,* an organism naturally found in the GI tract, also has been implicated in the pathogenesis of peptic ulcer disease.

Gastroesophageal varices develop when there is increased flow of blood through the portal venous system of the liver. If blood cannot flow easily through the liver because of obstructive disease, it is diverted to collateral channels. These channels are normally low-pressure vessels found in the distal esophagus (esophageal varices), the

TABLE 17–1. COMMON SOURCES OF UPPER GASTROINTESTINAL BLEEDING

Peptic Ulcer Disease
Gastric ulcer
Duodenal ulcer

Varices
Esophageal
Gastric

Pathologies of the Esophagus
Tumors
Mallory-Weiss syndrome
Inflammation
Ulcers

Pathologies of the Stomach
Cancer
Erosive gastritis
Stress ulcer
Tumors

Pathologies of the Small Intestine
Peptic ulcers
Angiodysplasia

---

veins in the proximal stomach (gastric varices), and in the rectal vault (hemorrhoids) (Figure 17–1). Acute upper GI hemorrhage occurs when esophageal and/or gastric varices rupture from increased portal vein pressure (portal hypertension). Portal hypertension is most commonly caused by primary liver disease (see next section), liver trauma, or thrombosis of the splenic or portal veins.

Mallory-Weiss syndrome is a linear, nonperforating tear of the gastric mucosa near the gastroesophageal junc-

AT THE BEDSIDE
▶ *Upper GI Bleeding*

Mr. B., a 45-year-old white male, is admitted with reports of an 8-hour history of nausea and vomiting of large amounts of "coffee ground secretions" and frequent "maroon colored" stools. Mr. B. reports a previous history of peptic ulcer disease diagnosed at age 35 years. He has been hospitalized twice in the past for active GI bleeding. A duodenal ulcer near the pylorus on the posterior wall of the stomach was diagnosed by endoscopy. Significant findings on his admission profile were:

Vital signs
Blood Pressure: 96/60 mm Hg lying;
                  82/50 mm Hg sitting
Heart Rate: 120 beats/minute; sinus tachy-
                  cardia with 2-mm ST-segment
                  elevation
Respiratory Rate: 32/minute, deep
Temperature: 99.2° F (oral)

Respiratory
   Breath sounds clear in all lung fields
Cardiovascular
   S_1/S_2 no murmurs
   Extremities cool, diaphoretic; pulses present but weak
Abdomen
   Distended with hyperactive bowel sounds in all four quadrants
   Tender right upper quadrant, no rebound tenderness
Neurological
   Alert, oriented
   Anxious
Genitourinary
   50 ml amber cloudy urine following Foley catheter insertion
   Stools liquid maroon, guaiac positive
Arterial blood gases

   pH: 7.49
   $PaCO_2$:   28 mm Hg
   HCO_3^-:   19 mEq/L
   PaO_2:   61 mm Hg on room air
   SaO_2:   89%
Hematocrit: 25%
Hemoglobin: 7.0 g/dl
White blood cell count: 17,000/mm^3
Prothrombin time: 11 seconds
Activated partial
   thromboplastin time: 30 seconds
Platelet count: 110,000/mm^3
Serum potassium: 3.5 mEq/L (decreased)

Serum sodium: 150 mEq/L
Serum glucose: 210 mg/dl
Serum blood urea nitrogen: 40
Serum creatinine: 0.9
Liver function: Within normal limits

tion. The tear is the result of pressure changes in the stomach that occur with vomiting. Alcohol abuse and inflammatory conditions of the stomach and esophagus are also associated with this disorder.

Hemorrhagic gastritis is a term used to describe gastric lesions which do not penetrate the muscularis mucosa. These are also referred to as stress ulcers. Onset of bleeding is sudden and is often the first symptom. The causes of gastritis are multifactorial (Table 17–2), most commonly associated with nonsteroidal antiinflammatory drug (NSAID) use, alcohol abuse, and physiologic conditions which cause severe stress (e.g., trauma, surgery, burns, severe medical problems). Alcohol and NSAIDs are known to directly disrupt the mucosal defense mechanisms of the stomach (Figure 17–2).

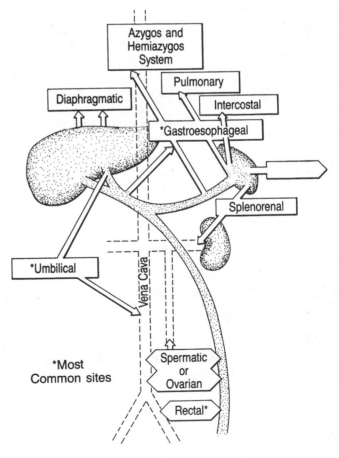

Figure 17–1. The liver with collateral circulation.

TABLE 17–2. CAUSES OF GASTRITIS

Alcohol abuse

Nonsteroidal antiinflammatory drug use
Aspirin
Ascriptin
Ecotrin
Ibuprofen
Naprozin

Severe physiologic stress
Burns (Curling's ulcer)
CNS disease (Cushing's ulcer)
Trauma
Surgery
Medical complications
   Sepsis
   Acute renal failure
   Hepatic failure
Long-term mechanical ventilation

Regardless of the etiology, upper GI bleeding that results in a sudden loss of blood volume decreases venous return to the heart, with a corresponding decrease in cardiac output (CO). The decrease in CO triggers the release of epinephrine and norepinephrine, causing intense vasoconstriction and tissue ischemia (Figure 17–3). The clinical signs and symptoms of upper GI hemorrhage are directly related

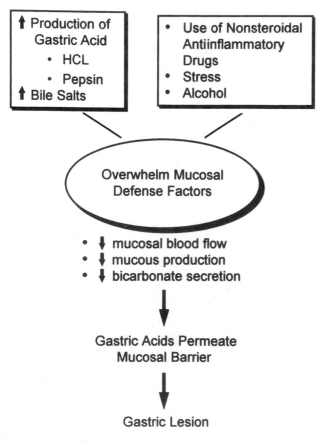

Figure 17–2. Pathogenesis of gastritis.

to the effects of the decrease in CO and of this vasoconstriction response, typical in hypovolemic shock. In addition, aldosterone and antidiuretic hormones are released, resulting in sodium and water retention.

Clinical Presentation

History
Individuals have a history of peptic ulcer disease, alcohol abuse, severe physiologic stress, NSAID use, or other GI bleeding causes.

Signs and Symptoms
The response of an individual to blood loss depends on the rate and amount of the loss, the patient's age and preexisting physiologic state, and the rapidity of treatment. Specific signs and symptoms include:

- Hematemesis: Bright red blood or coffee ground
- Melena or maroon-colored stools
- Nausea
- Epigastric pain
- Abdominal distension
- Bowel sounds increased or decreased
- If blood loss is greater that 25% of blood volume: Hypotension (orthostatic); altered hemodynamic values (decreased CVP, PCWP, MAP, CO)
- Rapid, deep respirations
- Tachycardia
- Fever
- Cold, clammy skin
- Dry mucous membranes
- Decreased pulses
- Weakness
- Decreased urine output
- Anxiety
- Mental status changes
- Restlessness
- ECG changes consistent with ischemia (e.g., ST-segment elevation, dysrhythmias)

Diagnostic Tests

- Hematocrit may be normal initially, then decreased with fluid resuscitation and blood loss.
- Hemoglobin may be normal initially, then decreased with fluid resuscitation and blood loss.
- WBC count is elevated.
- Platelet count is decreased depending on amount of blood loss.
- Serum sodium is usually elevated initially due to hemoconcentration.
- Serum potassium is usually decreased with vomiting.
- Serum BUN is elevated.

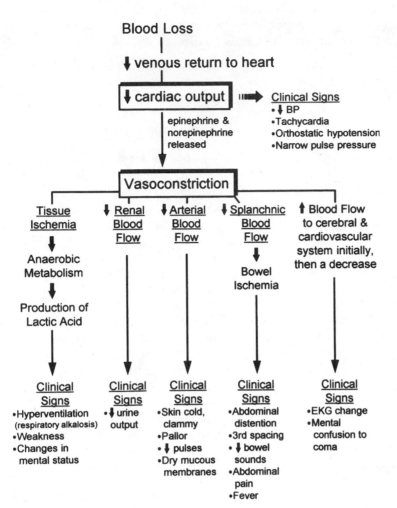

Figure 17–3. Hypovolemic shock.

- Serum creatinine is elevated.
- Serum lactate is elevated with severe bleeding.
- Prothrombin time (PT) is usually decreased.
- Activated thromboplastin time (APTT) is usually decreased.

- Arterial blood gases show respiratory alkalosis (early), metabolic acidosis with severe shock, and hypoxemia.
- Gastric aspirate shows normal or acidotic pH and is guaiac positive.

Patient Needs and Principles of Management

The management of the patient with an acute upper GI bleeding revolves around three major areas: hemodynamic stabilization, identification of the bleeding site, and initiation of definitive medical or surgical therapies to control or stop the bleeding. Measures to decrease anxiety in this patient population are also a focus due to the severity and sudden onset of GI bleeding.

► Hemodynamic Stabilization

The initial assessment of GI bleeding focuses on vital signs, which are the most reliable signs of the amount of blood loss. Resuscitation begins immediately in the presence of hemodynamic instability.

Patient Needs and Principles of Management, Cont.

1. Monitor and record cardiovascular status (blood pressure, heart rate including orthostatic changes), hemodynamics (CVP, PCWP, CO, MAP), and peripheral pulses.
2. Insert at least two large-bore intravenous (IV) catheters and begin fluid resuscitation with crystalloid solution (e.g., normal saline). Administer fluids to maintain MAP at 60 mm Hg or higher.
3. Obtain blood for hematocrit, hemoglobin, and clotting studies, as well as for typing and crossmatching for packed red blood cells. Usually at least 6 units are ordered. The hematocrit taken during the initial resuscitation rarely is useful for transfusion requirements. Estimates for the amount of blood loss are most reliably guided by vital sign values (Table 17–3).
4. Administer IV colloids, crystalloids, or blood products as prescribed until the patient is stabilized. Blood products may be considered in the initial resuscitation if the hemodynamic response is poor after administering 2 to 3 L of crystalloid fluids. Packed red blood cells (PRBC) are used to rapidly increase the hematocrit and with less volume than whole blood. Each unit of packed red blood cells increases the hematocrit by 2% to 3% and improves gas exchange. Up to 24 hours may be required for blood administration to be reflected in the hematocrit values to accurately reflect red blood cell counts, especially if large amounts of crystalloid solutions were administered during the resuscitation.
5. Monitor coagulation studies (e.g., PT/PTT, platelet count).
6. Monitor fluid balance and renal function (intake and output, daily weight, BUN, creatinine, and hourly urine output).
7. Insert a nasogastric (NG) tube if bleeding is massive (greater than 40% of blood volume) to assess for the rate of bleeding. Use of gastric lavage in upper GI hemorrhage is controversial. Proponents believe that removing blood clots by gastric lavage is useful in that it allows the stomach to contract and tamponade bleeding vessels. Removal of blood may give some indication of the rate of bleeding and may minimize the chance of pulmonary aspiration. If lavage is ordered, room temperature saline usually is used.
8. Position the patient in the left lateral decubitus position to minimize aspiration associated with hematemesis.
9. Monitor temperature and maintain normothermia. Rapid fluid resuscitation, particularly with blood products, can lead to hypothermia, with interference of normal coagulation. Warming of fluids may be required to prevent hypothermia if traditional measures are insufficient.

TABLE 17–3. ESTIMATING BLOOD LOSS FROM ACUTE GASTROINTESTINAL BLEEDING

Clinical Signs	Estimated Blood Loss
Systolic BP > 90 mm Hg Orthostatic hypotension Heart rate < 110 beats/minute	20%–25% total blood volume (approximately 1000 ml)

Systolic BP 70–90 mm Hg
Heart rate 110–130 beats/minute
Signs of moderate decreased tissue perfusion:
  Anxiety
  Cool, clammy skin
  Decreased urine output
  Hyperventilation
  Diminished pulses
	25%–40% total blood volume (approximately 1500–2000 ml)

Systolic blood pressure < 70 mm Hg
Mean arterial pressure < 60 mm Hg
Signs of severe decreased tissue perfusion:
  Impaired mental status
  Cold, clammy, diaphoretic skin
  Thready pulses
  Decreased urine output
  Metabolic acidosis
  ECG changes
  Heart failure
  Respiratory failure
	> 40% total blood volume

► Identify the Bleeding Site

Although the history and physical examination are used to differentiate between upper and lower GI bleeding, endoscopic examination is required to determine the exact site of the bleeding. Endoscopic visualization at the bedside is preferred to allow for early direct visualization of the upper tract during resuscitation measures.

1. Administer conscious sedation (e.g., Versed) as ordered and institute monitoring protocol.
2. Position patient in a left lateral decubitus position to prevent aspiration of GI contents during endoscopy. Have oral-tracheal suction available at the bedside before the procedure begins.
3. Monitor for cardiac ischemia during the exam [e.g., ST-segment changes (see Chapter 21, Advanced ECG Concepts), arrhythmias].

► Institute Therapies to Control or Stop the Bleeding

Definitive therapies to treat the bleeding differ depending on the cause. A treatment guideline is summarized in Figure

17–4. In nonvariceal upper GI bleeding, treatment may include endoscopic therapy, pharmacologic therapies, and surgical therapies. Sclerotherapy is the most commonly employed endoscopic therapy. It involves injecting the bleeding ulcer with a necrotizing agent which works by traumatizing the endothelial layer of the GI mucosa. This causes necrosis and eventual sclerosis of the bleeding vessel. Other endoscopic therapies include heater probe, laser therapy, and electrocoagulation. Treatment of variceal upper GI bleeding may include endoscopic therapy, tamponade therapy (e.g., Sengstaken-Blakemore tube), pharmacologic therapy to decrease portal hypertension, and surgical therapy to decompress the varices. Sclerotherapy is the treatment of choice for acute variceal bleeding.

1. Monitor for complications of endoscopic therapy and/or the sclerosing agents used to treat the ulcer or varix. Complications may include fever, pain due to esophageal spasm, motility disturbances of the esophageal sphincter, and perforation. Systemic complications of endoscopic therapy and/or sclerosing agents also may occur and predominantly affect the cardiovascular and respiratory systems.

Cardiovascular effects include heart failure, heart block, and pericarditis. Respiratory effects include mediastinitis, aspiration pneumonia, atelectasis, pneumothorax, embolism, and acute respiratory distress syndrome.

2. Institute pharmacologic therapies as prescribed to treat peptic ulcer disease or gastritis (stress ulcers). The most common pharmacologic agents and their actions are reviewed in Table 17–4.

3. Administer pharmacologic therapies as prescribed to treat variceal bleeding (Table 17–5). Pharmacologic agents exert their effect by constricting splanchnic blood flow and thereby reducing portal pressure. Monitor for side effects of systemic vasoconstriction and the cardiac effects of myocardial ischemia and bradycardia. Administer nitroglycerin titrated to maintain systolic blood pressure between 90 and 100 mm Hg to reduce these side effects and to further reduce portal pressure.

4. A tamponade tube, most commonly the Sengstaken-Blakemore tube (Figure 17–5) may be used to emergently decrease blood flow through the varix and to control bleeding so that endoscopy can be per-

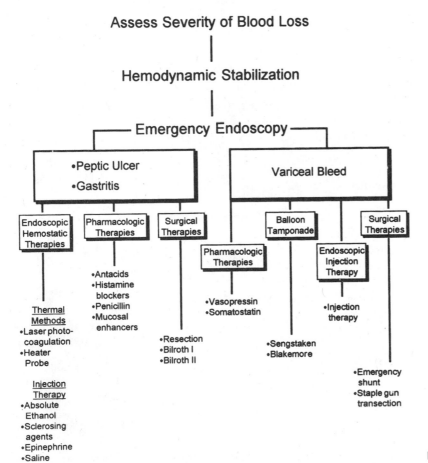

Assess Severity of Blood Loss

Hemodynamic Stabilization

Emergency Endoscopy

- Peptic Ulcer
- Gastritis

Variceal Bleed

Endoscopic Hemostatic Therapies

Pharmacologic Therapies

Surgical Therapies

Pharmacologic Therapies

Balloon Tamponade

Endoscopic Injection Therapy

Surgical Therapies

Thermal Methods
- Laser photocoagulation
- Heater Probe

Injection Therapy
- Absolute Ethanol
- Sclerosing agents
- Epinephrine
- Saline

- Antacids
- Histamine blockers
- Penicillin
- Mucosal enhancers

- Resection
- Bilroth I
- Bilroth II

- Vasopressin
- Somatostatin

- Injection therapy

- Sengstaken
- Blakemore

- Emergency shunt
- Staple gun transection

Figure 17–4. Upper GI bleeding treatment guide.

Patient Needs and Principles of Management, Cont.

TABLE 17–4. PHARMACOLOGIC THERAPIES FOR ULCER DISEASE/GASTRITIS

Agent	Action
Antacids	Acid neutralizers
Histamine blockers	Block production of gastric acid (pepsin, HCl) by inhibiting the action of histamine
Cimetidine	
Ranitidine	
Famotidine	
Nizatidine	
Sucralfate	Forms protective barrier over ulcer site
Mucosal barrier enhancers	Protect mucosa from injurious substances
Colloidal bismuth	
Prostaglandins	
Pencillins	Effective against *Helicobacter pylori*
Ampicillin	
Amoxicillin	
Mezlocillin	

TABLE 17–5. PHARMACOLOGIC THERAPIES FOR VARICEAL UPPER GI BLEEDING

Drug	Action	Administration
Vasopressin	Vasoconstricts splanchnic inflow and reduces portal pressure	Administered by continuous IV infusion at 0.2–0.6 units/minute
Somatostatin	Inhibits splanchnic blood flow	Administered by continuous IV infusion at 250 µg/hour
Octreotide	Vasodilates splanchnic vessels to decrease blood flow	IV infusion at 25 µg/hour
Nonselective beta-adrenergic blockers propranolol nadolol	Decreases cardiac output and reduces splanic flow (decreases portal hypertension)	Administered orally to reduce resting pulse by 20% or to 55–60 beats/minute

formed. Rebleeding is common after deflation or removal. Monitor for complications of this tube, including pulmonary aspiration, rupture of the esophagus, asphyxia, and erosion of the esophageal or gastric wall. Maintain esophageal suction to prevent aspiration. Keep a scissors at the bedside to cut and remove the tube if it becomes malpositioned and the tamponade balloon occludes the airway. Endotracheal intubation is usually recommended to prevent most pulmonary complications. Release pressure of the esophageal and or gastric balloons at regular intervals to prevent erosions. Administer frequent mouth care and monitor the skin around the tube to prevent necrosis from traction of the tube.

Surgical Therapies to Stop Bleeding

Surgery is considered for patients who have massive bleeding that is immediately life-threatening and for patients who continue to bleed despite aggressive medical therapies. Surgical therapies for peptic ulcer disease or stress ulcers include gastric resections such as antrectomy, gastrectomy, vagotomy, or combination procedures. An antrectomy or gastrectomy may be performed to decrease the acidity of the duodenum or stomach by removing gastric-acid secreting cells. A vagotomy decreases acid secretion in the stomach by dividing the vagus nerve along the esophagus. Combination procedures are common and include Billroth I, which is a vagotomy and antrectomy with anastomosis of the stomach to the duodenum. A Billroth II consists of a vagotomy, a resection of the antrum, and anastomosis of the stomach to the jejunum (Figure 17–6). The latter is preferred over the Billroth I because it prevents dumping syndrome. Gastric perforations can be treated by simple closure.

Surgical decompression of portal hypertension can be accomplished by a procedure called a *portal caval shunt*. This procedure connects the portal vein to the inferior vena cava, diverting blood from the liver into the vena cava to decrease portal pressure. Liver transplantation also can relieve portal

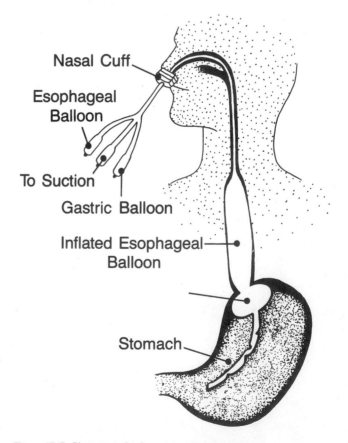

Figure 17–5. Placement of a Sengstaken-Blakemore tube.

Patient Needs and Principles of Management, Cont.

hypertension, but must be considered by weighing the risks versus the benefits in this patient population.

1. Monitor for fluid and electrolyte imbalances postoperatively due to intraoperative fluid loss and the drains inserted to decompress the stomach or to drain the surgical site.
2. Provide for adequate nutrition to promote wound healing.
3. Monitor the appearance of the incision and surrounding tissue.
4. Document and report all wound drainage (color, amount, odor) and complaints of pain or tenderness.
5. Culture any suspicious drainage.
6. Monitor white blood cell count and temperature trends.

New Therapies to Control Bleeding

A new procedure called the *transjugular intrahepatic portosystemic shunt* (TIPS) is a percutaneous option for creating a shunt between the portal and systemic venous systems within the liver, thereby relieving portal hypertension. The advantage of this procedure is that it can be performed in the radiology department. Vasopressin, a drug that vasoconstricts GI smooth muscle, lowering venous pressure and decreasing venous blood flow, is often administered concurrently.

1. Monitor blood pressure, ECG, and pulse oximetry throughout the procedure.

2. Administer preprocedure antibiotic coverage for gram-negative organisms as prophylaxis for sepsis.
3. Provide IV conscious sedation to treat anxiety.
4. Provide pain medication (e.g., fentanyl). Certain parts of the procedure, such as balloon dilation of the intrahepatic tract, can be painful.
5. Have lidocaine and atropine available to manage potential complications of the procedure. The vasopressin infusion can cause bradyarrhythmias. Due to the proximity of the hepatic vein to the right ventricle of the heart, ventricular ectopy can be induced during the procedure.
6. Have crystalloids, vasopressors, PRBCs, and fresh frozen plasma readily available to manage hypotension from sepsis, bleeding, or sedation.
7. Have continuous and intermittent suction ready to manage bleeding and airway patency.

▶ Reduction of Anxiety

1. Encourage communication with a calm, interested, and centered approach; e.g., "Mr. B., you look nervous (worried) to me. Can you tell me what is bothering you?"
2. Assess the patient's previous coping skills that were used in similar difficult situations (e.g., did family presence, watching TV or listening to music, or using relaxation techniques provide support?).
3. Offer appropriate reassurance, facts, and information as requested by the patient. Explain the ICU

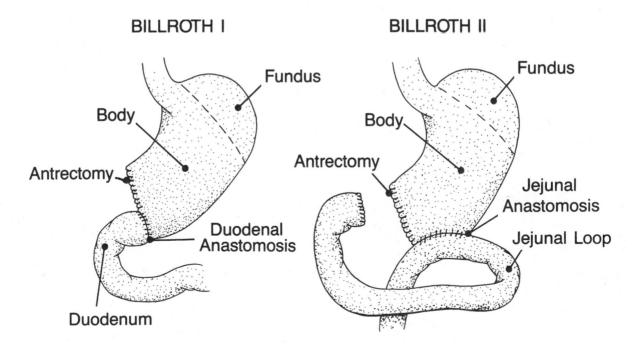

Figure 17–6. Billroth I and II procedures.

Patient Needs and Principles of Management, Cont.

routine and procedures to the patient. Present information in terms that the patient can understand. Repeat and rephrase the information as necessary.

4. Help the patient establish a sense of control. Assist the patient to make distinctions among those things he or she can (and should) control (e.g., bath time, working on reducing anxiety level) and those things that cannot be controlled (e.g., need for vasopressors and monitoring equipment).

5. Guide the patient in discovering that he or she has some control over anxiety and fear. Encourage the patient to participate in breathing and relaxation exercises as a strategy to control the current situation (Table 17–6).

TABLE 17–6. RELAXATION TECHNIQUE: BLENDING THE BREATH AND THOUGHT

Can you remember the last time you said "ahhhh" out loud to release some tension to calm yourself? The simple release of the breath and the "ahhhh" sound is an ancient way for your patients (or you) to release worries, fear, and pain, and evoke relaxation.

For centuries, the mystics have said that the breath connects consciousness to life. This practice of releasing the breath allows a space to emerge so that your patients can let go of emotions and pain. Blending the breath and thought facilitates a sensation of inner calm.

Use the following steps to help guide a patient in this technique.* At first, the "ahhhh" sound might be like an echoing of words, but staying with the sound allows releasing of tension, anxiety, and pain.

- Position yourself comfortably and close to the patient who is fearful or anxious. Sit by his or her side for a short time. A session may last for a few minutes or longer and later can be repeated by the patient as he or she feels necessary. Prepare whatever is necessary to maintain comfort for the patient (e.g., pillow, light blanket, closing the door or drapes). Families also may wish to participate.
- Suggest to the patient that watching the breath is an old method of calming the body and the mind. It is a method that can be used anytime, anywhere when he or she feels out of control or anxious. Instruct the patient to begin noticing the rise and fall of the abdomen with each breath in and out.
- Sitting at the patient's midsection, focus on the rise and fall of the abdomen with each inhalation and each exhalation. With focused intention, breathe in unison with the patient. At the top of the patient's exhalation, begin sounding softly and out loud the sound "ahhhh," matching the respiration of the patient. Encourage the patient to match the sound with the intensity and volume that seems right for him or her.
- Simple phrases such as "peaceful heart" or "releasing the breath and the tension" may be said occasionally. The fewer the words, however, the more powerful is the breath work in accomplishing its goal.

*Modified from: Boerstler R: Letting go. Watertown, MA: Associates in Thanatology, 1982.

AT THE BEDSIDE

Mr. B.: "I've had this trouble before. But this time, it's really bad. I feel like I might not make it."

Primary Nurse: "Although Mr. B. was alert and oriented, his body language, facial expression, and limited verbalization told me he was really scared and afraid he was going to die. I felt like I needed to do something with him on the spot to help lower his anxiety, so I guided him in a breathing technique called Blending the Breath and Thought (Table 17–6). It only took a few minutes. Mr. B.'s respiratory and heart rates slowed down, his facial expression was more relaxed, and he even fell asleep for a little while. I have noticed that the more anxious patients are, the better these relaxation techniques work."

AT THE BEDSIDE

Primary Nurse: "Mr. B.'s wife was at his side holding his hand and speaking softly. I could see she was a major source of support for him. I could tell that wild horses couldn't drag her away from his bedside, so, early on, I contracted with her about visitation. I explained our open visiting hours and our beeper system for communicating with families. When families leave the unit for meals or go home to sleep or rest, they check out one of our unit beepers. That way they can eat or sleep with some degree of confidence, knowing that if the patient's condition changes, or we need to talk to them about something, we will be able to contact them immediately no matter where they are. The beepers are not the fancy ones with digital readouts. They are just little boxes that beep. When the beepers sound off, families know it is us and they call in as soon as they can.

"Families have told us they love the beepers because they are not scared all the time that they will miss a phone call from the unit if they walk the dog, run an errand, or just go to the bathroom. It seems to give them the permission and the peace of mind to leave the hospital for a period of time to take care of themselves without the fear that something might happen and no one could contact them."

Liver Failure

The liver is a complex organ providing over 400 functions for the body. Disease processes in the liver can affect the liver cells, Kupffer's cells, bile ducts, and blood vessels. If severe, these processes can lead to fulminant liver failure. Liver dysfunction then potentially can be reversed. The liver has regenerative capability if the disease process in the liver does not adversely affect the structure of the cells. If the regeneration in liver tissue does not occur in a normal fashion (for example, with cirrhosis of the liver), fibrous tissue is laid down over time. These fibrotic changes are irreversible, resulting in chronic liver dysfunction and eventual end stage liver failure.

Etiology, Risk Factors, and Pathogenesis

Causes of liver failure include both inflammatory disease and processes which produce fibrosis of liver tissue (Table 17–7). Hepatitis is the most common form of inflammatory

AT THE BEDSIDE
▶ *Liver Failure*

Mr. C. is a 54-year-old admitted with a 3-day history of shortness of breath, increased confusion, vomiting, and weakness. He was hospitalized in the past year with upper GI bleeding from esophageal and gastric varices. He was diagnosed at that time as having Laënnec's cirrhosis, liver failure due to alcohol abuse. Significant findings on his admission profile were:

History

Complaints of decreased appetite for the past 2 months; also complaints of nausea and weakness.

Vital signs

Blood pressure: 98/50 lying; 90/54 sitting
Heart rate: Sinus tachycardia with frequent PVCs
Respiratory rate: 28/minute; shallow
Temperature: 100°F, orally

Cardiopulmonary

Rales and coarse rhonchi throughout all lung fields
Dyspneic; using accessory muscles
S_3/S_4; no murmurs
Extremities cool, weak pulses
3+ edema lower extremities

Neurologic

Alert, but disoriented to time and place
Irritable

Abdomen

Marked ascites, dull to percussion
Hyperactive bowel sounds in all four quadrants

Genitourinary

Urine dark, amber, and cloudy
Large hemorrhoid protruding from rectal vault
Liquid stool; black; guaiac positive

Laboratory data

Arterial blood gases on 2 L O_2 per nasal cannula
pH: 7.49
$PaCO_2$: 30 mm Hg
PaO_2: 54 mm Hg
SaO_2: 87%
Hematocrit: 30%
AST 80 IU/L
ALT 84 IU/L
Bilirubin: Total 10 mg/dl
Prothrombin time: 18 seconds
Activated thromboplastin time: 35 seconds
Fibrinogen: 158 mg/dl
Albumin: 3.0
Potassium: 3.2 mEq/L
Sodium: 130 mEq/L
Creatinine: 2.8 mg/dl
Blood urea nitrogen: 40 mg/dl
Glucose: 220 mg/dl
Urine electrolytes: Sodium 5 mEq/L/day; potassium 10 mEq/L/day

TABLE 17–7. COMMON CAUSES OF LIVER FAILURE

Inflammatory Liver Disease
Viruses
  Hepatitis A, B, C, D, and E
  Herpes simplex
  Epstein-Barr
  Cytomegalovirus
  Adenovirus
Parasites
Liver tumors
Toxic ingestion of drugs
  Acetaminophen
  Halothane
  Methyldopa
Toxic ingestion of chemicals and poisons
  Chlorinated hydrocarbons
  Phosphorus
Cirrhosis of the Liver
Alcohol ingestion
Biliary disease
Cardiac disease
Hepatitis

TABLE 17–8. VIRAL HEPATITIS

Type of Hepatitis	Mode of Transmission	Potential Complications
A; formerly called infectious hepatitis	Fecal-oral, person-to-person contact; also by uncooked shellfish, fruits, and vegetables, and contaminated water	Acute fulminant hepatitis relapse
B; formerly called serum hepatitis	Blood or body fluids; sexual contact; contaminated needles; and perinatal transmission	Acute fulminant hepatitis, chronic liver disease, cirrhosis, cancer of the liver
C; formerly non-A, non-B hepatitis	Blood	Chronic liver disease, cirrhosis, cancer of the liver
D	Blood and body fluids, sexual contact, and perinatal transmission	Chronic liver disease
E	Fecal-oral	High mortality in pregnant women

disease of the liver, with at least five different types identified to date. Each type of viral hepatitis has a different mode of transmission and complications (Table 17–8). Hepatitis B is the most serious of these and is vaccine-preventable. Health care providers are at risk for contracting this form of hepatitis. The liver is an important site of drug metabolism. Toxic ingestions of drugs, chemicals, or poisons may also initiate an acute inflammatory process in the liver, causing it to fail.

Alcohol abuse is the most common cause of cirrhosis of the liver. Alcohol is directly toxic to liver cells, causing them to die. Liver cells are replaced by fibrous tissue which causes the liver progressively to fail.

When the liver fails, the clinical manifestations are directly related to failure of the liver to perform important metabolic processes (Table 17–9). Complications of liver failure include ascites, hepatic encephalopathy, acute respiratory distress syndrome, electrolyte and acid-base imbalances, and hepatorenal syndrome.

Ascites

Impaired handling of salt and water by the kidney, as well as alterations in fluid homeostasis, causes the patient to accumulate fluid in the peritoneum. This complication is most problematic because it can impair movement of the diaphragm and cause an ineffective breathing pattern.

Hepatic Encephalopathy

One of the liver's major functions is detoxification. Normally, the liver detoxifies ammonia which is produced by bacteria in the bowel and converts it to urea for excretion. When the liver fails, this function of the liver is impaired, allowing ammonia to directly enter the central nervous system. Because ammonia is neurotoxic, as serum ammonia levels rise, the patient often exhibits signs of impaired cerebral functioning or encephalopathy. These signs can range from minor sensory-perceptual changes such as muscle tremors, slurred speech, or slight mental status changes to marked confusion or profound coma.

Acute Respiratory Distress Syndrome

The major pulmonary complication in liver failure is arterial hypoxemia. The cause has been linked to vascular dilatation in the lung and acute respiratory distress syndrome. Pulmonary edema is also a common finding.

Electrolyte Imbalance

A variety of electrolyte imbalances occur in liver failure. Hypoglycemia develops due to massive hepatic cell necrosis, leading to loss of glycogen stores and diminished glucose release. Hyponatremia is common due to the reduced capacity of the kidneys to excrete free water, leading to a dilutional hyponatremia. Hypokalemia may occur from inadequate oral intake, increased potassium losses from vomiting, or from medical interventions (e.g., NG suction or diuretic therapy). Hypomagnesemia commonly occurs in conjunction with hypokalemia as there is a close relationship between the movement of these electrolytes. Hypocalcemia is a complication of blood transfusions because the citrate used to anticoagulate stored blood causes calcium depletion. Hypophosphatemia also is commonly associated with acute liver failure. The exact mechanisms remain unknown.

TABLE 17–9. SEQUELAE OF LIVER FAILURE

Sequelae	Outcome	Clinical Manifestations
Impaired splanchnic hemodynamics	Portal hypertension	Varices
	Hyperdynamic circulation	Increased CO, decreased SVR
Reduced liver metabolic processes	Altered fat, protein, and carbohydrate metabolism	Malnutrition, impaired healing
	Decreased phagocytic function of Kupffer cells	Infection
	Decreased synthesis of blood clotting components	Bleeding
	Decreased removal of activated clotting factors	Emboli
	Decreased metabolism of vitamins and iron	Impaired skin integrity
	Impaired detoxification	Increased ammonia, mental status changes, increased drug levels
Impaired bile formation and flow	Impaired bilirubin metabolism	Jaundice

Acid-Base Disturbance
Hepatocellular necrosis results in the accumulation of organic acids, primarily lactic acid, causing a metabolic acidosis. Hypoventilation from ascites may complicate this disorder.

Hepatorenal Syndrome
Acute renal failure that occurs with liver failure is called hepatorenal syndrome. The pathophysiology of this functional renal failure is not well understood.

Acute GI Bleeding
Bleeding from varices related to portal hypertension is a life-threatening complication (see previous section).

Clinical Presentation

History

- Exposure to contaminated food, water
- Exposure to blood, body fluids
- Alcohol abuse

Signs and Symptoms

IMPAIRED THOUGHT PROCESSES

- Mental status changes (confusion, lethargy)
- Behavioral changes
- Delirium
- Seizures
- Coma

IMPAIRED GAS EXCHANGE

- Hypoxemia
- Pulmonary edema

FLUID VOLUME DEFICIT/EXCESS

- Hypotension

- Skin cool, pale, and dry
- Urine output less than 30 ml/hour
- Tachycardia
- Dry mucous membranes

HYPERDYNAMIC CIRCULATION

- Dysrhythmias
- Fever
- Palmar erythema (flushed palms)
- Jugular vein distension
- Rales
- Murmur
- Increased CO
- Decreased SVR

ALTERED NUTRITION

- Decreased appetite
- Decreased weight
- Nausea and vomiting

IMPAIRED LIVER METABOLISM

- Jaundice
- Dry skin
- Ascites

Diagnostic Tests

- Total bilirubin greater than 1 mg/dl
- AST greater than 36 IU/L
- ALT greater than 24 IU/L
- Prothrombin time (PT) greater than 13 seconds
- Activated thromboplastin time (APTT) greater than 45 seconds
- Fibrinogen less than 200 mg/dl
- Albumin less than 3.2 g/dl
- Ammonia greater than 45 μg/dl

Patient Needs and Principles of Management

The management of the patient with liver failure is centered on decreasing the metabolic requirements of the liver, supporting cardiopulmonary status, supporting hematologic and nutritional functions of the liver, and preventing and treating complications.

▶ Decrease Metabolic Requirements of the Liver

1. Place the patient on bedrest to decrease the metabolic needs of the liver. Position the head of the bed

at 45 degrees at all times to minimize complications related to ascites. Institute measures to prevent skin breakdown.
2. Monitor drugs that are metabolized by the liver, especially narcotics and sedatives.

▶ Support Cardiopulmonary Status

1. Monitor fluid balance. The patient may have a fluid volume deficit related to portal hypertension, third spacing of peritoneal fluid, GI bleeding, or

coagulation abnormalities. Fluid overload may be a problem related to sodium excess and hypoalbuminemia.
2. Monitor respiratory status and correlate with ABG results. Administer oxygen as ordered. Administer sedatives and analgesics cautiously. Assist the patient with maneuvers to improve oxygenation. Monitor abdominal girth when ascites is present.

▶ Support Hematologic and Nutritional Functions of the Liver

1. Monitor for signs of bleeding (e.g., gastric contents, stools, urine) and test for occult blood. Observe for petechiae and bruising. Monitor hematologic profile.
2. Administer blood and blood products as ordered.
3. Institute measures for variceal bleeding as needed.
4. Institute measures to provide for safety and to minimize tissue trauma. Provide for frequent mouth care. Avoid use of rectal tubes.
5. Limit protein intake; provide calories with carbohydrates and fats. Consider enteral nutrition if oral intake is insufficient.
6. Monitor for signs and symptoms of infection. Maintain sterility of invasive lines and tubes. Maintain aseptic technique when performing procedures.

▶ Prevent and Treat Complications

The most common complications of liver failure are hepatic encephalopathy, fluid and electrolyte imbalances, and hepatorenal syndrome.

1. Observe for changes in mentation. Institute safety measures during periods of mental status changes.
2. Administer cleansing enemas and cathartics to keep the bowel empty. Administer oral nonabsorbent antibiotics (neomycin) to decrease bacteria in the colon. Administer lactulose to decrease intestinal pH and increase ammonia excretion. Monitor patient response to therapy through neurologic assessments and by monitoring serum ammonia levels. Monitor the use of medications metabolized by the liver.

AT THE BEDSIDE

Primary Nurse: "Mr. C. was disoriented and irritable. We wanted to find a way to reduce his agitation. When his brother came to visit, I asked him whether Mr. C. liked music and what kind. As it turned out, Mr. C. was a big country-western fan, so we decided to try a short period of music therapy with him to assess whether it was effective in decreasing his agitation. I checked out a calm, soothing country music tape and a tape recorder and foam headset from our unit's music and relaxation library. At the bedside, I explained that I was going to play some music for him that would help him relax. I put in the tape, turned on the recorder, checked the volume, and put the headset on Mr. C. and the tape recorder under the mattress. It didn't take but 5 minutes for us all to notice a real difference. He stopped picking at the sheets, rattling his bedrails, and rolling his eyes. He just seemed to quiet down. We continued playing the tapes about 30 minutes at a time when Mr. C. needed some help in calming down."

Acute Pancreatitis

Acute pancreatitis is inflammation of the pancreas resulting from premature activation of pancreatic exocrine enzymes within the pancreas. The disease ranges in severity from a mild self-limiting form to a severe process where necrosis of pancreatic cells and release of substrates predominate. The substrates that are released not only cause a local pathology in and around the pancreas, but also can trigger systemic complications when released into the circulation. In the fulminant form, acute pancreatitis results in multisystem failure (see Chapter 14, Multisystem Problems).

Etiologies, Risk Factors, and Pathophysiology

The most common causes of acute pancreatitis are alcohol disease and biliary tract disease (stones). Some drugs also are associated with acute pancreatitis. Those most commonly used in critical care units include acetaminophen, cimetidine, furosemide, procainamide, and opiates. Pancreatitis also has been associated with shock states and following organ transplantation.

The pathogenesis of acute pancreatitis is not completely clear. The pancreas normally has a protective mechanism to prevent activating enzymes before they reach the duodenum, thereby preventing autodigestion of pancreatic cells. Regardless of the etiology, the process of premature activation of pancreatic enzymes is characteristic of pancreatitis.

Local inflammation and potential necrosis of the pancreas occur. The activated enzymes also can enter the systemic circulation via the portal vein and lymphatics. This is thought to activate complement and kinin systems. Multisystem failure can result, with a variety of complications (Table 17–10). Septic complications, particularly of the pancreas, also can occur. Pancreatic abscess, pseudocyst, and necrosis are not uncommon with fulminant forms of the disease.

Clinical Presentation

Signs and Symptoms

PANCREATIC INFLAMMATION

- Acute pain (severe, relentless, knifelike; midepigastrium or periumbilical)
- Abdominal guarding
- Nausea
- Vomiting
- Abdominal distention
- Hypoactive bowel sounds

FLUID VOLUME DEFICIT

- Hypotension
- Tachycardia
- Mental status changes
- Cool, clammy skin
- Decreased urine output

TABLE 17–10. COMMON MULTISYSTEM COMPLICATIONS OF ACUTE PANCREATITIS

Pulmonary
Atelectasis
Adult respiratory distress syndrome
Pleural effusions

Cardiovascular
Cardiogenic shock

Central Nervous System
Pancreatic encephalopathy

Metabolic
Metabolic acidosis
Hypocalcemia
Altered glucose metabolism

Hematologic
Disseminated intravascular coagulation
Gastrointestinal bleeding

Renal
Prerenal failure

IMPAIRED GAS EXCHANGE

- Decreasing PaO_2 (less than 60 mm Hg) and SaO_2 (less than 90%)

Diagnostic Tests

- Serum amylase greater than 85 IU/L
- Serum pancreatic isoamylase greater than 50%
- Serum lipase greater than 24 IU/dl
- Serum triglycerides greater than 150 mg/dl
- Urine amylase greater than 14 IU/hour
- Serum calcium less than 8.5 mg/dl
- Serum sodium less than 135 mEq/L
- Serum potassium less than 3.5 mEq/L
- Serum magnesium less than 1.5 mg/dl

Patient Needs and Principles of Management

The management of the patient with acute pancreatitis centers on disrupting the cycle of enzyme release of the pancreas and treating complications that can occur with multisystem disease. Principles of management include: fluid resuscitation, resting the pancreas, pain management, and supporting other organ systems that may fail because of mediators released during the inflammatory process.

▶ Fluid Resuscitation

Patients with acute pancreatitis may have fluid shifts of 4 to 12 L into the retroperitoneal space and peritoneal cavity due to inflammation. In fulminant acute pancreatitis, blood vessels in and around the pancreas may also become disrupted, resulting in hemorrhage.

1. Replace fluids with colloids, crystalloids, or blood products. Monitor outcomes of fluid replacement therapy including blood pressure, heart rate, intake and output, preload indicators (CVP, PCWP), skin turgor, capillary refill, and mucous membranes.
2. Monitor for signs and symptoms of hemorrhage (low hematocrit and hemoglobin levels). Cullen's sign is a bluish discoloration around the flanks, and Grey Turner's sign is a bluish discoloration around the umbilical area, indicating blood in the peritoneum. Monitor for increasing abdominal girths.
3. Monitor electrolytes for imbalances related to prolonged vomiting or fluid sequestration. Calcium, sodium, and potassium are most commonly affected. Hyperglycemia also may be present due to the stress response and from impaired secretion of insulin by the islet cells in the inflamed pancreas.

▶ Pain Management

Acute pain is the only universal sign of acute pancreatitis. It is caused by peritoneal irritation from activated pancreatic exocrine enzymes, edema or distention of the pancreas, or from interruption of the blood supply to the pancreas. Treatment of pain is a priority as it causes increased exocrine enzyme release by the pancreas, which may worsen the pathologic process.

1. Assess the degree of pain by having the patient use a pain-rating scale.
2. Administer pain analgesics. There is controversy about the use of opiate analgesics (e.g., morphine) because they may cause spasm of the sphincter of Oddi, which may worsen the pain. Use a pain-rating scale to assess patient outcomes regardless of what is prescribed. Consider scheduled doses or continuous infusion of pain medication for severe pain. Consider epidural analgesia for unrelieved acute pain.
3. Assess patient anxiety and administer sedatives with analgesics.
4. Assist the patient to a position which promotes comfort. The knee-to-chest position often decreases the intensity of the pain.

▶ Rest the Pancreas

Preventing stimulation of pancreatic exocrine secretion is a priority to interrupt the cycle of pancreatic inflammation.

1. Maintain the patient on NPO status. Avoiding the use of the GI tract is recommended until the patient no longer reports abdominal pain and the serum amylase has returned to normal. Intermittent NG suction also may be used to prevent GI secretions from stimulating the pancreas.
2. Provide nutrition parenterally. The solution is usually a mixture of hypertonic glucose and amino acids. The use of lipid emulsion is contraindicated during the acute phase because it increases pancreatic exocrine secretion.
3. Encourage bedrest. Bedrest decreases pancreatic exocrine secretion.
4. Administer pharmacologic agents as prescribed to block the secretion of pancreatic enzymes. These include anticholinergic agents, glucagon, cimetidine, calcitonin, and somatostatin.

▶ Treating Multisystem Failure

Cardiopulmonary complications are the most common multisystem problems. As mentioned previously, they are thought to be due to pancreatic enzyme–induced mediators. Pancreatic ischemia is also known to promote the release of myocardial depressant factor. This causes decreased myocardial contractility and CO. Surgical therapies such as a pancreatic resection may be performed to prevent systemic complications of acute necrotizing pancreatitis by removing necrotic or infected tissue. In some cases, a pancreatectomy may be performed, but it is associated with considerable mortality.

1. Administer oxygen therapy to maintain arterial oxygen tension and oxygen saturation.
2. Perform peritoneal lavage. Peritoneal lavage is used to clear activated mediators and enzymes from the peritoneal cavity. The procedure involves placement of a percutaneous peritoneal dialysis catheter and continuous infusion of isotonic solution. Close monitoring of respiratory status during fluid instillation is a priority. Characteristics of pancreatic lavage return should also be monitored.
3. Administer low-dose dopamine to support myocardial contractility. Dobutamine may also be considered if sepsis is not a complication.

Bowel Infarction/Obstruction

Major disorders of the intestine include intestinal ischemia which can lead to infarction, and intestinal obstruction. Both disorders can result in acute abdominal signs with or without peritoneal irritation.

Etiology, Risk Factors, and Pathophysiology

Intestinal ischemia develops from a decrease in blood flow, producing an inadequate oxygen concentration to meet the requirements of the splanchnic bed. Three major arterial trunks—the celiac axis, the superior mesenteric artery, and the inferior mesenteric artery—branch to form the vascular bed referred to as the splanchnic circulation. The splanchnic bed areas receive about 20% of the CO. Factors which can decrease splanchnic blood flow include abdominal distention, alpha-stimulating sympathomimetic amines (epinephrine, norepinephrine), cardiac glycosides, hypovolemia, and decreased CO. The ischemic bowel loses protein, electrolytes, and fluid into the lumen and wall of the bowel. The third-space extracellular fluid loss decreases the circulating blood volume. Bowel ischemia can lead to bowel necrosis and then gangrene of the bowel. Without surgical intervention, this condition usually is fatal.

Intestinal obstructions may be due to mechanical or functional causes. Obstruction of the bowel may cause circulation to the obstructed segment to be impaired. This may progress to gangrene and peritonitis. Mechanical obstruction involves a physical blockage of the bowel lumen. The most common causes are adhesions and strangulated hernias. The ileum is the most common site as it is the narrowest. A mechanical obstruction of the bowel results in the accumulation of intestinal secretions, ingested fluids, and gas proximal to the site of the obstruction. The increased intestinal secretions accumulating in the bowel deplete the extracellular fluid volume. Loss of electrolytes is also common and varies with the site of the obstruction.

A functional obstruction, or paralytic ileus, develops when there is a loss of peristalsis. Conditions that decrease or inhibit intestinal motility are abdominal surgery, intestinal distention, peritonitis, intestinal ischemia, hypokalemia, severe trauma, and severe medical disease.

Clinical Presentation

Ischemia	Obstruction
History	
CHF	Abdominal surgery
Shock	Hernia
Atrial fibrillation	
Signs and Symptoms	
Crampy umbilical pain	Abdominal pain (midabdominal)
Diarrhea	Cramping
Abdominal distention	Abdominal distention
Weight loss	Decreased bowel sounds
GI bleeding	Muscle guarding and tenderness
Ileus	
Rebound tenderness	Rebound tenderness
Vomiting	Obstipation
Abdominal guarding	
Muscle rigidity	
Fluid volume deficit	Fluid volume deficit

Patient Needs and Principles of Management

Patient priorities for both of these disorders revolve around treating the intravascular fluid volume deficit, treating pain related to inflammation and abdominal distension, and measures to decompress the bowel. Medical therapies for treating bowel infarction include relieving the mesenteric vasoconstriction and surgical therapies to resect necrotic bowel. Papaverine is the drug of choice in relieving mesenteric vasoconstriction. It is given intraarterially after the mesenteric artery is located via radiologic examination. Surgical therapy may also be required to treat bowel obstruction, including lysis of adhesions, reduction of hernias, bypass of obstructions, and excision of obstructions. A colostomy may be performed with left colonic obstructions.

1. Administer colloids and crystalloids to treat the fluid volume deficit. Monitor patient response to fluid resuscitation—hemodynamic parameters (MAP, heart rate), body weight, and intake and output.
2. Administer antimicrobial therapy to treat intraabdominal infection.
3. Position with head-of-bed elevated to promote lung expansion to relieve pressure from the distended

Patient Needs and Principles of Management, Cont.

abdomen. Assist with deep breathing exercises to promote lung expansion, mobilization of secretions, and relaxation.

4. Administer analgesics and sedatives for pain management. Insert an NG tube and apply and maintain suction to drain and decompress the upper GI tract. Avoid excess use of opiates to promote the return of peristalsis.

5. Monitor and report signs and symptoms of ongoing infection.

6. Provide nutrition as prescribed. Total parenteral nutrition may be required early in the course of therapy. Enteral therapy should be begun as early as possible as it promotes the return of peristalsis and may assist in maintaining the gut mucosal barrier function.

AT THE BEDSIDE
▶ *Thinking Critically*

You are caring for a patient with acute upper GI hemorrhage with the following patient orders:

- Monitor vital signs q 15 min until stable; then q 1 h
- Stat hemoglobin and hematocrit
- Administer 0.9 NS wide open until MAP is above 60; then call physician

Which of the above interventions will give you the best indication of the amount of blood lost? What do you expect to happen to the serum lab values with the administration of fluid?

SELECTED BIBLIOGRAPHY

What Heals: Gut Feelings and Intuition

Benner P, et al.: From beginner to expert: Gaining a differentiated clinical world in critical care nursing. *Advances in Nursing Science.* 1992;14:13–28.

Garrity PL: Perception in nursing: The value of intuition. *Holistic Nursing Practice.* 1987;1:63.

Jung C: *Psychological types.* New York: Harcourt, Brace, 1959.

Polanyi M: *Personal knowledge.* New York: Harper & Row, 1958.

Polanyi M: *The tacit dimension.* New York: Anchor Press, 1966.

Rew L: Intuition: Nursing knowledge and the spiritual dimension of persons. *Holistic Nursing Practice.* 1989;3(3):58.

Ruth-Sahd LA: A modification of Benner's hierarchy of clinical practice: The development of clinical intuition in the novice trauma nurse. *Holistic Nursing Practice.* 1993;7(3):10.

Schraeder BD, Fisher DK: Using intuitive knowledge in the neonatal intensive care nursery. *Holistic Nursing Practice.* 1987;1:47.

Slater VE: Modern physics, synchronicity, and intuition. *Holistic Nursing Practice.* 1992;6(4):20–25.

Young CE: Intuition and nursing process. *Holistic Nursing Practice.* 1987;1:52.

General Gastrointestinal

Russell S: Hypovolemic shock. *Nursing 94.* 1994;April:34–39.

Waite LG, Krumberger JM: *Noncardiac critical care nursing.* Albany, NY: Delmar, 1994.

Upper GI Bleeding

Adams L, Soulen MC: TIPS: A new alternative for variceal bleeding. *American Journal of Critical Care.* 1993; 2(3):196–200.

Bezarro ER: Changing perspectives of H_2 antagonists for stress ulcer prophylaxis. *Critical Care Clinics of North America.* 1993;5(2):325–331.

Chamberlain CE: Acute hemorrhagic gastritis. *Gastroenterology Clinics of North America.* 1993;22(4):843–865.

Goff JS: Gastroesophageal varices: Pathogenesis and therapy of acute bleeding. *Gastroenterology Clinics of North America.* 1993;22(4):779–796.

Gould SA, Sehgal LR, Sehgal HL, et al.: Hypovolemic shock. *Critical Care Clinics.* 1993;9(2):239–259.

Henderson JM, Carey WD, Vogt DP, et al.: Management of variceal bleeding in the 1990's. *Cleveland Clinic Journal of Medicine.* 1993;60(6):431–438.

Holsete A, Palitzsch KD, Scholmerich J: The role of drug treatment in variceal bleeding. *Digestion.* 1994;55:1–12.

Laine L: Rolling review: Upper gastrointestinal bleeding. *Alimentory Pharmacology and Therapeutics.* 1993;7:207–231.

Lieberman D. Gastrointestinal bleeding: Initial management. *Gastroenterology Clinics of North America.* 1993;22(8): 723–735.

Shigmann GV: Endoscopic management of esophageal varices. *Advances in Surgery.* 1994;27:209–231.

Steffes C, Fromm D: The current diagnosis and management of upper gastrointestinal bleeding. *Advances in Surgery.* 1992;25: 331–361.

Liver Failure

Bosche J, Pizcueta P, Feu F, Fernandez M, Garcia-Pagan JC: Pathophysiology of portal hypertension. *Gastroenterology Clinics of North America*. 1992;21(1):1–14.

Douglas D, Rakela J: Fulminant hepatitis. In Kaplowitz N (ed.): *Liver and biliary diseases*. Baltimore: Williams & Wilkins, 1992.

Kucharski SA: Fulminant hepatic failure. *Critical Care Nursing Clinics of North America*. 1993;5(1):141–151.

Shanna CG, Gollan JL: Fulminant hepatic failure. In Taylor MB, (ed.): *Gastrointestinal emergencies*. Baltimore: Williams & Wilkins, 1992.

Young LM: Managing the patient with liver failure. *Medical-Surgical Nursing*. 1993;2(4):275–281.

Acute Pancreatitis

Brown A: Acute pancreatitis. *Focus on Critical Care*. 1991; 18(2):121–130.

Krumberger JM: Acute pancreatitis. *Critical Care Nursing Clinics of North America*. 1993;5(1):185–202.

McFadden DW: Organ failure and multiple organ system failure in pancreatitis. *Pancreas*. 1991;6(1):S37–S43.

Intestinal Ischemia/Bowel Obstruction

Kaleya RN, Sammartano RT, Boley SJ: Aggressive approach to acute mesenteric ischemia. *Surgical Clinics of North America*. 1992;72(1):157–181.

McConnell EA: Loosening the grip of intestinal obstruction. *Nursing 94*. 1994;March:34–41.

Quinn DA: Acute mesenteric ischemia. *Critical Care Nursing Clinics of North America*. 1993;5(1):171–175.

Eighteen

Renal System

► Knowledge Competencies

1. Describe the etiology, pathophysiology, clinical presentation, patient needs, and principles of management of acute renal failure.

2. Differentiate between the three types of acute renal failure:

   • Prerenal
   • Intrarenal
   • Postrenal

3. Compare and contrast the pathophysiology, clinical presentation, patient needs, and management approaches of life-threatening electrolyte imbalances:

   • Sodium (Na^+)
   • Potassium (K^+)
   • Calcium (Ca^{++})
   • Magnesium (Mg^{++})
   • Phosphorous (PO_4^{--})

4. Differentiate between the indications for and the efficacy of the different types of renal replacement therapies.

5. Describe the nursing interventions for patients undergoing renal replacement therapy.

■ *What Heals: Intentional Touch*

Touch is a powerful way to share our presence with patients who are ill and in crisis. Physical touch done lovingly, freely, and with joy conveys through our hands what our hearts are feeling. As critical care nurses, we touch patients all the time. How often do you touch as part of a routine or procedure and how often do you touch with healing intention?

Touch with intention can be a healing force. When nurses touch with intention and for the purpose of the highest good, they are present with their patients in a healing way. Some of the special moments that critically ill patients remember that got them through the rough times are the fluffing of pillows or a straightening of sheets; a change in position, particularly in bony areas; or being given mouth care, a backrub, a foot massage, or light acupressure.

Encourage family or friends to participate in touch, explaining that it helps to connect them with their loved one and humanizes the technologic environment. Touch includes bathing, hair combing, feeding, and changing the patient's position, sheets, pillow, and sheepskins, as well as hugging and holding. Touch with intention is a powerful way to help patients shake loose the fear, guilt, and loneliness that often accompanies critical illness.

CED & BMD

Adapted from: Dossey BM, Guzzetta CE, Kenner CV: Critical care nursing: Body-mind-spirit, *3rd ed. Philadelphia: JB Lippincott, 1992, p. 231.*

SPECIAL ASSESSMENT TECHNIQUES, DIAGNOSTIC TESTS, AND MONITORING SYSTEMS

There are a wide variety of diagnostic tests available for use in determining the cause and location of renal dysfunction. The creatinine and blood urea nitrogen (BUN) levels are monitored closely, as these levels and their relationship to each other (BUN:creatinine ratio) provide valuable information about the kidney's filtering ability. The BUN level provides valuable information about the state of renal perfusion, while the creatinine level is more precise in evaluating actual tubular function. Urine Na^+ values vary as the kidneys attempt to retain or excrete water. Urine volume, specific gravity (SG), and osmolality are useful in identifying the kidney's ability to excrete and concentrate fluid. Comparisons of these test values as found in prerenal and intrarenal failure are shown in Table 18–1. These tests help to establish a firm diagnosis.

PATHOLOGIC CONDITIONS

Acute Renal Failure

The most common renal problem seen in critically ill patients is the development of acute renal failure (ARF). Acute renal failure is the abrupt reduction of renal function with progressive retention of metabolic waste products (e.g., creatinine and urea). Oliguria, urine output of <400 ml/day, is a common finding in acute renal failure. The development of acute renal failure in the critically ill patient has an estimated mortality of 65%. A history of chronic renal failure (CRF) complicates the clinical course of any critical illness.

TABLE 18–1. DIAGNOSTIC TESTS USED IN DIFFERENTIAL DIAGNOSIS OF ACUTE RENAL FAILURE

Test	Normal Values	Prerenal	Intrarenal
Urine			
Volume	1.0 to 1.5 L/day	<400 ml/day	<400 ml/day
Specific gravity	1.10 to 1.20	>1.020	<1.010
Osmolality	500 to 850 mOsm/kg	>500 mOsm/kg	<350 mOsm/kg
Sodium	40 to 220 mEq/L/24 hours	<20 mEq/L	>30 mEq/L
Serum			
BUN	10 to 20 mg/dl	>25 mg/dL	>25 mg/dl
Creatinine	0.6 to 1.2 mg/dl	Normal	>1.2 mg/dl
BUN: creatinine ratio	10:1	>20:1	10:1*

*both values elevated but ratio constant.

AT THE BEDSIDE
▶ Acute Renal Failure

Nancy V., a 62-year-old woman, was initially seen in the emergency department for reports of continued, intense abdominal pain with nausea and vomiting. Following ultrasound, she was taken to the operating room where surgical exploration revealed 5 feet of necrotic bowel, hemorrhagic ascites, and gross peritonitis. The bowel was excised and 460 ml of ascitic fluid was drained.

Upon admission to the critical care unit, Nancy was intubated and ventilated, had a pulmonary artery and Foley catheter in situ, and had a nasogastric tube for intermittent suction. Assessment revealed the following:

Skin:	Cool and moist
Neurologic:	Aroused easily to stimulation, moved all extremities to command
Cardiovascular:	Normal heart sounds, no edema or increased neck veins
Respiratory:	Diminished breath sounds with crackles bilaterally
Abdomen:	Distended, absent bowel sounds, NG drainage minimal (bloody, dark fluid)
Genitourinary:	<20 ml/hour of urine, dark gold in color

Vital signs

Heart rate:	130/minute (sinus tachycardia with occasional premature ventricular contractions)
Blood pressure:	90/60, labile
Respirations:	16/minute
Temperature:	39.5° C (rectal)

During the first 8 hours postoperatively, Nancy received 5 L of lactated Ringer's solution in an effort to stabilize her blood pressure and increase her urine output.

Aggressive fluid resuscitation was continued throughout her first postoperative day to manage her continued labile BP and poor urine output. Tests at that time revealed the following:

BUN:	33 mg/dl
Creatinine:	2.8 mg/dl
K^+:	6.2 mEq/L

Arterial blood gases

pH:	7.25
$PaCO_2$:	39 mm Hg
HCO_3	14 mEq/L
PaO_2:	94 mm Hg

Dopamine was started at 2.5 µg/kg/minute, along with dobutamine at 7.5 µg/kg/minute. Ventilator changes were made and 88 mEq of NaHCO₃ given IV.

On the second postoperative day CVVHD was initiated to correct her increasing renal failure and electrolyte imbalance (BUN 50 mg/dl; creatinine 2.8 mg/dl; K⁺ 5.8 mEq/L; arterial pH 7.26). The following day her blood pressure began to stabilize, with decreasing levels of BUN, creatinine, and K⁺ and an increase in pH to normal levels.

Etiology, Risk Factors, and Pathophysiology

ARF is best understood when the condition is considered in terms of the location of damage to the renal system: prerenal, intrarenal, or postrenal causes of failure. Each type of ARF has different etiologies, pathophysiology, laboratory findings, and clinical presentation.

Prerenal Failure

Physiologic conditions that lead to decreased perfusion of the kidneys, without intrinsic damage to the renal tubules, are identified as prerenal failure (Table 18–2). The decrease in renal arterial perfusion causes a decrease in the rate of filtration of blood through the glomerulus. When perfusion pressure falls below 70 mm Hg, the protection of autoregulation is lost, further decreasing glomerular filtration.

Renal tubular function, at this point, is still completely normal. As a result of the decreased glomerular filtration rate (GFR), the kidneys are unable to filter waste products from the blood. Consequently, more Na⁺ and water are reabsorbed, resulting in oliguria. If the decreased perfusion state persists, irreversible damage to the renal tubules may occur, resulting in intrarenal failure. Most forms of prerenal failure are easily reversed by treating the cause and increasing renal perfusion.

Intrarenal Failure

Physiologic conditions that damage the renal tubule, nephron, or renal blood vessels are identified as intrarenal failure (Table 18–1). Following prolonged decreases in renal perfusion, the kidneys gradually suffer damage that is not readily reversed with the restoration of renal perfusion. Intrarenal failure is commonly referred to as acute tubular necrosis.

When the insult to the kidney is nephrotoxic (from drugs or substances which cause direct damage to the kidney), the nephron damage occurs primarily at the epithelial layer. Since this layer has the ability to regenerate, rapid healing often occurs following nephrotoxic insults. When the insult is ischemic or inflammatory, the nephron's basement membrane is also damaged and regeneration is not possible. Ischemic and inflammatory insults are more likely to cause chronic renal failure than nephrotoxic insults.

TABLE 18–2. CAUSES OF ACUTE RENAL FAILURE

PRERENAL FAILURE
Hypovolemia
- Burns
- Excessive use of diuretics
- GI losses
- Hemorrhage
- Third spacing
- Shock

Altered Peripheral Vascular Resistance
- Anaphylactic reaction
- Antihypertensive medications
- Neurogenic shock
- Septic shock

Decreased Cardiac Output
- Arrhythmias
- Cardiac tamponade
- Cardiogenic shock
- Congestive heart failure
- Myocardial infarction
- Pulmonary embolism

INTRARENAL FAILURE
Ischemic
- Prolonged decreased renal perfusion
- Septic shock
- Transfusion reaction
- Trauma/crush injury

Nephrotoxic
- Antibiotics
- Fungicides
- Pesticides
- Radiographic dyes

Inflammatory
- Acute glomerulonephritis
- Acute vasculopathy
- Acute interstitial nephritis

POSTRENAL FAILURE
Mechanical
- Clots
- Stones
- Strictures
- Tumors

Functional
- Medications
- Neurological disorders

The underlying pathophysiologic abnormality in intrarenal failure is renal cellular damage. In healthy kidneys the glomerulus normally acts as a filter, preventing the passage of large molecules into the glomerular filtrate. Damage to the glomerulus allows protein and cellular debris to enter the renal tubules, leading to intraluminal obstruction.

Postrenal Failure

Physiologic conditions which partially or completely obstruct urine flow from the kidney to the urethral meatus can cause postrenal failure. Partial obstruction increases renal interstitial pressure, which in turn increases Bowman's capsule pressure and opposes glomerular filtration. Complete obstruction leads to urine backup into the kidney, eventually compressing the kidney. With complete obstruction, there is no urine output from the affected kidney. Postrenal failure is an uncommon cause of acute renal failure in critically ill patients. The treatment for postrenal failure is focused on removing the obstruction.

Clinical Phases

There are three clinical phases of ARF, seen primarily in intrarenal failure. The first, the oliguric phase, begins within 48 hours of the insult to the kidney. In intrarenal failure, the oliguric phase is accompanied by a significant rise in BUN and creatinine. The degree of elevation of these waste products is less pronounced in prerenal failure. The most common complications seen in this phase of renal failure are fluid overload and acute hyperkalemia. The oliguric phase will last from a few days to several weeks. The longer the oliguric phase continues, the poorer is the patient's prognosis.

The diuretic phase follows the oliguric phase. During this phase, there is a gradual return of renal function. Although the BUN and creatinine continue to rise, there is an increase in urine output. The patient's state of hydration prior to this phase determines the amount of urine output. A patient who was fluid overloaded may excrete up to 5 L of urine a day and have marked Na^+ wasting. The average time in this phase is 2 weeks. Patients must be observed carefully for risk of complications from fluid and electrolyte deficits.

The recovery phase marks the stabilization of laboratory values and can last 3 to 12 months. Some degree of residual renal insufficiency is common following ARF.

Some patients never recover renal function and progress to chronic renal failure.

Clinical Presentation

The diverse causes of renal failure determine the clinical presentation of the patient. Renal failure can cause multiple organ dysfunction and, therefore, manifests itself in a variety of ways. Uremia is the term used to describe the clinical syndrome that accompanies the detrimental effects of renal dysfunction on the other organ systems. The clinical presentation of the patient in uremia reflects the degree of nephron loss and, correspondingly, the loss of renal function.

Signs and Symptoms

- Oliguria (<400 ml/day) or anuria (<100 ml/day)
- Tachycardia
- Hypotension (prerenal)
- Hypertension (intrarenal)
- Flat neck veins (prerenal)
- Distended neck veins (intrarenal)
- Dry mucous membranes
- Cool, clammy skin
- Lethargy
- Deep, rapid respirations
- Vomiting
- Nausea
- Confusion

Diagnostic Tests

Laboratory tests are extremely important in diagnosing and evaluating the effectiveness of interventions in the ARF patient. Table 18–1 presents the usual laboratory values seen in prerenal and intrarenal failure.

Patient Needs and Principles of Management

A collaborative approach to the treatment of patients in renal failure begins with early recognition of patients at risk for renal failure. The focus is on the maintainence of adequate renal perfusion and avoiding renal compromise.

Much has changed in the prevention and treatment of ARF over the past several decades. These advances have focused on prompt correction of hypotension and the early use of renal replacement therapies (RRTs) before the development of uremia. Once the patient develops ARF, the goal is to quickly reestablish homeostasis by elimination of the underlying cause. Management of acute renal failure also includes correction of fluid imbalance, prevention and correction of life-threatening electrolyte imbalances, treatment

of acidosis, prevention of further renal damage, prevention and treatment of infection, and the improvement of nutritional status.

▶ Correction of Fluid Imbalance

Maintaining fluid balance in the renal failure patient is a challenge. A fine balance must be achieved in providing the fluid necessary for adequate renal perfusion while preventing fluid overload. It is often difficult to assess if the patient is volume depleted or overloaded. A pulmonary artery catheter may be inserted to assist with fluid status evaluation.

Patient Needs and Principles of Management, Cont.

1. Calculate daily fluid needs. In prerenal disease, fluid replacement must be matched with fluid loss, both in amount and composition. Insensible fluid losses must be considered in this calculation (Table 18–3). Normal saline volume loading (before a potential insult) of the patient at risk for renal dysfunction is a widely accepted practice. Additionally, volume expansion is certainly beneficial in preventing a volume-depleted patient from progressing from prerenal to intrarenal failure. While oliguric, patients can rarely tolerate more than 1000 ml of fluid per day, placing constraints on other therapies (e.g., IV drug administration, nutritional support). During the diuretic phase, the patient may require 1 to 4 L of fluid per day to prevent hypovolemia. The patient is frequently allowed to lose more fluid than is replaced in an effort to facilitate fluid movement from the interstitial and intracellular spaces into the vascular space.

2. Obtain accurate intake and output measurements. All insensible losses should be included in the measurements. Fluid therapy decisions will often be based on the patient's output.

3. Obtain daily weights. Body weight should be allowed to decrease by 0.2 to 0.3 kg/day as a result of catabolism. If the patient's weight is stable or increasing, volume expansion should be suspected. If weight loss exceeds these recommendations, volume depletion or hypercatabolism should be investigated.

4. Administer diuretics to evaluate the patient's response when the patient's fluid status is uncertain. Increasing dosages are used in an attempt to determine the optimal dose. This is often done by doubling the dose (e.g., first dose, 20 mg; second dose, 40 mg; third dose, 80 mg; etc.) every 30 to 60 minutes until diuresis is achieved or a maximum dose is reached. Once renal failure is established, diuretics may be used to avoid fluid overload and to potentiate the effects of antihypertensive medications. Potassium-sparing diuretics are typically avoided since K^+ elimination is diminished in renal failure. Two commonly used diuretics are mannitol and furosemide. Mannitol, an osmotic diuretic, is used in attempts to prevent ARF. It causes vasodilation of the renal vessels and expands vascular volume by enhancing movement of fluid from the interstitial space. The beneficial use of mannitol after ARF is established is not clear. Mannitol can contribute to fluid overload without excretory renal function and should be used cautiously. Furosemide, a loop diuretic, is the most common diuretic used in ARF. It works by blocking Na^+ reabsorption in the renal tubules, thereby enhancing excretion of Na^+ and water. It is often used to reduce fluid overload and dialysis frequency in ARF. Furosemide should be used cautiously in patients receiving aminoglycoside antibiotics since it potentiates the nephrotoxic effects of these medications.

5. Administer dopamine at low doses (2 to 5 μg/kg/minute) to increase renal vasodilation and blood flow. Renal dose dopamine is used both for prevention in the high-risk patient and for treatment of acute renal failure.

6. Institute renal replacement therapy (RRT) as needed. Until recently, patients in renal failure had either peritoneal dialysis or hemodialysis for assistance in maintaining fluid balance. A number of new continuous filtration devices are now available to increase fluid and metabolic waste product removal during acute renal failure. These newer therapies may be better tolerated in hemodynamically unstable patients than peritoneal dialysis or hemodialysis.

▶ Prevention and Treatment of Life-Threatening Electrolyte Imbalances

There are a number of electrolyte imbalances that can occur in renal failure, the most common being hyperkalemia, hypocalcemia, hypermagnesemia, and hyperphosphatemia. In ARF, the electrolyte status guides decisions about the type of fluid replacement and renal replacement therapy. The management of these electrolyte disorders is detailed later in this chapter.

▶ Treatment of Acidosis

Renal failure patients often develop metabolic acidosis, with a mild respiratory alkalosis compensation.

1. Administer sodium bicarbonate ($NaHCO_3$) as indicated. Treatment is usually not instituted until the serum bicarbonate level drops below 15 mEq/L. Even then, replacement of only half the base deficit is made to avoid overcorrection of the pH. Administration of excessive $NaHCO_3$ can cause metabolic alkalosis, tetany, and pulmonary edema.

TABLE 18–3. MINIMAL VOLUMES OF FLUID ASSOCIATED WITH INSENSIBLE FLUID LOSSES

Situation/Condition	Volume
Respiratory losses	500 to 850 ml/day (dependent on minute ventilation rate)
Fever (loss/degree C elevation over 38.0)	200 ml
Diaphoresis	500 ml
Diarrhea	50 to 200 ml/stool

2. If a patient is being dialyzed, using a dialysate containing bicarbonate will facilitate buffering of the patient's acidotic state.

▶ Prevention of Additional Kidney Damage

In acute renal failure, drugs which are metabolized or excreted by the kidney require adjustment to avoid excessive blood levels and potential nephrotoxicity. Particular attention must be given to medication scheduling related to renal replacement therapy schedules. Medications may be eliminated or have their actions potentiated by these therapies. A clinical pharmacist is a helpful resource on medication delivery during ARF.

1. Modify medication dosing. Since many medications are eliminated by the kidney, drug administration (dose and schedule) must be altered in the patient with renal failure. Medication dose and schedule decisions are based upon the drug and the patient's degree of renal dysfunction. The phase of renal failure and other concommitant treatments help determine the appropriate dose of medication.
2. Administer antihypertensive agents as needed. Hypertension is a major problem for many renal failure patients, often requiring concomitant use of several antihypertensive agents. Most antihypertensive agents are not removed by RRT. During hemodialysis, it is important to adjust the dosage schedule of antihypertensive agents to avoid hypotensive episodes during dialysis. Some antihypertensive agents, however, are eliminated by the kidney. Therefore, dialysis patients receiving these medications require alterations in their dose or dosing schedule.

▶ Prevention and Treatment of Infection

Renal failure patients are at high risk for infection and are commonly treated with antimicrobial agents. The antimicrobial agents need to be carefully selected and monitored, often needing dose adjustment. Careful monitoring of both renal function and drug levels during antimicrobial therapy is imperative to avoid further renal damage.

▶ Improvement of Nutritional Status

The challenge in managing the renal failure patient's nutrition is to provide a balance between sufficient calories and protein to prevent catabolism, yet not create problems such as fluid and electrolyte imbalances or increase the requirement for RRT. The typical renal failure patient is hypermetabolic, with caloric needs potentially twice normal. Additional stresses, related to being critically ill, can further elevate caloric requirements. Nausea and vomiting, common in uremia, further decrease oral caloric intake. Adequate nutrition is also important in preventing infection by helping to maintain the integrity of the immune system.

1. Restrict the patient's fluid, K^+, Na^+, and protein intake. Since these patients cannot eliminate wastes, fluid, or electrolytes, their dietary intake of these substances is typically restricted. The degree of restriction is dependent upon the cause and severity of their disease. For example, the level of Na^+ restriction is determined by the cause of the renal failure and the serum Na^+ level. Some causes lead to Na^+ wasting and others to Na^+ retention. Phosphorus may need to be restricted and Ca^{++} supplemented if the Ca^{++} level is low in conjunction with normal PO_4^{--} levels.
2. Administer necessary vitamin supplementation. Supplementation of folic acid, pyridoxine, and the water-soluble vitamins is most frequently necessary.
3. Consult a dietitian for a diet plan. Dietary requirements change for patients, depending upon their renal status and the severity of their underlying condition. Although the precise role of nutrition in ARF is controversial, malnutrition is thought to increase morbidity and mortality. Total parenteral nutrition, used in conjunction with daily RRT, is thought to improve survival and promote healing of renal tubular cells.

The usual approach to hypercatabolic states is to provide adequate proteins and carbohydrates to provide for resynthesis of damaged or lost tissue elements. Protein requirements may range initially from 0.5 to 1.0 g/kg/day and increase with RRT to 1.0 to 1.5 g/kg/day. Nonprotein calories, usually in the form of fat, are given for nonanabolic metabolic needs.

Life-Threatening Electrolyte Imbalances

The kidneys play a major role in the regulation of fluid and electrolyte balance in the body. Regulation of body fluids and electrolytes helps to ensure a stable internal environment, resulting in maximal intracellular function. Any renal dysfunction will result in abnormalities in both fluid and electrolyte balance.

For all of the electrolyte disorders, the indications for treatment vary from patient to patient. The signs and symptoms of any electrolyte imbalance are not necessarily determined by the degree of abnormality. Rather, the signs and symptoms are determined by the cause of the condition, as well as the magnitude and rapidity of onset. For many of the electrolyte imbalances it is difficult to determine at precisely what level signs or symptoms may occur.

Sodium Imbalance: Hyperosmolar Disorders

Etiologies, Risk Factors, and Pathophysiology

Serum osmolality, a measure of the number of particles in a unit of blood volume, is an important indicator of fluid status. Since serum osmolality is determined primarily by the serum Na^+ level, evaluation of Na^+ levels provides valuable information on serum osmolality and potential excesses or deficits of total body water. A quick estimate of serum osmolality can be calculated by simply doubling the serum Na^+ value. Normal serum osmolality values are 285 to 295 mOsm/kg. Abnormal serum Na^+ levels are classified as disorders of osmolality, with hyperosmolality referring to high Na^+ levels, indicative of water deficit, or hypoosmolality referring to low sodium levels, indicative of water excess.

Critically ill patients often are at risk for disorders of osmolality, with children and the elderly at highest risk. As a person ages, the hypothalamus becomes less sensitive to changes in osmolality and is, therefore, less able to alert the body to abnormalities through normal mechanisms. Additionally, the neurologic signs indicative of osmolality disorders often are ignored or related to age rather than to a physiologic abnormality.

Hyperosmolar disorders are the result of a deficit of water. The causes of hyperosmolality include inadequate intake of water, excessive loss of water, or conditions that cause an inhibition of antidiuretic hormone (ADH). In the critically ill patient, hyperosmolar disorders develop due to inadequate intake, usually related to loss of consciousness or endotracheal intubation, and ADH inhibition, as manifested by diabetes insipidus in a patient with a head injury. The signs and symptoms seen are the result of the ensuing cerebral dehydration. Water is pulled from the intracellular space to enhance intravascular volume, leaving the cells dehydrated.

Clinical Presentation

SIGNS AND SYMPTOMS

- Lethargy
- Restlessness
- Disorientation
- Delusions
- Seizures
- Oliguria
- Hypotension
- Thirst
- Tachycardia
- Dry mucous membranes
- Coma

Diagnostic Tests

- Serum Na^+ > 150 mEq/L
- Serum osmolality > 300 mOsm/kg
- Urine specific gravity > 1.024

Sodium Imbalance: Hypoosmolar Disorders

Hypoosmolality disorders are the result of an excess of water. The causes of hypoosmolality include excess intake or impaired secretion of water, excess ADH as in syndrome of inappropriate ADH (SIADH), replacement of volume loss with pure water, and salt wasting disorders. Hypoosmolar disorders are extremely common in critically ill patients, most often related to the use of D5W IV solutions. As these patients have often lost some volume, balanced fluid replacement is extremely important. The signs and symptoms seen with hypoosmolar disorders are related to cerebral intracellular swelling, as water moves from the intravascular to the intracellular spaces.

Clinical Presentation

SIGNS AND SYMPTOMS

- Confusion
- Delirium
- Seizures
- Muscle twitching
- Nausea
- Weight gain
- Headache
- Personality changes
- Coma
- Anorexia
- Vomiting

Diagnostic Tests

- Serum Na^+ <130 mEq/L
- Serum osmolality <280 mOsm/kg
- Urine specific gravity <1.010

Potassium Imbalance: Hyperkalemia

Etiologies, Risk Factors, and Pathophysiology

There are three primary causes of hyperkalemia: increased intake, decreased excretion, and redistribution of K^+ from intracellular to extracellular fluid. Rarely is increased intake a sole cause of hyperkalemia, but it is commonly found in combination with decreased K^+ excretion. The most common causes of hyperkalemia in the critically ill are ARF, cellular destruction (e.g., from crush injuries), and excess supplementation. As cardiac tissue is sensitive to K^+ levels, hyperkalemia often manifests first in changes to the electrical conduction, demonstrated by changes on ECG tracings. Elevated serum K^+ levels alter the conduction of electrical impulses, particularly in cardiac and muscle tissue. These conduction abnormalities can lead to serious cardiac arrhythmias and death.

Clinical Presentation

Since K^+ impacts normal neuromuscular and cardiac function, these systems should be carefully evaluated when hyperkalemia is suspected. It is important to note that a patient may be experiencing hyperkalemia and have no ECG or rhythm changes.

Signs and Symptoms

- Vague muscle weakness
- Decreased deep tendon reflexes
- Flaccid paralysis
- Mental confusion
- Nausea
- Diarrhea
- Cramping

ECG Changes

- Tall, tented T waves
- QT interval may shorten
- Intraventricular conduction is slowed
- Widened QRS
- Wide P waves
- Bradycardia
- First-degree atrioventricular (AV) block
- Advanced AV block with ventricular escape rhythms, ventricular fibrillation, or asystole

Diagnostic Tests

- Serum $K^+ > 5.5$ mEq/L

Potassium Imbalance: Hypokalemia

Etiologies, Risk Factors, and Pathophysiology

The causes of hypokalemia include decreased intake, increased excretion or impaired conservation of potassium, excess or abnormal loss, and increased movement into the cells. In the critically ill patient, hypokalemia is often related to use of diuretics and excess losses through the gastrointestinal tract. Muscle weakness, including cardiac muscle, is the hallmark sign of hypokalemia. Asystole can result from severe hypokalemia. Depressed levels of serum K^+ lead to increased irritability of cardiac muscle and neuromuscular cells. Serious cardiac arrhythmias, and death, may result from hypokalemia.

Clinical Presentation

Signs and Symptoms

- Weakness
- Respiratory muscle weakness, hypoventilation
- Paralytic ileus
- Abdominal distention
- Cramping
- Confusion, irritability
- Lethargy

ECG Changes

- Ventricular ectopy and flat, inverted T waves
- QT-interval prolongation
- U-wave development
- ST-segment shortening and depression

Diagnostic Tests

- Serum $K^+ < 3.5$ mEq/L

Calcium Imbalance: Hypercalcemia

Etiologies, Risk Factors, and Pathophysiology

The causes of hypercalcemia are threefold: increased Ca^{++} release from the bone, increased Ca^{++} absorption from the GI tract, and decreased Ca^{++} excretion.

Clinical Presentation

Signs and Symptoms

- Somnolence
- Stupor
- Nausea
- Anorexia
- Polyuria
- Lethargy
- Coma
- Vomiting
- Constipation
- Renal calculi

ECG Changes

- Arrhythmias
- Prolonged QT interval
- Prolonged ST segment
- Flat, inverted T waves

Diagnostic Tests

- Serum Ca^{++}>10.5 mg/dl

Calcium Imbalance: Hypocalcemia

Etiologies, Risk Factors, and Pathophysiology

True hypocalcemia is rare. The causes of hypocalcemia are classified into three categories: decreased absorption of Ca^{++}, increased loss of Ca^{++}, and decreased amounts of physiologically active Ca^{++}. Critically ill patients develop hypocalcemia infrequently, most often related to either gastrointestinal losses or malabsorption. The low Ca^{++} levels result in muscle contraction, seen as tetany, and bronchospasm.

Clinical Presentation

Signs and Symptoms

- Positive Chvostek's sign (twitching of the upper lip in response to tapping of the facial nerve)
- Positive Trousseau's sign (carpopedal spasm in response to occlusion of circulation to the extremity for 3 minutes)
- Tetany
- Seizures
- Respiratory arrest
- Bronchospasms
- Stridor
- Wheezing
- Paralytic ileus
- Diarrhea

ECG Changes

- Arrhythmias
- Shortened QT interval
- ST-segment sagging and shortening
- T-wave inversion

Diagnostic Tests

- Serum Ca^{++}<8.5 mg/dl

Magnesium Imbalance: Hypermagnesemia

Etiologies, Risk Factors, and Pathophysiology

Hypermagnesemia is most commonly seen in renal failure patients with an inability to excrete Mg^{++} or with increased intake of Mg^{++} from antacid. ARF is the most common etiology of hypermagnesemia in critically ill patients. Both neuromuscular and cardiac depression are observed. Hypermagnesemia may also develop in non-renal-failure situations when Mg^{++} intake is increased, excretion is decreased, or adrenal insufficiency or hyperparathyroidism causes increased Mg^{++}.

Clinical Presentation

Signs and Symptoms

- Respiratory depression
- Diminished deep tendon reflexes
- Flaccid paralysis
- Drowsiness
- Lethargy

ECG Changes

- Cardiac arrest
- Prolonged PR and QT intervals
- Widened QRS
- Increased T-wave amplitude
- Bradycardia

Diagnostic Tests

- Serum Mg^{++}>2.5 mEq/L

Magnesium Imbalance: Hypomagnesemia

Etiologies, Risk Factors, and Pathophysiology

Hypomagnesemia frequently occurs in alcoholic and critically ill patients and is often associated with hypocalcemia and hypokalemia. Hypomagnesemia can be caused by decreased intake, increased excretion, such as with diuretic therapy, and excessive loss of body fluids. The hypomagnesemia seen in the critically ill is most often the manifestation of a compromised nutritional status, secondary to starvation and malabsorption.

Clinical Presentation

Signs and Symptoms

- Hyperreflexia
- Positive Chvostek's and Trousseau's signs
- Nystagmus
- Seizures
- Tetany

ECG Changes

- Prolonged PR and QT intervals
- Broad, flat T waves
- Ventricular arrhythmias

Diagnostic Tests

- Serum $Mg^{++} < 1.5$ mEq/L

Phosphate Imbalance: Hyperphosphatemia

Etiologies, Risk Factors, and Pathophysiology

The most common cause of hyperphosphatemia in all patients, including the critically ill, is renal failure since the regulation of phosphate in the body is regulated by the kidneys. Hyperphosphatemia is also seen in hypoparathyroidism, excessive intake of alkali or vitamin D, Addison's disease, and with bone tumors or fractures. Hypophosphatemia is often associated with hypocalcemia.

Clinical Presentation

Signs and Symptoms

- Muscle cramps
- Joint pain
- Seizures

Diagnostic Tests

- Serum phosphate > 4.5 mg/dl

Phosphate Imbalance: Hypophosphatemia

Etiologies, Risk Factors, and Pathophysiology

Hypophosphatemia is caused by hyperparathyroidism, hyperinsulinism, administration of IV glucose, and conditions that cause bone deterioration, such as osteomalacia. This condition is not often seen in critically ill patients. When seen, it is frequently in conjunction with hypercalcemia.

Clinical Presentation

Signs and Symptoms

- Muscle weakness and wasting
- Fatigue
- Confusion
- Oliguria
- Tachycardia
- Anorexia
- Dyspnea
- Cool Skin

Diagnostic Tests

- Serum phosphate < 3.0 mg/dl

Patients Needs and Principles of Management

Hyperosmolar Disorders

1. Administer free water. Fluid replacement can be given orally, if feasible or with intravenous administration of D5W also can be used. The goal is to normalize the serum Na^+ level over a 48- to 72-hour period. Gradual return to normal will avoid cellular overhydration.
2. Monitor Na^+ and serum osmolality level frequently. Care must be taken to correct the Na^+ and osmolality level gradually. Correcting these levels too quickly may precipitate hypoosmolar conditions and seizures.
3. Administer desmopressin (nasally) or vasopressin (IV, IM, SC) in diabetes insipidus. These medications work on the kidney to inhibit the action of ADH.

Hypoosmolar Disorders

1. Restrict water intake. Mild, asymptomatic hyponatremia often is not treated, or is treated only with a water restriction.
2. Institute RRT. RRT is indicated for severe fluid overload in the presence of renal failure.
3. Administer hypertonic saline. Hypertonic saline may be needed to correct Na^+ levels below 115 mEq/L when the patient is symptomatic. Careful, slow administration of hypertonic saline is important to avoid sudden shifts in serum osmolality and subsequent hyperosmolality.
4. Monitor Na^+ and serum osmolality levels frequently. Care must be taken to correct these levels gradually. Rapid correction can precipitate hyperosmolar conditions and seizures.

Hyperkalemia

Of all the potential electrolyte disorders, hyperkalemia is considered the most life-threatening because of potassium's profound impact on the electrophysiology of the heart. Hyperkalemia is also the most common reason for initiation of hemodialysis in the ARF patient.

1. Initiate cardiac monitoring. Since hyperkalemia does affect cardiac tissue, continuous ECG monitoring will assist in recognizing cardiac manifestations of altered K^+ levels.
2. Restrict dietary intake of K^+ to 40 mEq/day. A dietary restriction is considered conservative management and is usually instituted in conjunction with

other therapies aimed at removing K^+ from the body.

3. Administer cation-exchange resins. Kayexalate is used to increase K^+ excretion and is administered by mouth or enema with sorbitol. Sorbitol acts to draw fluid into the bowel where the Kayexalate causes an exchange between Na^+ and K^+ ions. The K^+ is then eliminated from the body through feces.

4. Administer hypertonic (50%) glucose and regular insulin. Insulin acts to drive K^+ into the cells on a temporary basis, thereby protecting the heart from the effect of the elevated serum (extracellular) K^+ level.

5. Administer $NaHCO_3$. The administration of sodium bicarbonate causes movement of K^+ into the cell, encouraging the exchange of hydrogen (H^+) ion inside the cells with the excess K^+ ion outside the cell.

6. Administer calcium salts, such as calcium gluconate. Calcium elevates the stimulation threshold, protecting the patient from the negative myocardial effects of hyperkalemia. The administration of calcium does not change the level of K^+ in the extracellular fluid.

7. Institute RRT. Hemodialysis may be necessary when the patient's K^+ level cannot be controlled by other methods of rapidly removing K^+.

Hypokalemia

1. Administer K^+ supplementation. Depending on the severity of the deficit, oral or IV replacements can be utilized. Ideally, supplementation of K^+ is given through a central IV line due to the irritating nature of K^+ to the tissues. Potassium replacement should be given in at least 50 ml of fluid with no more than 20 mEq replaced per hour. It is not uncommon for patients to be unable to tolerate more than 10 mEq/hour if the supplementation is given peripherally. Some institutions mix lidocaine into their K^+ supplements to decrease discomfort during administration. Since K^+ is primarily an intracellular cation, allow at least 1 hour after administration for the movement of the K^+ into the cells before evaluating the serum K^+ level. A level obtained too quickly after supplementation is completed may reflect an artificially high serum value.

2. Evaluate the patient's diuretic therapy.

Hypercalcemia

1. Administer normal saline IV and diuretics. In the presence of normal renal function, normal saline infusions given with diuretics will increase the GFR and enhance Ca^{++} excretion from the kidneys.

2. Administer corticosteroids. Corticosteroids decrease absorption of Ca^{++} from the GI tract.

3. Administer plicamycin. Plicamycin increases the bone uptake and storage of Ca^{++}.

4. Administer oral phosphate (PO_4^{--}) supplementation. PO_4^{--} binds Ca^{++} so that it will be excreted in stool.

Hypocalcemia

1. Administer Ca^{++} supplementation. Calcium-containing antacids may be used. Often Ca^{++} supplementation is done concurrently with the administration of PO_4^{--} binders, such as aluminum hydroxide. There is a reciprocal relationship between Ca^{++} and PO_4^{--} levels in the body. Calcium may be given orally in the form of antacids or intravenously as calcium gluconate or calcium chloride when symptoms are serious.

2. Administer vitamin D supplementation. Vitamin D is necessary for Ca^{++} to be absorbed from the GI tract.

3. Institute seizure precautions. Patients with hypocalcemia are at risk for developing tetany and seizures.

Hypermagnesemia

1. Institute RRT. See below.

2. Discontinue use of Mg^{++}-containing antacids.

3. Administer normal saline and diuretics. If the patient has normal renal function, the administration of saline and diuretics will increase GFR and enhance excretion of Mg^{++}.

Hypomagnesemia

1. Administer Mg^{++} supplementation. Oral administration or Mg^{++} sulfate IM or IV. IV Mg^{++} should not be given faster than 150 mg/minute. Total daily replacement should not exceed 30 to 40 g.

2. Reduce auditory, pressure, and visual stimuli.

Hyperphosphatemia

1. Administer aluminum hydroxide binding gels. These gels bind with phosphate in the intestine, limiting the absorption, promoting excretion, and decreasing the serum level.

2. Institute RRT. If the patient is symptomatic, hemodialysis is the most effective choice to rapidly decrease the serum levels.

3. Administer acetazolamide. Acetazolamide increases the urinary excretion of phosphate.

Hypophosphatemia

1. Administer phosphate supplementation. Supplementation can be administered by mouth or IV.

2. Discontinue use of phosphate binding gels.

Renal Replacement Therapy

For many years hemodialysis (HD) and peritoneal dialysis (PD) were the only therapies available to manage renal failure and/or fluid overload situations. Many critically ill patients cannot tolerate the rapid fluid and electrolyte shifts associated with traditional hemodialysis because of hemodynamic instability and cardiac arrhythmias. Peritoneal dialysis, an option for patients who cannot tolerate the hemodynamic changes associated with hemodialysis, is limited to patients without recent abdominal incisions, respiratory distress, or bowel perforations.

Several alternative therapies to manage acute fluid and electrolyte problems have been introduced during the past 2 decades, beginning with continuous arteriovenous hemofiltration (CAVH). A number of additional continuous renal replacement therapies (CRRTs) have been introduced, offering more treatment options for the critically ill patient with renal failure and/or fluid overload. Using CRRT, many of the desirable outcomes of HD can be accomplished without the associated hemodynamic instability.

The goal of any type of RRT is the removal of excess fluid and uremic toxins and correction of electrolyte imbalances. Each of the RRT methods are able to accomplish that goal, with varying levels of success. These homeostatic corrections are accomplished through three processes: diffusion, osmosis, and filtration. Diffusion, the process by which substrates move from an area of high concentration to one of a lesser concentration, provides for movement of fluids and electrolytes from the body into the filtrate. Through osmosis, water from an area of lesser solute concentration moves to an area of greater solute concentration, becoming part of the filtrate. Filtration also occurs, allowing for movement of water and solute as a result of a difference in hydrostatic pressure.

RRTs are grouped into two general categories: those requiring arteriovenous (AV) access and those requiring venous access only (Table 18–4). RRT is applied for periods of 4 hours or more, with some requiring continuous use. Except for PD, all of the RRT devices require extracorporeal blood flow. This flow is accomplished through the use of two catheters, one arterial and one venous, or through a double-lumen venous catheter. Filtration and dialysis occur as the blood moves through a dialyzer or hemofilter.

Access

Before any type of RRT can be performed, access to the bloodstream or peritoneum is necessary. The type of access is determined by the reason for initiation and method of renal replacement. It can be either temporary or permanent.

Peritoneal Access

Peritoneal catheters are made of silastic tubing, with multiple perforations to allow for fluid exchange, and an attached cuff, soft disk, or balloon to anchor the catheter. When PD needs to be initiated immediately, a rigid stylet, designed for single acute use only, is inserted. Both types of catheters are inserted through small incisions in the abdomen and threaded into the peritoneal space.

Permanent Vascular Access

Originally, external arteriovenous shunts, such as the Scribner shunt, were the access of choice for HD. These shunts are rarely used today. These catheters were surgically placed between the radial artery and an adjacent vein. Many

TABLE 18–4. SUMMARY OF RENAL REPLACEMENT THERAPIES

Type	Indications	Contraindications	Complications
Arterial Venous Access			
Hemodialysis	Life-threatening fluid/electrolyte imbalances Renal failure	Hemodynamic instability Hypovolemia Coagulation disorders	Blood loss
CAVH, CAVU, SCUF	Fluid overload Acute renal failure	Inadequate blood pressure	Filter clotting Worsening uremia
CAVHD	Fluid/electrolyte imbalances Acute renal failure	Inadequate blood pressure	Filter clotting
Venous Access			
CVVH (continuous venovenous hemofiltration) CVVHD (continuous venovenous hemodialysis)	Fluid overload Fluid/electrolyte imbalances Renal failure		
Peritoneal Access			
PD (peritoneal dialysis)	Fluid/electrolyte imbalances Renal failure	Recent abdominal surgery Abdominal adhesions Peritonitis Respiratory distress Pregnancy	Peritonitis

problems were encountered in trying to maintain these shunts, including clotting and infection. Additionally, their life span was relatively short (6 to 12 months).

Permanent access is achieved by placement of either an AV fistula or graft. A fistula is a surgically created anastomosis between an artery, usually the radial, brachial, or femoral, and an adjacent vein. This anastomosis allows arterial blood to flow through the vein, causing venous enlargement and engorgement. Permanent access is necessary for patients requiring chronic dialysis.

Arteriovenous grafts are placed in patients who do not have adequate vessels to create a fistula. A prosthetic graft is implanted subcutaneously and used to anastomose an artery to a vein. A period of maturation, usually 2 to 3 weeks, is necessary before the access can be used. This maturation time allows for the venous side to dilate and the vessel wall to thicken, permitting repeated insertion of dialysis needles.

Temporary Vascular Access

Temporary access to the bloodstream is obtained through cannulation of an artery and/or a large-diameter vein, with a large-bore, double- or single-lumen catheter specifically designed for dialysis. These catheters are inserted and maintained similarly to other arterial and central venous devices, but are used primarily for dialysis treatments. A double-lumen catheter is more commonly used than a single-lumen, single-vessel catheter to maximize the filtration and dialysis capabilities of the renal replacement devices. These catheters can be used for extended periods of time with meticulous attention to sterile technique. One of the longest lasting temporary catheters is a surgically placed central venous catheter with a cuff at the skin exit site. This catheter has greater stability and can be left in place for several months. The location for catheter placement is chosen to maximize blood flow and prevent kinking of the catheter with patient movement.

In order to initiate continuous arteriovenous ultrafiltration (CAVU), hemofiltration (CAVH), or hemodialysis (CAVHD), two 14- to 16-gauge catheters are placed, one in an artery and one in a vein. The femoral artery and vein are commonly used. Occasionally, the subclavian vein and the axillary artery are used. In some centers, Scribner shunts are placed as access. If present, internal AV fistulas or AV shunts can be utilized. When either continuous venovenous hemofiltration (CVVH) or hemodialysis (CVVHD) is instituted, a 14- to 16-gauge, double-lumen catheter is placed in the subclavian or femoral vein.

Dialyzer/Hemofilters/Dialysate

There are a variety of dialyzers and hemofilters available for use. The type of dialyzer or hemofilter chosen is determined by the patient's condition and desired outcomes of the RRT. All dialyzers have a blood and dialysate compartment, separated by a semipermeable membrane. The dialyzer has two inlet ports and two outlet ports, one each for blood and dialysate. During use for dialysis, blood and dialysate are pumped through the dialyzer in opposite directions.

Hemofilters are made of highly permeable hollow fibers or plates. These fibers or plates are surrounded by an ultrafiltrate space and have arterial and venous blood ports. Plasma water and certain solutes are separated from the blood by the hemofilter and drain into a collection device.

Dialysate solution, used in any therapy that has dialysis as a component, is specifically designed to create concentration gradients so that optimal removal of wastes, acid-base and electrolyte balance, and maintenance of extracellular fluid balance can be achieved. The specific solution is determined by the patient's condition and desired outcomes. While standard solutions may initially be used, they can be tailored to meet the individual patient's needs and will contain varying concentrations of Na^+, K^+, Mg^+, Ca^{++}, Cl^-, glucose, and buffers.

Procedures

Hemodialysis

Initiation of HD through a temporary access is accomplished utilizing a procedure called coupling. During coupling, the dialysis catheter and the dialysis circuitry are connected, utilizing sterile technique. To initiate dialysis through a permanent access, two 14- or 16-gauge needles are inserted into the dilated vein of the fistula or the graft portion of the synthetic graft. One needle is considered arterial, used for blood outflow, and the other is considered venous, used for blood return.

The basic components of a hemodialysis system are shown in Figure 18–1. Blood, leaving the patient through the arterial needle, is pumped through the circuitry and returned to the patient through the venous needle. A blood pump moves the blood through the dialysis circuitry and dialyzer, allowing for different flow rates. Both arterial and venous pressures are monitored in the circuitry.

Peritoneal Dialysis

PD is accomplished through a series of cycles or exchanges. The dialysate, administered into the peritoneal cavity, remains in the cavity for a preset amount of time (dwell time) and then is drained. Each set of these activities is called a cycle or exchange. Dialysate flows into the peritoneal cavity by gravity, taking approximately 10 minutes for 2 L of fluid to infuse. During the dwell time, diffusion, osmosis, and ultrafiltration occur. Typically, dwell times range from 10 to 30 minutes. With an optimally functioning catheter, it takes 2 L of fluid 10 minutes to drain from the abdomen.

CRRT

In CRRT, the blood lines are primed with a saline and heparin solution and then attached to the appropriate vascu-

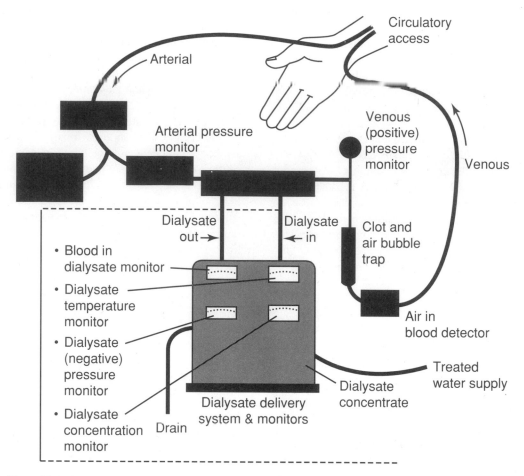

Figure 18–1. Components of a hemodialysis system. *(From: Thompson JM, McFarland GK, Hirsch JE, et al. (eds.): Mosby's manual of clinical nursing. St. Louis, MO: CV Mosby, 1989, p. 592.)*

lar access catheter (venous or arterial). Blood flow begins at the arterial side and passes through the hemofilter. The blood returns to the body via the venous tubing after fluid and electrolytes are moved into the ultrafiltrate. The ultrafiltrate is collected in a bag after removal. The process for CVVH and CVVHD is similar except the venous catheter serves as the "arterial" catheter. This requires the use of a pump within the circuit to augment blood flow through the filter and back to the patient.

In CAVHD and CVVHD, blood leaves the patient through the arterial catheter and flows or is pumped through a dialyzer rather than a hemofilter. Wastes and fluid are removed and drain into an ultrafiltrate bag. The blood is then returned to the body through the venous catheter. The dialysate flows through the dialyzer countercurrent to blood flow, pumped slowly with an IV pump by gravity drainage.

Indications and Efficacy of RRT Modes

Each type of RRT is indicated for different clinical situations and achieves different goals. The goals of therapy should be clearly delineated before selection of the type of therapy.

Hemodialysis

HD is implemented when aggressive therapy is indicated in acute situations. HD is contraindicated in patients with hemodynamic instability, hypovolemia, coagulation disorders, or vascular access problems.

HD is the most effective of all of the RRTs. Fluid and uremic wastes can be eliminated from the body during a 4- to 6-hour treatment. Approximately 200 ml of blood is utilized in the circuit, which can add to a patient's unstable condition. HD is the gold standard for the treatment of acute and chronic renal failure.

Peritoneal Dialysis

Most often, PD is indicated for critically ill patients who need dialysis but are unable to tolerate the hemodynamic changes associated with HD. PD may also be performed in a critical care unit for a patient who is on chronic PD and presently hospitalized with an acute illness.

PD is contraindicated in patients who have had recent or extensive abdominal surgery; who have abdominal adhesions, peritonitis, or respiratory distress; or who are pregnant.

Utilizing the peritoneal membrane as the dialyzer, effective elimination of fluid and waste products can be achieved. PD is slower and less effective than HD.

Continuous RRT

Patients appropriate for CRRT are chosen after evaluating their clinical diagnosis, hemodynamic parameters, and metabolic status. The specific type of CRRT is selected after considering the patient's fluid and electrolyte status, metabolic needs, and severity of uremia. The most commonly used forms of CRRT are CAVU, CAVH, and CAVHD, with CVVH and CVVHD, newer therapies, being used with increasing frequency.

CONTINUOUS ARTERIOVENOUS ULTRAFILTRATION

When slow continuous ultrafiltration is desired, CAVU or slow continuous ultrafiltration (SCUF) will be the therapies of choice. These therapies are primarily for use in patients with a fluid volume excess and some degree of renal function. Because fluid removal is the primary goal, these procedures are performed without simultaneous fluid replacement. There is a minimal impact on the urea and creatinine levels.

CONTINUOUS ARTERIOVENOUS HEMOFILTRATION

The main objective of CAVH is fluid removal (Figure 18–2). While large changes in blood chemistries are not expected, it is possible for a patient to achieve and maintain a stable volume and composition of electrolytes in his or her extracellular fluid. Since large volumes of fluid can be removed, the health care team has more flexibility in treating patients. Nutrition, a problem in many critically ill patients, can often be enhanced in these patients as total parenteral nutrition can be used without fear of fluid overload.

CAVH, in some institutions, has become the treatment of choice when patients have contraindications to HD or PD. Fluid shifts in CAVH are less rapid than with hemodialysis, making use in hemodynamic instability possible. Other patients that may benefit from CAVH are patients with uncontrolled congestive heart failure, pulmonary edema, or hepatorenal syndrome. Patients can be maintained on CAVH for several weeks until either long-term HD can be initiated or there is return of renal function. There are no absolute contraindications for CAVH.

CONTINUOUS ARTERIOVENOUS HEMODIALYSIS

CAVHD combines the principles of hemofiltration with a slow form of dialysis (Figure 18–3). More aggressive removal of fluid and solute is possible than with CAVH. Dialysate is infused through a dialyzer, countercurrent to the patient's blood flow.

The indications for CAVHD are similar to those for HD. Selection of CAVHD is generally made because a patient is unstable and not able to tolerate the rapid fluid and electrolyte shifts that occur with HD. CAVHD provides an avenue for these hemodynamically unstable patients to

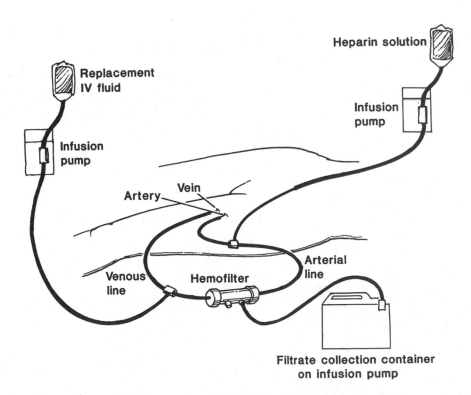

Figure 18–2. Components of a CAVH System. *(From Wright J, Shelton B:* Desk reference for critical care nursing. *Boston, MA: Jones and Bartlett, 1993, p. 803.)*

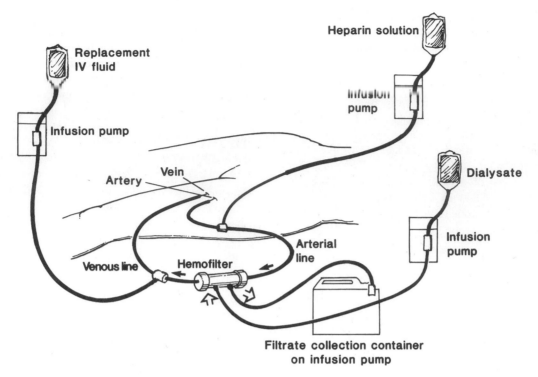

Figure 18–3. Components of a Continuous Arteriovenous Hemodialysis (CAVHD) System. *(From Wright J, Shelton B: Desk reference for critical care nursing. Boston, MA: Jones and Bartlett, 1993, p. 804.)*

achieve a stable fluid and electrolyte balance without further compromise of their status.

There are no absolute contraindications for CAVHD. Patients with a systolic BP less than 80 mm Hg will often not be good candidates since the AV pressure difference is crucial to maintaining adequate blood flow. Maintaining patency of the dialyzer is also key to successful CAVHD. Patients with coagulopathies will need special monitoring.

CONTINUOUS VENOVENOUS HEMOFILTRATION

CVVH is one of the newest forms of CRRT. While similar to CAVH, CVVH is pump-assisted instead of using the arterial blood pressure to circulate blood through the filter. The major advantage being suggested of CVVH to CAVH is a decrease in access-related complications.

CONTINUOUS VENOVENOUS HEMODIALYSIS

CVVHD, similar to CAVHD, is also a pump-assisted rather than a blood-pressure-assisted technique (Figure 18–4). It

requires only a venous access and so provides therapy for patients with only venous access who cannot tolerate traditional HD.

General RRT Interventions

The frequency of RRT as a therapy in critical care units is on the rise. Some practitioners feel CRRT will replace HD as the therapy of choice for ARF in the critically ill patient.

Although each therapy has unique characteristics, all require similar interventions. Careful observations and interventions are essential, as is accurate fluid management. Close monitoring of mean arterial pressure (MAP), urine output, cardiac output, central venous pressure, pulmonary capillary wedge pressure, daily weights, and state of anti-coagulation are critical. Careful monitoring of acid-base and serum chemistries is mandatory. The critical care nurse assumes a primary responsibility for early recognition and initial interventions for patient and system problems.

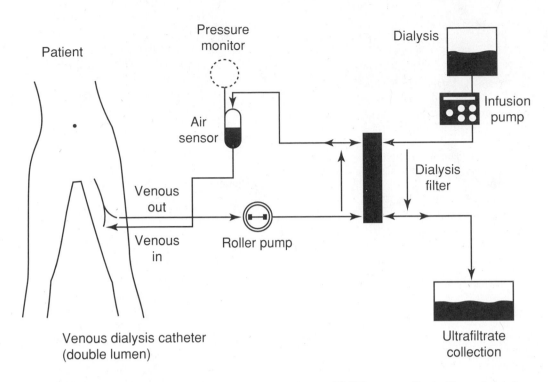

Figure 18–4. Components of a continuous venovenous hemodialysis (CVVHD) system. *(Used with permission from: Strohschein BL, Caruso DM, Greene KA: Continuous venovenous hemodialysis.* American Journal of Critical Care. *1994;3:95.)*

AT THE BEDSIDE
■ *Thinking Critically*

R.J., a 60-year-old gentleman, was admitted through the ED following the onset of severe abdominal and back pain. On arrival to the ED, BP was 80/60, and pulse was 120 and regular. He was slightly dyspneic. His abdomen was large and rigid, and bowel tones were absent. Within an hour, he received 1200 ml of albumin and 1500 ml of NS. When his BP did not respond to the fluid challenge, he was placed on a dopamine drip at 5 μg/kg/minute. A Foley catheter was placed with only 35 ml of urine output. After a CAT scan, he was taken to the OR for repair of a ruptured aortic aneurysm. Estimated blood loss was 12,000 ml, with replacement of 11,000 ml of whole blood, 600 ml of fresh frozen plasma, and 1250 ml of albumin. He was admitted to the critical care unit following surgery with no urine output.

- What therapies would you consider for R.J. at this time?
- Would initiation of a diuretic be appropriate?

R.J.'s BP continued to be low (80/60). A pulmonary artery catheter was placed to assist in evaluation of his fluid status. Pulmonary artery pressures were 20/7 mm Hg, with a PAWP of 8 mm Hg.

- What type of fluid therapy should R.J. be given?

While his BP was gradually increased using fluids and dopamine, R.J. continued to have a rocky course. By his third postoperative day, he still had a low urine output. His creatinine had climbed quickly to 7.5 mg/dl and BUN to 90 mg/dl. His potassium was 5.8 mEq/L. Hemodialysis was instituted.

- What special considerations should be made for R.J.'s medication therapy while he is being treated with dialysis?
- What should the team consider to meet R.J.'s increased caloric demands?

After 2 weeks on dialysis, R.J.'s urine output began to gradually increase. His wound bleeding stopped, and he became hemodynamically more stable. He had been started on TPN, which was stopped as soon as he started eating an adequate diet. Seven weeks after the rupture, R.J. was ready for discharge. His urine output was averaging 1200 ml/day; BUN and creatinine were 28 and 1.9 mg/dl, respectively.

SELECTED BIBLIOGRAPHY

General Renal

Baer CL: Fluid and electrolyte balance. In Kinney M, Packa D, Dunbar S (eds.): AACN's clinical reference for critical care Nursing, 3rd ed. St. Louis, MO: CV Mosby, 1993, pp. 173–208.

Baer CL, Lancaster LE: Acute renal failure. *Critical Care Nursing Quarterly.* 1992;14(4):1–21.

Brezis M, Rosen S, Epstein FH: Acute renal failure. In Brenner J, Rector W (eds.): *The kidney.* 4th ed. Philadelphia: WB Saunders, 1991, pp. 993–1061.

Carlson KK: Acute renal failure. In Urban N, Greenlee K, Krumberger J, Winkleman C (eds.): *Guidelines for critical care nursing.* St. Louis, MO: CV Mosby, 1995.

Stark JL: The renal system. In Alspach G (ed): *Core curriculum for critical care nursing,* 4th ed. Philadelphia: WB Saunders, 1991, pp. 472–608.

Nutrition in the Acute Renal Failure Patient

Wolfson M, Kopple JD: Nutritional management of acute renal failure. In Lazarus L, Brenner J (eds.): *Acute renal failure,* 3rd ed. New York: Churchill Livingston, 1993, pp. 467–485.

Renal Replacement Therapy—General

Boggs RL, Wooldridge M (eds): *AACN procedure manual for critical care.* Philadelphia: WB Saunders, 1993.

Peritoneal Dialysis

Carlson KK: Peritoneal dialysis. In Urban N, Greenlee K, Krumberger J, Winkleman C (eds.): *Guidelines for critical care nursing.* St. Louis, MO: CV Mosby, 1995.

Keen M, Lancaster L, Binkley L: Concepts and principles of hemodialysis. In Lancaster L (ed.): *Core curriculum for nephrology nursing.* Pitman, NJ: American Nephrology Nurse's Association, 1990.

Prowant B, Gallagher NM: Concepts and principles of peritoneal dialysis. In Lancaster L (ed.): *Core curriculum for nephrology nursing.* American Nephrology Nurse's Association, 1990.

Hemodialysis

Carlson KK: Hemodialysis. In Urban N, Greenlee K, Krumberger J, Winkleman C (eds.): *Guidelines for critical care nursing.* St. Louis, MO: CV Mosby, 1995.

Ismail N, Hakim R: Hemodialysis. In Levine DZ (ed.): *Care of the renal patient,* 2nd ed. Philadelphia: WB Saunders, 1991, pp. 220–246.

Thompson JM, McFarland GK, Hirsch JE, et al. (eds.). *Mosby's manual of clinical nursing.* St. Louis, MO: CV Mosby, 1989.

Continuous Renal Replacement Therapies

Bellomo R, Parkin G, Love J, et al.: A prospective comparative study of continuous arteriovenous hemodiafiltration and continuous venovenous hemodiafiltration in critically ill patients. *American Journal of Kidney Diseases.* 1993;21(4):400–404.

Bosworth C: SCUF/CAVH/CAVHD: Critical differences. *Critical Care Nursing Quarterly.* 1992;14(4):45–55.

Carlson KK: Continuous renal replacement therapies. In Urban N, Greenlee K, Krumberger J, Winkleman C (eds.): *Guidelines for critical care nursing.* St. Louis, MO: CV Mosby, 1995.

Lawyer LA, Velasco A: Continuous arteriovenous hemodialysis in the ICU. *Critical Care Nursing.* 1989;9(1):29–41.

Macias WL, Mueller BA, Scarim SK, et al.: Continuous venovenous hemofiltration: An alternative to continuous arteriovenous hemofiltration and hemodiafiltration. *American Journal of Kidney Diseases.* 1991;18(4):451–458.

Nahman NS, Middendorf DF: Continuous arteriovenous hemofiltration. *Medical Clinics of North America.* 1990; 74(4):975–984.

Price CA: Continuous renal replacement therapy: The treatment of choice for acute renal failure. *American Nephrology Nurse's Association Journal.* 1991;18(3):239–244.

Price CA: An update on continuous renal replacement therapies. *AACN Clinical Issues in Critical Care Nursing.* 1992; 3(3):597–604.

Price CA: Continuous renal replacement therapies. In Burrows-Hudson S (ed.): *Standards of clinical practice for nephrology nursing.* Pitman, NJ: American Nephrology Nurse's Association, 1993.

Strohschein BL, Caruso DM, Greene KA: Continuous venovenous hemodialysis. *American Journal of Critical Care.* 1994; 3:92–101.

Endocrine System

■ What Heals: Bio-psycho-social-spiritual Unity

Nurses and physicians have long observed that periods of psychologic stress often precede the onset or exacerbation of endocrine diseases. It also is well known that many endocrine diseases can cause significant psychologic symptoms. Agitation, anxiety, paranoia, and depression can be observed during the course of illness.

The question then is, "Is the emotional instability associated with the endocrine problem a cause or an effect?" Does emotional stress worsen the illness or does the illness state itself result in the psychologic disturbances? This discussion about cause or effect is fueled by popular assumptions about disease:

• A disease is primarily either functional or organic in origin (i.e., either the mind or the body is at fault).
• A disease is a process that affects primarily either the mind or the body.

• Therapy, therefore, should be directed toward the mind (psychotherapeutic interventions) or toward the body (medical or surgical interventions), depending on whether the mind or body is primarily at fault in the particular disease.

These assumptions are so ingrained in our thinking that they often escape our attention. They operate unconsciously, but they determine in major ways our attitudes towards patients and illness. As critical care nurses, we must question and see beyond the traditional either/or assumptions of disease. Disease is not a state of malfunction of either the mind or the body. It affects and is affected by both. It is this unity that operates in every person in every disease process that we must strive to uncover.

CEG & BMD

SPECIAL ASSESSMENT TECHNIQUES, DIAGNOSTIC TESTS, AND MONITORING SYSTEMS

Blood Glucose Monitoring (BGM)

Frequent assessments of blood glucose levels in the critically ill patient commonly are performed at the bedside by placing a drop of blood on a chemical reagent strip and observing color changes to estimate glucose levels by simple visual observation or with a glucometer (Figure 19–1). Bedside glucose monitoring allows more rapid treatments of glucose abnormalities than laboratory analysis.

Large discrepancies between laboratory serum blood glucose and capillary BGM results should be investigated. Most authors recommend that BGM readings be within a 20% to 30% variance of the laboratory values to be acceptable. Clinical signs and symptoms of the patient always need to be considered when interpreting results.

Equipment-Related Discrepancies

Capillary BGM instruments require a drop of whole blood. Before using serum blood on the reagent strip, it is important to check the manufacturer's instructions to determine if the test result displayed is for whole blood glucose or if the test result has been corrected by the meter to a serum glucose value. Serum glucose values are generally 10% to 15% greater than the whole blood value, and this needs to be taken into consideration when interpreting glucose levels. There also may be variations between the laboratory and BGM results depending on the source of blood (capillary, venous, or arterial). Obtaining a simultaneous laboratory sample and bedside BGM reading periodically will identify discrepancies and allow for more accurate interpre-

TABLE 19–1. CLINICAL SITUATIONS THAT MAY AFFECT THE ACCURACY OF BEDSIDE BLOOD GLUCOSE MONITORING

Blood glucose levels > 500 mg/dl
Hct < 30% or > 55%
Inadequate tissue perfusion
   Hypovolemia
High blood levels of acetaminophen
Use of vasoactive drugs
Patients requiring control of hypoglycemic or hyperglycemic states
Neonates

tation of the bedside BGM reading. In general, a capillary BGM result of greater than 500 mg/dl should always be checked with a laboratory specimen, as BGM meters are not considered reliable for serum glucose levels above 500 mg/dl.

Patient-Related Discrepancies

Several clinical conditions may also influence bedside BGM measurements (Table 19–1). The presence of hypovolemia or abnormal hematocrit values (<30% or >55%) fall outside the BGM instrument's hematocrit range and may cause inaccurate results. Higher than normal hematocrit levels result in underestimation of the blood glucose. Lower than normal hematocrit levels will result in overestimating blood glucose. In addition, conditions which lead to inadequate tissue perfusion in the fingers, such as hypotensive shock or edema, make unreliable any capillary BGM done by fingerstick (underestimation of the blood glucose). Finally, patients receiving large doses of acetaminophen may cause a chemical reaction on some BGM strips which

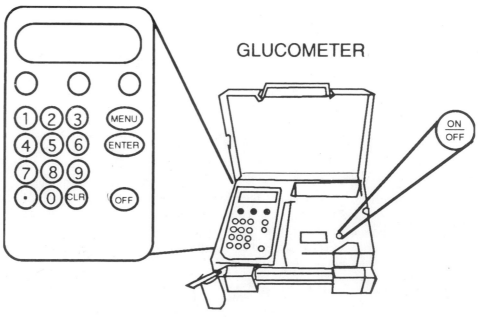

Figure 19–1. Reagent strip and glucometer for bedside testing of blood glucose levels.

GLUCOMETER

REAGENT STRIPS

TABLE 19–2. TIPS FOR BGM USE

- Review the manufacturer's guidelines for specific procedures related to the use of your BGM device. User error is the most common reason for inaccurate readings.
- Ensure that the BGM device is calibrated and clean before using.
- Do not use alcohol to clean the machine.
- For patients with cold hands, let the hand hang down below the level of the heart so that blood can flow to the fingertips.
- Obtain a large drop of blood and let it drop down onto the reagent pad. Distribute evenly over the entire pad, but do not smear the blood.
- Use the side of the finger rather than the underside as it has fewer nerve endings (therefore is less painful) and more capillaries (will get larger drop of blood).
- Correlate the BGM device reading with the clinical assessment of the patient.
- Use universal precautions during the entire procedure.

also may introduce error into the result. Tips for BGM are reviewed in Table 19–2.

Patient Teaching

The specific procedure for BGM needs to be taught to the patient. The goal of treatment is to maintain a fasting glucose less than 140 mg/dl. Higher serum glucose target values for older patients may be more appropriate as they are more vulnerable to hypoglycemia. Patients on insulin should be encouraged to test their glucose before each meal and at bedtime to evaluate the effectiveness of their insulin dose. If this is not feasible, patients should be encouraged to test at least two times a day at alternating times so they can track glucose patterns at all four times of day. For non-insulin-dependent diabetics, BGM is recommended before breakfast and 2 hours before, during, and after exercise and whenever they experience signs and symptoms of hyperglycemia. They should also check more frequently during any illness or major changes in eating patterns. Patients should also be instructed to test their meter control at least once per week.

PATHOLOGIC CONDITIONS

Hyperglycemic Emergencies

Two most common endocrine crises which require critical care admission are: diabetic ketoacidosis (DKA) and hyperosmolar hyperglycemic nonketotic coma (HHNC). Diabetic ketoacidosis is defined as acute hyperglycemia with acidosis, and HHNC is classified as acute hyperglycemia without acidosis.

The common feature of these hyperglycemic emergencies is diabetes mellitus (DM). Diabetes mellitus is a metabolic disease that is caused by ineffective uptake of glucose by cells. There are several types of diabetes, the two most common being insulin-dependent DM (Type I, IDDM) and

AT THE BEDSIDE
▶ *Diabetic Ketoacidosis*

Mary K., 18 years old, was admitted to the MICU with a diagnosis of diabetic ketoacidosis. She was diagnosed with insulin-dependent diabetes mellitus (IDDM) 9 months earlier. Mary's roommate reported that she had consumed approximately six or seven beers at a school party when she "passed out" and was difficult to arouse. Her friend also reported that Mary had been complaining of flulike symptoms (vomiting, diarrhea) for 2 or 3 days prior to admission. On arrival in the ER, Mary was alert, but confused. Significant findings on her admission profile were:

Respiratory rate:	38/minute, deep ("fruity" breath)
Blood pressure:	98/50 mm Hg;
Heart rate:	110 beats/minute; sinus tachycardia
Skin:	Warm and flushed
Arterial blood gases:	pH 7.08
	$Paco_2$ 24 mm Hg
	Pao_2 60 mm Hg
	HCO_3^- 12 mEq/L
	Sao_2 91%
Serum glucose:	440 mg/dl
Serum ketones:	3+
Serum osmolality:	310 mOsm/kg
Anion gap:	22 mEq/L
Serum potassium:	5.8 mEq/L
Serum blood urea nitrogen:	28 mg/dl
Serum creatinine:	1.5 mg/dl
Serum sodium:	128 mEq/L
Serum magnesium:	1.1 mg/dl
Serum phosphate:	2.2 mg/dl
Serum chloride:	94 mEq/L
White blood cell count:	14,000 / mm^3
Urine glucose:	Positive
Urine ketone:	Positive

non-insulin-dependent DM (Type II, NIDDM). Type I IDDM usually has a juvenile or early adult onset and is characterized by little or no insulin being produced by pancreatic beta cells. Type II DM usually occurs in older adults and is associated with below normal, normal, or above normal insulin production. Although hyperglycemia is the common feature, the etiology, risk factors, pathophysiology, and management priorities vary considerably for each of these disorders.

Etiology, Risk Factors, and Pathophysiology

Insulin is normally released from the pancreas by beta cells of the islets of Langerhans in response to increases in blood

AT THE BEDSIDE

▶ *Hyperosmolar Hyperglycemic Nonketotic Coma*

Mr. H., 72 years old, was admitted to the MICU with a diagnosis of hyperglycemic crisis. Mr. H. lives with his small dog. His daughter dialed 911 after finding her father nonarousable at his home. She reported that he had complained of flulike symptoms 3 weeks earlier. Mr. H.'s history is significant for congestive heart failure and adult onset Type II IDDM. His daily medications included: Digoxin 0.25 mg po qd, Lasix 10 mg po bid, KCl 20 mEq po qd, and glyburide 10 mg po bid. On arrival in the ER Mr. H. was comatose. Significant findings on his admission profile were:

Blood pressure:	82/44 mm Hg; MAP 56 mm Hg
Heart rate:	121 beats/minute
Respiratory rate:	14/minute, shallow
Skin:	Dry, poor turgor; dry mucous membranes
Arterial blood gases on 2L/minute O_2 per nasal cannula:	pH 7.35 $PaCO_2$ 49 mm Hg PaO_2 56 mm Hg HCO_3^- 22 mEq/L SaO_2 88%
Serum glucose:	1100 mg/dl
Serum osmolality:	362 mOsm/kg
Serum potassium:	2.8 mEq/L
Serum blood urea nitrogen:	41 mg/dl
Serum creatinine:	2.2 mg/dl
Serum sodium:	152 mEq/L
Serum phosphate:	2.0 mg/dl
Serum chloride:	121 mEq/L

glucose. Insulin is necessary for cellular uptake of glucose by most cells in the body (except brain and liver cells). Without insulin, the glucose fails to enter cells and accumulates in the blood, resulting in hyperglycemia. Cells without glucose begin to starve and begin to use existing stores of fat and protein to provide energy for body processes (gluconeogenesis). This triggers a complex series of physiological processes which account for the major signs and symptoms associated with DKA and HHNC.

Diabetes Ketoacidosis

The most common causes of DKA include previously undiagnosed IDDM, infections, and omission of insulin (Table 19–3). The initiating event in DKA is an insufficient or absent level of circulating insulin. This insulin deficiency results in increased fatty acid metabolism, increased liver gluconeogenesis (formation of glucose from amino acids

and proteins), and increased secretion of counterregulatory hormones, including glucagon and the stress hormones (catecholamines, cortisol, and growth hormone). The pathophysiology of DKA can be organized into two main components: fluid volume deficit and acid-base imbalance (Figure 19–2).

Fluid Volume Deficit

Because of the insulin deficiency, there is both hyperglycemia and increased amino acid release from cells. The stress response in the body leads to metabolic decompensation, and stress hormones further trigger a rise in plasma glucose and ketones. The hyperglycemia causes an osmotic diuresis, leading to fluid volume deficits (intracellular and extracellular) and electrolyte losses. As serum glucose exceeds the renal threshold, glycosuria results. In the absence of insulin, protein stores are also broken down by the liver into amino acids and then into glucose for energy. This further increases serum blood glucose, increases urine glucose, and worsens the osmotic diuresis and ketonemia. Urinary losses of water, sodium, magnesium, calcium, and phosphorous cause an increase in serum osmolality and decreased electrolyte levels. Potassium levels may be increased or decreased depending on the amount of nausea and vomiting, the acid-base balance, and the fluid status of the patient. This hyperosmolality causes additional fluid shifts from the intracellular to the extracellular space, increasing dehydration. Hypovolemic shock can result from severe fluid losses in DKA (see Chapter 12, Cardiovascular System). Volume depletion decreases glomerular filtration

TABLE 19–3. CAUSES OF DIABETIC KETOACIDOSIS (DKA)

Initial presentation of previously undiagnosed patients with DM

Type I IDDM who omits insulin dose, decreases dose, does not adhere to diet, or experiences severe stress or increased exercise without adequate insulin adjustment

Type II NIDDM with severe medical problems or stress

Stressors
  Infections
  Trauma
  Surgery
  Pregnancy
  Acute illness
  Renal failure
  Myocardial ischemia

Impairment of glucose metabolism by drugs
  Thiazide diuretics
  Phenytoin
  Beta blockers
  Calcium channel blockers
  Steroids
  Epinephrine
  Analgesics
  Psychotropics

Intoxication
  Alcohol
  Salicylate

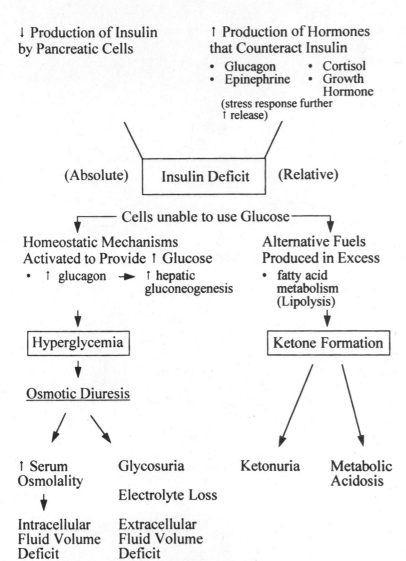

↓ Production of Insulin
by Pancreatic Cells

↑ Production of Hormones
that Counteract Insulin
- Glucagon   • Cortisol
- Epinephrine   • Growth
          Hormone
(stress response further
↑ release)

(Absolute)   Insulin Deficit   (Relative)

Cells unable to use Glucose

Homeostatic Mechanisms
Activated to Provide ↑ Glucose
- ↑ glucagon → ↑ hepatic
          gluconeogenesis

Alternative Fuels
Produced in Excess
- fatty acid
  metabolism
  (Lipolysis)

Hyperglycemia

Ketone Formation

Osmotic Diuresis

↑ Serum
Osmolality

Glycosuria

Electrolyte Loss

Ketonuria

Metabolic
Acidosis

Intracellular
Fluid Volume
Deficit

Extracellular
Fluid Volume
Deficit

Figure 19–2. Pathogenesis of diabetic ketoacidosis.

of glucose and creates a cycle of progressive hyperglycemia. The increase in serum osmolarity also is thought to further impair insulin secretion and promote insulin resistance. The altered neurological status frequently seen in these patients is due primarily to cellular dehydration and serum hyperosmolarity.

Acid-Base Imbalance

Cells without glucose will starve and begin to use existing stores of fat and protein to provide energy for body processes (gluconeogenesis). Fats are broken down faster than they can be metabolized in the liver, which will result in an accumulation of ketone acids. Ketone acids accumulate in the blood stream where hydrogen ions (H^+) will dissociate, causing a metabolic acidosis. Acetone also is formed during this process and is responsible for the "fruity breath" found in these patients.

This acidosis may be worsened with severe fluid volume deficits because hypovolemia results in hypoperfusion

and production of lactic acids from anaerobic metabolism. Excess lactic acid results in what is called increased anion gap (increased body acids). Sodium, potassium, chloride, and bicarbonate are responsible for maintaining a normal anion gap in the body which is normally less than 12 to 14 mEq/L (Table 19–4). Ketone accumulation, a byproduct of gluconeogenesis, will cause an increase in the anion gap above 14 mEq/L.

The normal physiologic response to metabolic acidosis is to produce bicarbonate to buffer the ketones and H^+ ions. The patient with DKA often has diminished bicarbonate

TABLE 19–4. CALCULATION OF ANION GAP (NORMAL <12 MEQ/L)

$Na^+ - (Cl^- + HCO_3^-)$ = anion gap
Example from DKA case study:
    128 − (94 + 12) = 22 mEq/L (anion gap acidosis)
Example from HHNK case study:
    152 − (121 + 22) = 10 mEq/L (no anion gap)

levels because of the osmotic diuresis. The respiratory system will attempt to compensate by eliminating acids by blowing off carbon dioxide to restore normal blood pH. This explains the deep rapid breathing, called Kussmaul's respirations, seen in these patients.

Metabolic acidosis also results in potentially life-threatening electrolyte imbalances. Serum potassium is elevated initially in DKA probably due to potassium shifts from the intracellular to the extracellular space because of the acidosis. Later, hypokalemia is common due to increased urinary excretion of potassium with the osmotic diuresis.

Hyperosmolar Hyperglycemic Nonketotic Coma

There is no clear-cut differentiation between DKA and HHNC. It is classified as hyperglycemia without ketosis. The onset of hyperglycemia in HHNC is progressive because many patients have a history of Type II IDDM with some circulating insulin levels. The extremely severe hyperglycemia in HHNC results in profound extracellular fluid volume contraction, marked intracellular dehydration, and excessive loss of electrolytes. In addition, because there is some insulin, lipolysis is suppressed; therefore, there is no production of ketones and no specific physical signs and symptoms of ketosis (i.e. no Kussmaul's respiration, renal excretion of ketones, abdominal pain, nausea, vomiting, or anorexia). Because of the lack of these signs and symptoms, many of these patients do not seek early treatment. Sustained osmotic diuresis results, leading to massive volume losses, electrolyte imbalance, and central nervous system (CNS) dysfunction. Mortality rates, therefore, are higher with HHNC, both because of the severe volume loss and because it occurs more frequently in a more elderly population. Death results from CNS depression of vital body functions (cardiac and respiratory centers in the brain are depressed), cerebral edema, cardiovascular collapse, renal shutdown, and vascular embolism.

Clinical Presentation

History	DKA	HHNC
	Younger with history of Type I IDDM or previously undiagnosed; Preexisting infection common	Elderly with history of Type II IDDM, and preexisting chronic illnesses which are associated with decreased renal glucose excretion, concurrent illness frequently precipitates viral infections or pneumonia

Signs and Symptoms	Nonspecific: polyuria, polydipsia, weakness; Specific: nausea, vomiting, anorexia, Kussmaul's respiration, fruity breath	Nonspecific: polyuria, polydipsia, weakness; Specific: none

Diagnostic Tests

	DKA	HHNC
Serum glucose	250 to 800 mg/dl	At least 600 mg/dl, often greater than 1000 mg/dl
Serum osmolality	Less than 330 mOsm/kg/H_2O	Greater than 350 mOsm/kg/H_2O
Ketoacidosis	Marked pH < 7.30 HCO_3^- less than 15 mEq/L Serum ketones above 2+ Positive urine ketones Kussmaul's respirations Acetone breath Positive anion gap	Not a feature pH greater than 7.30 HCO_3^- greater than 15 mEq/L Serum ketones below 2+ Minimal urine ketones
Dehydration	Volume depletion (intracellular and extracellular)	Severe volume depletion (intracellular and extracellular)
Renal function	Increased BUN: creatinine ratio	Marked increased BUN: creatinine ratio
Neurological impairment	Common	Common due to serum osmolality
Electrolyte depletion	Potassium Magnesium Phosphate	Potassium Magnesium Phosphate Sodium

AT THE BEDSIDE

Mary K.: "I didn't want to admit that I had a problem. I thought it would just go away. I mean, I'm too young to have something like this. I just started college. I just wanted to be like everyone else. I feel like I have lost control over my body. I don't ever want this to happen again."

Patient Needs and Principles of Management

The management of the patient in acute DKA and HHNC revolves around six primary areas: fluid replacement, treatment of hyperglycemia, electrolyte replacement, treatment of any underlying disorders, prevention and management of complications, and patient/family teaching.

▶ Fluid Replacement

Treatment of intracellular and extracellular fluid volume deficits is a priority for both DKA and HHNC to restore intravascular volume and prevent cardiovascular collapse.

1. Administer normal saline (0.9%) or one-half normal saline (0.45%). The choice of intravenous (IV) fluid depends on the initial blood pressure readings and the serum sodium level. The presence of hyperglycemia and dehydration masks the true serum sodium level, requiring a correction of serum sodium levels prior to IV fluid selection (Table 19–5). IV fluids are generally infused at rapid rates (1000 to 2000 ml in the first hour, 1000 ml in the second hour, and then at 500 ml/hour) until fluid volume is restored.

2. Titrate the rate of infusion based on urine output, mean arterial blood pressure, and central venous pressure measurements. Typically, the patient with HHNC has more profound fluid volume deficits, but because the patient is older and often has other underlying medical problems, the rate of fluid replacement needs to be carefully titrated. Serum glucose will fall with initiation of fluids alone. It is critical that insulin therapy not be started without simultaneously correcting the fluid deficit. Otherwise, the result is an acute loss of vascular volume, worsening of the hypernatremia, shock, and increased risk of mortality.

▶ Treatment of Hyperglycemia

In both DKA and HHNC some insulin replacement will be needed, although the requirements in HHNC are typically low.

1. Initiate low-dose IV insulin at a rate of 0.1 to 0.2 units/kg/hour via constant infusion to achieve a smooth and steady decrease in serum glucose levels. Low-dose insulin is recommended even with severe hyperglycemia to minimize the risks of hypo-

glycemia and hypokalemia. The goal is to decrease the serum glucose 50 to 100 mg/dl per hour. If this does not occur, the rate of insulin administration can then be increased. Some patients may require as much as 50 units/hour to achieve this goal.

2. Monitor serum glucose levels closely and titrate insulin infusion accordingly. Once the serum glucose reaches 250 mg/dl, the insulin infusion should be decreased to a rate of 2 to 4 units/hour and the IV fluids changed to half normal saline with glucose (D5-$\frac{1}{2}$NS). This will ensure that hypoglycemia does not occur during ongoing treatment of the acute condition. It is essential that insulin therapy continues in the patient with DKA until the serum pH is corrected in order to avoid intracellular hypokalemia. Additional glucose may be needed to keep the insulin drip infusing to achieve this outcome. Glucose-containing solution should also be started in the patient with HHNC when serum glucose reaches 250 to 300 mg/dl to protect against cerebral edema.

▶ Electrolyte Replacement

Electrolyte deficits are usually present in both DKA and HHNC due to the osmotic diuresis.

1. Administer potassium supplements according to serum levels. Replacement of potassium is a priority during the correction of hyperglycemia to avoid hypokalemia during rehydration, when potassium moves into the cell along with glucose. Potassium chloride replacement should begin when insulin therapy is started, with the rate of infusion adjusted according to frequently monitored serum potassium and the urine output.

2. Monitor magnesium, calcium, and phosphate levels during rehydration. Hemodilution may further decrease serum levels of these electrolytes. Magnesium and calcium replacements will be given based on serum levels. Total body phosphorous levels are depleted due to osmotic diuresis. This may result in impaired cardiac and respiratory functions. The administration of potassium phosphate 20 mEq/L is the best method of phosphate replacement as it replaces both potassium and phosphate simultaneously. Phosphate replacements should not be administered in patients with renal failure. If hypokalemia is refractory to potassium replacement, magnesium replacement should be considered.

3. Administer bicarbonate as indicated. Bicarbonate administration rarely is indicated in the treatment of

TABLE 19–5. CORRECTION OF SERUM SODIUM LEVELS IN THE PRESENCE OF HYPERGLYCEMIA

$$\text{Corrected sodium} = (\text{serum sodium}) + 1.6 \times \left[\frac{\text{glucose (mg/dl)} - 100}{100} \right]$$

Patient Needs and Principles of Management, Cont.

DKA hyperosmolar coma unless the serum pH is less than 6.9 to 7.10. In fact, bicarbonate administration may be harmful as each ampule delivers 44 mEq of sodium, an amount that will acutely raise the serum sodium. This will worsen the patient's hyperosmolar state. Bicarbonate should be given if there are clinical complications of acidosis (ventricular dysrhythmias, decreased myocardial contractility) or to treat acute hyperkalemia with DKA. Bicarbonate, if given, should be given by IV push or added to a hypotonic solution and administered by continuous IV infusion.

▶ Treatment of Underlying Disorders

The precipitating cause for the hyperglycemic emergency needs to be determined. Underlying infection is a common precipitating factor in both DKA and HHNC.

1. Investigate precipitating factors through the following tests: urinalysis, complete blood count, ECG, chest x-ray, and appropriate cultures. Administer antibiotics as appropriate if infection is suspected.
2. Obtain history from patient and family about the possibility of missed insulin doses.

▶ Prevention and Management of Complications

1. Monitor serum glucose, electrolytes (sodium and potassium), and ABGs (DKA only) for 2 hours until normal levels are approached.
2. Measure serum phosphate and magnesium initially and repeat as necessary.
3. Monitor temperature, blood pressure, pulse, respiratory rate, pulse oximetry, urinary output, and central venous pressure at frequent intervals.
4. Evaluate neurological status at frequent intervals. Institute seizure precautions if cerebral edema is suspected. Institute measures to avoid aspiration in patients with altered mental status. Administer dexamethasone and mannitol if appropriate.
5. Titrate fluid replacement carefully to prevent congestive heart failure. Auscultate lung sounds frequently during fluid replacement.
6. Administer anticoagulants as ordered. Hyperosmolar patients are at great risk of thrombosis.

▶ Patient and Family Education

Particularly in Type I IDDM, the key to prevention of recurrent DKA is adequate patient education regarding diabetes management. Teach the skills needed to manage diabetes. Table 19–6 outlines the required skills for diabetic management. Return demonstrations by the patient or designated caregiver are essential. Instruction regarding the need for routine medical follow-up and the availability of hospital and community resources is also an important component of the diabetes management plan.

AT THE BEDSIDE

Primary Nurse: "Mary K. said it all in just a few words. She had been diagnosed with IDDM just about the time she left for college. I would guess the diagnosis of diabetes and the emotional stress of leaving home and getting through her freshman year was pretty overwhelming. It was clear that she did not see herself with a chronic, permanent illness that would affect many areas of her new life. It also was clear that this hospitalization was effective in replacing denial with a desire to learn about her illness. She wanted to know how she could prevent this complication from occurring in the future. We arranged for her to participate in our diabetic management education classes as soon as she was stable. She was eager and ready to learn this time. You know, readiness to learn is a fascinating thing. All we had to do for Mary K. was listen and answer her questions. She did the rest—she was in charge."

TABLE 19–6. SKILLS FOR DIABETIC MANAGEMENT

Blood glucose monitoring

Insulin administration

Diet therapy

Meal planning

Exercise therapy

Urine ketone testing

Sick day management

Recognition of signs and symptoms of hypoglycemia and hyperglycemia

Proper treatments for hypoglycemia and hyperglycemia

Expected Outcomes
1. The patient or caregiver will be able to verbalize essential aspects of diet therapy, meal planning, exercise therapy, sick day management, signs and symptoms of hypoglycemia and hyperglycemia, and proper treatments for hypoglycemia and hyperglycemia.
2. The patient or caregiver will be able to demonstrate blood glucose monitoring, insulin administration, and urine ketone testing.

AT THE BEDSIDE

Primary Nurse: "When Mr. H. woke up he was pretty quiet and withdrawn, but seemed to be comforted by having his daughter in the room. His daughter later told me that she knew of a remedy that would help speed her father's recovery. The remedy was Mr. H.'s dog. It took a little doing to get old Sparky in our unit, but it wasn't too hard because we have had pet visitation in our unit from time to time in the past. Sparky was as glad to see Mr. H. as he was to see him. Sparky visited for several more days until Mr. H. was out of the unit. Mr. H.'s daughter had been correct. It was the right thing to do, and we all knew it the minute we saw Mr. H.'s face. It was a pretty powerful remedy, and I'm convinced that it did help in his recovery. I know that Mr. H. would agree."

Acute Hypoglycemia

Hypoglycemia is defined as a blood glucose level less than 40 to 50 mg/dl and is a common endocrine emergency. Of the acute complications, hypoglycemia is most common in insulin-dependent diabetics, but it also can occur with Type II diabetics who are treated with insulin or oral hypoglycemic agents, such as chlorpropamide (Diabinese).

Etiology, Risk Factors, and Pathophysiology

Hypoglycemia can be divided into two categories: fasting hypoglycemia (more than 5 hours after a meal) and postprandial hypoglycemia (1 to 2 hours after a meal) (Table 19–7). Fasting hypoglycemia occurs when the normal physiologic response to a falling glucose level is altered and there is an imbalance in glucose production and use. Hypoglycemia in a diabetic person is most commonly caused by excessive insulin or oral hypoglycemic agent, too much exercise, or not enough food. Excessive insulin doses usually result from errors in administration technique, especially in diabetics with decreased visual acuity. The most common cause of postprandial hypoglycemia is gastric surgery because after this surgery, food passes more rapidly through the small intestine, causing glucose levels to fall.

Physiologically, hypoglycemia is inadequate glucose delivery to the central nervous system (CNS) because the CNS is the tissue most sensitive to acute glucose deprivation. The CNS relies primarily on glucose for energy, cannot store glucose, and cannot convert quickly to alternative fuels, for example, ketones. As blood glucose declines rapidly, epinephrine, glucagon, glucocorticoids, and growth hormones are released. Patients will exhibit adrenergic symptoms, i.e., tachycardia, anxiety, sweating, trembling, and hunger. These symptoms can occur even if the blood glucose is normal but there is a sudden acute decline (i.e., blood glucose level decrease from 180 to 90 mg/dl). In moderate to severe hypoglycemic reactions, the CNS is affected, signifying that the brain is being deprived of the glucose it needs. Hypoglycemia unawareness is the term for diabetics whose first manifestations of hypoglycemia may be the CNS symptoms, at which time it may be too late for self-treatment.

Clinical Presentation

Signs and Symptoms
Mild hypoglycemic symptoms (adrenergic response):

- Tremors
- Shakiness
- Tachycardia
- Paresthesias
- Pallor
- Excessive hunger
- Anxiety
- Diaphoresis

Moderate to severe hypoglycemic symptoms (CNS or neuroglycopenic symptoms):

- Headache
- Inability to concentrate
- Mood changes
- Drowsiness
- Irritability
- Confusion
- Impaired judgement
- Slurred speech
- Staggering gait
- Double or blurred vision
- Morning headaches
- Nightmares
- Psychosis (late)
- Seizures
- Coma

Diagnostic Tests

- Serum blood glucose level for fingerstick glucose less than 50gm/dl

---

TABLE 19–7. CAUSES OF HYPOGLYCEMIA (PARTIAL LISTING)

Fasting Hypoglycemia
Excessive insulin dosage
Decreased need for insulin
   Decreased food intake
   Increased exercise
   Renal failure
   Liver failure
   Congestive heart failure
Drugs
   Oral hypoglycemic agents
   Alcohol
   Salicylates
   Beta-adrenergic blockers

Postprandial Hypoglycemia
Excessive insulin effect
Post gastric surgery

Patient Needs and Principles of Management

The management of the patient with acute hypoglycemia depends on the severity of the reaction. Principles of management include normalization of blood glucose concentrations and patient teaching.

► Normalization of Blood Glucose Concentrations

Treatment of the hypoglycemia depends on its severity. With a mild reaction (conscious person or mild symptoms):

1. Administer 10 to 15 g carbohydrate (Table 19–8). Follow in 10 minutes with another 10 to 15 g if the condition does not improve.
2. Obtain a blood glucose measurement.
3. If the next meal is more than 2 hours away, provide the patient with a complex carbohydrate (i.e., 4 oz milk).

TABLE 19–8. EXAMPLES OF FOODS WITH 10 TO 15 GRAMS OF CARBOHYDRATE EQUIVALENTS FOR TREATMENT OF MILD HYPOGLYCEMIC REACTIONS

4 oz orange juice
6 oz regular (nondiet) cola
3 glucose tablets
6 to 8 oz 2% fat or skim milk
3 graham-cracker squares
6 to 8 Lifesavers
6 jelly beans
2 tbsp. raisins
1 small (2-oz) tube of cake icing

4. If patient is not alert enough to swallow or unable to do so, inject 1 mg glucagon. If the patient cannot swallow and has a feeding tube, administer a liquid source of glucose, i.e., soda.

With moderate and severe reactions:

1. Administer IV glucose. The initial bolus is 50% dextrose (equivalent of 25 g glucose) followed by a continuous IV infusion until oral replacement is possible.
2. Provide for patient rest.
3. Monitor glucose levels frequently for several hours.

► Patient Teaching

The best treatment for hypoglycemia is prevention.

1. Teach the early signs and symptoms of hypoglycemia. Instruct the patient to always carry a source of fast-acting carbohydrate (Table 19–8).
2. Advise the patient not to skip or delay meals and snacks more than 30 minutes; to limit alcohol to no more than 2 oz liquor, 8 oz wine, or 24 oz beer per week; and to never drink on an empty stomach.
3. Evaluate the patient's pattern of blood glucose self-monitoring.
4. Teach the patient and family or friends how to give glucagon for severe reactions.
5. Stress the importance of wearing visible health identification.
6. Assess the patient's exercise pattern.

Disorders of Antidiuretic Hormone Secretion

Antidiuretic hormone (ADH), also known as arginine vasopressin, is produced by the hypothalamus and is stored in the posterior pituitary gland. In response to changes that occur in the blood osmolality and blood volume, ADH exerts its effect on the kidney, causing concentration of the urine and body water conservation. Syndrome of inappropriate antidiuretic hormone (SIADH) and diabetes insipidus (DI) are the most common disorders that affect ADH secretion in the critically ill.

Syndrome of Inappropriate Antidiuretic Hormone Secretion

Etiology, Risk Factors, and Pathophysiology

The syndrome of inappropriate antidiuretic hormone (SIADH) is characterized by excessive release of ADH unrelated to the plasma osmolality, or the concentration of electrolytes and other osmotically active particles. Normal mechanisms which control ADH secretion fail, causing impaired water excretion and profound hyponatremia.

There are many causes of SIADH (Table 19–9). Vasopressin can be produced by a variety of malignancies, most commonly oat cell carcinoma of the lung. Therefore, patients who develop "idiopathic" SIADH are screened for malignant tumors. SIADH is also commonly associated with pulmonary diseases or conditions, disorders of the CNS, and drugs, particularly chlorpropamide (Diabinese), thiazide diuretics, narcotics, and barbiturates.

Surgical patients are also at risk because many operative procedures are followed by increased vasopressin secretion, usually during the first 3 to 4 days postoperatively.

TABLE 19–9. ETIOLOGIES OF SIADH (PARTIAL LISTING)

Malignancies
Lung
Lymphoma
GI

Pulmonary diseases/conditions
Positive pressure ventilation
Asthma
Pneumonia
COPD
Acute respiratory failure
Tuberculosis

Disorders of the CNS
Head trauma
Meningitis, encephalitis
Cerebrovascular accidents
Brain tumors
Guillian-Barré syndrome

Drugs
Vasopressin
Desmopressin
Thiazide diuretics
Narcotics
Barbiturates
Nicotine
Antineoplastic drugs
Tricyclic antidepressants

Clinically, SIADH is distinguished by hyponatremia and water retention that progresses to water intoxication. The seriousness of the patient's signs and symptoms depends on how low the serum sodium falls and how rapidly the fluid accumulates. As water intoxication progresses and the serum becomes more hypotonic, brain cells swell, causing neurological problems. Without treatment, irreversible brain damage and death can occur.

Clinical Presentation

Signs and Symptoms
Early:

- Urine volume decreased and concentrated
- Headache
- Dulled sensorium
- Anorexia
- Weight gain
- Dyspnea
- Nausea
- Vomiting
- Impaired taste
- Muscle weakness and cramps
- Adventitious breath sounds
- Increased CVP, PCWP

Late:
- Confusion
- Aberrant respirations
- Coma
- Hostility
- Hypothermia
- Convulsions

Diagnostic Tests
- Serum Na$^+$ less than 135 mEq/L
- Serum osmolality less than 280 mOsm/kg
- Increased urine osmolality
- Urine sodium above 20 mEq/L
- Blood urea nitrogen and creatinine decreased (hemodilution)

Patient Needs and Principles of Management

Principles of management depend on the severity and duration of the hyponatremia. Generally, treatment will focus on restricting fluids, replenishing sodium deficits, and in severe cases of hyponatremia, inhibiting antidiuretic actions. Treatment of the underlying disorder is also a priority.

▶ Fluid Restriction

Fluid restriction is the mainstay of treatment and, to be effective, a negative water balance must be achieved.

1. Restrict fluids to the sum of the urine output. In most cases, this will be below 1000 ml/day. In severe hyponatremia, fluid may be limited to less than 250 ml/day. Concentrate all infusions and antibiotics to minimize fluids. Maintain strict intake and output and weigh the patient at the same time each day. Once serum sodium is within normal range, fluid intake can be increased to urine output plus insensible losses.

2. Assess cardiovascular and respiratory functions

closely to evaluate the effects of the excess volume on these systems. Right and left ventricular volumes may increase, causing heart failure. Tachypnea, reports of shortness of breath, and fine crackles are indicators of fluid overload and impending heart failure.

3. Administer diuretics as prescribed. Diuretics decrease the effectiveness of ADH and promote water excretion.

4. Provide for patient comfort with limited fluid intake. Provide for frequent mouth care. Explain why fluid is being restricted and allow the patient to develop the schedule for allotted fluid intake. If the patient complains of nausea, administer an antiemetic prior to meals.

► Replenish Sodium Deficits

1. In severe symptomatic hyponatremia, infuse 3% saline at a rate of 0.1 ml/kg/minute for 2 hours to raise plasma sodium. Monitor closely for signs of hypernatremia, fluid overload, and heart failure as this treatment causes a transient increase in the serum sodium.

2. Monitor neurological status closely and protect the patient from harm. Institute seizure precautions as necessary. Monitor respiratory status closely.

► Inhibit Antidiuretic Hormone Actions

In cases where SIADH does not resolve within 1 to 2 weeks, drugs which interfere with the renal effect of vasopressin, such as demeclocycline (Declomycin), may be ordered. The full effect of these drugs may take as long as 1 or 2 weeks, and therefore they are unsuitable for acute management of the syndrome.

Diabetes Insipidus

Etiology, Risk Factors, and Pathophysiology

Diabetes insipidus (DI) results from a group of disorders in which there is an absolute or relative deficiency of ADH (called central DI) or an insensitivity to its effects on the renal tubules (called nephrogenic DI)(Figure 19–3). Diabetes insipidus may complicate the course of the critically ill patient and can result in acute fluid and electrolyte disturbances.

There are many causes of DI (Table 19–10). Neurogenic DI results from damage to the hypothalamic system. An absolute deficiency of ADH results in impaired urine-concentrating ability, polyuria, and a subsequent tendency to dehydration. Patients with head trauma or those who have had neurosurgery must be watched closely for at least 7 to 10 days after the injury for evidence of DI. Nephrogenic DI is characterized by renal tubule insensitivity to ADH and develops because of structural or functional changes in the kidney. This results in an impairment in urine-concentrating ability and free water conservation.

Regardless of the etiology, in DI the ability of the body to increase ADH secretion or respond to ADH is impaired. A persistent output of dilute urine despite increasing hemoconcentration is the hallmark of DI. Signs and symptoms of dehydration are present in those patients in whom the thirst mechanism has been impaired (neurogenic DI), or in whom there is inadequate fluid replacement. In addition, if a hyperosmolar state exists, intracellular brain volume depletion occurs as water moves from within the brain cells to the plasma.

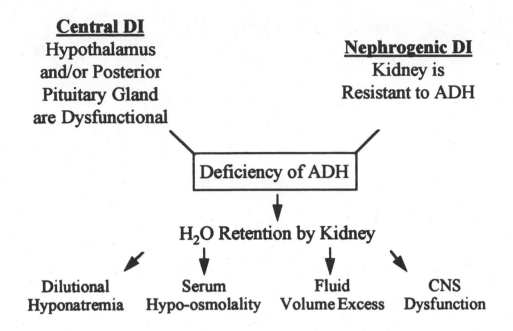

Figure 19–3. Pathogenesis of diabetes insipidus.

Clinical Presentation

Signs and Symptoms
Deficiency of ADH:

- Polydipsia (if alert)
- Polyuria (5 to 20 L in 24 hours)

Fluid volume deficit:

- Orthostatic hypotension
- Weight loss
- Tachycardia
- Decreased CVP, PCWP
- Poor skin turgor
- Dry mucous membranes

Intracellular brain volume depletion:

- Confusion
- Restlessness
- Lethargy
- Irritability
- Seizures
- Coma

Diagnostic Tests

- Serum sodium greater than 145 mEq/L
- Serum osmolality greater than 295 mOsm/kg/H_2O
- Urine osmolality inappropriately low with high serum osmolality
- Urine specific gravity decreased
- BUN and creatinine increased (hemoconcentration)

TABLE 19–10. CAUSES OF DIABETES INSIPIDUS

ADH Insufficiency (Neurogenic DI)
Familial (hereditary)
Trauma
Neoplasms
Infections
   Tuberculosis
   Cryptococcosis
   Syphilis
   CNS infections
Vascular
   Cerebrovascular hemorrhage
   Aneurysm (circle of Willis)
   Cerebral thrombosis

ADH Insensitivity (Nephrogenic DI)
Familial (hereditary)
Drug-induced
   Lithium
   Demeclocycline
   Glyburide
   Colchicine
   Amphotericin B
   Gentamicin
   Furosemide
Electrolyte disorders
   Hypokalemia
   Hypercalcemia
Renal disease

Excessive Water Intake (Secondary DI)
Excessive IV fluid administration
Psychogenic polydipsia (lesion in thirst center)

Patient Needs and Principles of Management

The management of the patient in DI is directed at correcting the profound fluid volume deficit and electrolyte imbalances associated with this condition. If fluid losses are not replaced, hypovolemic shock can rapidly develop (see Chapter 12, Cardiovascular System). In some cases of DI, vasopressin or agents that simulate ADH release and renal response to ADH are prescribed to treat the disorder. As with other disorders, location and treatment of the cause of DI are priorities.

▶ Fluid Volume Replacement

If the patient is alert and the thirst mechanism is not impaired, allow the patient to drink water to maintain normal serum osmolality. In many critically ill patients, this is not possible.

1. Administer dextrose in water IV as prescribed to restore fluid volume. The administration of normal saline to replace volume is usually contraindicated as it presents an added renal load, promoting osmotic diuresis and worsening dehydration. In severe DI, where large amounts of fluid replacement are required, the IV intake is usually titrated to urine output. For example, 400 ml of urine output for 1 hour is replaced with 400 ml IV fluid the next hour. Hypotonic saline solutions are usually used (quarter-strength or half-strength saline) because the solutions are hypotonic.

2. Monitor fluid status: intake and output, daily weight, and urine specific gravity. Monitor for signs of continuing fluid volume deficit. Expected outcomes for the patient with DI are listed in Table 19–11.

3. Monitor neurological status continuously. An altered level of consciousness indicates intracellular dehydration and hypovolemia.

▶ Vasopressin Administration

Exogenous vasopressin, or Pitressin, which replaces the absent or reduced ADH may be used to restore normal serum ADH levels. Carbamazepine or chlorpropamide may be used to enhance the release of ADH and increase the renal response to ADH.

1. Administer 5 to 10 units Pitressin SQ or IM. Major side effects to watch for include headache, abdominal cramps, vasoconstrictive effects, or allergic reactions. Monitor for overmedication, which may precipitate hypervolemia. Signs and symptoms of fluid volume excess include dyspnea, hypertension, weight gain, and angina.

2. For central DI, administer vasopressin and carbamazepine as prescribed and monitor for fluid overload.

3. For nephrogenic DI, administer chlorpropamide (Diabinese). Because of this agent's antidiabetic properties, monitor for hypoglycemia.

TABLE 19–11. EXPECTED OUTCOMES FOR THE PATIENT WITH DIABETES INSIPIDUS

Adequate fluid balance is maintained/restored as evidenced by:
  Blood pressure within 10 mm Hg of patient baseline
  Heart rate 60 to 100 beats/minute
  Normal skin turgor
  Peripheral pulses return to baseline
  CVP and PCWP within patient norms
  Serum osmolality 275 to 295 mOsm/kg
  Serum sodium 135 to 145 mEq/L
  Urine osmolality appropriate for serum osmolality

AT THE BEDSIDE
■ *Thinking Critically*

You are caring for a patient in acute diabetic ketoacidosis with the following interventions and laboratory results:

- 0.9 NS with 20 mEq KCl at 150 mL/hour
- Insulin (regular) drip at 20 units/hr
- Oxygen 6 L/minute by nasal cannula
- Arterial blood gases

pH:	7.16
$PaCO_2$:	24 mm Hg
PaO_2:	59 mm Hg
SaO_2:	89%
HCO_3:	14 mEq/L

Which intervention is most important in correcting the acidosis in this case? Why isn't sodium bicarbonate ordered to correct the acidosis?

SELECTED BIBLIOGRAPHY

General Endocrine

Loriaux TC, Drass JA: Endocrine and diabetic disorders. In Kinney MR, Packa DR, Dunbar SB (eds.): *AACN's clinical reference for critical care nursing,* 3rd ed. St. Louis, MO: CV Mosby, 1993, pp. 927–959.

Waite LG, Krumberger JM: *Noncardiac critical care nursing.* Albany, NY: Delmar, 1994, pp. 13–52.

Blood Glucose Monitoring

Harding K: A comparison of four glucose monitors in a hospital medical surgical setting. *Clinical Nurse Specialist.* 1993;7(1):13–16.

Kestel F: Using blood glucose meters: What you and your patient need to know (Part I). *Nursing 93.* 1993;March:34–41.

Kestel F: Using blood glucose meters: What you and your patient need to know (Part II). *Nursing 93.* 1993;April:50–53.

Pressly K, Batteiger TH, Barnett DZ, Woodie ME: Use of arterial blood for glucose measurement by reflectance. *Nursing Research.* 1990;39(6):371–372.

Sylvain H, Pokomy ME, English SM, et al.: Accuracy of fingerstick glucose values in shock patients. *American Journal of Critical Care.* 1995;4(1):44–88.

Walker EA: Quality assurance for blood glucose monitoring. *Nursing Clinics of North America.* 1993;28(1):61–68.

DKA and HHNC

Brody GM: Diabetic ketoacidosis and hyperosmolar hyperglycemic nonketotic coma. *Topics in Emergency Medicine.* 1992;14(1):12–22.

Drass J: Insulin injections. *Nursing 92.* 1992;November:40–43.

Fish LH: Diabetic ketoacidosis. *Postgraduate Medicine.* 1994; 96(3):75–93.

Lipsky MS: Management of diabetic ketoacidosis. *American Family Physician.* 1994;49(7):1607–1612.

Marshall SM: Hyperglycemic emergencies. *Care of the Critically Ill.* 1993;9(5):220–223.

Reising DL: Acute hyperglycemia. *Nursing 95.* 1995;February:33–40.

Sauve DO, Kessler CA: Hyperglycemic emergencies. *AACN Clinical Issues.* 1992;3(2):350–360.

Siperstein MD: Diabetic ketoacidosis and hyperosmolar coma. *Endocrinology and Metabolism Clinics of North America.* 1992;21(2):415–432.

Steil C, Deakins DA: Oral hypoglycemics. *Nursing 92.* 1992; November:34–39.

Tal A: Clinical and metabolic characteristics of diabetic ketoacidosis. *Journal of the Tennessee Medical Association.* 1992; 85(1):12–16.

Hypoglycemia

Arbour R: Acute hypoglycemia. *Nursing 94.* 1994;January:33.

Comi RJ: Approach to acute hypoglycemia. *Endocrinology and Metabolism Clinics of North America.* 1993;22(2):247–260.

Hollander P: Intensified insulin regimens. *Postgraduate Medicine.* 1994;93(3):63–72.

Macheca MK: Diabetic hypoglycemia: How to keep the threat at bay. *American Journal of Nursing.* 1993;April:26–30.

Malone ML, Klos SE, Gennis VM, Goodwin JS: Frequent hypoglycemia episodes in the treatment of patients with diabetic ketoacidosis. *Archives of Internal Medicine.* 1992;152:2472–2477.

Malcahy K: Hypoglycemic emergencies. *AACN Clinical Issues.* 1992;3(2):361–369.

Reising DL. Acute hypoglycemia. *Nursing 95.*1995; February:41–48.

Disorders of Antidiuretic Hormone Secretion

Batcheller J: Disorders of antidiuretic hormone secretion. *AACN Clinical Issues.* 1992;3(2):370–378.

Blevins LS, Wand GS: Diabetes insipidus. *Critical Care Medicine.* 1992;20(1):69–78.

Bryant WP, O'Marcaigh AS, Ledger GA, Zimmerman D: Aqueous vasopressin infusion during chemotherapy in patients with diabetes insipidus. *Cancer.* 1994;74(9):2589–2592.

Buonocore CM, Robinson AG: The diagnosis and management of diabetes insipidus during medical emergencies. *Endocrinology and Metabolism Clinics of North America.* 1994;22(2):411–422.

Holtzman EJ, Ausiello DA: Nephrogenic diabetes insipidus: Causes revealed. *Hospital Practice.* 1994;March 15:89–104.

Kovacs L, Robertson GL: Syndrome of inappropriate antidiuresis. *Endocrinology and Metabolism Clinics of North America.* 1992;21(4):859–875.

Lindaman C: S.I.A.D.H.: Is your patient at risk? *Nursing 92.* 1992;June:60–63.

Secki JR, Dunger DB. Diabetes insipidum *Drugs.* 1992;44(2): 216–224.

Stawron D, Lewison L, Marks J, Turner G, Levin D: Brain death in pediatric intensive care unit patients: Incidence, primary diagnosis, and the clinical occurrence of Turner's triad. *Critical Care Medicine.* 1994;22(8):1301–1304.

Twenty

Trauma

▶ Knowledge Competencies

1. Describe the mechanisms of traumatic injury and relate them to accurate assessment of obvious and subtle injuries.

2. Discuss the common physiologic and psychosocial effects on the patient and family due to major trauma.

3. Identify the unique aspects of the trauma patient in the critical care unit.

4. Apply selected management principles to treat trauma patients with chest, abdominal, and musculoskeletal trauma.

■ What Heals: Correct Biologic Images in Wound and Bone Healing

Patients who are given specific information about the role of body-mind connections, correct biologic healing images, and stress management strategies can assist in enhancing their own recovery. The nurse elicits from the patient images and symbols that have special healing meaning and value, and then makes an audiocassette for the patient that includes correct biologic images, specific concrete objective information, specific symbols, and specific types of imagery (see Chapter 8, Alternative Therapies in Critical Care, for guidelines on making an audiocassette tape and establishing an audio/video library).

It may seem that the following scripts may appear suitable for well-educated, sophisticated individuals, but this is not the case. It is necessary, however, for the nurse to assess the individual's education level and adapt these scripts to fit the person's needs, cultural beliefs, and symbols. Imagery is an important tool, particularly for those patients who do not read.

WOUND HEALING

To teach the normal wound healing process with the correct biologic images, the nurse explains the following:

- *Reaction.* Fluid leaks into tissue at the time of the injury, causing swelling and inflammation; white blood cells migrate to the wound. Inflammation continues for 72 hours from the time of injury (Figure 20–1A).
- *Regeneration.* Granulation and deposit of fibrous collagen protein tissue continue for as long as 3 weeks following the injury (Figure 20–1B).
- *Remodeling.* Healing of a wound takes from 3 weeks for a minor wound to 2 years for a severe wound (Figure 20–1C).

A wound healing intervention may last 20 to 30 minutes.

Script: Focus on calmness and rhythmic breathing . . . and become aware of your ritual . . . for

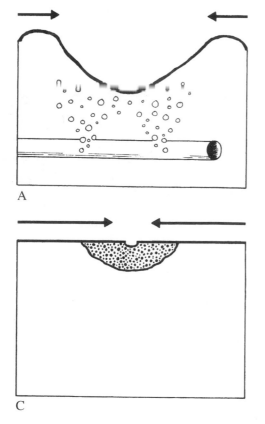

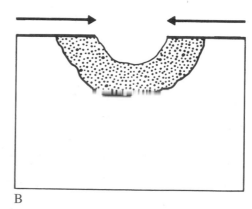

Figure 20–1. A. Reaction: inflammation and stabilization of wound (from time of injury for 72 hours). B. Regeneration: granulation and deposition of fibrous collagen protein tissue (up to 3 weeks). C. Remodeling: healed wound (3 weeks to 2 years). *(From: Achterberg J, Dossey B, Kolkmeier L:* Rituals of healing. *New York: Bantam Books, 1994.)*

cleansing your wound. Let it be done slowly . . . without hurry. To avoid holding your breath, . . . take several rhythmic breaths prior to cleansing your wound. When you are ready to begin the cleansing of your wound . . . take a breath in . . . and, on the exhale, place the hydrogen peroxide or other solutions on the wound and surrounding area or along suture lines. Next, on the area that has been cleaned and patted dry, place the ointment in the same area to help speed the healing process. Now is the time to place a clean dressing on the wound.

Allow yourself to imagine a natural process that is occurring within your body. New cells are being made in the open skin area . . . to allow a stable place for repair and new growth. Now your blood flow is surging to this area. Special white blood cells, your macrophages, are recognizing any foreign material and carrying it away. Remember . . . be with the special healing process of your wound. If your wound is superficial, it heals from the edges toward the center. A deep wound will heal from the inside to the outside.

A beautiful area is now forming . . . you might imagine it like looking down into a lovely shallow bowl. Within this area . . . your body now places soft, healthy, delicate fibrous protein tissue . . . like a network of beautiful lights . . . the beginning of a strong scar that starts below the surface of the skin.

Become more aware . . . of the fact . . . that your own special cells, the fibroblasts, are producing this collagen protein. Many small buds of new tissue continue to be laid down and grow stronger and fuller, creating healthy new skin and scar tissue. The opening shrinks and becomes smaller as healing occurs. Let an image or feeling of the new healed skin surface emerge. Your skin has healed from the inside to the outside. See, hear, and feel your healed, smooth, new skin that is strong and healthy.

BONE HEALING

An imagery exercise for bone healing may be done in 20 to 30 minutes. Prior to imagery, to teach basic biologic process of bone healing, the nurse explains the following:

- *Reaction (cellular proliferation).* Within the hematoma surrounding the fracture, cells and tissues proliferate and develop into a random structure (Figure 20–2A).
- *Regeneration (callus formation).* At 10 to 14 days after the fracture, the cells within the hematoma become organized in a fibrous lattice. With sufficient organization, the callus becomes clinically stable. The callus obliterates the medullary canal and surrounds the

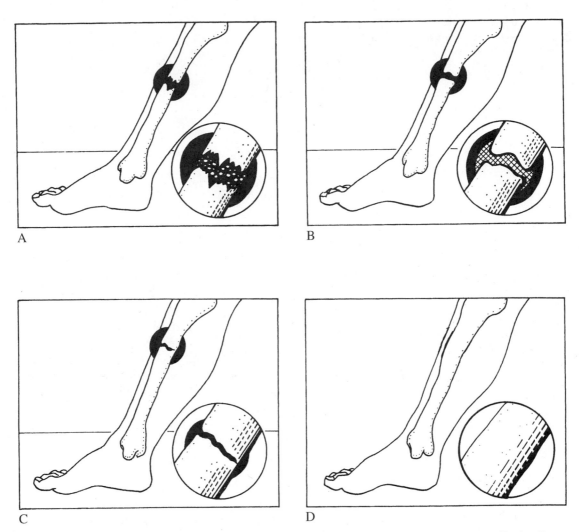

Figure 20–2. A. Reaction: hematoma and cellular proliferation. B. Regeneration. C. Remodeling: calcium ossification. D. Healed bone. *(From: Achterberg J, Dossey B, Kolkmeier L: Rituals of healing. New York: Bantam Books, 1994.)*

two ends of bone by irregularly surrounding the fracture defect (Figure 20–2B).

- *Remodeling (new bone formation).* Approximately 25 to 40 days after the fracture, calcium is laid down within the bone that has spicules perpendicular to the cortical surface (Figure 20–2C). Osteonal bone gradually replaces and remodels fiber bone. The fracture has been bridged over by new bone (Figure 20–2D). Conversion and remodeling continue up to 3 years following an acute fracture.

Script: In your relaxed state, (name), allow yourself to imagine a natural process that is occurring within your body. New cells are gathering very fast at the site of your fracture (cellular proliferation). This is an important process as it lays the foundation for your bone healing. With your next breath in . . . become aware of the fact . . . that right now your body is allowing those new

cells to multiply rapidly (truism). Your blood cells . . . at the site of your fracture, are arranging themselves in a special healing pattern (reaction). You can relax . . . even more . . . if you want to . . . as you continue with this very natural healing process (embedded command).

In a few days . . . your wise body will begin to create a strong lattice network of new bone (regeneration). This will allow your bone to become stable, bridging the new bone that is forming. As you focus in a relaxed way . . . you help in your healing . . . for relaxation increases this natural process (linkage). Imagine your relaxation to be like a gentle breeze of wind that flows over and throughout your body (metaphor).

In a few more weeks, your new bone will be formed . . . natural deposits of calcium from your body will be taken into the place of healing (remodeling). Allow an image to come to your mind now of beautiful, healed bone. In about 6 weeks, you will have a beautiful bridge where the calcium has formed new bone (remodeling). Can you imagine the healing colors that are within you right now, and seeing sounds (synesthesia)? *Just five a few minutes more . . . allow yourself*

. . . to relax into the healing process . . . feel . . . as you breathe into this healing movement.

CEG & BMD

Reproduced with permission from: Achterberg J, Dossey BM, Kolkmeier L: Rituals of healing. New York: Bantam Books, 1994, pp. 78.5 186 and 100 102.

SPECIALIZED ASSESSMENT TECHNIQUES, DIAGNOSTIC TESTS, AND MONITORING SYSTEMS

Critically ill trauma patients are unlike other hospitalized patients and require specialized assessment and monitoring. For the trauma victim, admission to the critical care setting is sudden and unplanned, with no time for psychological preparation or the stabilizing of chronic conditions. Trauma patients are often young; however, trauma in the elderly is increasing. Traumatic injuries may be subtle, and complications are common (Table 20–1). Alcohol or drug abuse plays a major role in the cause of the trauma and subsequent treatment. Rehabilitation is often needed after injury, and quality of life may never return to normal. This is especially true for severe head and spinal cord injuries; however, even in lower extremity trauma, it may take a full year for an individual to return to work. Trauma takes a significant emotional and financial toll on the patient, family, and society.

Management of traumatic injury in the initial phases of care occurs in tandem with assessment. For example, the administration of fluids, the insertion of an airway, and pain medication may all be provided before the site of bleeding is identified and controlled. One of the most important aspects of assessing the traumatically injured patient is to determine the mechanism of injury. Based upon this information, an "index of suspicion" regarding specific injuries is developed to ensure that no injuries are overlooked.

AT THE BEDSIDE
▶ *Trauma*

Joe was a 27-year-old white male driver with his seat belt on who was involved in a high-speed, head-on motor vehicle collision on Super Bowl Sunday. The passenger in Joe's car and the driver of the oncoming vehicle were dead at the scene. Both were unbelted and had been ejected from their vehicles.

Joe was found unconscious and required a long extrication time due to the significant vehicle damage and the suspicion of spinal cord injury. The prehospital providers were meticulous about moving him. He arrived at the emergency department 3 hours after the collision with the following assessment:

Primary Assessment

Airway	Spontaneous respirations
Breathing	Respiratory rate 32 breaths/minute, shallow and labored
Circulation	Heart rate 127/minute and irregular
Deformity	Lacerations on forehead and both knees, right thigh grossly edematous
Exposure	No other injuries noted upon exposing patient

Primary and Secondary Trauma Survey Assessment

The life-threatening nature of trauma requires a reorganization of the traditional assessment priorities (Tables 20–2 and 20–3). The primary and secondary surveys reveal immediate life-threatening injuries and direct the trauma team toward an individualized resuscitation. This approach ensures that common causes of tissue injury are rapidly identified so appropriate therapeutic interventions can be started.

Diagnostic Peritoneal Lavage

Diagnostic peritoneal lavage (DPL) is performed to detect free blood in the peritoneal cavity and if positive, may indicate the need for exploratory surgery. The test is especially important in the blunt, multiple trauma patient who is unconscious or unable to verbalize abdominal pain upon palpation.

Under local anesthetic, a lavage catheter is percutaneously placed into the abdomen. If no blood or fluid is aspirated, a liter of normal saline solution is instilled and then drained. Bloody return or drainage with red blood cells

TABLE 20–1. MAJOR COMPLICATIONS IN TRAUMA

Complication	Associated Conditions	What To Look For	Nursing Interventions
Hypovolemia	Internal hemorrhage Multiple-system injuries Fractures of major bones Coagulopathies	Decreased blood pressure Tachycardia, tachypnea Cool, clammy skin Pallor Decreased urine output Frank hemorrhage Anxiety Obtunded sensorium	Notify physician immediately Type and cross-match patient's blood Check amount of blood on hand in blood bank Administer transfusion as ordered Elevate patient's legs while patient is supine, with head elevated as necessary to facilitate respiration Administer medications as ordered Monitor vital signs q 15 minutes
Sepsis	Systemic infection Peritonitis	Increased WBCs Increased or decreased temperature Tachycardia Sudden hypotension Increased serum glucose Decreased platelets, decreased Pao_2 Confusion/disorientation Diaphoresis/flushed face	Monitor ABGs Notify physician Monitor VS q 15 minutes Administer fluid replacement and medications as ordered Monitor arterial blood gases (ABGs), electrolytes, and CBC Maintain normothermia
Neurogenic shock	Spinal cord injury	Hypotension Hypothermia with absence of sweating below injury level Flaccid paralysis below injury level Bradycardia	Notify physician Administer medications and IV fluids as ordered Monitor VS q 15 minutes Insert Foley catheter and nasogastric tube as ordered
Pulmonary embolism	Immobility Fracture of the long bones, pelvis, or ribs Improper handling of fractures before and during admission	Chest pain Shortness of breath Sudden disorientation Petechiae over axillae and chest (fat) Decreased Pao_2 Tachycardia	Notify physician Assist with transport to lung scan Monitor ECG Administer O_2 Draw ABGs STAT and serially Assist ventilation as ordered
Adult respiratory distress syndrome (ARDS)	Chest trauma Sepsis Multiple transfusions Brain injuries Multiple-system injuries	Decreased $Paco_2$, decreased Pao_2 Decreased lung compliance Decreased tidal volume Increased airway pressures Increased WBC	Assess chest, monitor lung volumes and compliance Draw serial ABGs Administer O_2 or ventilator therapy as ordered Suction PRN Administer medications as ordered Monitor ECG
Pneumonia	Blunt chest trauma Immobility Atelectasis Endotracheal intubation	Increased temperature Increased WBC Decreased breath sounds Rales, some bronchi on auscultation Radiologic changes Positive sputum cultures	Assess chest Use sterile suction technique and chest physiotherapy for pulmonary hygiene PRN Supplemental O_2 PRN Serial chest x-rays as ordered
Wound dehiscence	Abdominal surgery Wound infection Poor nutritional status	Pink serous wound exudate Poor wound edge approximation	Notify physician Have sterile saline and dressings on hand Prevent/correct abdominal distention
Gastrointestinal fistula	Penetrating abdominal trauma Sepsis	Bile, fecal, or pancreatic drainage from wounds or drain sites	Monitor amount, odor, and color of drainage Meticulous skin care around drainage sites Perform dressing changes as necessary
Stress ulcers	Multiple-system trauma Patient kept NPO for prolonged periods Head injury Sepsis Continuous mechanical ventilation Prolonged ICU	NG aspirate hemopositive Decreased pH of NG aspirate Stools hemopositive Decreased hematocrit Melena	Administer medications as ordered Chilled saline lavage until clear Administer transfusions, medications, and fluid replacement as ordered
Pneumothorax (simple)	Mechanical ventilation	Decreased or absent breath sounds Radiologic evidence Decreased Pao_2, cyanosis Unequal chest expansion Hyperresonance over affected area	Notify physician Administer supplemental O_2 Assist with chest tube insertion or thoracentesis
Pneumothorax (tension)	PEEP Improper CVP line placement	Decreased Pao_2, cyanosis Decreased tidal volume, unequal chest expansion Decreased lung compliance Breath sounds absent Tracheal deviation Increased airway pressures Restlessness Hyperresonance over affected area Hemodynamic instability	Notify physician STAT Insert 18-gauge needle into 2nd intercostal space laterally if certified Assist with chest tube insertion If chest tubes in place, check for patency and suction Monitor VS q 15 minutes
Renal failure	Prolonged hypotension Sepsis Ruptured aorta Toxic drug reaction ARDS	Increased serum BUN and creatinine Decreased urine output, decreased specific gravity Increased serum potassium Increased confusion Uremic frost	Record hourly intake and output Foley catheter care daily Monitor lab values Administer hemodialysis or peritoneal dialysis as ordered Daily weights
Bronchoesophageal fistula	Prolonged tracheostomy Overinflation of cuff balloon Prolonged need for NG tube	Gastric contents suctioned through tracheostomy Radiologic confirmation Respiratory distress	Maintain NPO Maintain proper positioning of endotracheal tube to maintain ventilation Administer feedings as ordered via gastrostomy or jejunostomy
Diabetes insipidus	Brain injuries	Increased urine output Decreased urine specific gravity Decreased urine osmolality Severe thirst	Record hourly intake and output, check urine specific gravity q4h Maintain fluid balance Replace urine output as ordered Administer Pitressin as ordered
Ruptured innominate artery	Tracheostomy Tracheal tube too long Inadvertent traction on tracheal tube when moving patient Prolonged overinflation of tracheal tube cuff	Visible pulsation of trachea Frank bleeding from trachea	Elevate tracheal flange with 4 × 4's if arterial pulsations present If rupture occurs, slide finger down outside of outer cannula and attempt to tamponade innominate artery against clavicle
Atelectasis	Immobility Prolonged anesthesia Blunt chest trauma Pain Endotracheal intubation	Radiologic changes Decreased Pao_2 Inability to cough Decreased breath sounds	Provide pulmonary hygiene and chest physiotherapy Turn and position q 1-2h Kinetic therapy Encourage coughing and deep breathing Draw serial ABGs Administer O_2 PRN Incentive spirometer
Empyema	Blunt chest trauma Pneumonia Prolonged atelectasis Pleural effusion Open chest wound	Purulent chest drainage Increased temperature Increased WBC Generalized malaise Radiologic confirmation Sepsis	Monitor amount and consistency of chest tube drainage as ordered Culture chest tube drainage as ordered Maintain chest tube patency Provide pulmonary hygiene and chest physiotherapy
Aspiration	Unconscious patients Spinal cord injury Sudden vomiting Malfunctioning NG tube Decreased gag reflex Prolonged endotracheal intubation	Suctioning of gastric contents from tracheal tube or ET tube Radiologic confirmation Increased temperature and WBCs Decreased Pao_2	Notify physician immediately Take chest x-ray STAT Turn patient to side or suction if vomits Elevate head of bed when giving tube feedings
Meningitis	Brain injury Skull fracture Maxillofacial trauma Intraventricular catheter placement	Increased temperature Increased WBC Positive spinal fluid cultures Changes in neurological status	Administer medications as ordered Monitor VS q1h Do neurological checks q1h Assist with spinal tap Draw serial WBCs
Sensory deprivation/ ICU psychosis	Prolonged stay in ICU Sleep deprivation	Confusion Disorientation Hallucinations Restlessness Combativeness	Arrange for psychiatric consult if necessary Provide quiet environment Plan nursing care in blocks of time to promote sleep Administer medications as ordered Use consistent nursing approach to orient to reality

From: Cardona VD, Hurn PD, Mason PJB, Scanlon AM, Veise-Berry SW (eds.): Trauma nursing from resuscitation through rehabilitation. Philadelphia: WB Saunders, 1994, pp. 840–841.

TABLE 20–2. PRIMARY TRAUMA SURVEY ASSESSMENT

Assessment	Observations Indicating Impaired ABCDs
Airway: Open and patent, maintain cervical spine immobilization	Shallow, noisy breathing Stridor Cyanosis Nasal flaring Accessory muscle use Inability to speak Drooling Anxiety Decreased level of consciousness Trauma to face, mouth, neck Debris or foreign matter in mouth or pharynx
Breathing: Presence and effectiveness	Asymmetric rise and fall of chest Absent, decreased, or unequal breath sounds Open sucking chest wounds Blunt chest injury Dyspnea Cyanosis Respiratory rate < 8 to 10/minute or > 40/minute Accessory muscle use Anxiety Tracheal shift Distended neck veins Paradoxical chest wall motion
Circulation: Presence of major pulses; external hemorrhage	Weak, thready pulse > 120/minute Moisture, color, temperature of skin Capillary refill > 2 seconds Obvious external hemorrhage Decreased level of consciousness Distended neck veins
Disability: Gross neurologic status; pupil size, equality, and reactivity to light	Glasgow Coma Scale < 15

From: Sparger G, Shea S, Selfridge J: Patients with trauma. In Clochesy J, Breu C Cardin S, Rudy E, Whittaker A: Critical care nursing. Philadelphia: WB Saunders, 1993, p. 1230.

greater than 100,000 cells/mm^3 demonstrates a positive DPL. Retroperitoneal injuries, such as pancreatic injury, will not show up as positive with a lavage. Computerized tomography (CT) is a good alternative to DPL in the stable trauma patient. Ultrasound is increasingly being used for abdominal screening to detect injury.

Cervical Spine X-Ray

A cervical spine (C-spine) x-ray is one of the first priorities of assessment after the primary survey. All trauma patients are presumed to have a C-spine injury until all seven cervical vertebrae have been cleared or visualized as intact on x-ray. A cervical collar to immobilize the neck is applied until the C-spine is cleared.

Serial Examinations

Trauma patients require frequent reexamination to prevent injuries from being missed which can create pain, disability, and or increased mortality. Head trauma and abdominal injuries are examples where repeated assessments by the same provider are recommended. Having a high degree of suspicion for traumatic injuries comes from a knowledge of mechanism of injury and the specific injuries created by destructive blunt or penetrating forces.

Mechanism of Injury

The principles of mechanism of injury (MOI) help the trauma team "make sense" of the injuries sustained by the patient. How an injury occurred, the nature of the forces involved, and suspected tissue and organ damage are all important aspects of MOI. This knowledge is required when assessing a trauma patient at the scene and in the emergency department, as well as in the critical care unit.

Injuries result when a body is exposed to an uncontrolled outside source of energy that disrupts the body's integrity or functional ability. This energy can come from a variety of sources, and can be kinetic, chemical, thermal, electrical, or radiating energy. The severity of the resultant injury is determined by several factors: the force or speed of impact, the length of the impact or exposure, the total surface area exposed, and related risk factors such as age, gender, preinjury health, alcohol/drug ingestion, and geographical location of the injury. Kinetic energy injuries are the most common in trauma patients.

Kinetic Forces

Trauma victims sustain injuries from kinetic sources when motion is either abruptly halted or initiated from an outside force, for example, from a fall, moving vehicle, or other object. The types of force that cause injury include acceleration/deceleration, shearing, and compression. Acceleration/deceleration forces are those that abruptly increase or decrease velocity of movement, such as motor vehicle collisions and falls. Shearing injuries are sustained when force or energy is applied within the same plane as the impacted area, such as skin burns caused by having a limb dragged on a rough surface, which might occur in motorcycle trauma. Compression forces are those which apply direct energy to an area. For example, a compression injury to the spine can occur when a person jumps from a high distance and lands directly on the feet.

Mechanism of injury investigation provides clinicians with the patterns of injury. These common patterns are helpful when assessing trauma patients who cannot speak to indicate areas of pain. Common patterns offer the trauma team an index of suspicion and direction, indicating which diagnostic tests to perform in what order to identify each of the patient's injuries. For example, in motor vehicle crashes, the key impact areas for the unrestrained driver include head, pelvis, chest, and musculoskeletal areas (e.g., hip, ankle, and foot trauma) (Figure 20–3A). Thoracic trauma is often due to impact with a steering wheel. Injuries to unrestrained passengers demonstrate an increased incidence of craniofacial trauma from hitting the head on the windshield (Figure 20–3B). Fractures of the clavicle and

TABLE 20–3. SECONDARY TRAUMA SURVEY ASSESSMENT

Area	Inspection	Palpation	Percussion	Auscultation

Head:
  Scalp
  Skull
  Face
  Eyes/ears
  Nose
  Mouth
	Soft tissue injury
	Deformities
	Edema
	Asymmetry of face
	Open bite
	Periorbital
	Otorrhea
	Rhinorrhea
	Bloody drainage
	Extraocular movements
	Subcutaneous air
	Gross vision
	Eye injuries
		Bony deformities of facial bones or skull
		Scalp wounds
		Subcutaneous air
		Crepitus
		Pain
		Decreased sensation of face		

Neck	Soft tissue injury Tracheal position Distended neck veins Ask about pain, hoarseness, dysphagia	Crepitus Subcutaneous air Tracheal position Cervical spine tenderness or deformities		
Chest	Soft tissue injury Open sucking wound Subcutaneous air Intercostal retractions Symmetry of chest Respiratory rate, effort Seatbelt marks Impaled objects	Crepitus Subcutaneous air Bony deformities Chest wall excursion	Dullness Hyperresonance	Absent or diminished breath sounds Distant heart or gastric sounds
Abdomen and flanks*	Soft tissue injury Distention Seatbelt marks Impaled objects Contour Discolorations	Rigidity Distention Pain: diffuse or localized	Dullness Hyperresonance	Bowel sounds in all four quadrants
Pelvis or perineum	Soft tissue injury External genitalia injury Blood at urinary meatus Vaginal bleeding Rectal bleeding Suprapubic masses Priapism	Pelvic instability Femoral pulses Rectal sphincter tone Prostate position Vaginal integrity Open fractures		
Extremities	Soft tissue injury Amputation Crush injury Deformity: open or closed Motor/sensory	Diminished or absent pulses Crepitus Pain or tenderness		
Back	Soft tissue injury Buttock Posterior thighs Flanks	Thoracic, lumbar, sacral spine pain, tenderness, deformity		

*NOTE: The sequence of examination of the abdomen is inspection, auscultation, palpation, and percussion.
From: Sparger G, Shea S, Selfridge J: Patients with trauma. In Clochesy J, Breu C, Cardin S, Rudy E, Whittaker A: Critical care nursing. Philadelphia: WB Saunders, 1993, p. 1231.

humerus are more frequent in passengers, possibly due to the defensive reflex action of raising the arms prior to impact. Similar patterns of injury have been identified for victims of falls and pedestrians struck by motor vehicles (Figure 20–4). Knowledge of these patterns of suspected injuries also helps to prevent further damage or complications during the resuscitation efforts. For example, if a patient has sustained a head injury with a high suspicion of basilar skull fracture, a nasogastric tube should not be inserted because it could be passed through the fracture directly into the brain. A Foley catheter should not be inserted if the MOI suggests bladder rupture or trauma.

Mechanisms of injury are divided into two major categories: blunt and penetrating. Blunt trauma is defined as injuries without communication with the environment and penetrating as injuries where the tissue has been pierced.

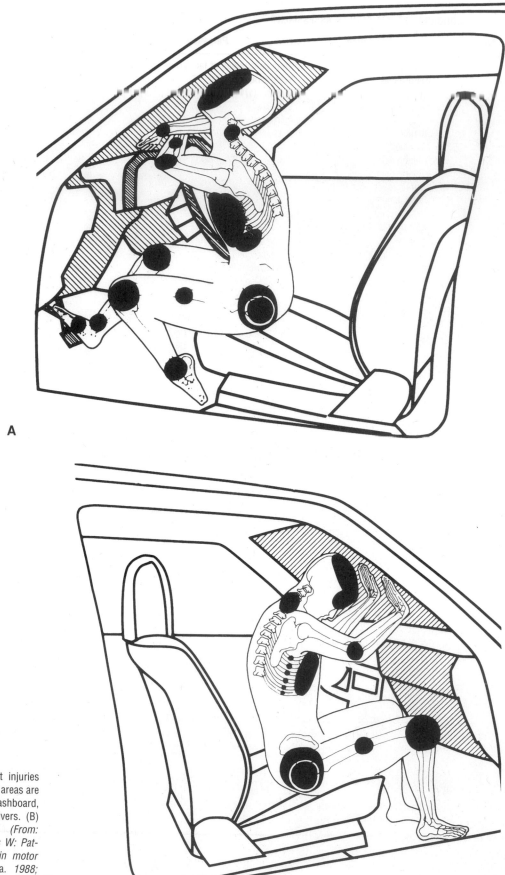

A

B

Figure 20–3. Major areas of impact injuries (solid dark areas). The "hostile" contact areas are striped (windshield, steering column, dashboard, and foot pedals). (A) Unrestrained drivers. (B) Unrestrained front seat passengers. *(From: Daffner R, Deeb Z, Lupetin A, Rothfus W: Patterns of high speed impact injuries in motor vehicle occupants. Journal of Trauma. 1988; 28:499–500.)*

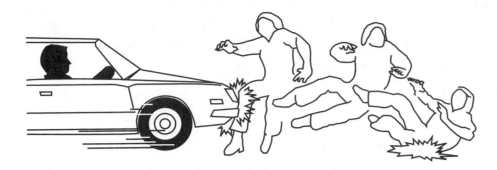

Figure 20–4. Waddell's triad in adult pedestrians. Impact (1) with the bumper or hood and lateral rotation (2) produce injury to the upper and/or lower leg (3). *(From: Weigelt J, Klein J: Mechanism of injury. In Cardona VD, Hurn PD, Mason PJB, Scanlon AM, Veise-Berry SW (eds.): Trauma nursing from resuscitation through rehabilitation. Philadelphia: WB Saunders, 1994, p. 94.)*

Blunt trauma usually results from motor vehicle or motorcycle collisions, assaults, falls, contact sports injuries, or pedestrian/vehicle collisions. Assessment strategies useful in diagnosing blunt traumatic injuries include: physical assessment, x-ray, angiography, diagnostic peritoneal lavage, CT scanning, and blood count and blood chemistry analysis. Penetrating trauma is commonly caused by bullets or knives in urban areas and by farm or industrial equipment in rural areas. Penetrating injuries are easier to diagnose because they are more easily identified. However, blunt trauma is frequently more life-threatening because multiple organ systems may be injured and diagnosis takes longer.

Mechanism of injury assessment is critical for accurate patient assessment, preventing complications, and monitoring for secondary injuries. Application of this knowledge will decrease morbidity and mortality in the critical care setting. The case study below presents an injured patient with typical multiple trauma from a car crash.

Social Impact of Trauma

Trauma patients typically experience a cascade of common physiologic and psychosocial responses to trauma. Although each patient presents as an individual with unique concerns, trauma patients as a group are very different from other hospitalized patients. They have a higher incidence of substance abuse, are often under the age of 44, and typically receive minimal to no preoperative teaching due to the emergent nature of many injuries. Family members experience the trauma as a major crisis.

AT THE BEDSIDE

Joe was driving his brother home from a Super Bowl Party at their eldest brother's home. Joe has a high school education and works as a construction contractor. He is self-employed and does not have health insurance. He is married with one small child. His wife did not return to work after the birth of their child 3 years ago. This is his fourth "driving while intoxicated" (DWI) incident, but the first where anyone was injured.

PHYSIOLOGIC CONSEQUENCES OF TRAUMA

Traumatic injury creates fractures, wounds, and crushed tissues that may not be readily visible. Once the ABCs or primary trauma survey is completed and management begins, the head-to-toe in-depth assessment, known as the secondary survey, is initiated as depicted in the case study below. This is where evidence accumulates for the detailed diagnosis of multiple trauma and definitive care is planned. A high index of suspicion is needed to link patterns of trauma, mechanism of injury, and physiologic consequences. The critical care nurse assists in stabilizing the patient with fluids and ventilatory and circulatory support, and provides emotional support during diagnostic tests or while rushing the patient to the operating room.

Priorities include supporting tissue oxygenation through hemodynamic stability and ventilatory control. Pain and anxiety are treated at the same time as wounds are assessed, and positioning is maximized for optimal oxygenation and comfort. Traumatic injury unleashes a cascade of vasoactive mediators, such as various hormones, prostaglandins, and cytokines, that serve a protective func-

AT THE BEDSIDE

Primary Nurse: "When I heard I was getting Joe, a motor vehicle trauma admission with multiple injuries, the first things I asked was what was the mechanism of injury, was he wearing a seat belt, and did he lose consciousness? When I learned that his brother died in the accident, I knew first to expect major injuries due to the probable force of the trauma and secondly, what a very emotional crisis this will be for the family I expect to meet soon. With the potential for major chest trauma, I know that Joe will likely be on a ventilator, have chest tubes, and need a great deal of pain medication. The most important thing I plan to do as I admit Joe is a very systematic head-to-toe assessment, making sure that I understand the injuries and their severity, and that nothing was missed in the resuscitation. Missed injuries are actually pretty common when multiple systems are involved, and I need to share my initial assessment with the trauma team."

AT THE BEDSIDE
▶ *Trauma: Secondary Survey*

System	Secondary Assessment	Injury/Test Result
Neurological	Glasgow Coma Score = 8 Pupils 3 cm, sluggish to react to light Does not follow commands or have spontaneous movement Strong gag and corneal reflex Stabilized on backboard with cervical collar in place	Head CT was negative for any injuries, bleeding, or fractures
Respiratory	Respiratory rate 32/minute, shallow and labored Arterial blood gas: PaO_2 76 mm Hg, $PaCO_2$ 50 mm Hg, pH 7.25, SaO_2 82% Chest x-ray taken	Fractured ribs 3–7 on right Hemopneumothorax on right Bilateral infiltrates
Cardiovascular	Heart rate 127 beats/minute Blood pressure 86/40 mm Hg Color pale Rhythm: sinus tachycardia with premature ventricular contractions Pulses weak in both arms and left leg; no popliteal, dorsalis pedal, or posterior tibial pulses on right leg	12-lead ECG: mild ischemia leads V_4–V_6 (lateral leads) Cardiac contusion
Gastrointestinal	Abdomen round and firm to touch No gross deformities, lacerations, or markings noted Nasogastric tube placed with bile drainage and some blood present DPL performed	DPL grossly positive Exploratory laparotomy performed and lacerated liver was repaired and a ruptured spleen removed
Extremity	Laceration on center forehead, 7 cm and bleeding Right thigh edema, firm and warm to touch Bilateral knee superficial lacerations	Laceration on forehead required six sutures Knee laceration did not require sutures Right femur complex fracture; surgery for open reduction and internal fixation; placed in skeletal traction
Laboratory	Hemoglobin/hematocrit 6 mg/dl and 18% Blood alcohol content 150 mg/dl CPK 1258 MB bands 25%	Resuscitation in ED and OR 10 units PRBC 7 units FFP 6 units Platelets 5 L of LR

tion via the stress response. However, in severe multisystem trauma, these same mediators that help the trauma patient survive the initial injury may prolong the stress response and contribute to complications and even death. This response is best limited by enhancing the patient's healing ability through attention to physiologic and psychosocial care.

Consequences of traumatic injury include blood loss, tissue destruction, intense pain due to damaged tissues, and altered oxygenation and ventilation. Fluid balance, airway management, aggressive pain control, and wound care are major priorities. Stabilization of fractures and surgical repair of injured organs are accomplished in the early operative period. The priority for care in the early phases of trauma is to optimize tissue oxygenation. Although patients

in critical care settings frequently have more than one injured system, a focus on one body system at a time assists in providing an organized management plan.

COMMON INJURIES IN THE CRITICALLY ILL TRAUMA PATIENT

Chest Trauma

Etiology and Pathophysiology

Blunt trauma to the chest commonly includes injuries created by fractured ribs and crushed or punctured lung tissue. Mechanism of injury is frequently a motor vehicle crash

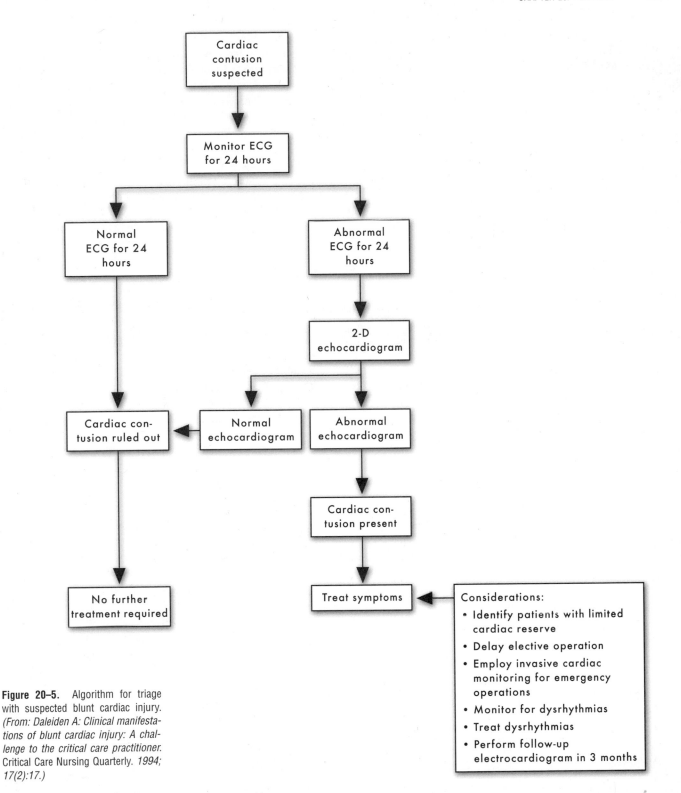

Figure 20–5. Algorithm for triage with suspected blunt cardiac injury. *(From: Daleiden A: Clinical manifestations of blunt cardiac injury: A challenge to the critical care practitioner. Critical Care Nursing Quarterly. 1994; 17(2):17.)*

where the torso is crushed between the steering wheel and the front seat, especially in the unbelted driver. A hemopneumothorax, blood and air in the pleural space, may result, requiring the insertion of chest tubes. Fractures to the first and second ribs are considered most serious because of the degree of force and the potential for damage to the great vessels. An initial chest x-ray demonstrating a widened mediastinum often confirms this suspicion, and the patient requires further tests, such as an aortagram, and perhaps an emergent trip to the operating room for repair of the aorta.

Fractured lower ribs can damage the liver or spleen, while upper rib fractures puncture lung tissue. All patients with rib fractures are suspected of having a pulmonary contusion which leads to alveolar capillary membrane disruption. Depending on the severity of the contusion, hypoxemia occurs, which may worsen several days after the injury, progressing to respiratory failure and adult respiratory distress syndrome (ARDS).

Clinical presentation includes dyspnea, tachypnea, and chest pain. A flail chest may occur when three or more adjacent ribs are fractured in two segments, creating a "floating segment" that may puncture the lung. Diagnosis of a flail chest is made by observing inward movement of the chest during inspiration and outward movement during expiration. This is best assessed when the patient is breathing spontaneously. The paradoxical motion of the chest wall creates hypoxemia from a decreased tidal volume and atelectasis. Because patients are unable to take a deep breath without pain, pneumonia and respiratory failure may ensue. Cardiac contusion results from damage to the myocardium without involving the coronary arteries and may occur with blunt chest trauma. Diagnosis is based on ECG changes suggestive of ischemia, elevation of CPK-MB isoenzymes, and by the use of echocardiography (Figure 20–5). These tests do not always demonstrate changes, but cardiac contusion always should be anticipated in major trauma to the chest. Arrhythmias such as sinus tachycardia, atrial fibrillation, and premature ventricular contractions are the chief concern in myocardial contusion in the first 12 hours after injury.

Patient Needs and Principles of Management

Management of the patient with trauma to the chest includes four basic principles: ventilatory support to prevent hypoxemia, monitoring chest tubes for drainage, providing optimal pain control, and positioning to promote adequate oxygenation (Tables 20–4 and 20–5).

▶ Ventilatory Support

Management of thoracic trauma emphasizes assessment of chest structure and function using physical assessment and diagnostic tests. Severe and multiple rib fractures with large pulmonary contusions are often treated with mechanical ventilation to stabilize the chest and prevent the persistent hypoxemia from the paradoxical breathing of a flail chest. Care of the patient with flail chest includes ventilator support to stabilize the chest wall.

▶ Monitoring Chest Tubes

Chest tubes are inserted for patients with chest wall injuries and punctured lung tissue. Care of the patient with chest tubes includes observing for drainage characteristics, signs of a resolving air leak, and prevention of infection with meticulous attention to sterile dressings. Trauma patients may have draining wounds adjacent to the chest tube site and, therefore, ensuring sterile dressing changes as needed is essential.

▶ Pain Control

Pain control, both systemic and local, is needed and may even preempt the need for mechanical ventilation in patients with milder degrees of chest trauma. For example, when patients are able to breathe deeply and cough without severe chest discomfort, smaller airways remain open, atelectasis is avoided, and healing can occur. Patient-controlled analgesia, epidural narcotic infusions, or local anesthetics can be used for aggressive pain control in the trauma patient.

Patients report that chest tubes, suctioning, and turning are all more painful than caregivers imagine. Attacking a patient's pain aggressively is not only a humane concern, but it allows the patient to focus energy on healing. Pain

TABLE 20–4. SUMMARY OF TRAUMA TIPS FOR SELECTED INJURIES

Chest	Abdominal	Musculoskeletal
Watch for flail chest	Use the enteral route for nutritional support within 24 to 48 hours after injury when possible	Early operation for stabilizing fractures decreases blood loss
Administer appropriate pain control		Monitor for compartment syndrome
Watch for worsening hypoxemia due to pulmonary contusion days after injury	Infection may be inevitable	Assess neurovascular status of all extremities at frequent intervals
	Salvage of the spleen when possible is advocated to support immune function	
Position patient with the good lung down	Reoperation is often necessary to explore/debride	Pain control using PCA if possible abscesses
Monitor for pulmonary or fat embolism	If pain not resolving, further bleeding or an abscess may be developing	Mobilize patient out of bed at earliest point in time
	Observe for pancreatitis	

Patient Needs and Principles of Management, Cont.

can be controlled through narcotics that act centrally, locally, or regionally, and through drugs that act at the periphery to interrupt the painful stimulus (see Chapter 7, Pain Management in Critical Care). Nonpharmacologic approaches can also operate at the central level through cognitive distraction or relaxation, and peripherally by using positioning or application of heat and cold (see Chapter 8, Alternative Therapies in Critical Care).

Patient-controlled analgesia (PCA) is designed for the awake patient with an injury to provide control over the dose needed to relieve pain. Epidural PCA is used with success in patients with rib fractures and may eliminate the need for mechanical ventilation, an important benefit in older trauma patients. Careful monitoring of the patient's response to PCA is needed to ensure the technology is adequate. For example, an epidural catheter may migrate and not provide pain relief at all. A patient's report of pain relief needs to be requested by the nurse at hourly intervals initially as it is the only reliable measurement for pain.

A variety of nonpharmacologic pain-reducing strategies are useful in patients with trauma, and the nurse needs to combine these with drug therapy for maximal gain. Because narcotics have side effects, combining them with a nonsteroidal antiinflammatory agent (Toradol/ketorolac) and a cognitive intervention may offer the patient the best pain reduction possible. Cognitive interventions for pain include relaxation, guided imagery, music therapy, and hypnosis, among others. Clear documentation of what strategies or combinations work best for the individual is needed. This requires an established communication system between patient and nurse. Anxiety and sleeplessness contribute to the pain response and should be addressed by asking the patients how they typically try to relax and by eliminating as much environmental noise as possible. Encouraging rest and sleep and limiting patient interruptions will provide a better healing environment.

▶ Positioning

Early mobilization assists in promoting oxygenation. This includes positioning the patient in and out of bed. Positioning of the good lung down is especially important to maximize oxygenation if there is unilateral lung disease or injury to one side of the chest. Knowledge of daily chest x-ray results is essential for accurate positioning of the patient. An example of how the concept of therapeutic positioning can be used by the nurse is to position the patient and observe pulse oximetry, peak inspiratory pressures, and if applicable, SvO_2 data for improvement.

TABLE 20–5. FIFTEEN CARDINAL RULES IN MULTIPLE TRAUMA

1. All patients with head and facial trauma have a cervical spine injury.
2. All patients with an altered level of consciousness have a head injury.
3. All young, healthy patients lacking a palpable radial pulse are in shock.
4. Hypotension, tachycardia, and pallor indicate bleeding into the chest, abdomen, or pelvis if no obvious external injuries are present.
5. All patients with chest trauma are presumed critical.
6. All patients with distended neck veins have a pericardial tamponade or tension pneumothorax.
7. Penetrating wounds at or below the nipple line involve the chest and abdomen.
8. Systolic blood pressure is estimated to be:
   Palpable radial pulse = 80 to 100 mm Hg
   Palpable femoral pulse = 70 mm Hg
   Palpable carotid pulse = 60 mm Hg
9. Presence of multiple rib fractures increases the likelihood of other injuries and complications.
10. Do not place intravenous lines in limbs with soft tissue damage.
11. Do not insert a nasogastric tube in a patient with a basilar skull fracture.
12. A Foley catheter should not be inserted in a suspected ruptured bladder. A rectal exam should be performed before a Foley catheter insertion.
13. Treatment of a pregnant trauma victim is directed at the mother as you are more likely to save the baby if the mother survives.
14. Mechanism of injury should guide investigation of injuries after ABCs.
15. Fluid resuscitation is the primary treatment for most traumatic injuries.

Abdominal Trauma

Etiology and Pathophysiology

Trauma to the abdomen may occur to organs in three distinct abdominal regions: peritoneal cavity, retroperitoneum, and pelvis. Trauma to the spleen or liver, peritoneal organs, is diagnosed by pain in the awake patient or by positive DPL. Retroperitoneal trauma occurs when the pancreas or kidneys are injured and cannot be discovered with DPL. Bladder trauma is an example of pelvic area trauma and can accompany fractures of the pelvis. Depending on the mechanism of injury, identification of the injured organs is accomplished through history, taking serial physical examinations, CT scans, and DPL where appropriate. Trauma to the spleen is one of the most frequently encountered

abdominal injuries after a motor vehicle crash. Depending on severity of splenic injury, interventions range from nonoperative observation and bedrest with mild lacerations to removal of a massively ruptured spleen. Liver trauma runs the spectrum from minor injury to severe laceration requiring operative repair and packing.

Presenting signs and symptoms in abdominal trauma include pain and hypovolemia, as massive blood loss can occur. Kehr's sign is severe left shoulder pain at times accompanying a ruptured spleen. Complications due to abdominal trauma are directly linked to the function of the gastrointestinal tract and include metabolic/nutritional alterations, infections such as peritonitis, and pancreatitis. Patients may require extensive dressing changes if the wound is open or frequent trips to the operating suite.

Patient Needs and Principles of Management

Selected principles of caring for the patient with abdominal trauma include: monitoring for bleeding and infection, providing optimum wound care, and initiating early (within 24 to 48 hours) nutritional support (Tables 20–4 and 20–5).

▶ Monitoring for Infection

Salvage of the spleen by performing a splenorrhaphy, repair of the spleen, or watchful waiting is increasing in popularity. The goal is to allow the spleen to heal and preserve the valuable immunoprotective function. Overwhelming postsplenectomy sepsis can occur as a serious complication years after removal of the spleen and efforts to optimally care for the damaged spleen, especially in children, are warranted. If splenectomy is indicated due to massive injury, patients are given polyvalent pneumococcal vaccine within 72 hours after surgery to prevent infection due to pneumococci. Management also includes monitoring for rebleeding during 3 days of bedrest and preventing the complications of immobility.

▶ Wound Care

Wound care for the patient with a large abdominal wound is directed by the type of wound (open or closed) and the

degree of contamination. Keep drainage away from skin using drain care products as appropriate. Consult an enterostomal therapist for complex draining wounds.

▶ Nutritional Support

Enteral nutrition is encouraged whenever possible at the earliest time after injury. Even a small amount of nutrition delivered via tube feeding to the gut is believed to limit the translocation of bacteria from the bowel, the suspected cause of many trauma infections. A variety of metabolic derangements in the hypermetabolic trauma patient make nutritional

TABLE 20–6. METABOLIC SUPPORT RECOMMENDATIONS FOR TRAUMA PATIENTS IN THE INTENSIVE CARE UNIT

General Nutrient Recommendations
Total calories: 25 to 30 kcal/kg/day
Glucose: up to 5 g/kg/day
Long-chain omega-6 fatty acid triglycerides: 1 to 1.5 g/kg/day
Protein: 1.5 to 2 g/kg/day to achieve nitrogen equilibrium; the modified amino acids are more efficient

Route
Early enteral feeds with a feeding tube distal to the pylorus are most effective
Use of a formula designed for immunonutrition is most efficacious

Monitor Effectiveness and Complications for 5 to 7 Days
Nitrogen balance
Rising visceral proteins
Blood urea nitrogen < 120 mg/dl
Blood sugar 150 to 200 mg/dl
Respiratory quotient < 0.9 (when necessary)
Liver and renal function

From: Goins WA, Wiles CE, Cerra FB: Pharmacology, monitoring, and nutritional support. Critical Care Clinics. *1993;9:689–713.*

AT THE BEDSIDE

Primary Nurse: "Joe has been in the unit for 48 hours now and the trauma team is debating when to start feeding. The nutritionist has calculated his energy needs and even though he has minimal bowel sounds, the plan is to slowly begin feeding Joe today using a feeding tube into the duodenum."

support an early imperative (Table 20–6). Insertion and maintenance of small-bowel feeding tubes, percutaneous gastrostomy tubes, or jejunostomy tubes is often required after injury until the patient can be orally fed. Total parenteral nutrition is recommended only if the gastrointestinal tract is unable to tolerate adequate nutrients. Accurate nutritional assessment in collaboration with the nutritionist is essential, as trauma patients are at risk of complications from overfeeding as well as underfeeding. Diarrhea, inappropriate withholding of tube feedings, and the potential for increased aspiration are issues that need to be addressed for trauma patients.

Musculoskeletal Trauma

Etiology and Pathophysiology

Trauma to the musculoskeletal system is the most common type of injury. Patients in the critical care setting with extremity or pelvic fractures often have other injuries. Motor vehicle trauma, falls, sports injuries, and industrial trauma are all causes of musculoskeletal trauma. Motorcycle victims frequently have severe fractures with extensive soft tissue damage. Massive blood loss, edema of tissues, tissue destruction, and pain are all common features.

Compartment syndrome is a serious complication of extremity trauma as a result of contused tissue swelling in a specific muscle compartment. This may lead to blood loss and nerve compression in the area. Muscle compartments are located in the forearm, leg, hand, foot, and thigh. As pain may or may not be present, measuring compartment pressures with a specialized needle is indicated for major fractures. Even open fractures may have significantly increased compartment pressures (normal pressure 0 to 8 mm Hg). A fasciotomy entails opening the skin and fascia to relieve the pressure in a muscle compartment and is the treatment of choice to treat and prevent compartment syndrome.

Patient Needs and Principles of Management

Management of extremity trauma focuses on early stabilization of fractures to prevent further bleeding and increased incidence of pulmonary emboli, pain control to promote mobility, and assessment of neurovascular status (Tables 20–4 and 20–5).

Fractures are repaired early after a traumatic injury to decrease further bleeding and to limit pulmonary complications. External fixation is used for pelvic fractures and lower limb fractures. Frequent sensation, movement, and vascular checks on affected extremities are essential. If the presence of pulses is in doubt, Doppler ultrasound should be used at the bedside.

Pain control is best achieved with an individualized strategy of medications and nonpharmacologic therapies. Patients respond best when strict attention is paid to pain control and their own unique coping style is used. Patients are expected to move in bed and get out of bed as soon as possible after an injury. Titrated pain medication is required to achieve this goal using PCA optimally or continuous infusion. Nurses need to spend time determining patient anxieties regarding the trauma and promote adequate sleep and rest. Sleep deprivation from a noisy environment, constant worry, and needless pain only make the patient perceive a more intense pain.

AT THE BEDSIDE

Joe's wife: "I am really worried about Joe—he seems to be in a lot of pain and I know he is upset and guilty about the accident because of his drinking. He wrote me notes, because he has that tube in his mouth, that he is afraid to go to sleep because he has nightmares. Luckily, the nurses let me stay at the bedside as long as I want, but I wish there was something else I could do. They asked me what he likes to do at home to relax. One nurse suggested that we try playing some music that he likes during his dressing changes in addition to his pain medication."

COMPLICATIONS OF TRAUMATIC INJURY IN SEVERE MULTISYSTEM TRAUMA

The key to survival for patients with multiple trauma is to limit the extent of complications experienced and increase the delivery of oxygen to the tissues during the initial phase of trauma. When oxygen and blood flow are provided at supernormal levels, the frequency of complications decreases. Heart rate and blood pressure are not considered adequate parameters to judge the effectiveness of resuscitation, as they indicate only the body's compensation to the stress of trauma and not real-time tissue oxygenation. Appropriate measurement of successful oxygen delivery requires pulmonary artery catheterization. Variables to assess for adequate tissue oxygenation include oxygenation transport, delivery, and utilization. Serum lactate is an additional diagnostic indicator of the adequacy of tissue oxygenation.

Common complications of trauma are infection, adult respiratory distress syndrome (ARDS), and systemic inflammatory response syndrome (SIRS) (see Chapter 13, Respiratory System, and Chapter 14, Multisystem Problems). Patients with SIRS experience a persistent inflammatory response to a stressor such as multiple trauma. This can lead to acute lung injury and multiple organ dysfunction syndrome. Delivering supernormal oxygen to the tissues by maintaining increased blood flow is believed to decrease the incidence of an oxygen debt and these often lethal complications. Oxygen debt occurs when resuscitation is delayed or inadequate and refers to the body's unmet and continuous need for oxygen. Similar to a bank debt, survival without consequences only can occur when the debt is repaid with interest. Providing an elevated or supernormal oxygen delivery to the tissues repays this debt interest.

To achieve adequate oxygen delivery to the tissues, massive fluid resuscitation and/or transfusion are needed. Trauma patients are at risk of experiencing several complications after massive transfusion. Massive transfusion is defined as the infusion of more than 10 units of whole blood or packed red blood cells within 24 hours, replacing the patient's total blood volume. Knowledge of and agreement on therapeutic endpoints, for example an oxygen delivery of greater than 600 ml/minute/m$_2$, is crucial for the entire health care team. The same treatment, massive fluid/blood replacement, believed to prevent the complications of an oxygen debt, has specific consequences the clinician needs to monitor. Coagulopathy, acidosis, electrolyte imbalances, pulmonary dysfunction, and edema are potential complications associated with massive fluid/blood replacement.

ARDS

The complications of ARDS, infections, and SIRS are interrelated in the trauma patient but require specific monitoring and treatment. Patients with trauma have an increased incidence of the severe respiratory dysfunction known as ARDS. Precipitating factors for ARDS include massive fluid resuscitation, a significant lung injury, and an infectious process, among others. Patients with rib fractures and large pulmonary contusions often develop respiratory failure and ARDS.

Standard treatment for ARDS includes mechanical ventilation, oxygen titrated to maintain Pao$_2$ above 60 mm Hg, and positive and expiratory pressure (PEEP) (see Chapter 13, Respiratory System). ARDS treatment in the trauma patient differs from other critically ill patients in that the positioning for optimal oxygenation with multiple injuries may be a challenge. For example, the patient with an unstable pelvic fracture, or the patient with bilateral lower extremity fractures, may have difficulty turning.

Infections

Trauma patients are at high risk of developing an infection due to the nature of the injury, the nonsterile conditions in which invasive devices may have been initially placed, and the multiple invasive techniques necessary for trauma management. All invasive devices placed in the emergency department should be replaced within the first 24 hours. Fever and identification of a source of infection are variable and may not be present in the trauma patient, especially the elderly patient. Meticulous attention to sterile technique and hand washing is essential.

SIRS

Management of SIRS requires knowledge of the underlying inflammatory process (see Chapter 14, Multisystem Problems). Mediators from injured tissue may lead to a sustained state of intense systemic inflammation. Assessment criteria for SIRS includes two or more of the following: temperature greater than 38° or less than 36° C, heart rate greater than 90 beats/minute, respiratory rate greater than 20/minute, Paco$_2$ less than 32 mm Hg, and white blood cell count greater than 12,000/mm^3 or less than 4000/mm^3. Other cardiopulmonary changes typical in SIRS include high cardiac output, decreased systemic vascular resistance, and elevated oxygen consumption.

Goals for managing the patient with SIRS are to provide the essential materials necessary for maintaining body processes such as oxygenation and nutrition, limit known stressors such as pain, and support organ system integrity. Inotropic support to maximize the heart's ability to generate the work needed to sustain the patient through SIRS is often needed.

The individual's response to SIRS may be prolonged and destructive, leading to a common problem in severe trauma, multiple organ dysfunction syndrome. Patients may require maximal ventilatory support and hemodialysis, for example. Mortality remains high for this syndrome, requiring increased attention to prevention of early oxygen debts. In trauma care, what the critical care team does in the first 24 hours of injury often determines survival.

PSYCHOLOGIC CONSEQUENCES OF TRAUMA

The clinician's ability to understand, accept, and intervene in the patient's psychologic response to the traumatic event may assist in the successful return of the patient to optimal functioning. The presence of clinicians who are calmly supportive and empathetic encourages the patient to do the hard work of recovery from trauma even during the critical care phase of care. Common responses to trauma include anxiety, fear, grief, loss, guilt, and sleeplessness.

Fear begins immediately as the awake trauma patient is transported from the scene via ambulance or air. Fear is related to the unknown, the specifics of the injuries, and impact on the patient's future, including body image, family, and career. Loss typifies the experience of trauma and can be characterized as loss of physical functioning, loss of quality of life, or even loss of significant others due to the traumatic event. Guilt may ensue as the patient may perceive responsibility for the event, and this can be overwhelming. Patient responses to guilt may include a spectrum from withdrawing to increased agitation. The provision of support and information is essential to assist the patient. While providing competent technologic care, clinicians should make interpersonal connections through eye contact, sitting at the bedside and encouraging the patient to communicate through appropriate methods, and offering opportunities to be with the patient as needed.

Fear creates anxiety in the trauma patient, and unrelieved pain may worsen anxiety. As the intense monitoring and frequent care interruptions proceed in the critical care environment, sleep becomes impossible. A vicious cycle is thus initiated whereby sleeplessness leads to an increased perception of pain, which in turn creates needles anxiety and inhibits sleep. The importance of viewing these responses as cyclical emphasizes that the critical care nurse may intervene anywhere in the cycle of responses and make a major impact on all three. For example, providing pain-relieving strategies that permit sleep will automatically decrease anxiety. A focus on information sharing may ease the patient's mind so that sleep can occur and pain perception will decrease. The nurse has a significant role in intervening to stop this vicious cycle through a variety of holistic strategies.

All families of trauma patients experience a crisis. Families may have no idea of how to act or what the health care team expects of them. Clinicians have a key role in providing the right amount of support and information to meet family needs, and in identifying family coping mechanisms. Knowing the phases of family emotional response and suggested interventions is useful (Table 20–7). Early assessment of family system structure, relationship process, and family functioning are keys to effective management of the psychosocial needs of the patient and family. Getting to know and work with family members in trauma care is essential and can be best facilitated with a flexible visiting policy where family members are wanted and expected by the patient and the nurse.

TABLE 10–7. PHASES AND MANIFESTATIONS OF STRESS AND NURSING INTERVENTIONS FOR FAMILIES OF TRAUMA PATIENTS

Phase	Manifestions	Interventions
High anxiety	Restlessness Fainting Nausea High-pitched voice	Encourage ventilation of feelings Provide accurate information
Denial	Families commonly state, "Everything will be all right" Refusing to discuss reality	Reiterate the facts of the situation
Anger	Verbal abuse directed toward health care staff	Active listening Allow ventilation of angry feelings Help to refocus on the real cause of anger
Remorse	Elements of guilt and sorrow "If only" stage	Listen to family's expressions of remorse Interject reality
Grief	Intense period of sadness Crying	Encourage flow of tears Provide empathetic gestures such as silent physical closeness, holding a trembling hand, embracing limp shoulders

From: Hopkins AG: The trauma nurse's role with families in crisis. Critical Care Nurse. 1994;14(2):37; and Epperson M: Families in sudden crisis: Process and intervention in a critical care center. Social Work in Health Care. 1977;2:265–273.

Selected Bibliography

General Trauma

Abou-Khalil B, Scalea TM, Trooskin SZ, Henry SM, Hitchcock R: Hemodynamic responses to shock in young trauma patients: Need for invasive monitoring. *Critical Care Medicine.* 1994; 22:633–639.

ACCP-SCCM Consensus Conference Committee: Definitions for sepsis and organ failure and guidelines for the use of innovative therapies in sepsis. *Chest.* 1992; 101:1644–1655.

Davis A: Trauma. In Kinney M, Packa D, Dunbar S (eds.): *AACN's clinical reference for critical-care nursing.* 3rd ed. St. Louis, MO: CV Mosby, 1993, pp. 1243–1282.

Fontaine DK: Physical, personal, and cognitive responses to trauma. *Critical Care Nursing Clinics.* 1989;1:11–22.

Prentice D, Ahrens T: Pulmonary complications of trauma. *Critical Care Nursing Quarterly.* 1994;17(2):24–33.

Romito RA: Early administration of enteral nutrients in critically ill patients. *AACN Clinical Issues.* 1995;6:242–256.

Scanlon AM: Psychosocial responses of the human spirit: The journey of trauma. In Cardona VD, Hurn PD, Mason PJB, Scanlon AM, Veise-Berry SW (eds.): *Trauma nursing from resuscitation through rehabilitation.* Philadelphia: WB Saunders, 1994, pp. 179–198.

Sparger G, Shea S, Selfridge J: Patients with trauma. In Clochesy J, Breu C, Cardin S, Rudy E, Whittaker, A: *Critical care nursing*. Philadelphia: WB Saunders, 1993, pp. 1219–1244.

Von Rueden KT, Dunham CM: Sequelae of massive fluid resuscitation in trauma patients. *Critical Care Nursing Clinics*. 1994; (6).160 170.

Wachtel T L: Critical care concepts in the management of abdominal trauma. *Critical Care Nursing Quarterly*. 1994;17(2):34–50.

Mechanism of Injury

Cayten G, Stahl W, Agarwal N, Murphy J: Analyses of preventable deaths by mechanism of injury among 13,500 trauma admissions. *Annals of Surgery*. 1991;214(4):510–521.

Daffner R, Deeb Z, Lupetin A, Rothfus W: Patterns of high speed impact injuries in motor vehicle occupants. *Journal of Trauma*. 1988;28:494–501.

Halpern J: Mechanisms and patterns of trauma. *Journal of Emergency Nursing*. 1989;15(9):380–388.

Knopp R, Yanagi A, Kallsen G, Geehring L: Mechanism of injury and anatomic injury as criteria for prehospital trauma triage. *Annals of Emergency Medicine*. 1988;17:895–902.

Weigelt J, Klein J: Mechanism of injury. In Cardona VD, Hurn PD, Mason PJB, Scanlon AM, Veise-Berry SW (eds.): *Trauma nursing from resuscitation through rehabilitation*. Philadelphia: WB Saunders, 1994, pp. 91–113.

Advanced Concepts in Caring for the Critically Ill Patient and Family

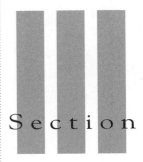

Section III

Advanced ECG Concepts

▶ **Knowledge Competencies**

1. Identify ECG characteristics and treatment approaches for each of the following advanced arrhythmias:

    - Supraventricular tachycardias
    - Wide QRS beats and rhythms

2. Using the 12-lead electrocardiogram, determine the following:

    - Bundle branch blocks
    - Axis of the heart
    - Patterns of myocardial ischemia, injury, and infarct

3. Identify ECG characteristics of single- and dual-chamber pacemakers during normal and abnormal functioning.

■ *What Heals: Enhancing Cardiovascular Health with Interpersonal Communication*

Studies evaluating the association between coronary-prone (type A) behavior pattern and coronary heart disease (CHD) have focused on cardiovascular reactivity. Cardiovascular reactivity represents the acute change in a cardiovascular variable (e.g., heart rate [HR] or blood pressure [BP] that is attributed to a behavioral stimulus. Exaggerated and chronic cardiovascular reactivity to various types of stressors among CHD and hypertensive patients have been implicated in the cause and progression of the disease. Rapid speech is associated with coronary-prone behavior patterns and with increased cardiovascular responses. On the other hand, social support, a known contributor to cardiovascular health, acts as a buffer of psychologic and physical stressors. An essential component of social support is interpersonal communication (e.g., speech).

Recent research has demonstrated the striking consequences of verbalization on cardiovascular responses. Calm conversations or reading aloud can cause BP and HR to increase by 50% within 1 minute of the verbalization and to fall back to baseline 1 minute after cessation of speech. Modifying one component of type A behavior, rapid speech, can cause significant decreases in cardiovascular reactivity for both coronary-prone and noncoronary-prone patients during verbal communication.

Modifying extreme reactivity during verbal communication, a common daily activity, may have important health benefits. Thus, as clinicians, we need to assist patients in developing and expressing social support in ways that enhance rather than diminish cardiovascular health. For our acute cardiac patients, we need to make the time to listen to our patients' concerns without giving the impression that we are sprinting through our conversations. We can encourage patients to speak at a slower pace and try to reduce stressful conversations, foster short dialogues that include periods of listening (allowing cardiovascular responses to return to baseline), and ensure periods of restful silence. Teaching patients relaxation techniques and deep breathing is an essential intervention. We can use HR and BP monitors as biofeedback equipment to provide the patient with cardiovascular readings to demonstrate the effects of

their rapid versus slow speech. With such feedback, patients can learn to recognize not only the effects of their verbalizations on their body but also to alter the rate of their speech.

CEG & BMD

From: Guzzetta CE: Comments. Capsules and Comments in Critical Care Nursing. *1995;3:148–149.*

THE 12-LEAD ELECTROCARDIOGRAM (ECG)

Introduction

The 12-lead ECG records electrical activity as it spreads through the heart from 12 different leads, which are in turn recorded by electrodes placed on the arms and legs and in specific spots on the chest. Each lead represents a different "view" of the heart and consists of two electrodes. A *bipolar* lead has two poles—one positive and one negative. A *unipolar* lead has one positive pole and a reference pole that is a point in the center of the chest that is mathematically determined by the ECG machine. The standard 12-lead ECG consists of six frontal plane limb leads that record electrical activity traveling up/down and right/left in the heart, and six precordial leads that record electrical activity in the horizontal plane traveling anterior/posterior and right/left. Limb leads are recorded by electrodes placed on the arms and legs, while precordial leads are recorded by electrodes placed on the chest (Figure 21–1).

A camera analogy makes the 12-lead ECG easier to understand. Each lead of the ECG represents a picture of the electrical activity in the heart taken by the camera. In any lead, the positive electrode is the recording electrode or the camera lens. The negative electrode tells the camera which way to "shoot" its picture and determines the direction in which the positive electrode will record. When the positive electrode sees electrical activity traveling toward it, it records an upright deflection on the ECG. When the positive electrode sees electrical activity traveling away from it, it records a negative deflection (Figure 21–2). If the electrical activity travels perpendicular to a positive electrode, either a diphasic deflection or no activity is recorded. The ECG records three bipolar frontal plane leads (lead I, lead II, and lead III) and three unipolar frontal plane leads (aVR, aVL, and aVF). In addition, there are six unipolar precordial leads: V_1, V_2, V_3, V_4, V_5, and V_6.

The three bipolar frontal plane leads are illustrated in Figure 21–3A. In each lead, the camera represents the positive pole of the lead. In lead I, the positive electrode is on the left arm and the negative electrode is on the right arm. Any electrical activity in the heart that travels toward the positive electrode (camera lens) on the left arm is recorded as an upright deflection and any traveling away from it is recorded as a negative deflection. In lead II, the positive electrode is on the left leg and the negative electrode is on the right arm. Any electrical activity traveling toward the left leg electrode (camera lens) is recorded as an upright deflection and any traveling away from it toward the right arm electrode is recorded as a negative deflection. In lead III, the positive electrode is on the left leg and the negative electrode is on the left arm. Any electrical activity coming toward the left leg electrode (camera lens) is recorded upright and any traveling away from it toward the left arm is recorded negative. The view of the heart by the bipolar leads can be compared to a wide-angle camera lens.

The three unipolar frontal plane leads, aVR, aVL, and aVF, are illustrated in Figure 21–3B. The camera represents the location of the positive electrode: on the right shoulder for aVR, on the left shoulder for aVL, and at the foot for aVF. The "negative end" of the unipolar lead is a reference spot in the center of the chest that is mathematically determined by the ECG machine. The same principles apply to unipolar leads: any electrical activity traveling toward the positive electrode is recorded as an upright deflection and any traveling away from it is recorded as a negative deflection. The six unipolar precordial leads are recorded from their locations on the chest as shown in Figure 21–3C. The view of the heart by unipolar leads can be compared to a telephoto lens on the camera, "zooming in" on the electrical activity in the heart.

The *hexaxial reference system* (or axis wheel) is formed when the six frontal plane leads are moved together in such a

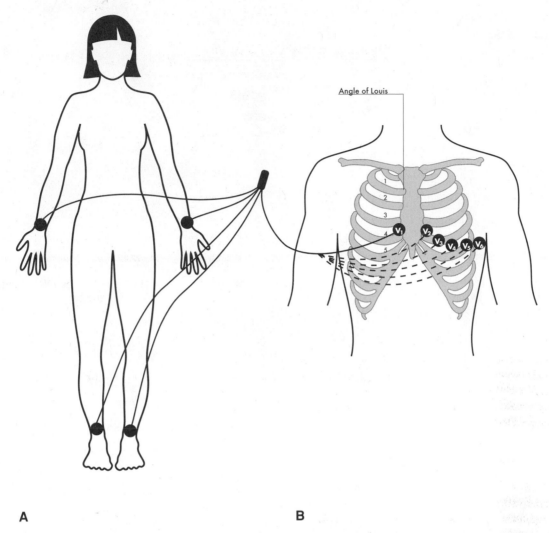

Figure 21–1. (A) Limb electrodes can be placed anywhere on arms and legs. Standard placement is shown here on wrists and ankles. (B) Chest electrode placement. V_1 = fourth intercostal space to right of sternum; V_2 = fourth intercostal space to left of sternum; V_3 = halfway between V_2 and V_4 in a straight line; V_4 = fifth intercostal space at midclavicular line; V_5 = same level as V_4 at anterior axillary line; V_6 = same level as V_4 at midaxillary line.

way that they bisect each other in the center (Figure 21–4A). Each lead is labeled at its positive end to make it easy to remember where the positive electrode is. In Figure 21–4B, the hexaxial reference system is superimposed over a drawing of the heart to illustrate how each lead views the heart.

The normal sequence of depolarization through the heart begins with an electrical impulse originating in the sinus node, high in the right atrium, and spreading leftward through the left atrium and downward toward the AV node low in the right atrium (Figure 21–5A). Leads I and aVL, with their positive electrodes (camera lens) on the left side of the body, record this leftward electrical activity as an upright P wave, and leads II, III, and aVF, with their positive electrodes at the bottom of the heart, record the downward spread of activity as upright P waves. Lead aVR, with its positive electrode on the right shoulder, sees the electrical activity moving away from it and records a negative P wave.

As the impulse spreads through the AV node, no electrical activity is recorded because the AV node is too small to be recorded by surface leads. As the impulse exits the AV node, it moves through the bundle of His and enters the right and left bundle branches. The left bundle branch sprouts some Purkinje fibers high on the left side of the septum that carry the impulse into the septum and cause it to depolarize first in a left-to-right direction. The electrical impulse then enters the Purkinje system of both ventricular free walls simultaneously and depolarizes them from endocardium to epicardium, as shown by the small arrows through the ventricular wall in Figure 21–5A. The millions of electrical forces travel through the heart in three dimensions simultaneously, but if averaged together they move downward, leftward, and posteriorly toward the large left ventricle, as indicated by the large arrow in the same figure. This large arrow represents the *mean axis,* which is the net

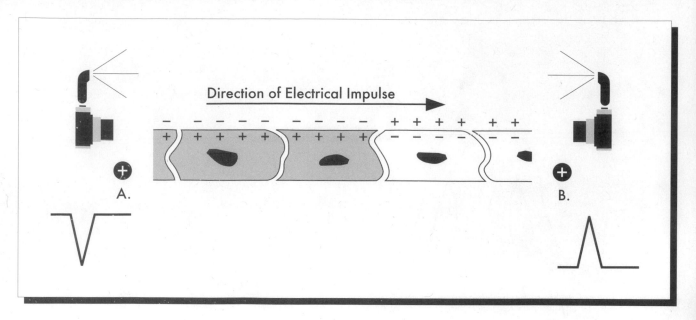

Figure 21–2. A strip of cardiac muscle depolarizing in the direction of the arrow. A positive electrode at *B* sees depolarization coming toward it and records an upright deflection. A positive electrode at *A* sees depolarization going away from it and records a negative deflection.

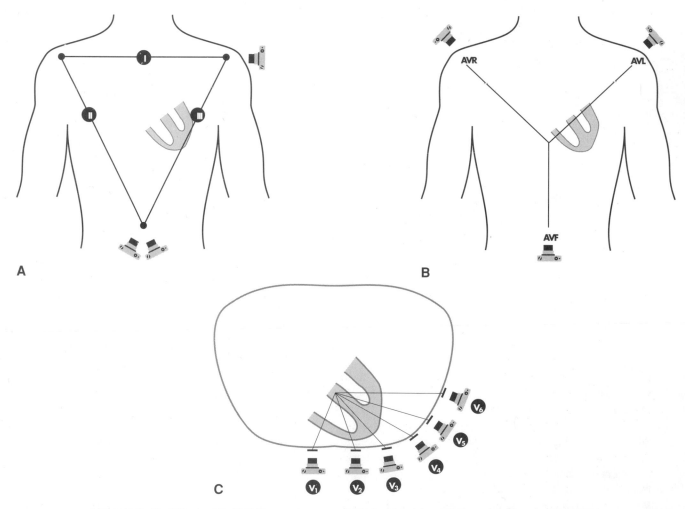

Figure 21–3. The 12 leads of the ECG. The camera represents the location of the positive, or recording, electrode in each lead. (A) Bipolar frontal plane leads I, II, and III. (B) Unipolar frontal plane leads aVR, aVL, and aVF. (C) Unipolar precordial leads V1 to V6.

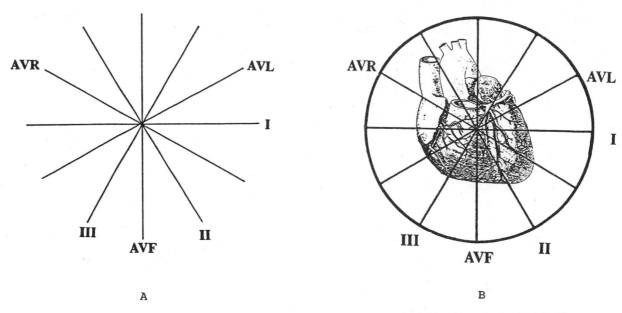

A   B

Figure 21–4. Hexaxial reference system (or axis wheel). (A) All six frontal plane leads bisecting each other. Each lead is labeled at its positive end. (B) The axis wheel superimposed on the heart to demonstrate each lead's view of the heart. Leads I and aVL face the left lateral wall; leads II, III, and aVF face the inferior wall.

direction of electrical depolarization through the ventricles when all the smaller arrows are averaged together.

The QRS complex is recorded as the ventricles depolarize. Leads I and aVL, with their positive electrodes on the left side of the body, see the septum depolarizing away from them and record a small negative deflection (Q wave). These leads then see the large left ventricular free wall depolarizing toward them and record an upright deflection (R wave). Leads II, III, and aVF, with their positive electrodes at the bottom of the heart, may not see septal activity at all and record no deflections. However, if these leads see septal electrical activity coming slightly toward them, they record a positive deflection. As the forces continue moving downward toward leads II, III, and aVF, an upright deflection (R wave) will be recorded. Lead aVR, positive on the right shoulder, sees all activity moving away from it and records a negative deflection (QS complex). Figure 21–5B illustrates how the six precordial leads record normal electrical activity as it spreads through the ventricles.

The six precordial leads record electrical activity traveling in the horizontal plane. Figure 21–5B illustrates the position of the precordial leads and how they record electrical activity as it spreads through the ventricles. Lead V_1 is located on the front of the chest and records a small R wave as the septum depolarizes toward it from left to right. It then records a deep S wave as depolarization spreads away from it through the thick left ventricle. As the positive electrode is moved across the precordium from the V_1 to the V_6 position it records progressively more left ventricular forces and the R wave gets progressively larger. Lead V_6 is located on the left side of the chest and usually records a small Q wave as the septum depolarizes from left to right

away from the positive electrode, and it records a large R wave as electrical activity spreads toward the positive electrode through the thick left ventricle.

In addition to P waves and QRS complexes, the ECG records T waves as the ventricles repolarize. Normal T waves are slightly asymmetrical with an ascending limb that is more gradual than the descending limb. T waves are usually upright in leads I, II, and V_{3-6}, and negative in lead aVR. T waves can vary in other leads. A normal T wave is not taller than 5 mm in a limb lead and 10 mm in a chest lead. Tall T waves can indicate hyperkalemia or myocardial ischemia or infarction.

The ST segment begins at the end of the QRS complex (the J point) and ends at the beginning of the T wave. It is normally at the baseline (the isoelectric segment between the T wave and the next P wave), and should not stay on the baseline for longer than 0.12 second (Figure 21–6). The ST segment should gently curve upward into the T wave without forming a sharp angle. Normal ST-segment elevation and depression is discussed under "ST-Segment Monitoring" later in this chapter.

The U wave is sometimes seen following the T wave, and when present it should be smaller than the T wave and point in the same direction as the T wave. U waves are thought to represent either repolarization of the terminal portion of the Purkinje system or of the papillary muscles. Large U waves can be seen in hypokalemia and with certain drugs, like quinidine. Inverted U waves can indicate myocardial ischemia.

Figure 21–7 shows a normal 12-lead ECG. Normal sinus rhythm is present, and the axis is +45°. P waves are normal (they are flat in V_2, but this is not necessarily abnormal), and

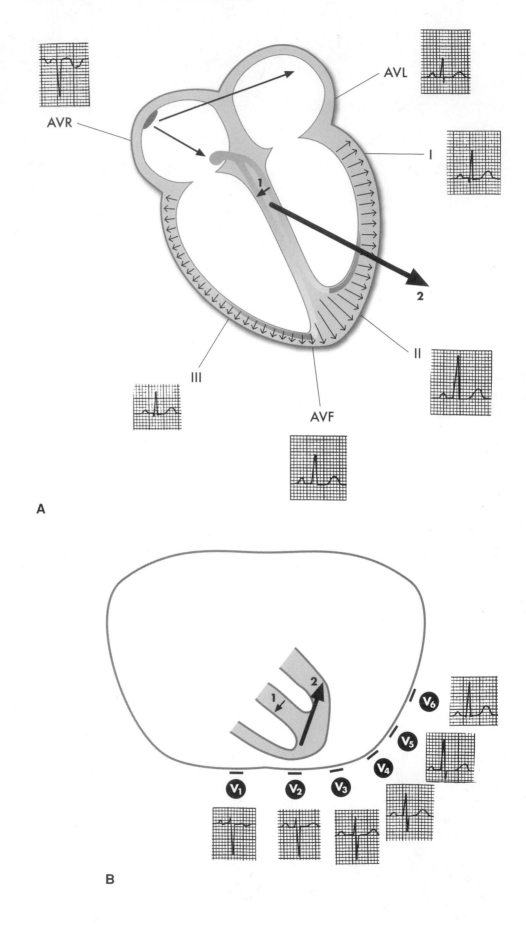

Figure 21–5. (A) Normal sequence of depolarization through the heart as recorded by each of the frontal plane leads. (B) Cross section of the thorax illustrating how the six precordial leads record normal electrical activity in the ventricles. The small arrow (1) shows the initial direction of depolarization through the septum, followed by the direction of ventricular depolarization, indicated by the larger arrow (2).

Lead II   Lead V_I

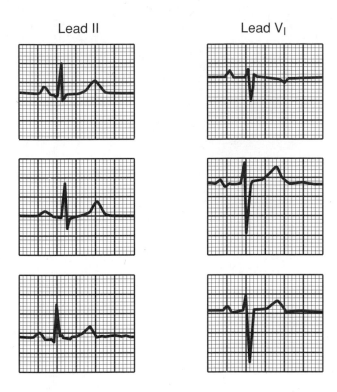

Figure 21–6. Normal ST segment and T waves.

T waves are normal. The QRS complex is normal (0.08 second wide), there are no abnormal Q waves, and R-wave progression is normal across the precordium. The ST segment is at baseline in all leads. This ECG can be used for comparison as abnormalities are discussed throughout this chapter.

Axis Determination

The hexaxial reference system (axis wheel) forms a 360° circle surrounding the heart that by convention is divided into 180 positive degrees and 180 negative degrees (Figure 21–8). The normal QRS axis is defined as −30° to +110°

because most of the electrical forces in a normal heart are directed downward and leftward toward the large left ventricle. Left axis deviation (LAD) is defined as an axis of −31° to −90° and occurs when most of the forces move in a leftward and superior direction, as can happen in a variety of conditions, such as left ventricular hypertrophy, left anterior fascicular block, inferior myocardial infarction, or left bundle branch block (Table 21–1). Right axis deviation (RAD) is defined as +110° to +180° and occurs when most of the forces move rightward, as can happen in conditions such as right ventricular hypertrophy, left posterior fascicular block, and right bundle branch block (Table 21–1). When most of the forces are directed superior and rightward between −90° and −180°, the term indeterminate axis is used. This axis can occur with ventricular tachycardia and occasionally with bifascicular block.

The mean frontal plane QRS axis can be determined in a number of ways. The most accurate method is to average the forces moving right and left with those moving up and down. Since this represents the frontal plane, lead I is the "pure" right/left lead and lead aVF is the "pure" up/down lead; it is easiest to use these two perpendicular leads to calculate the mean axis. Figure 21–9A shows the frontal plane leads of a 12-lead ECG. Leads I and aVF are shown enlarged along with the axis wheel with small hash marks along the axes of lead I and lead aVF (Figure 21–9B). These hash marks represent the small 1-mV boxes on the ECG paper. To determine the mean QRS axis, follow these steps:

1. Look at the QRS complex in lead I and count the number of positive and negative boxes. Mark the net vector along the appropriate end of lead I on the axis wheel. In Figure 21–9B, the QRS complex in lead I is 5 boxes positive and 2 boxes negative, resulting in a net 3 boxes positive, or +3. Count 3 hash marks towards the positive end of lead I and put a mark on the axis wheel at that spot.

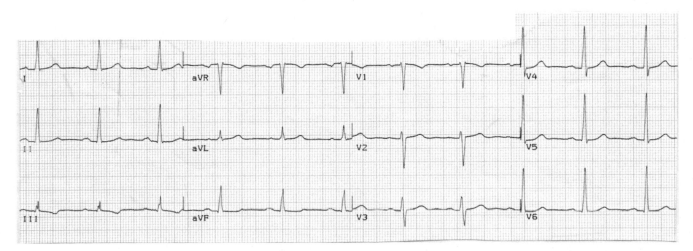

Figure 21–7. Normal 12-lead ECG.

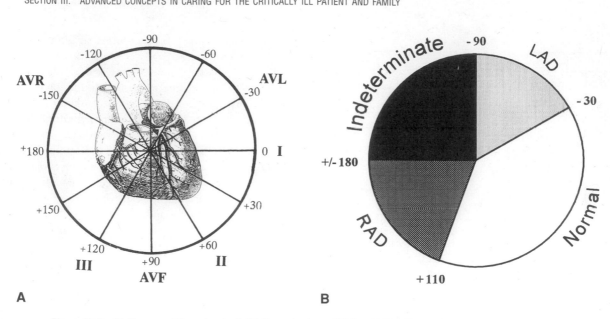

Figure 21–8. (A) Degrees of the axis wheel. (B) Normal axis = –30° to +110°; LAD = –30° to –90°; RAD = +110° to +180°; indeterminate axis = –90° to –180°.

2. Look at the QRS complex in aVF and follow the same procedure as above. In this example, the QRS complex in aVF is 8 boxes positive and has two very small negative deflections that equal approximately 1 box when added together, resulting in a net +7. Count 7 hash marks along the positive end of aVF's axis and place a mark at that spot.

3. Draw a perpendicular line down from the mark on lead I's axis and a perpendicular line across from the mark on aVF's axis.

4. Draw a line from the center of the axis wheel to the spot where the two perpendicular lines meet. This line represents the mean QRS axis. In the example in Figure 21–9B, the axis is about +65°.

TABLE 21–1. SUMMARY OF CAUSES OF AXIS DEVIATIONS

Axis: –30° to +110°
- Normal

Left Axis Deviation: –31° to –90°
- Left ventricular hypertrophy
- Left anterior fascicular block
- Inferior myocardial infarction
- Left bundle branch block (LBBB)
- Congenital defects
- Ventricular tachycardia
- Wolff-Parkinson-White syndrome

Right Axis Deviation: +110° to +180°
- Right ventricular hypertrophy
- Left posterior fascicular block
- Right bundle branch block (RBBB)
- Dextrocardia
- Ventricular tachycardia
- Wolff-Parkinson-White syndrome

Intermediate Axis: –90° to –180°
- Ventricular tachycardia
- Bifascicular block

A quick but less accurate method of axis determination is to place the axis in its proper quadrant of the axis wheel by looking at leads I and aVF, since these leads divide the wheel into four quadrants. As illustrated in Figure 21–10, if both of these leads are positive, the axis falls in the normal quadrant, 0° to +90°. If lead I is positive and aVF is negative, the axis falls in the left quadrant, 0° to –90°. If lead I is negative and aVF is positive, the axis falls in the right quadrant, +90° to +180°. If both leads are negative, the axis falls in the indeterminate quadrant or "no-mans-land," –90° to –180°. Locating the correct quadrant is sometimes adequate, but since 30° of the left quadrant is considered normal, it is necessary to be more precise in describing the axis when it falls in the left quadrant. To "fine-tune" the axis quickly, find the limb lead with the smallest or most biphasic QRS complex. This lead must not be seeing much electrical force if it is the smallest; therefore, its perpendicular lead must be seeing most of the forces. Locate the perpendicular lead (leads I and aVF, leads II and aVL, leads III and aVR) and see if the QRS is positive or negative in that lead. If it is positive, the axis is directed toward the positive end of the lead; if it is negative, the axis is directed toward the negative end of the lead. Using the ECG in Figure 21–9A do the following:

1. Place the axis in its correct quadrant by looking at leads I and aVF. Since both leads are positive, the axis is in the normal quadrant.

2. Find the smallest or most diphasic limb lead. Lead aVL is the most diphasic lead in this example.

3. Find the lead that is perpendicular to the diphasic lead and note if it is positive or negative. Lead II is perpendicular to aVL and lead II is positive in this example. Therefore, the axis is directed toward the positive end of lead II, which is +60°.

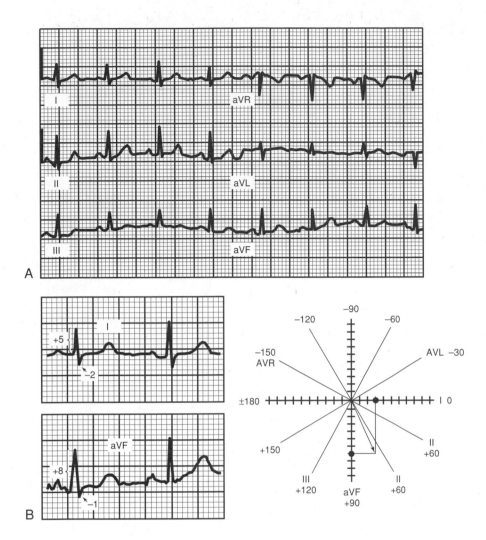

Figure 21–9. Calculating the mean QRS axis. (A) The six frontal plane leads of an ECG. (B) Leads I and aVF enlarged. See the text for instructions on calculating the axis using leads I and aVF on the axis wheel.

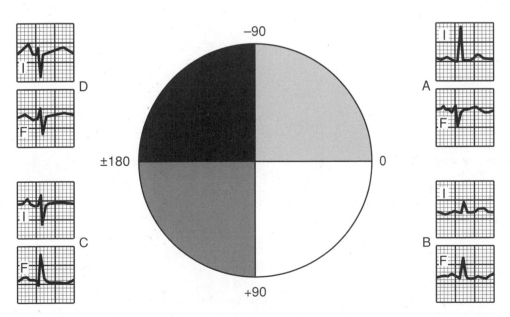

Figure 21–10. The four quadrants of the axis wheel. (A) Left axis deviation quadrant; lead I is positive and lead aVF is negative. (B) Normal axis quadrant; leads I and aVF are both positive. (C) Right axis deviation quadrant; lead I is negative and lead aVF is positive. (D) Indeterminate axis quadrant; leads I and aVF are both negative. *(With permission from: Marriott, HJL:* Practical electrocardiography, *8th ed. Baltimore: Williams & Wilkins, 1988, p. 35.)*

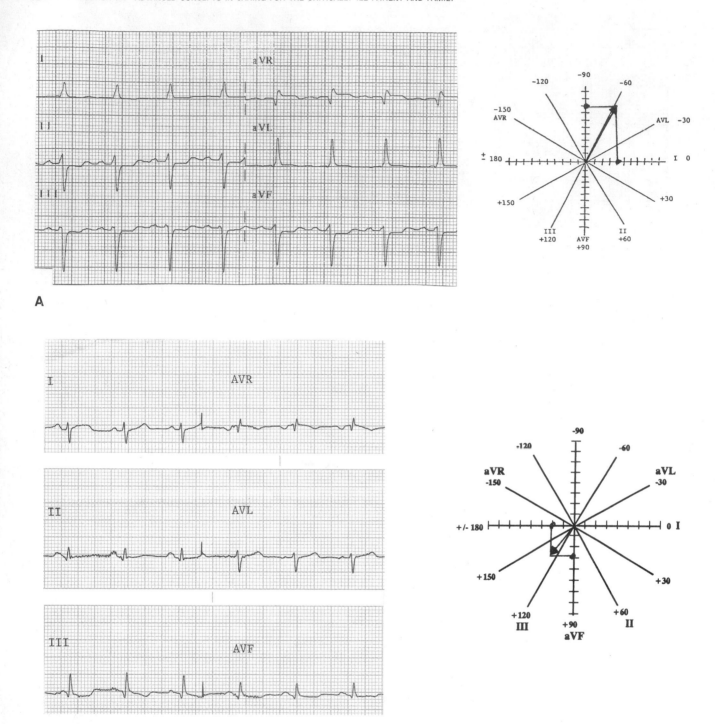

Figure 21–11. (A) Frontal plane leads demonstrating left axis deviation. Lead I is 5 boxes positive; aVF is 2 boxes positive and 10 boxes negative for a net of −8. The axis is −60°. (B) Frontal plane leads demonstrating right axis deviation. Lead I is 2 boxes positive and 5 boxes negative for a net of −3; lead aVF is 2 boxes positive. The axis is +150°.

Using the ECG in Figure 21–11A, first place the axis in the appropriate quadrant by using leads I and aVF. Lead I is upright and aVF is negative, placing the axis in the left quadrant. However, since 30° of the left quadrant is considered normal, we need to fine-tune the axis to determine where within the left quadrant it actually falls. Lead aVR is the most biphasic lead in this ECG, which means that most of the electrical force is moving perpendicular to aVR. Lead III is perpendicular to aVR, and lead III is negative in this ECG, indicating that the axis is directed toward the negative pole of lead III. The axis is −60°. The axis wheel shows how to count boxes in this example.

Using the ECG in Figure 21–11B, place the axis in the appropriate quadrant. Since lead I is negative and aVF is positive, the axis is in the right quadrant. The most diphasic lead is aVR, and lead III is perpendicular to aVR. Since lead III is positive, the axis is directed toward the positive pole of lead III, or +150°. The axis wheel shows how boxes are counted in this example.

Bundle Branch Block

When one of the bundle branches is blocked, the ventricles depolarize asynchronously. Bundle branch block is characterized by a delay of excitation to one ventricle and an abnormal spread of electrical activity through the ventricle whose bundle is blocked. This delayed conduction results in widening of the QRS complex to 0.12 second or more and a characteristic pattern best recognized in precordial leads V_1 and V_6 and limb leads I and aVL.

Normal ventricular depolarization as recorded by leads V_1 and V_6 is illustrated in Figure 21–12. The positive electrode for V_1 is located on the front of the chest at the fourth intercostal space to the right of the sternum, close to the right ventricle. The positive electrode for V_6 is located in the left midaxillary line at the fifth intercostal space, close to the left ventricle. Lead V_1 records a small R wave as the septum depolarizes from left to right toward the positive electrode. It then records a negative deflection (S wave) as the main forces travel away from the positive electrode toward the left ventricle, resulting in the normal rS complex in V_1. Lead V_6 records a small Q wave as the septum depolarizes left to right away from the positive electrode. It then records a tall R wave as the main forces travel toward the left ventricle,

resulting in the normal qR complex in V_6. When both ventricles depolarize together, the QRS width is <0.12 second.

Right Bundle Branch Block (RBBB)

The presence of a block in the right bundle branch causes a different spread of electrical forces in the ventricles and thus a different pattern to the QRS complex. Three separate forces occur, as seen in Figure 21–13A.

1. Septal activation occurs first from left to right (arrow 1), resulting in the normal small R wave in V_1 and small Q wave in V_6.
2. The left ventricle is activated next through the normally functioning left bundle branch. Depolarization spreads normally through the Purkinje fibers in the left ventricle (arrow 2), causing an S wave in V_1 as the impulse travels away from its positive electrode and an R wave in V_6 as the impulse travels toward the positive electrode in V_6.
3. The right ventricle depolarizes late and abnormally as the impulse spreads via cell-to-cell conduction through the right ventricle (arrow 3). This abnormal activation causes a wide second R wave (called R prime, R′) in V_1 as it travels toward the positive electrode in V_1 and a wide S wave in V_6 as it travels away from the positive electrode in V_6. Since muscle cell-to-cell conduction is much slower than conduction through the Purkinje system, the QRS complex widens to 0.12 second or greater.

Right bundle branch block can be recognized by a wide rSR′ pattern in V_1 and a wide qRs pattern in V_6, I, and

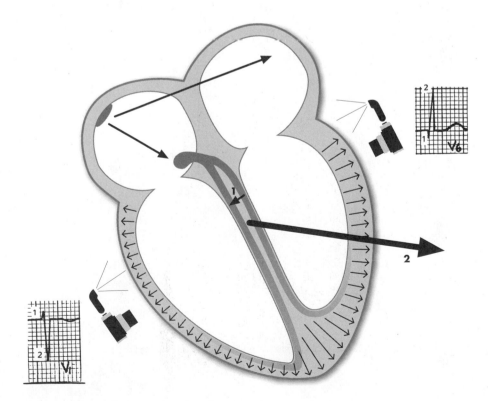

Figure 21–12. Normal ventricular activation as recorded by leads V_1 and V_6. See the text for discussion.

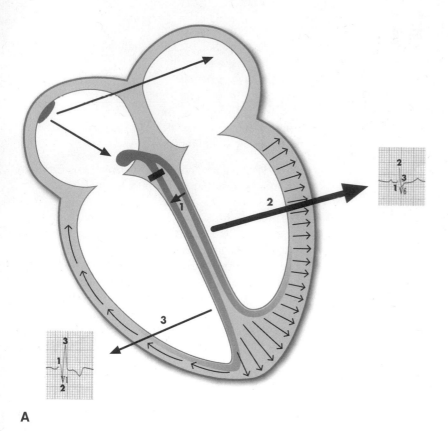

A

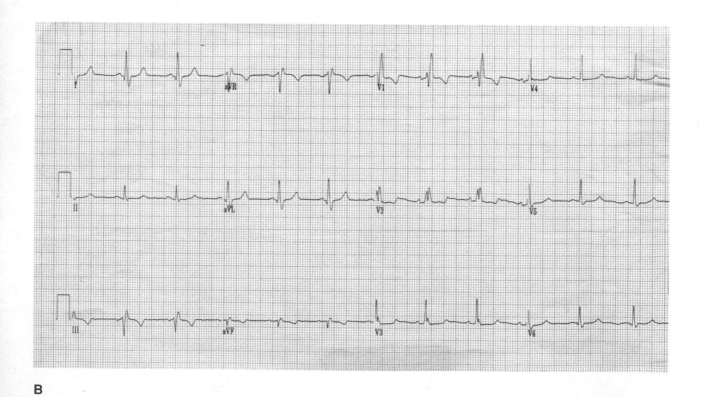

B

Figure 21–13. (A) Ventricular depolarization with right bundle branch block as recorded by leads V$_1$ and V$_6$. See the text for details. (B) 12-lead ECG illustrating RBBB.

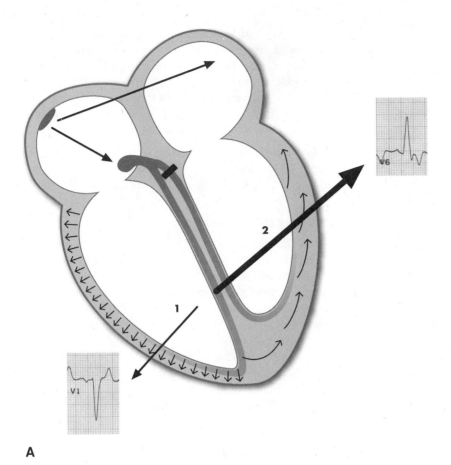

A

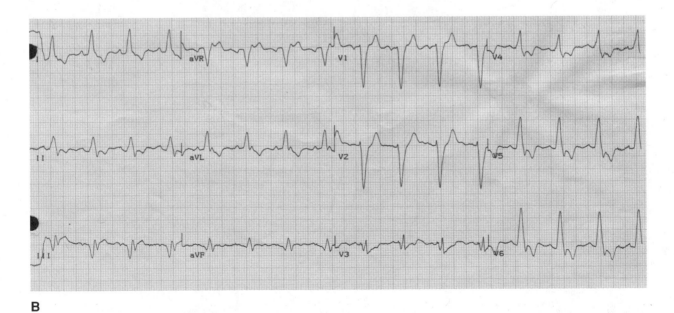

B

Figure 21–14. (A) Ventricular depolarization with left bundle branch block as recorded by leads V_1 and V_6. See the text for details. (B) 12-lead ECG illustrating LBBB.

aVL, since the positive electrode in these two limb leads is located on the left side of the body. The ECG in Figure 21–13B illustrates RBBB.

Left Bundle Branch Block (LBBB)

Figure 21–14 illustrates the spread of electrical forces through the ventricles when the left bundle branch is blocked. In LBBB the septum does not depolarize in its normal left-to-right direction since the block occurs above the Purkinje fibers that normally activate the left side of the septum. This results in the loss of the normal small R wave in V_1 and loss of the Q wave in V_6, I, and aVL. Two main forces occur in LBBB:

1. The right ventricle is activated first through the Purkinje fibers (arrow 1). Since the right ventricular free wall is so much thinner than that of the left ventricle, forces traveling through it are often not recorded in V_1. Sometimes a small, narrow R wave is recorded in V_1 during LBBB, and this is most likely the result of forces traveling through the right ventricular free wall.
2. The left ventricle depolarizes late and abnormally as the impulse spreads via cell-to-cell conduction through the thick left ventricle (arrow 2). This

causes V_1 to record a wide negative QS complex as the impulse travels away from its positive electrode. The lateral leads V_6, I, and aVL record a wide R wave as the impulse travels through the large left ventricle toward their positive electrodes. The QRS widens to 0.12 second or greater due to the slow cell-to-cell conduction in the left ventricle.

Left bundle branch block can be recognized by a wide QS complex in V_1 and wide R waves with no Q waves in V_6, I, and aVL. The ECG in Figure 21–14B illustrates LBBB.

Myocardial Ischemia, Injury, and Infarction

Myocardial ischemia is the result of an imbalance between myocardial O_2 supply and demand and is a reversible process if blood flow is restored before cellular damage occurs. If ischemia is severe and blood flow is not restored relatively soon, cellular injury and eventually necrosis (infarction) results. When infarction does occur, there are three "zones" of tissue involvement, each of which produces characteristic changes on the ECG (Figure 21–15).

Myocardial ischemia can result in several changes on the ECG (Figure 21–16). The most familiar patterns of ischemia are ST-segment depression of 0.5 mm or more and T-wave inversion. Other indicators of ischemia include an

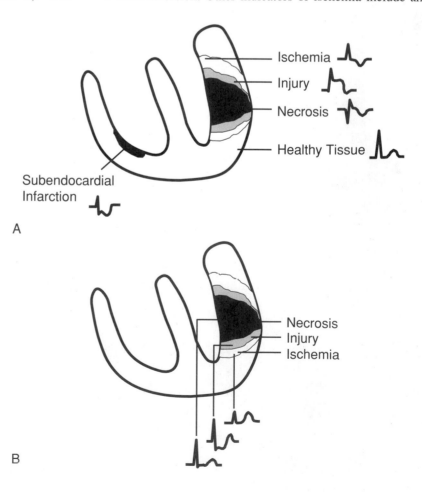

Figure 21–15. Zones of myocardial ischemia, injury, and infarction with associated ECG changes. (A) Indicative changes of ischemia, injury, and necrosis seen in leads facing the injured area. (B) Reciprocal changes often seen in leads not directly facing the involved area.

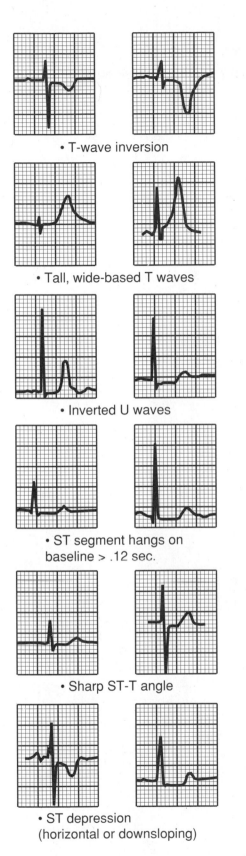

- T-wave inversion

- Tall, wide-based T waves

- Inverted U waves

- ST segment hangs on
baseline > .12 sec.

- Sharp ST-T angle

- ST depression
(horizontal or downsloping)

Figure 21–16. ECG patterns associated with myocardial ischemia.

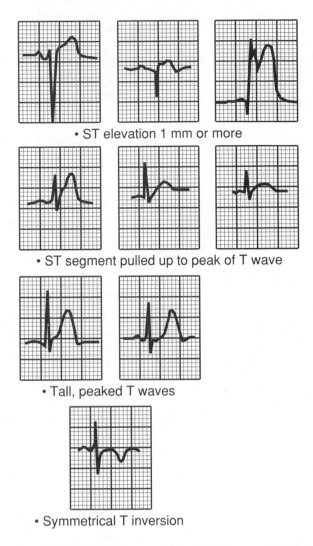

- ST elevation 1 mm or more

- ST segment pulled up to peak of T wave

- Tall, peaked T waves

- Symmetrical T inversion

Figure 21–17. ECG patterns associated with acute myocardial injury.

ST segment that remains on the baseline longer than 0.12 second, an ST segment that forms a sharp angle with the T wave, tall, wide-based T waves, and inverted U waves.

Myocardial injury is most often indicated by ST-segment elevation of 1 mm or more above the baseline (Figure 21–17). Other signs of acute injury include an ST segment that slopes up to the peak of the T wave without spending any time on the baseline, tall, peaked T waves, and symmetrical T-wave inversion.

Necrosis or death of myocardial tissue is indicated on the ECG by development of Q waves that are >0.03 second wide. Infarction Q waves are also deeper than normal, with criteria ranging from 2 mm deep to 25% of the R-wave amplitude (see Figures 21–5A and 21–9 for normal Q waves and Figures 21–18 and 21–19 for abnormal Q waves). Traditionally, it was taught that the presence of Q waves indicates transmural MI extending through the entire thickness of the muscle, and that subendocardial infarction involving less than the entire thickness of the muscle does not produce Q waves. Now it is thought that Q waves can develop transiently with severe ischemia and that infarction can occur without the development of Q waves. Subendocardial infarction is recognized by decreased amplitude of R waves, ST depression, and T-wave inversion. The newer terms *Q-wave* and *non-Q-wave* MI are replacing the older terms of *transmural* and *subendocardial* infarction. In any case, the presence of Q waves is still considered indicative of myocardial necrosis.

The ECG reflects the evolution of the infarction from the acute stage through the fully evolved stage. Very early MI often causes peaking and widening of the T waves, followed within minutes by ST-segment elevation. ST elevation can persist for hours to several days but resolves more quickly with successful reperfusion. Once the ST segment has returned to baseline, ECG evidence of the acute infarction stage is lost. Q waves appear within hours of pain onset and usually remain forever, although sometimes Q waves disappear over the years following infarction. T-wave inversion occurs within hours after infarction and can last for months. T waves often return to their previous upright position within a few months after acute MI. Thus an "evolving" infarct is one in which the ECG shows ST segments returning toward baseline, the development of Q waves, and T-wave inversion. The term "old" infarction or "infarct of indeterminate age" is used when the first ECG recorded shows Q waves, ST segment at baseline, and T waves either inverted or upright, indicating that an MI occurred at some point in the past.

TABLE 21–2. ECG CHANGES ASSOCIATED WITH MYOCARDIAL INFARCTION

Location of MI	Indicative Changes	Reciprocal Changes
Anterior	V_1 to V_4	I, aVL, II, III, aVF
Septal	V_1, V_2	I, aVL
Inferior	II, III, aVF	I, aVL, V_1 to V_4
Posterior	None	V_1 to V_4
Lateral	I, aVL, V_5, V_6	II, III, aVF, V_1, V_2
Right ventricle	V_3R to V_6R	

Locating the Infarction From the ECG

ST-segment elevation, Q waves, and T-wave inversion are recorded in leads facing the damaged myocardium and are called the *indicative changes* of infarction. Leads not facing the involved tissue often show changes related to the loss of electrical forces (depolarization and repolarization) in the damaged tissue. These leads record mirror-image changes that are called *reciprocal changes*. Figure 21–13 illustrates indicative and reciprocal changes associated with MI, and Table 21–2 lists leads in which indicative and reciprocal changes are found in each of the major types of MI.

Anterior wall MI is recognized by indicative changes in leads facing the anterior wall precordial leads V_1 to V_4 (Figure 21–18). Reciprocal changes are often recorded in the lateral leads I and aVL, as well as in the inferior leads II, III, and aVF. Inferior wall MI is diagnosed by indicative changes in leads II, III, and aVF (Figure 21–19). Re-

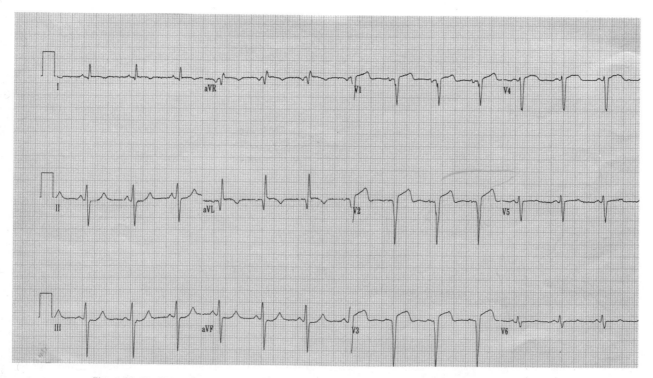

Figure 21–18. 12-lead ECG demonstrating acute anterior wall MI. Q waves are present in V_1 to V_3 and ST-segment elevation is present in V_1 to V_4. An abnormal Q wave is also present in aVL.

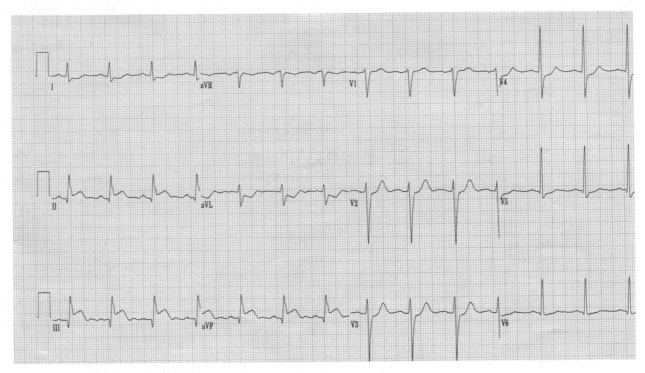

Figure 21–19. 12-lead ECG demonstrating acute inferior wall MI. ST elevation is present in II, III, and aVF; reciprocal ST depression is present in I, aVL, and V_2 to V_4. Q waves can be seen in III and aVF.

ciprocal changes are often seen in leads I and aVL and/or the V leads. Lateral wall MI presents with indicative changes in leads I, aVL, and sometimes V_5 and V_6, with reciprocal changes in inferior or anterior leads (Figure 21–20). Posterior wall MI is less obvious because in the standard 12-lead ECG there are no leads that face the posterior wall, and therefore there are no indicative changes recorded (Figure 21–21). The diagnosis is made by observing reciprocal changes in the anterior leads, especially V_1 and V_2 but often all the way to V_4. Reciprocal changes seen in these leads include a taller R wave than normal (mirror image of the Q wave that would be recorded over the posterior wall), ST-segment depression (mirror image of the ST elevation from the posterior wall), and upright, tall T waves (mirror image of the T-wave inversion from the posterior wall).

Right ventricular MI occurs in up to 45% of inferior MIs; therefore, it usually is associated with indicative changes in the inferior leads II, III, and aVF (Figure 21–22). In addition, it is not uncommon to see ST elevation in V_1 as well, since V_1 is the chest lead that is closest to the right ventricle. ST elevation in V_1, together with ST elevation in the inferior leads, is suspicious for right ventricular MI. Another clue is discordance between the ST segment in V_1 and the ST segment in V_2. Normally, when the ST segment in V_1 is elevated, it is related to anterior

or septal MI, in which case the ST in V_2 is also elevated. Discordance means that the ST segments do not point in the same direction—V_1 shows ST elevation while V_2 is either normal or shows ST depression. This finding is suspicious of right ventricular MI. When right ventricular MI is suspected, right-sided chest leads should be obtained (Figure 21–23). Leads V_{3R} through V_{6R} develop ST elevation when acute right ventricular MI is present. Lead V_{4R} is the most sensitive and specific lead for recognition of right ventricular MI.

Preexcitation Syndromes

Preexcitation means early activation of the ventricle by supraventricular impulses that reach the ventricle through an accessory conduction pathway faster than they travel through the AV node. Many people have tracts of tissue, often referred to as "bypass tracts" or "accessory pathways," that can carry electrical impulses directly from atria to ventricles, bypassing the delay in the AV node and causing early and abnormal depolarization of the ventricles. These accessory pathways can be found anywhere around the tricuspid or mitral valve rings. The most common type of preexcitation syndrome is the Wolff-Parkinson-White (WPW) syndrome, in which the impulse travels down the accessory pathway from the atria directly into the ventricles, completely bypassing AV node delay. Lown-Ganong-

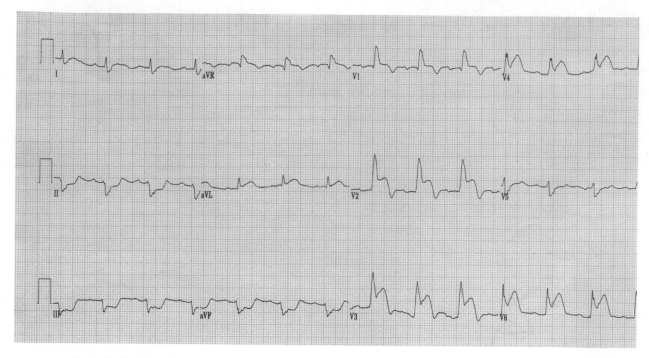

Figure 21–20. 12-lead ECG demonstrating acute anterolateral wall MI. ST elevation is present in I, aVL, V_2 to V_4, and V_6. Reciprocal ST depression is present in III, aVF, and aVR.

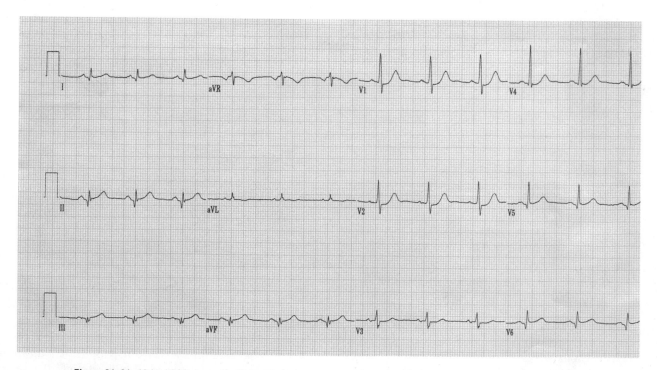

Figure 21–21. 12-lead ECG demonstrating posterior wall MI. Large R waves and ST depression are present in V_1 and V_2. Q waves and wide-based T waves in II, III, and aVF probably indicate inferior infarction as well.

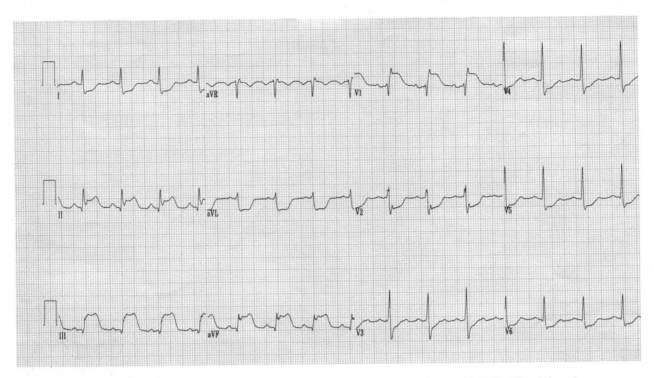

Figure 21–22. 12-lead ECG demonstrating acute right ventricular MI. ST elevation is present in II, III, aVF, and V_1; reciprocal ST depression is present in all other leads. Note the discordant ST elevation in V_1 and ST depression in V_2.

Levine (LGL) syndrome involves an accessory pathway that carries the impulse from the atria to a point low in the AV node or bundle of His, bypassing the AV node delay but entering the normal conduction system rather than the ventricular myocardium.

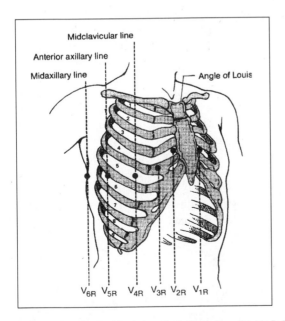

Figure 21–23. Right side chest lead placement. *From: Drew BJ, Ide B: Right ventricular infarction.* Progress in Cardiovascular Nursing. *1995;10:54–46.*

Wolff-Parkinson-White Syndrome

In Wolff-Parkinson-White syndrome, the ventricle is stimulated prematurely by an electrical impulse traveling through the accessory pathway while the impulse simultaneously descends normally through the AV node (Figure 21–24A). Impulses travel faster through the accessory pathway because they bypass the normal AV node delay. Part of the ventricle receives the impulse early via the accessory pathway and begins to depolarize before the rest of the ventricle is activated through the His-Purkinje system. Early stimulation of the ventricle results in a short PR interval and a widened QRS complex as the impulse begins to depolarize the ventricle via muscle cell-to-cell conduction. Premature stimulation of the ventricle causes a characteristic slurring of the initial part of the QRS complex, called a *delta wave*. The remainder of the QRS complex is normal since the rest of the ventricle is depolarized normally through the Purkinje system. This preexcitation results in ventricular fusion beats as the ventricles are depolarized simultaneously by the impulse coming through the accessory pathway and through the normal AV node. The degree of preexcitation varies, depending on the relative rates of conduction down the accessory pathway and through the AV node, and it determines the length of the PR interval and size of the delta wave (Figures 21–24A to 21–24C).

Wolff-Parkinson-White syndrome is recognized on the ECG by the presence of a short PR interval, <0.12 second, and delta waves in many leads. Figure 21–25 shows two

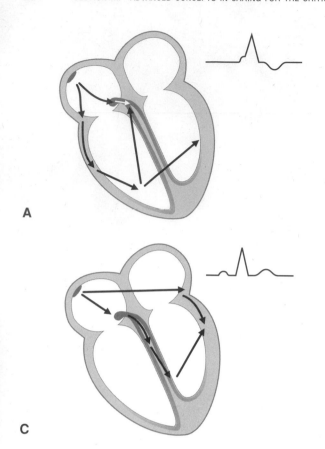

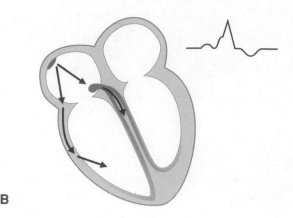

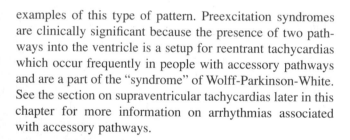

Figure 21–24. Varying degrees of preexcitation. (A) Maximal preexcitation when the ventricles are activated totally by the accessory pathway. (B) Less than maximal preexcitation when the ventricles are activated by the impulse traveling through both the accessory pathway and the normal AV conduction system. (C) Concealed accessory pathway. The ventricles are activated through the normal AV conduction system with no participation of the accessory pathway, resulting in a normal PR interval and normal QRS complex.

examples of this type of pattern. Preexcitation syndromes are clinically significant because the presence of two pathways into the ventricle is a setup for reentrant tachycardias which occur frequently in people with accessory pathways and are a part of the "syndrome" of Wolff-Parkinson-White. See the section on supraventricular tachycardias later in this chapter for more information on arrhythmias associated with accessory pathways.

Lown-Ganong-Levine Syndrome

Lown-Ganong-Levine syndrome is a preexcitation pattern that involves an accessory pathway that originates in the atrium and inserts below the area of physiologic delay in the AV node or in the bundle of His. Since the supraventricular impulse bypasses the AV node delay, the PR interval is short, as it is in Wolff-Parkinson-White syndrome. However, since the tract terminates within the normal conduction system rather than in ventricular myocardium, there is no delta wave as there is in Wolff-Parkinson-White. Lown-Ganong-Levine syndrome is recognized on the ECG by a short PR interval (<0.12 second) and a normal QRS (Figure 21–26). People with Lown-Ganong-Levine syndrome are prone to the same types of tachycardias as occur Wolff-Parkinson-White syndrome.

Treatment

Wolff-Parkinson-White syndrome and Lown-Ganong-Levine syndrome do not require treatment unless they are associated with symptomatic tachycardias. Specific therapy depends on the mechanism of the tachyarrhythmia, the effect of drugs on conduction through the AV node and the accessory pathway, and on the patient's tolerance of the arrhythmia. The section on supraventricular tachycardias later in this chapter discusses drug treatment of tachycardias associated with accessory pathways.

Radio-frequency (RF) catheter ablation of the bypass tract provides a cure for the tachyarrhythmias associated with accessory pathways in many patients. RF ablation is an invasive procedure that requires the introduction of several catheters into the heart through the venous and sometimes arterial systems. An electrophysiology (EP) study is done first to record intracardiac signals and determine the mechanism of the tachycardia. The EP study confirms the presence and location of the accessory pathway, participation of the pathway in maintaining the tachycardia, and conduction characteristics of the accessory pathway. A special ablation catheter is then positioned next to the bypass tract and RF energy is delivered through the catheter to the tract, destroying the tissue and preventing it from being able to conduct. Permanent tissue damage in the accessory pathway is the goal of RF ablation, and when successful, it prevents further episodes of tachycardia.

ADVANCED ARRHYTHMIA INTERPRETATION

The study of cardiac rhythms provides a never-ending challenge to those interested in learning about arrhythmias. In

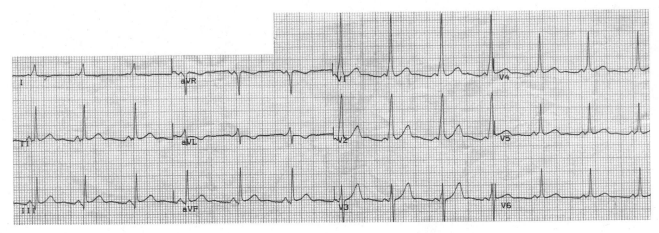

A

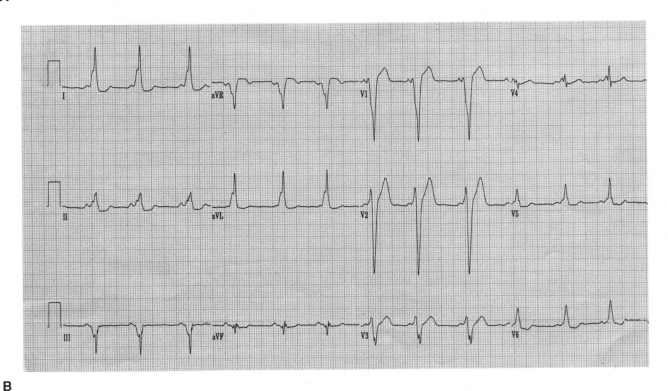

B

Figure 21–25. (A) 12-lead ECG demonstrating Wolff-Parkinson-White syndrome with short PR interval and delta waves. Lead V$_1$ is positive, sometimes called Type A Wolff-Parkinson-White syndrome, indicating a posterior accessory pathway. *(From: Jacobson C: Arrhythmias and conduction disturbances. In Woods SL, et al. (eds.):* Cardiac nursing, *3rd ed. Philadelphia: JB Lippincott, 1995, p. 338.)* (B) Wolff-Parkinson-White syndrome with short PR and delta waves with a negative V$_1$, sometimes called Type B Wolff-Parkinson-White syndrome, indicating an anterior or right-sided accessory pathway.

most basic ECG classes the content presented is limited to basic rhythms originating in the sinus node, atria, AV junction, and ventricles, and to basic AV conduction abnormalities. Rarely does time permit the inclusion of more advanced concepts. This section discusses some of the more advanced concepts of arrhythmia interpretation and provides clues to aid in recognition of selected arrhythmias not usually covered in a basic course.

Supraventricular Tachycardias

The term *supraventricular tachycardia,* or SVT, is used to describe a rapid rhythm that arises above the level of the ventricles (atria or AV junction) but whose exact origin is not known. Usually, the term supraventricular tachycardia is used to describe a narrow QRS tachycardia where atrial activity (P waves) cannot be identified, and therefore the origin of the tachycardia cannot be determined from the surface ECG. The

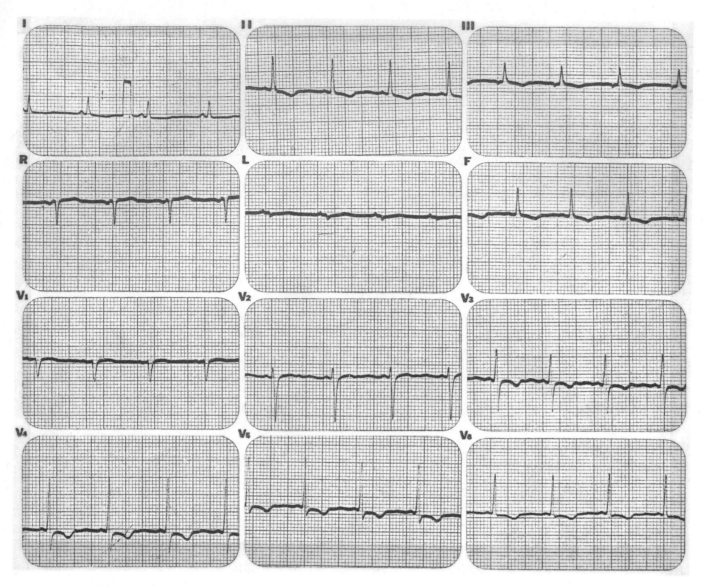

Figure 21–26. Lown-Ganong-Levine (LGL) syndrome with short PR interval and normal QRS. *(From: Jacobson C: Arrhythmias and conduction disturbances. In Woods SL, et al. (eds.): Cardiac nursing, 3rd ed. Philadelphia: JB Lippin-cott, 1995, p. 339.)*

presence of the narrow QRS indicates the supraventricular origin of the rhythm and conduction through the normal His-Purkinje system into the ventricles. Sometimes supraventricular tachycardia conducts with bundle branch block, which results in a wide QRS but does not change the fact that the rhythm is supraventricular in origin. Thus, the term supraventricular tachycardia can be used for narrow QRS tachycardias whose mechanism is uncertain or for wide QRS tachycardias that are known to be coming from above the ventricles.

Supraventricular tachycardias can be classified into those that are AV nodal passive and those that are AV nodal active. *AV nodal passive* supraventricular tachycardias are those in which the AV node is not required for the maintenance of the tachycardia but serves only to passively conduct supraventricular impulses into the ventricles. Exam-

ples of AV nodal passive arrhythmias include atrial tachycardia, atrial flutter, and atrial fibrillation, all of which originate within the atria and do not need the AV node to sustain the atrial arrhythmia. In these rhythms the AV node passively conducts the atrial impulses into the ventricles but does not participate in the maintenance of the arrhythmia itself. *AV nodal active* tachycardias require participation of the AV node in the maintenance of the tachycardia. The two most common causes of a regular, narrow QRS tachycardia are AV nodal reentry tachycardia and circus movement tachycardia using an accessory pathway, both of which require the active participation of the AV node in maintaining the tachycardia.

Atrial fibrillation is a supraventricular rhythm that is usually easily recognized due to its irregularity, but atrial tachycardia, atrial flutter, junctional tachycardia, AV nodal reentry tachycardia, and circus movement tachycardia can all present as regular narrow QRS tachycardias whose mechanism often cannot be determined from the ECG. Since AV nodal reentry tachycardia and circus movement tachycardia are the most common causes of a regular narrow QRS tachycardia, and since they are the two least likely to be presented in a basic ECG class, they are discussed in detail here.

Atrioventricular Nodal Reentry Tachycardia

In people with AV nodal reentry tachycardia (AVNRT), the AV node has two pathways that are capable of conducting the impulse into the ventricles. One pathway conducts more rapidly and has a longer refractory period than the other pathway (Figure 21–27A). In AVNRT, a reentry circuit is set up within the AV node, usually using the slow pathway as the antegrade limb into the ventricle and the fast pathway as the retrograde limb back into the atria (Figure 21–27C).

The sinus impulse normally conducts down the fast pathway into the ventricles, resulting in a normal PR interval of 0.12 to 0.20 second. If a PAC occurs and enters the AV node before the fast pathway with its longer refractory

period has recovered its ability to conduct, the impulse conducts down the slow pathway into the ventricle because of its shorter refractory period (Figure 21–27B). This slow conduction causes the PR interval of the PAC to be longer than the PR interval of sinus beats. The long conduction time through the slow pathway allows the fast pathway time to recover, making it possible for the impulse to conduct backward through the fast pathway into the atria. This returning impulse may then reenter the slow pathway, which is again ready to conduct antegrade due to its short refractory period, thus setting up a reentry circuit within the AV node and resulting in AVNRT. Figure 21–27C illustrates the mechanism of the most common type of AVNRT in which antegrade conduction occurs over the slow pathway and retrograde conduction over the fast pathway. The resulting rhythm is usually a narrow QRS tachycardia because the ventricles are activated through the normal His-Purkinje system. P waves are either not seen at all or are barely visible peeking out at the tail end of the QRS complex because the atria and ventricles depolarize almost simultaneously (Figure 21–28). In the presence of preexisting bundle branch block or rate-dependent bundle branch block, the QRS in AVNRT is wide.

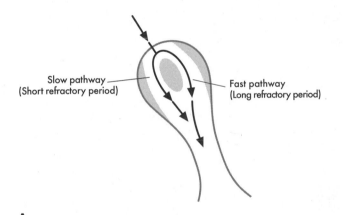

Slow pathway
(Short refractory period)

Fast pathway
(Long refractory period)

A

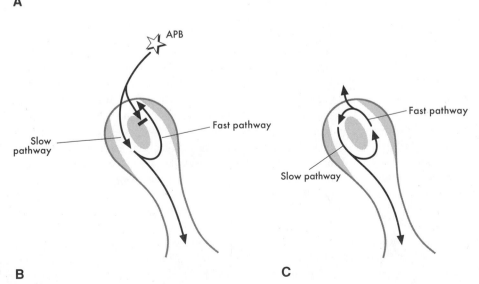

APB

Slow pathway

Fast pathway

B

Fast pathway

Slow pathway

C

Figure 21–27. (A) Illustration of two conduction pathways within the AV node. The fast conducting pathway has a longer refractory period than the slow conducting pathway. Normal conduction occurs through the fast pathway. (B) A PAC finds the fast pathway still refractory so it conducts to the ventricle through the slow pathway, resulting in a long PR interval. Slow conduction through the slow pathway allows the fast pathway to recover and allows retrograde conduction. (C) Reentry within the AV node using the slow pathway as the antegrade limb and the fast pathway as the retrograde limb of the circuit, resulting in AV nodal reentry tachycardia. Atrial and ventricular depolarization occur simultaneously. *(From: Marriott HJL, Conover M: Advanced concepts in arrhythmias, 2nd ed. St. Louis, MO: CV Mosby, 1989, p. 121–123.)*

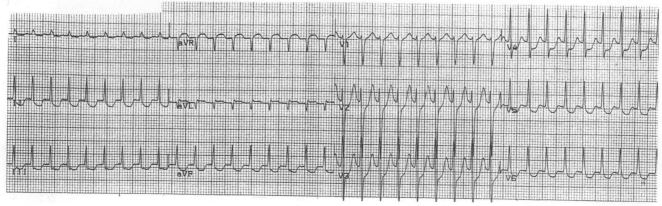

A

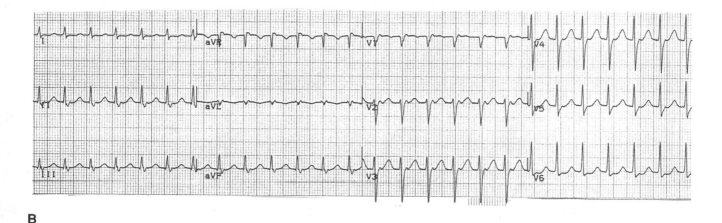

B

Figure 21–28. (A) AV nodal reentry tachycardia (AVNRT), rate 214. No P waves are visible. (B) AVNRT, rate 150. P waves distort the end of the QRS complex in leads II, III, aVF, and V$_1$ to V$_3$. *(From: Jacobson C: Arrhythmias and conduction disturbances. In Woods SL, et al. (eds.):* Cardiac nursing, *3rd ed. Philadelphia: JB Lippincott, 1995, p. 341.)*

In about 4% of cases of AVNRT, the impulse conducts antegrade into the ventricle through the fast pathway and retrograde into the atria through the slow pathway, reversing the circuit within the AV node. This reversal of the circuit in the AV node results in P waves that appear immediately in front of the QRS because atrial activation is delayed due to slow conduction backward through the slow pathway. These P waves are inverted in inferior leads because the atria depolarize in a retrograde direction.

Treatment

AVNRT is an AV nodal active SVT since the AV node is required for the maintenance of the tachycardia. Therefore, anything that causes block in the AV node, such as vagal stimulation or drugs like adenosine, beta blockers, or calcium channel blockers, can terminate the rhythm. AVNRT is usually well tolerated unless the rate is extremely rapid. Episodes can become frequent and, if not controlled with drugs, can interfere with lifestyle. Many people learn to stop the rhythm by coughing or breath holding, which stimulates the vagus nerve. Acute medical treatment involves administering any drug that blocks AV node conduction,

but adenosine is usually used first because of its rapid effect, short duration of action, and lack of significant side effects. Radio-frequency ablation can destroy the slow pathway and prevent recurrence of the arrhythmia.

Circus Movement Tachycardia

Circus movement tachycardia is an SVT that occurs in people who have accessory pathways (see the section on preexcitation syndromes above). The term AV reentrant tachycardia (AVRT) is also used to describe this arrhythmia, but to avoid confusion between AVRT and AVNRT, the term circus movement tachycardia is used here.

In circus movement tachycardia, an impulse travels a reentry circuit that involves the atria, AV node, ventricles, and accessory pathway. The term *orthodromic* is used to describe the most common type of circus movement tachycardia, in which the impulse travels antegrade through the AV node into the ventricles and retrograde back into the atria through the accessory pathway (Figure 21–29A). The result is a regular narrow QRS tachycardia because the ventricles are activated through the normal His-Purkinje system. In the presence of bundle branch block a wide QRS

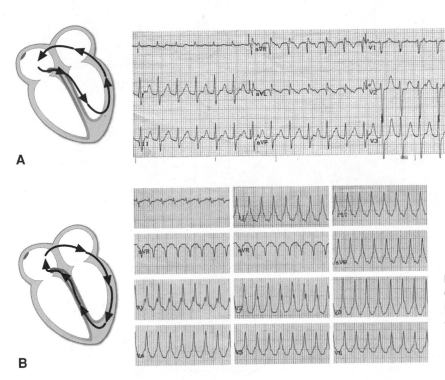

Figure 21–29. (A) Orthodromic circus movement tachy-cardia. P waves are visible on the upstroke of the T wave in leads II, III, aVF, and V_1 to V_3. *(From: Jacobson C: Arrhythmias and conduction disturbances. In Woods SL, et al. (eds.):* Cardiac nursing, *3rd ed. Philadelphia: JB Lippincott, 1995, p. 342.)* (B) Antidromic circus move-ment tachycardia.

pattern is present. Because the atria and ventricles depolar-ize separately, P waves, if visible at all, are seen following the QRS complex in the ST segment or between two QRS complexes, usually closest to the first QRS.

The term *antidromic* is used for the rare form of circus movement tachycardia in which the accessory pathway conducts the impulse from atria to ventricles and the AV node conducts it retrograde back to the atria (Figure 21–29B). Antidromic circus movement tachycardia is a reg-ular wide QRS tachycardia because the ventricles depolar-ize abnormally through the accessory pathway. This form of supraventricular tachycardia is indistinguishable from ventricular tachycardia on the ECG.

Treatment

Circus movement tachycardia is an AV nodal active tachy-cardia since the AV node is necessary for maintenance of the arrhythmia. Vagal maneuvers and drugs that block AV conduction can be used to terminate an episode of tachy-cardia. Acute treatment is aimed at slowing conduction through the AV node with adenosine, beta blockers, or cal-cium channel blockers, or at slowing accessory pathway conduction with drugs like procainamide or quinidine. Radio-frequency ablation is used to destroy the accessory pathway and permanently prevent recurrence of circus movement tachycardia.

Atrial Fibrillation in Wolff-Parkinson-White Syndrome

Atrial fibrillation occurs more frequently in people with accessory pathways than in the general population and can

be life-threatening. Atrial flutter and fibrillation are espe-cially dangerous in the presence of an accessory pathway because the pathway can conduct impulses rapidly and without delay into the ventricles, resulting in dangerously fast ventricular rates (Figure 21–30). These rapid ventricu-lar rates can degenerate into ventricular fibrillation and result in sudden death. When atrial fibrillation is the mech-anism of the tachycardia in Wolff-Parkinson-White syn-drome, the QRS complex is wide and bizarre due to con-duction of the impulses into the ventricle through the bypass tract. The ventricular response to the atrial fibrilla-tion is irregular and very rapid, often approaching rates of 300 beat/minute or more due to lack of delay in conduction through the accessory pathway. Atrial fibrillation with accessory pathway conduction must be recognized and dif-ferentiated from atrial fibrillation conducting through the AV node because treatment is different for the two situa-tions. When accessory pathway conduction is known or suspected, the drug of choice is procainamide because it prolongs the refractory period of the accessory pathway and slows ventricular rate. Verapamil often is used to slow AV conduction in atrial fibrillation conducting into the ventri-cles through the AV node but can be very dangerous and even lethal when used in the presence of an accessory path-way. Digitalis, verapamil, diltiazem, and similar calcium channel blocking agents can shorten the refractory period in the accessory pathway, resulting in even faster ventricular rates and degeneration into ventricular fibrillation. In addi-tion, the hypotensive effects of these agents may intensify the hypotension related to the arrhythmia's rapid ventricu-lar rate.

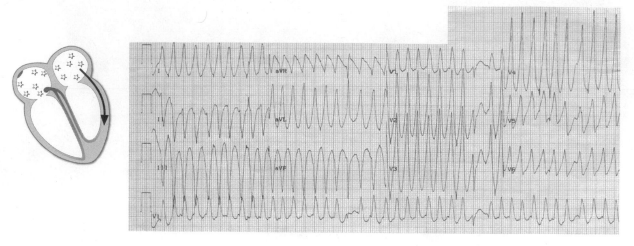

Figure 21–30. Atrial fibrillation conducting into the ventricle through an accessory pathway. Note the extremely short RR intervals in the V leads. QRS is fast, wide, and irregular.

Differentiating Wide QRS Beats and Rhythms

Determining the origin of a wide QRS beat or a wide QRS tachycardia is one of the most common problems encountered when caring for monitored patients. A supraventricular beat with abnormal, or aberrant, conduction through the ventricles, can look almost identical to a beat that originates in the ventricle. The problem with aberration is that it can mimic ventricular arrhythmias, which require different therapy and carry a different prognosis than aberrancy. Aberrancy is always secondary to some other primary disturbance and does not itself require treatment. Nurses must be able to identify accurately which mechanism is responsible for the wide QRS rhythm being observed whenever possible, initiate appropriate treatment when needed, and avoid inappropriate treatment.

Mechanisms of Aberration

Aberrancy is the temporary abnormal intraventricular conduction of supraventricular impulses. Aberration occurs whenever the His-Purkinje system or ventricle is still partly refractory when a supraventricular impulse attempts to travel through it. The refractory period of the conduction system is directly proportional to preceding cycle length. Long cycles are followed by long refractory periods, while short cycles are followed by short refractory periods. An early supraventricular beat, such as a PAC, may enter the conduction system during a portion of its refractory period, forcing conduction through the ventricles to occur in an abnormal manner. Beats that follow a sudden lengthening of the cycle may conduct aberrantly because of the increased length of the refractory period that occurs when the cycle lengthens (Figure 21–31). The right bundle

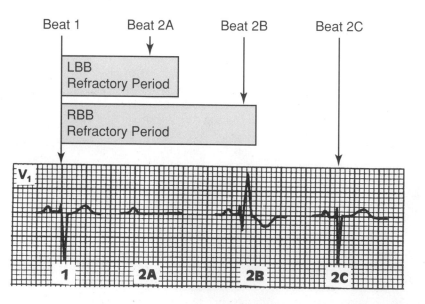

Figure 21–31. Diagram of refractory periods in the bundle branches and the effect of cycle length on conduction. The right bundle has a longer refractory period than the left. Beat 2A occurs so early that it cannot conduct through either bundle branch. Beat 2B encounters a refractory right bundle and conducts with RBBB. Beat 2C falls outside the refractory period of both bundles and is able to conduct normally.

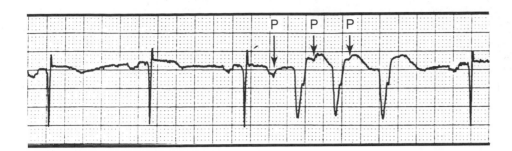

Figure 21–32. Sinus rhythm with PACs and three wide QRS beats that could be mistaken for ventricular tachycardia. The second beat in the strip is a PAC that conducts normally. Note the P waves preceding the wide QRS complexes, indicating aberrant conduction. *(From: Jacobson C: Arrhythmias and conduction disturbances. In Woods SL, et al. (eds.): Cardiac nursing, 3rd ed. Philadelphia: JB Lippincott, 1995, p. 346.)*

branch has a longer refractory period than the left; therefore, aberrant beats tend to conduct most often with a RBBB pattern, although LBBB aberration is common in people with cardiac disease.

Electrocardiographic Clues to the Origin of Wide QRS Beats and Rhythms

P Waves

If P waves can be seen during a wide QRS tachycardia, they are very helpful in making the differential diagnosis of aberration versus ventricular ectopy. Atrial activity, represented by the P wave on the ECG and preceding a wide QRS beat or run of tachycardia, strongly favors a supraventricular origin of the arrhythmia. Figure 21–32 shows three wide QRS beats that could easily be mistaken for PVCs if not for the obvious presence of the early P wave initiating the run.

An exception to the preceding P-wave rule occurs with end-diastolic PVCs. End-diastolic PVCs are those that occur at the end of diastole, after the sinus P wave has been recorded but before it has a chance to conduct through the AV node into the ventricle. Figure 21–33 shows sinus rhythm with an end-diastolic PVC occurring immediately after the sinus P wave. Here, the P wave preceding the wide QRS is merely a coincidence and does not indicate aberrant conduction. The PR interval is much too short to have conducted that QRS complex. In addition, the P wave preceding the wide QRS is not early—it is the regularly scheduled

sinus beat coming on time. Thus, early P waves that precede early wide QRS complexes are usually "married to" those QRSs and indicate aberrant conduction, while "on time" P waves in front of end-diastolic PVCs are not early and do not cause the wide QRS.

P waves seen during a wide QRS tachycardia also can be very helpful in making the differential diagnosis between supraventricular tachycardias with aberration and ventricular tachycardia. If P waves are seen associated with every QRS, the rhythm is supraventricular in origin (Figure 21–34A). P waves that occur independently of the QRS and have no consistent relationship to QRS complexes indicate the presence of AV dissociation, which means that the atria and the ventricles are under the control of separate pacemakers and strongly favors ventricular tachycardia (Figure 21–34B).

QRS Morphology

The shape of the QRS complex is very helpful in determining the origin of a wide QRS rhythm. When using QRS morphology clues, it is extremely important to examine the correct leads and apply the criteria only to leads that have been proven helpful. Many practitioners prefer to monitor with lead II because usually it shows an upright QRS complex and clear P wave. Lead II, however, has no value in determining the origin of a wide QRS rhythm. The single best arrhythmia monitoring lead is V_1, followed by V_6 and V_2 in certain situations.

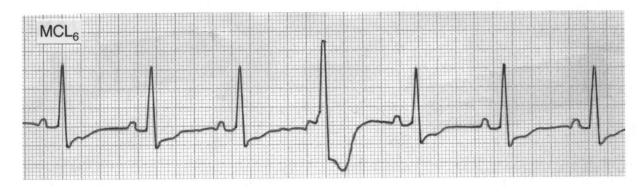

Figure 21–33. Sinus rhythm with an end-diastolic PVC. The P wave preceding the PVC is the sinus P wave that coincidentally occurs just before the PVC. *(From: Jacobson C: Arrhythmias and conduction disturbances. In Woods SL, et al. (eds.): Cardiac nursing, 3rd ed. Philadelphia: JB Lippincott, 1995, p. 347.)*

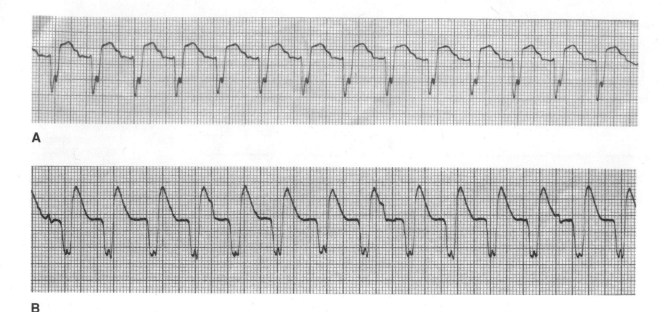

Figure 21–34. Two very similar wide QRS tachycardias. (A) Sinus tachycardia, rate 115. P waves can be seen on the downslope of the T wave preceding each QRS, indicating a supraventricular origin of the tachycardia. (B) P waves are independent of QRS complexes, indicating AV dissociation which favors ventricular tachycardia. *(From: Jacobson C: Arrhythmias and conduction disturbances. In Woods SL, et al. (eds.):* Cardiac nursing, *3rd ed. Philadelphia: JB Lippincott, 1995, p. 347.)*

When applying QRS morphology criteria for wide QRS rhythms, it is helpful to first decide whether the QRS complexes have a right bundle branch block (RBBB) morphology or a left bundle branch block (LBBB) morphology (Figure 21–35). RBBB morphology rhythms have an upright QRS in lead V_1, while LBBB morphology rhythms have a negative QRS complex in V_1.

When dealing with a wide QRS rhythm of RBBB morphology (upright in V_1), follow these steps to evaluate QRS morphology (Figures 21–35 and 21–36A):

1. Look at V_1 and determine if the upright QRS complex is monophasic (R wave), diphasic (qR), or triphasic (rsR′). Monophasic and diphasic complexes favor a ventricular origin, while the triphasic rsR′ is typical of RBBB aberration in V_1.
2. Look at V_6 and determine if the QRS is monophasic (all negative QS), diphasic (rS), or triphasic (qRs). A monophasic or diphasic complex in V_6 favors a ventricular origin, while the triphasic qRs complex is typical of RBBB aberration in V_6.
3. If the QRS in V_1 has "rabbit ears" (two peaks), determine if the left or the right rabbit ear is taller. A taller left rabbit ear favors a ventricular origin, while a taller right rabbit ear does not favor either diagnosis.

If the QRS has a LBBB morphology (negative in V_1), follow these steps to evaluate morphology (Figures 21–35 and 21–36B):

1. Look at V_1 or V_2 (both are helpful in this case) and determine if the R wave (if present) is wide or narrow. A wide R wave of >0.03 second favors a ventricular rhythm, while a narrow R wave favors a supraventricular origin with LBBB aberration.
2. Next look at the downstroke of the S wave in V_1 or V_2. Slurring or notching on the downstroke favors a ventricular origin. LBBB aberration typically slurs on the upstroke if it slurs at all.
3. Measure from the onset of the QRS complex to the deepest part of the S wave in V_1 or V_2. A measurement of >0.06 second favors a ventricular rhythm and a narrower measurement favors LBBB aberration. Note that this measurement can be prolonged due to either a wide R wave or slurring on the downstroke of the S wave, either one of which favors the ventricular origin of the rhythm.
4. Look at V_6 and determine if a Q wave is present. Any Q wave (either a QS or qR complex) favors a ventricular origin.

Concordance

The term *concordance* means that all the QRS complexes across the precordium from V_1 through V_6 point in the same direction; positive concordance means they are all upright, and negative concordance means they are all negative (Figure 21–37A). Negative concordance favors a diagnosis of ventricular tachycardia when it occurs in a wide QRS tachycardia, while positive concordance favors ven-

RBBB MORPHOLOGY

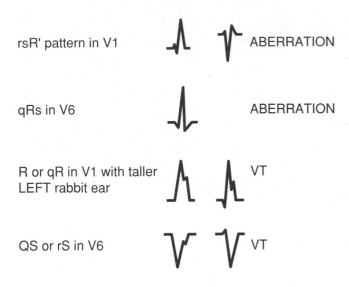

rsR' pattern in V1   ABERRATION

qRs in V6   ABERRATION

R or qR in V1 with taller
LEFT rabbit ear   VT

QS or rS in V6   VT

LBBB MORPHOLOGY

In Leads V1 or V2:

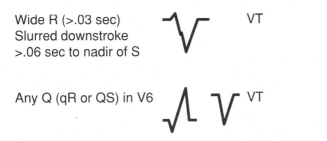

Wide R (>.03 sec)
Slurred downstroke
>.06 sec to nadir of S   VT

Any Q (qR or QS) in V6   VT

Figure 21–35. Morphology clues for wide QRS beats and rhythms with RBBB and LBBB patterns. *(From: Jacobson, C: Arrhythmias and conduction disturbances. In Woods SL, et al. (eds.): Cardiac nursing, 3rd ed. Philadelphia: J.B. Lippincott, 1995, p. 348.)*

tricular tachycardia as long as Wolff-Parkinson-White syndrome can be ruled out.

Fusion and Capture Beats
Ventricular *fusion beats* occur when the ventricles are depolarized by two different wavefronts of electrical activity at the same time. Fusion often results when a supraventricular impulse travels through the AV node and begins to depolarize the ventricles at the same time that an impulse from a ventricular focus depolarizes the ventricles. When two different impulses contribute to ventricular depolarization, the resulting QRS shape and width are determined by the relative contributions of both the supraventricular and the ventricular impulses. In the presence of a wide QRS tachycardia, the presence of fusion beats indicates AV dissociation,

which means that the atria and ventricles are under the control of separate pacemakers. *Capture beats* occur when the supraventricular impulse manages to conduct all the way into and through the ventricle, depolarizing ("capturing") the ventricle and resulting in a normal QRS in the midst of the wide QRS tachycardia. The presence of fusion and capture beats in a wide QRS tachycardia is strong evidence supporting the diagnosis of ventricular tachycardia, but they occur rarely and cannot be counted on to make the diagnosis. Figure 21–37B shows fusion beats in a wide QRS tachycardia. Helpful ECG clues for differentiating aberrancy from ventricular ectopy are summarized in Table 21–3.

ST-SEGMENT MONITORING

Many bedside monitors have software programs that allow for continuous monitoring of the ST segment in addition to routine arrhythmia monitoring. Continuous ST-segment monitoring can detect ischemia related to reocclusion of the involved artery in patients with acute MI who have received thrombolytic therapy, angioplasty, or other interventional cardiologic procedures aimed at opening occluded coronary arteries. ST-segment monitoring is also useful in detecting silent ischemia (ischemic episodes that occur in the absence of chest pain or other symptoms) that would otherwise go unnoticed with symptom and arrhythmia monitoring alone. Early detection of ischemic changes is critical in identifying patients who need interventions to reestablish blood flow to myocardium before permanent damage occurs.

ST elevation in leads facing damaged myocardium is the ECG sign of myocardial injury. ST depression is often recorded as a reciprocal change in leads that do not directly face involved myocardium. In addition, ST depression can be recorded in leads facing ischemic tissue. Therefore, either ST elevation or ST depression indicates myocardium at risk for infarction and a patient potentially at risk for complications related to infarction. The sooner the artery is opened and blood flow reestablished to ischemic or injured tissue, the more myocardium is salvaged and the fewer complications and deaths occur.

Measuring the ST Segment

Clinically significant ST-segment deviation is defined as ST elevation or depression 1 mm or more from the baseline, or isoelectric line, measured 80 ms (0.08 second) after the J point. The J point is the point at which the QRS ends and the ST segment begins. Some sources recommend measuring the ST segment 60 ms (0.06 second) after the J point, but this may lead to more false-positive ST changes when there is no myocardial ischemia. Figure 21–38 illustrates a normal ST segment and ST-segment elevation and depression.

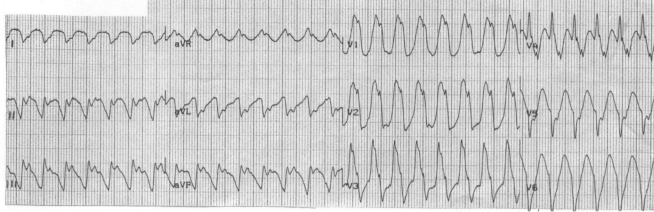

A

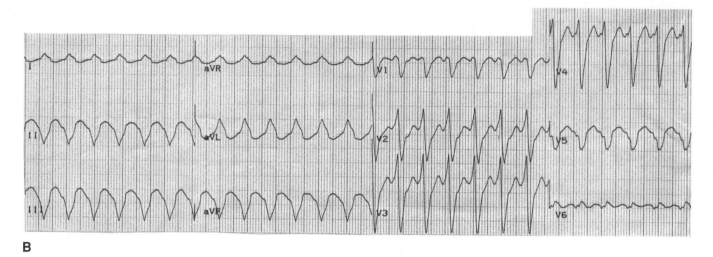

B

Figure 21–36. 12-lead ECG of ventricular tachycardia. (A) With RBBB morphology. Note monophasic R wave with taller left rabbit ear in V_1 and QS complex in V_6. (B) With LBBB morphology. Note wide R wave in V_1 and V_2, and qR pattern in V_6.

ST-segment monitoring software in newer bedside monitors defines the baseline and the ST-segment measuring point. It also sets default alarm parameters so the equipment can audibly notify the nurse when the patient's ST segment falls outside the defined parameters. Most monitors allow the user to redefine the baseline, reset the J point, choose where the ST segment is measured, and change the alarm parameters to account for individual patient variations. The monitor then displays the ST segment measurement in millimeters on the screen, and most monitors also allow for trending of the ST segment over specified time intervals.

Choosing the Best Leads for ST-Segment Monitoring

Most newer-generation bedside monitors offer at least two leads for simultaneous ECG monitoring and some offer three leads. The single best lead for arrhythmia monitoring is V_1, with V_6 being next best. Using two or three leads for ST-segment monitoring is optimal since a single lead may

miss significant ST-segment deviations. Since current bedside monitors allow for the use of only one V lead at a time, use V_1 as the arrhythmia monitoring lead (or V_6 if V_1 is not available due to dressings, etc). This means that only limb leads are available for use in ST-segment monitoring. The best limb leads are discussed below.

The best way to choose leads for ST-segment monitoring is to know the patient's "ischemic fingerprint." To determine the patient's ischemic fingerprint, obtain a 12-lead ECG during a pain episode or with inflation of the balloon during angioplasty and note which leads show the most ST-segment displacement (either elevation or depression) during the acute ischemic event. Choose the lead or leads with the most ST-segment displacement as the bedside ST-segment monitoring leads.

If no ischemic fingerprint is available, use a lead or leads that have been determined through research to be best for the artery involved (Table 21–4). The limb leads that

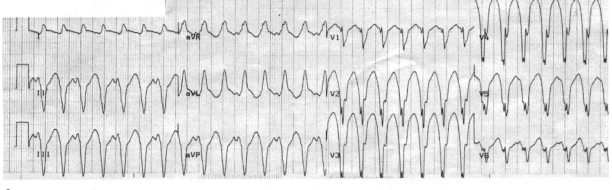

A

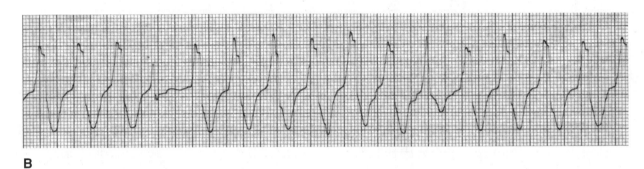

B

Figure 21–37. (A) 12-lead ECG of ventricular tachycardia with negative concordance. (B) Rhythm strips of ventricular tachycardia with fusion beats.

have been shown to best detect ischemia related to all three major coronary arteries (right coronary, left anterior descending, and circumflex) are leads III and aVF. In the case of the right coronary artery (RCA), leads III and aVF directly face the inferior wall supplied by this artery and record ST elevation with inferior wall injury. The left anterior descending (LAD) and circumflex artery supply the anterior and lateral walls, respectively. Since these walls are not directly faced by leads III and aVF, ST-segment depression is recorded as a reciprocal change when anterior or lateral wall injury occurs.

CARDIAC PACEMAKERS

Chapter 4 describes the components of a temporary pacing system and basic pacemaker operation. This section discusses single-chamber and dual-chamber pacemaker function and evaluation of pacemaker rhythm strips for appropriate capture and sensing.

Cardiac pacemakers are classified by a standardized five-letter pacemaker code that describes the location of the pacing wire(s) and the expected function of the pacemaker. Table 21–5 illustrates the five-letter code. The first letter in

TABLE 21–3.   ECG CLUES FOR DIFFERENTIATING ABERRATION FROM VENTRICULAR ECTOPY

	Aberrancy	Ventricular Ectopy
P Waves	Precede QRS complexes	Dissociated from QRS or occur at rate slower than QRS; if 1:1 V-A conduction is present, retrograde P waves follow every QRS
Precordial QRS concordance	Positive concordance may occur with WPW	Negative concordance favors VT; positive concordance favors VT if WPW ruled out
Fusion or capture beats		Strong evidence in favor of VT
QRS axis	Often normal; may be deviated to right or left	Indeterminate axis favors VT; often deviated to left or right
RBBB QRS morphology	Triphasic rsR′ in V_1; triphasic qRs in V_6	Monophasic R wave or diphasic qR complex in V_1; left "rabbit ear" taller in V_1; monophasic QS or diphasic rS in V_6
LBBB QRS morphology	Narrow R wave (<0.04 second) in V_1; straight downstroke of S wave in V_1 (often slurs or notches on upstroke); usually no Q wave in V_6	Wide R wave (>0.03 second) in V_1 or V_2; slurring or notching on downstroke of S wave in V_1; delay of greater than 0.06 second to nadir of S wave in V_1 or V_2; any Q wave in V_6

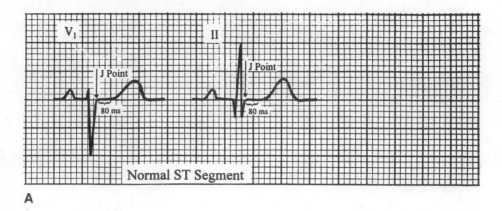

A

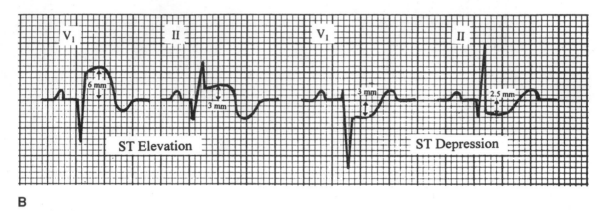

B

Figure 21–38. (A) Normal ST segment on the baseline in leads V_1 and II. (B) ST-segment elevation and ST-segment depression.

the pacemaker code describes the chamber that is paced (A = atrium, V = ventricle, D = dual [atrium and ventricle], O = none). The letter in the second position describes the chamber where intrinsic electrical activity is sensed (A = atrium, V = ventricle, D = dual, 0 = none). The letter in the third position describes the pacemaker's response to sensing of intrinsic electrical activity (I = inhibited, T = triggered, D = dual [inhibited or triggered], 0 = none). The fourth letter describes programmable functions of the pacemaker or the presence of rate modulation, and the fifth letter describes antitachycardia pacing functions. In order to know how a pacemaker should function, it is necessary to know at a minimum the first three letters of the code, which describe where the pacemaker is supposed to pace, where it is supposed to sense, and what it should do when it senses. The last two codes, representing advanced pacemaker function, are not covered in this text. See the recommended references at the end of the chapter.

Three types of temporary pacing are commonly used in the critical care setting. The first is transvenous pacing through a wire introduced into the apex of the right ventricle via a peripheral or central vein and set in the demand mode (sensitive to intrinsic ventricular activity). Ventricular pacing is always done in the demand mode to avoid the delivery

of pacing stimuli into the vulnerable period of the cardiac cycle, which could induce ventricular tachycardia or fibrillation (see Chapter 4, Basic Cardiac Rhythms). This type of pacing is described by the pacemaker code as a VVI pacemaker—it paces the ventricle, senses intrinsic ventricular electrical activity, and inhibits its output when sensing occurs.

The second type of pacing done in critical care is temporary epicardial pacing (either atrial, ventricular, or dual-chamber) via pacing wires attached to the atria and/or ventricles during cardiac surgery. If atrial pacing is done with no sensing of atrial electrical activity, also called asynchronous

TABLE 21–4. RECOMMENDED LEADS FOR CONTINUOUS ECG MONITORING

Purpose	Best Leads
Arrhythmia detection	V_1 or MCL_1 (V_6 or MCL_6 next best)
RCA ischemia, inferior MI	III, AVF
LAD ischemia, anterior MI	V_2, V_3, V_4 (III, aVF best limb leads)
Circumflex ischemia, lateral MI	III, aVF, V_2
RV infarction	V_4R
Wellens warning	V_2 or V_3
Axis shifts	I and aVF together

TABLE 21–5. PACEMAKER CODES

First Letter: Chamber Paced	Second Letter: Chamber Sensed	Third Letter: Response to Sensing	Fourth Letter: Programmability, Rate Modulation	Fifth Letter: Antitachycardia Pacing Functions
0 = None	0 = None	0 = None	0 = None	0 = None
A = Atrium	A = Atrium	I = Inhibited	P = Simple programmable	P = Pacing (Antitachycardia)
V = Ventricle	V = Ventricle	T = Triggered	M = Multiprogrammable	S = Shock
D = Dual (A&V)	D = Dual (A&V)	D = Dual (I&T)	C = Communicating	D = Dual (P&S)
			R = Rate modulation	

mode, the pacemaker operates as an AOO pacemaker—it paces the atria, does not sense, and therefore does not respond to sensing. If atrial pacing is done with sensing of atrial electrical activity, also called the demand mode, the pacemaker operates as an AAI pacemaker—it paces the atria, senses atrial activity, and inhibits its output when it senses. Dual-chamber pacing can be done in several modes involving pacing and sensing functions in one or both chambers and described by the pacemaker code according to the mode chosen. The two most common dual-chamber modes used with temporary epicardial pacing (and occasionally with temporary transvenous pacing) are DVI (paces atria and ventricles, senses only in the ventricle, and inhibits pacing output when sensing occurs) and DDD (paces both chambers, senses both chambers, and either triggers or inhibits pacing output in response to sensing). The common dual-chamber pacing modes are listed in Table 21–6.

The third type of temporary pacing is external (transcutaneous) pacing. External pacing is done in emergency situations requiring immediate pacing when placement of a temporary transvenous pacing wire is not feasible. External pacing is not as reliable as transvenous or epicardial pacing and is used as a temporary measure until transvenous pacing can be instituted. External pacing is briefly described in Chapter 4, Interpretations and Management of Basic Cardiac Rhythms.

Evaluating Pacemaker Function

Evaluating pacemaker function requires knowledge of the mode of pacing expected (VVI, AAI, etc.); the minimum rate of the pacemaker, or pacing interval; and any other programmed parameters in the pacemaker. The basic functions of a pacemaker include *stimulus release, capture,* and *sensing.* Stimulus release refers to pacemaker output, or the

ability of the pacemaker to generate and release a pacing impulse. Capture is the ability of the pacing stimulus to result in depolarization of the chamber being paced. Sensing is the ability of the pacemaker to recognize and respond to intrinsic electrical activity in the heart. Pacemaker operation is evaluated according to these three functions. Single-chamber pacemaker evaluation is much less complicated than dual-chamber evaluation. Since single-chamber ventricular pacing is a very common type of temporary pacing in critical care and telemetry units, VVI pacemaker evaluation is discussed here.

VVI Pacemaker Evaluation

Stimulus release, capture, and sensing must all be assessed when evaluating VVI pacemakers. A VVI pacemaker is expected to pace the ventricle at the set rate unless spontaneous ventricular activity occurs to inhibit pacing. The set rate of the pacemaker, or pacing interval, is measured from one pacing stimulus to the next consecutive stimulus. Pacemakers have a refractory period, which is a period following either pacing or sensing in the chamber, during which the pacemaker is unable to respond to intrinsic activity. During the refractory period, the pacemaker in effect has its eyes closed and is not able to see spontaneous activity. In a normally functioning VVI pacemaker, pacing spikes occur at the set pacing interval and each spike results in a ventricular depolarization (capture). If spontaneous ventricular activity occurs (either a normally conducted QRS or a PVC), that activity is sensed and the next pacing stimulus is inhibited. Figure 21–39 shows normal VVI pacemaker function.

Stimulus Release

Stimulus release depends on a pacemaker with enough battery power to generate the electrical impulse, and on an

TABLE 21–6. DUAL-CHAMBER PACING MODES

Mode	Chamber(s) Paced	Chamber(s) Sensed	Response to Sensing
DVI	Atrium and ventricle	Ventricle	Inhibited
VDD	Ventricle	Atrium and ventricle	Atrial sensing triggers ventricular pacing
			Ventricular sensing inhibits ventricular pacing
DDI	Atrium and ventricle	Atrium and ventricle	Inhibited
DDD	Atrium and ventricle	Atrium and ventricle	Atrial sensing inhibits atrial pacing, triggers ventricular pacing
			Ventricular sensing inhibits atrial and ventricular pacing

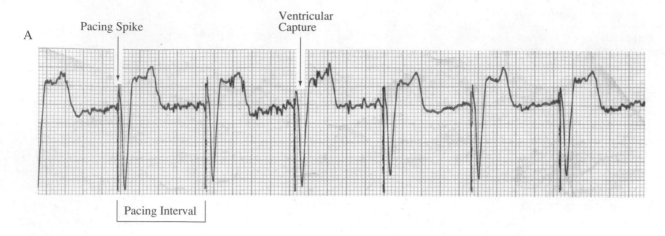

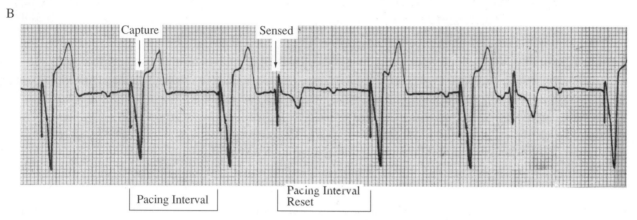

Figure 21–39. Normal VVI pacemaker function. (A) Pacing electrical activity ("pacer spike") followed by a wide QRS complex indicating ventricular capture. Pacemaker sensing cannot be evaluated since no intrinsic QRS complexes are present. (B) Pacemaker capture and sensing both normal. Intrinsic QRS complexes are sensed, inhibiting ventricular pacing output, and resetting the pacing interval. Absence of intrinsic ventricular electrical activity causes pacing to occur with capture.

intact pacemaker lead system to deliver the electrical stimulus to the heart. The presence of a pacer spike on the rhythm strip or monitor indicates that the stimulus was released from the generator and entered the body. The presence of the spike does not indicate where the stimulus was delivered (e.g., atria or ventricles), only that it entered the body somewhere. Total absence of pacing stimuli, when they should be present, can indicate a faulty pulse generator or battery, or a break or disconnection in the lead system.

Pacing stimuli also can be absent when pacing is inhibited by the sensing of intrinsic electrical activity. Figure 21–40 illustrates total loss of stimulus release in a patient whose pacemaker battery was dead.

Capture
Capture is indicated by a wide QRS complex immediately following the pacemaker spike and represents the ability of the pacing stimulus to depolarize the ventricle. Loss of cap-

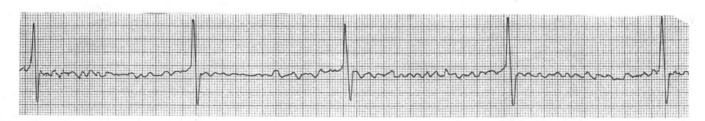

Figure 21–40. Absence of stimulus release in a patient with a permanent pacemaker. Underlying rhythm is atrial fibrillation with complete AV block and a very slow ventricular rate. The battery in the pacemaker generator was dead.

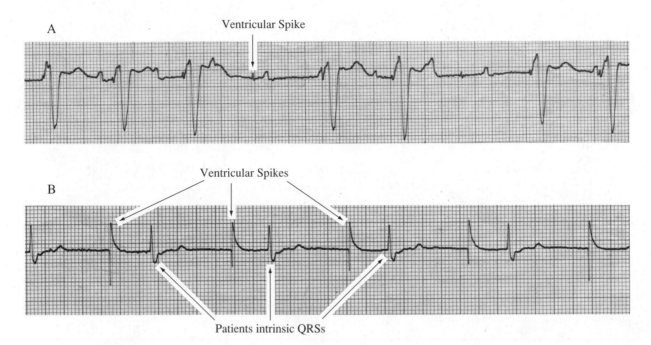

A — Ventricular Spike

B — Ventricular Spikes / Patients intrinsic QRSs

Figure 21–41. (A) VVI pacemaker with intermittent loss of capture. (B) VVI pacemaker with total loss of capture.

ture is recognized by the presence of pacer spikes that are not followed by paced ventricular complexes (Figure 21–41). Causes of loss of capture include:

- Inadequate stimulus strength, which can be corrected by increasing the electrical output of the pacemaker (turning up the milliampere level).
- Pacing wire out of position and not in contact with myocardium, which can be corrected by repositioning the wire and sometimes by repositioning the patient.
- Pacing lead positioned in infarcted tissue, which can be corrected by repositioning the wire to a place where the myocardium is not injured and is capable of responding to the stimulus.
- Electrolyte imbalances or drugs that alter the ability of the heart to respond to the pacing stimulus.
- Delivery of a pacing stimulus during the ventricles refractory period when the heart is physiologically unable to respond to the stimulus. This problem occurs with loss of sensing (undersensing) and can be corrected by correcting the sensing problem (Figure 21–43A).

Sensing

Sensing of intrinsic ventricular electrical activity inhibits the next pacing stimulus and resets the pacing interval. Sensing cannot occur unless the pacemaker is given the opportunity to sense. It must be in the demand mode and there must be intrinsic ventricular activity that occurs in order for the pacemaker to have an opportunity to sense. In Figure 21–39A, sensing cannot be evaluated because there is no intrinsic ventricular activity that occurs, and therefore the pacemaker is not given an opportunity to sense. In Figure 21–39B, the occurrence of two spontaneous QRS complexes provides the pacemaker with an opportunity to sense. In this example, sensing occurred normally, as indicated by the absence of the next expected pacing stimulus and resetting of the pacing interval by the intrinsic QRS complex.

Two sensing problems can occur: undersensing and oversensing. *Undersensing,* also called "failure to sense" or "loss of sensing," can be due to:

- Asynchronous (fixed rate) mode in which the sensing circuit is off. This problem can be corrected by turning the sensitivity control to the demand mode.
- Pacing catheter out of position or lying in infarcted tissue, which can be corrected by repositioning the wire. Pacing wire repositioning must be done by a physician; however, turning the patient onto his or her side sometimes temporarily works when the pacing wire loses contact with the ventricle.
- Intrinsic QRS voltage too low to be sensed by the pacemaker. Turning the sensitivity control clockwise or decreasing the sensitivity number increases the sensitivity of the pacemaker and makes it able to "see" smaller intrinsic electrical signals. Repositioning the wire sometimes helps.
- Break in connections, battery failure, or faulty pulse generator. Check and tighten all connections along the pacing system, and replace the battery if it is low. A chest x-ray may detect wire fracture. Change the pulse generator if problems cannot be corrected any other way.

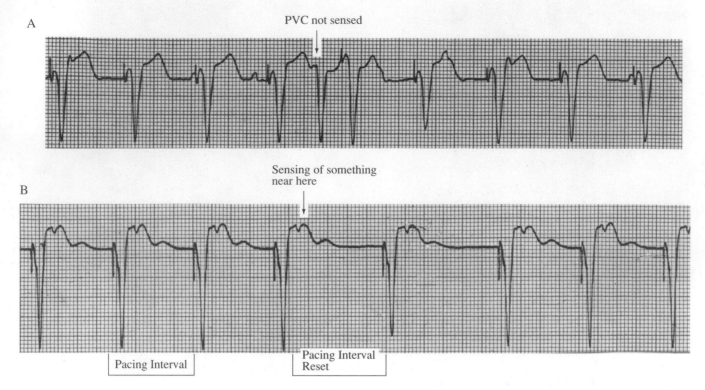

Figure 21–42. (A) Undersensing in a VVI pacemaker. The PVC is not sensed and pacing occurs at the programmed pacing interval, resulting in a pacemaker spike on the T wave of the PVC without capture. (B) Oversensing in a VVI pacemaker. The pacing rate slows for two intervals, presumably due to sensing of something near the T wave which resets the pacing interval from the point where sensing occurred.

- Intrinsic ventricular activity falling in the pacemaker's refractory period. If a spontaneous QRS complex occurs during the time the pacemaker has its eyes closed, the pacemaker cannot see it. This event occurs when the pacemaker fails to capture, which can allow an intrinsic QRS to occur during the pacemaker's refractory period. This problem is due to loss of capture and does not reflect a sensing malfunction (Figure 21–43).

Oversensing means that the pacemaker is so sensitive that it inappropriately senses internal or outside signals as QRS complexes and inhibits its output. Common sources of outside signals that can interfere with pacemaker function include electromagnetic or radio-frequency signals, or electronic equipment in use near the pacemaker. Internal sources of interference can include large P waves, large T-wave voltage, local myopotentials in the heart, or skeletal muscle potentials (Figure 21–42B). Since a VVI pacemaker is programmed to inhibit its output when it senses, oversensing can be a dangerous situation in a pacemaker-dependent patient, resulting in ventricular asystole. Oversensing is usually due to the sensitivity control being set too high, which can be corrected by turning the sensitivity dial counterclockwise and reducing the pacemaker's sensitivity. It is recommended that the sensitivity control be set between the 1 o'clock and 3 o'clock positions on the dial rather than all

the way to the right, unless a higher sensitivity is required to make the pacemaker sense QRS complexes.

Stimulation Threshold Testing

The stimulation threshold is the minimum output of the pacemaker necessary to capture the heart consistently. The stimulation threshold changes over time; when the pacing lead is first placed, the stimulation threshold is usually very low. Over time, the threshold increases and it takes more output to result in capture. When caring for a patient with a temporary pacemaker, stimulation threshold testing should be done every shift until a stable threshold is reached. Once the threshold has been determined, set the output two to three times higher than threshold to ensure an adequate safety margin for capture. To determine the stimulation threshold, follow these steps:

- Verify that the patient is in a paced rhythm. The pacing rate may need to be temporarily increased to override an intrinsic rhythm.
- Watch the monitor continuously while slowly decreasing output by turning the output control counterclockwise.
- Note when the pacing stimulus no longer captures the heart (a pacing spike not followed by a paced beat).
- Slowly increase the output until 1:1 capture resumes. This is the stimulation threshold.

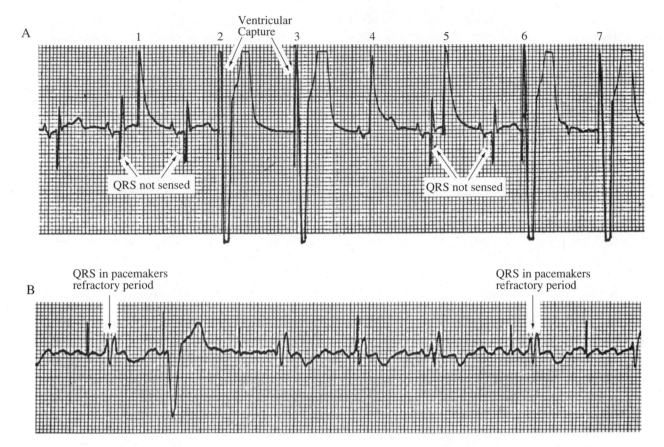

Figure 21–43. (A) Intermittent loss of sensing in a VVI pacemaker. Delivery of the pacing stimulus during the heart's refractory period makes it appear that capture is lost as well. Since the heart is physiologically unable to respond to the pacing stimulus when it falls in the refractory period, this is not a capture problem. Pacer spikes 1, 2, 5, and 6 should not have occurred; their presence is due to loss of sensing. Pacer spike 4 occurred coincident with the normal QRS complex, resulting in a "pseudofusion" beat, and does not represent loss of sensing. (B) Loss of capture in a VVI pacemaker. Only one pacer spike captures the ventricle. Two QRS complexes occur during the pacemaker's refractory period and thus are not sensed. This does not represent loss of sensing because the pacemaker has its "eyes closed" during the time intrinsic ventricular activity occurred.

- Set the output two to three times higher than threshold (i.e., if threshold is 2 mA, set output between 4 and 6 mA).

DDD Pacemaker Evaluation

Dual-chamber pacemakers have become very complicated, with multiple programmable parameters and varying functions depending on the manufacturer. It is impossible to present dual-chamber pacemaker function in detail in a single chapter. In order to understand dual-chamber pacemaker function, it is necessary to understand the timing cycles involved in dual-chamber pacing. This information is best obtained in a class sponsored by a pacemaker manufacturer or from a pacemaker technical manual. In this section, the major timing cycles are defined and basic DDD pacemaker evaluation is covered in a very generic manner, since each pacemaker is different depending on the manufacturer. Dual-chamber pacemakers can function in a variety of modes (Table 21–5). Since the DDD mode is most commonly used, basic DDD function is described here.

According to the pacemaker code, DDD means that both chambers (atria and ventricles) are paced, both chambers are sensed, and the mode of response to sensed events is either inhibited or triggered, depending on which chamber is sensed. When atrial activity is sensed, pacing is triggered in the ventricle after the programmed AV delay. When ventricular activity is sensed, all pacemaker output is inhibited.

The following timing cycles determine dual-chamber pacemaker function:

- Pacing interval (or lower rate limit): the base rate of the pacemaker, measured between two consecutive atrial pacing stimuli. The pacing interval is a programmed parameter.
- AV delay (or AV interval): the amount of time between atrial and ventricular pacing, or the "elec-

tronic PR interval." This is measured from the atrial pacing spike to the ventricular pacing spike and is a programmed parameter.

- Atrial escape interval (or VA interval): the interval from a sensed or paced ventricular event to the next atrial pacing output. The VA interval represents the amount of time the pacemaker waits after it paces in the ventricle or senses ventricular activity before pacing the atrium. The atrial escape interval is not a programmed parameter, but is derived by subtracting the AV delay from the pacing interval. Its length can be estimated by measuring from a ventricular spike to the next atrial pacing spike.

- Total atrial refractory period (TARP): the period of time following a sensed P wave or a paced atrial event during which the atrial channel will not respond to sensed events (i.e., "has its eyes closed"). The TARP consists of the AV delay and the PVARP (see below).

- Post ventricular atrial refractory period (PVARP): the period of time following an intrinsic QRS or a paced ventricular beat during which the atrial channel is refractory and will not respond to sensed atrial activity. PVARP is a programmable parameter but is not evident on a rhythm strip.

- Blanking period: the very short ventricular refractory period that occurs with every atrial pacemaker output. The ventricular channel "blinks its eyes" so it won't sense the atrial output and inappropriately inhibit ventricular pacing. The blanking period is a programmable parameter but is not evident on a rhythm strip.

- Ventricular refractory period (VRP): the period of time following a paced ventricular beat or a sensed QRS during which the ventricular channel ignores intrinsic ventricular activity (i.e., "has its eyes closed"). VRP is a programmable parameter but is not evident on a rhythm strip.

- Maximum tracking interval (or upper rate limit): the maximum rate at which the ventricular channel will track atrial activity. The upper rate limit prevents rapid ventricular pacing in response to very rapid atrial activity, such as atrial tachycardia or atrial flutter. The maximum tracking interval is a programmable parameter and usually is set according to how active a patient is expected to be and how fast a ventricular rate is likely to be tolerated.

Since a dual-chamber pacemaker has both atrial and ventricular pacing and sensing functions, evaluation includes assessing atrial capture, atrial sensing, ventricular capture, and ventricular sensing. In order to evaluate dual chamber pacemaker function accurately, it is necessary to know the following information: mode of function (DDD, DVI, etc.), minimum rate, upper rate limit, AV delay, and atrial and ventricular refractory periods. In the real world of bedside nursing, this information is not always available, so we do the best we can with what we have. The following sections briefly discuss the issues of assessing atrial and ventricular capture and sensing in a dual-chamber pacing system.

Atrial capture

Atrial capture, unlike ventricular capture, is not always easy to see. Often, the atrial response to pacing is so small

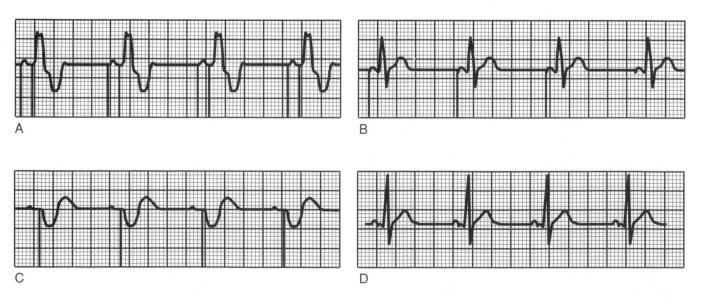

Figure 21–44. Four states of DDD pacing. (A) Atrial and ventricular pacing (AV sequential pacing state). (B) Atrial pacing, ventricular sensing. (C) Atrial sensing, ventricular pacing (atrial tracking state). (D) Atrial and ventricular sensing (inhibited pacing state).

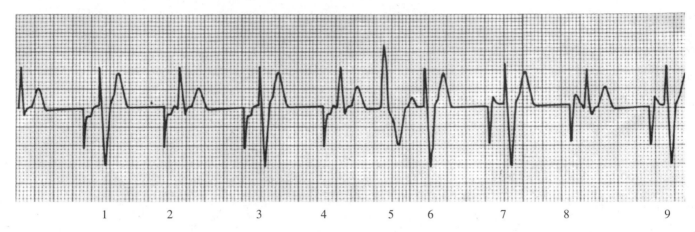

Figure 21–45. DDD pacemaker operating in all four states of pacing. Beat 1 = AV sequential pacing; beat 2 = atrial pacing, ventricular sensing; beat 3 = AV sequential pacing; beat 4 = atrial pacing, ventricular sensing; beat 5 = PVC; beat 6 = atrial sensing, ventricular pacing; beat 7 = AV sequential pacing; beat 8 = atrial pacing, ventricular sensing; beat 9 = AV sequential pacing. *Atrial capture* is proven by beats 2, 4, and 8 (atrial spike followed by normal QRS within the programmed AV delay). *Atrial sensing* is proven by beat 6 (normal P followed by paced V at end of AV delay). *Ventricular capture* is verified by beats 1, 3, 6, 7, and 9 (wide paced QRS following ventricular pacing spike). *Ventricular sensing* is proven by beats 2, 4, and 8 (atrial spike followed by normal QRS which inhibited ventricular pacing spike).

that it cannot be seen in many monitoring leads, so we cannot rely on the presence of a P wave following every atrial pacer spike as evidence of atrial capture. If a clear P wave is present after every atrial pacemaker spike, atrial capture can be assumed. In the absence of a clear P wave, atrial capture can only be assumed when an atrial pacer spike is followed by a normally conducted QRS complex within the programmed AV delay. If the atrial spike captures the atrium and there is intact AV conduction, the presence of the normal QRS indicates that the atrium must have been captured in order for conduction to have occurred into the ventricles before the ventricular pacing stimulus was delivered. Since a DDD pacemaker paces the ventricle at a preset AV interval following atrial pacing, the presence of a ventricular paced beat following an atrial paced beat does not verify capture, since the ventricle will pace at the end of the AV delay whether atrial capture occurs or not. Therefore, atrial capture can only be assumed when there is an obvious P wave after every atrial pacing spike or when an atrial pacing spike is followed by a normal QRS within the programmed AV delay.

Atrial sensing

Atrial sensing is verified by the presence of a spontaneous P wave that is followed by a paced ventricular beat at the end of the programmed AV delay. If a P wave is sensed, it starts the AV delay and ventricular pacing is triggered at the end of the AV delay unless AV conduction is intact and results in a normal QRS. The presence of a normal P wave

followed by a normal QRS only proves that AV conduction is intact, not that the P wave was sensed by the pacemaker. Therefore, atrial sensing is verified by a spontaneous P wave followed by a paced QRS.

Ventricular capture

Ventricular capture is recognized by a wide QRS immediately following a ventricular pacing spike. Ventricular capture is much easier to recognize than atrial capture and is no different than with single-chamber ventricular pacing.

Ventricular sensing

Ventricular sensing can only be verified if there is spontaneous ventricular activity present for the pacemaker to sense. Ventricular sensing is verified by an atrial pacer spike followed by a normal QRS that inhibits the ventricular pacing spike, which is the same event that proves atrial capture. If a QRS is sensed before the next atrial pacing spike is due, both the atrial and ventricular pacing stimuli are inhibited and the VA interval (atrial escape interval) is reset.

Dual-chamber pacemakers are capable of operating in four states of pacing: atrial and ventricular pacing, atrial pacing with ventricular sensing, atrial sensing with ventricular pacing, and atrial and ventricular sensing. All four states of pacing can occur within a short period of time, and the timing cycles determine which state of pacing is done. Figure 21–44 shows the four states of dual-chamber pacing, and Figure 21–45 illustrates the basic principles of dual-chamber pacemaker evaluation.

SELECTED BIBLIOGRAPHY

What Heals: Enhancing Cardiovascular Health with Interpersonal Communication

Thomas SA, Friedmann E: The cardiovascular effects of rate of verbal communication. *Journal of Cardiovascular Nursing.* 1994;9:16–26.

Thomas SA, Liehr P: Cardiovascular reactivity during verbal communication: An emerging risk factor. *Journal of Cardiovascular Nursing.* 1995;9:1–11.

General Electrocardiography

Conover MB: *Understanding electrocardiography,* 6th ed. St. Louis, MO: Mosby Year-Book, 1992.

Davis D: *How to quickly and accurately master ECG interpretation,* 2nd ed. Philadelphia: JB Lippincott, 1992.

Gilmore SB, Woods SL: Electrocardiography and vectorcardiography. In Woods SL, et al. (eds.): *Cardiac nursing,* 3rd ed. Philadelphia: JB Lippincott, 1995.

Marriott HJL: *Practical electrocardiography,* 8th ed. Baltimore: Williams & Wilkins, 1988.

Wagoner GS: *Marriott's practical electrocardiography,* 9th ed. Baltimore: Williams & Wilkins, 1994.

Wellens HJJ, Conover MB: *The ECG in emergency decision making.* Philadelphia: WB Saunders, 1992.

ST-Segment Monitoring

Drew B, Tisdale LA: ST segment monitoring for coronary artery reocclusion following thrombolytic therapy and coronary angioplasty: Identification of optimal bedside monitoring leads. *American Journal of Critical Care.* 1993;2:280–292.

Tisdale LA, Drew B: ST segment monitoring for myocardial ischemia. *AACN Clinical Issues.* 1993;4:34–43.

Cardiac Pacing

Furman S, Hayes D, Holmes D: *A practice of cardiac pacing,* 3rd ed. New York: Futura, 1993.

Moses HW, Schneider JA, Miller BD, Taylor GJ: *A practical guide to cardiac pacing,* 3rd ed. Boston: Little, Brown, 1991.

Siemens Pacesetter: Pacemaker technology for nurses and allied health professionals. Norcross, Georgia: Siemens Pacesetter Education Department.

Advanced Arrhythmia Interpretation

Jacobson C: Arrhythmias and conduction disturbances. In Woods SL, et al. (eds.): *Cardiac nursing,* 3rd ed. Philadelphia: JB Lippincott, 1995.

Marriott HJL, Conover M: *Advanced concepts in arrhythmias,* 2nd ed. St. Louis, MO: CV Mosby, 1989.

Advanced Cardiovascular Concepts

22

► **Knowledge Competencies**

1. Describe the etiology, pathophysiology, clinical presentation, patient needs, and principles of management of:
   - Cardiomyopathy
   - Valvular disease
   - Pericarditis
   - Aortic aneurysm
   - Cardiac transplantation

2. Compare and contrast the pathophysiology, clinical presentation, patient needs, and management approaches of:
   - Cardiomyopathy
   - Valvular disease
   - Pericarditis
   - Aortic aneurysm
   - Cardiac transplantation

3. Identify indications for, complications of, and nursing management of patients receiving intraaortic balloon pump and ventricular assist device therapy.

■ *What Heals: Integrity of the Family Unit in the Midst of Death*

When technology cannot reverse the death process, creating a place of peace, love, compassion, and openness for the patient and family is needed to foster the integrity of the family unit in the midst of death. Each patient, family, and situation will be different. The following are examples of moments when nurses facilitated this process:

- Lynn, a 30-year-old mother of three children, was dying with end-stage heart disease. She asked her nurse whether guitar music could be played in her critical care room. The nurse arranged to meet Lynn's last request. Three hours before her death, the nurse tended to Lynn as a friend played guitar, the family sang her favorite songs, and her husband held her in his arms. Lynn died with her children, hus-

band, parents, and three friends surrounding her in the critical care unit.

- Jack, a 26-year-old dying with hypertrophic cardiomyopathy, never made it off of the ventilator following resuscitation from his cardiac arrest. However, when he was still conscious, he wrote a note to his nurse that said, "Call mom and ask her to bring my collection of bandannas and my country music tapes." Nothing else could be done. The physicians and nurses knew that death was imminent. As the nurse continued to care for Jack, his mother, father, brother, and sister stayed close to him. During this dying time, Jack wore a brightly colored bandanna across his forehead and he and his family listened to his music.

The last gesture Jack made was to smile as he tied another bandanna around the palm of his hand; he made a fist and raised his arm, indicating being a winner. With a smile on his face, he lost consciousness, went into bradycardia, and died within a few minutes.

Jack's critical care bed was needed for another patient from the emergency room. However, the nurse realized that this family needed more time to be with Jack. All life support equipment and intravenous lines were removed, and the family and Jack's body were moved to a private room at the end of the critical care unit. The family stayed for another hour with their deceased son. When the nurse discussed the steps necessary in preparing their son for transport to the funeral home, the mother asked if she could help. The nurse agreed. Tears fell down the mother's cheeks as she stroked her son's upper body and held him on his side for the nurse to finish her care. Tears also flowed down the nurse's cheeks as she completed her work and then embraced the mother. The room was filled with love and healing in the midst of death.

CEG & BMD

Adapted from: Dossey BM, Guzzetta CE, Kenner CV: Critical care nursing: Body-mind-spirit, *3rd ed. Philadelphia: JB Lippincott, 1992, p. 443.*

PATHOLOGIC CONDITIONS

Cardiomyopathy

Cardiomyopathy is a disease which involves destruction of the cardiac muscle fibers, leading to impaired cardiac function. The cause of cardiomyopathy is often unknown. Cardiomyopathy commonly is classified into three types: dilated, hypertrophic, and restrictive (Figure 22–1).

The two case studies below involve patients with dilated cardiomyopathy. As is typical with this type of cardiomyopathy, myocardial contractility is impaired and ventricular filling pressures are increased. Dilated cardiomyopathy is the most common type of cardiomyopathy, frequently affecting men during midlife.

AT THE BEDSIDE
▶ *Cardiomyopathy*

Mr. Grahm, 56 years old, was admitted to the emergency room with shortness of breath. His chest x-ray revealed an enlarged heart and pulmonary congestion. His 12-lead ECG was consistent with left ventricular hypertrophy. His rhythm was atrial fibrillation with a ventricular rate of 102. Clinical findings included bilateral rales auscultated one-third up from the bases, bilateral lower extremity 4+ pitting edema to the midcalf, jugular vein distention, an S_3, and a systolic murmur heard best at the apex. An emergency echocardiogram showed limited contractility of a dilated left ventricle.

AT THE BEDSIDE
▶ *Cardiomyopathy*

Andrea, 32 years old, was admitted to the high-risk perinatal unit at 31 weeks' gestation with dyspnea and fatigue. She had bilateral, basilar rales and her oxygen saturation via pulse oximetry was 88%. An echocardiogram showed a markedly dilated left ventricle with diffuse hypokinesis and an ejection fraction of 20% to 25%.

A pulmonary artery catheter was placed with the following parameters obtained:

RA: 12 mm Hg
PA: 48/26 mm Hg
PCW: 24 mm Hg
CO: 3.7 L/minute
CI: 1.8 L/minute/m^2

A dobutamine infusion was initiated at 5 µg/kg/minute and oxygen was applied at 6 L/minute via nasal cannula.

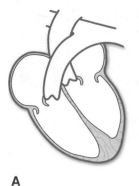
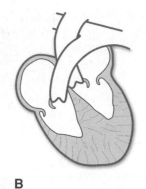
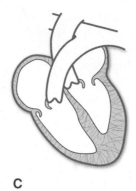

A   **B**   **C**

Figure 22–1. Types of cardiomyopathies. (A) Dilated (cardiac dilatation and impaired contractility). (B) Hypertrophic (decreased size of ventricular chambers and increased ventricular muscle mass). (C) Restrictive (decreased ventricular compliance).

Hypertrophic cardiomyopathy may occur in both the young and the elderly. Hypertrophic cardiomyopathy often is categorized as obstructive or nonobstructive. Ventricular hypertrophy occurs in both types. The diagnosis of obstructive hypertrophic cardiomyopathy is made if hypertrophy of the intraventricular septum is also present. The hypertrophied septum obstructs left ventricular ejection.

Restrictive cardiomyopathy is the least common type. A classic finding for this type of cardiomyopathy is ventricular fibrosis. The fibrosis causes the ventricles to become rigid, thus limiting their compliance or ability to distend.

Etiology and Pathophysiology
The etiology of cardiomyopathy is unclear. It is postulated that a variety of conditions may cause or contribute to the development of cardiomyopathy (Table 22–1).

Pathophysiology of Dilated Cardiomyopathy
Dilated cardiomyopathy begins with gradual destruction of the myocardial fibers, limiting the ability of cardiac muscle to forcefully contract. As the disease progresses, left ventricular dilatation occurs, with increases of blood volume in the left ventricle. This causes increased filling pressures and a decrease in cardiac output. Left atrial volume and pressure eventually increase as the atrium struggles to eject blood into a fluid-overloaded left ventricle. Increased left atrial pressure may lead to increased pulmonary vascular pressure as blood backs up into the pulmonary system. Right-sided heart failure may result from increased pulmonary vascular pressure or due to destruction of right atrial and ventricular myocardial fibers. Lastly, the atrioventricular valves (mitral and tricuspid) may develop insufficiency due to the increased ventricular pressures.

Pathophysiology of Hypertrophic Cardiomyopathy
Patients with hypertrophic cardiomyopathy have a greatly enlarged ventricular wall (Figure 22–1). It is not uncommon for the ventricular chamber size to be dramatically reduced from the hypertrophy. In obstructive cardiomyopathy the intraventricular septum is also involved in the hypertrophic process, whereas in nonobstructive cardiomyopathy the septum is relatively normal. This excessive myocardial muscle development causes the ventricle to become rigid, leading to decreased ventricular compliance and distensibility. This causes a decrease in the force of each myocardial contraction. As the strength of myocardial contractions decreases, left ventricular ejection into the aorta and cardiac output also decrease. Left ventricular systolic ejection may be further compromised by obstruction of the outflow tract as the anterior leaflet of the mitral valve presses against an enlarged intraventricular septum (obstructive cardiomyopathy).

TABLE 22–1. ETIOLOGY OF CARDIOMYOPATHY

Dilated Cardiomyopathy
Idiopathic
Toxins, such as lead, alcohol, cocaine
Muscle dystrophy
Myotonic dystrophy
Hypophosphatemia
Hypocalcemia
Hypokalemia
Viral, bacterial, or fungal infections
Lupus erythematosus
Peripartum or postpartum status
Rheumatoid disease
Scleroderma
Hypertension
Thiamine deficiency
Microvascular spasm

Hypertrophic Cardiomyopathy
Idiopathic
Genetic transmission
Friedreich's ataxia
Hypoparathyroidism

Restrictive Cardiomyopathy
Idiopathic
Myocardial fibrosis
Infiltration
Hypertrophy
Amyloidosis
Hemochromatosis
Glycogen deposition
Scleroderma

Stress is placed on the left atrium as it attempts to propel blood forward into the stiff left ventricle. It is not uncommon for left atrial enlargement to develop as the left atrium is forced to contract against high left ventricular resistance. In addition, mitral insufficiency may occur as elevated left ventricular end-diastolic pressure places added stress and pressure on the closed mitral valve.

Similar changes may occur on the right side of the heart. These may produce changes in the right atrium, right ventricle, and tricuspid valve.

Pathophysiology of Restrictive Cardiomyopathy

The ventricles of patients with restrictive cardiomyopathy become rigid as fibrotic tissue infiltrates the myocardium. This stiffness of the ventricles decreases the compliance, or distensibility, of the ventricles, thus decreasing ventricular filling and increasing end-diastolic pressures. The strength of the myocardial contraction is diminished, leading to decreases in cardiac output. As with the other types of cardiomyopathy, atrial workload is increased as the atria attempt to propel blood forward into stiff ventricles. It is not uncommon for atrioventricular valve insufficiency to develop, and for fluid to back up into the pulmonary and venous systems.

Clinical Presentation

Patients may be asymptomatic for lengthy periods of time (months to years) prior to being diagnosed with cardiomyopathy. By the time patients develop symptoms, significant cardiac dysfunction already may have occurred.

An increase in heart rate may occur initially as the heart attempts to maintain an adequate cardiac output. As the disease progresses and/or during physical exertion, the dysfunctional myocardium is usually unable to maintain an increase in heart rate and cardiac output begins to decrease.

Dilated Cardiomyopathy

1. Inability to maintain adequate cardiac output
   - Fatigue
   - Weakness
   - Sinus tachycardia (ST)
   - Pulses alternans
   - Narrowed pulse pressure
   - Decreased cardiac output (CO)
2. Increased left ventricular filling pressures
   - Dyspnea
   - Orthopnea
   - Paroxysmal nocturnal dyspnea
   - Rales
   - S_3/S_4
   - Arrhythmias
   - Systolic murmur with mitral valve insufficiency
   - Abnormal hemodynamic profile:

Increased pulmonary artery systolic (PAS) and diastolic (PAD) pressures
Elevated pulmonary capillary wedge (PCW) pressures
Increased systemic vascular resistance (SVR)
Elevated V wave on PCW waveform with mitral valve insufficiency

3. Increased right ventricular filling pressures
   - Peripheral edema
   - Jugular vein distention
   - Hepatomegaly
   - Elevated V wave on the right atrial (RA) waveform and systolic murmur with tricuspid valve insufficiency
4. Increased atrial pressure
   - Palpitations
   - S_4 may develop as the atria attempt to eject blood into rigid ventricles
   - Atrial arrhythmias may occur, such as premature atrial contractions (PACs) or atrial fibrillation (AF), due to the increase in atrial pressure
   - Elevated A wave on PCW waveform
   - Elevated RA pressures
   - Elevated A wave on the RA waveform

Hypertrophic Cardiomyopathy

1. Inability to maintain adequate cardiac output
   - Angina
   - Syncope
   - Fatigue
   - Sinus tachycardia
   - Ventricular fibrillation
   - Cardiac output is initially normal, then decreases
2. Increased ventricular filling pressures
   - Dyspnea
   - Orthopnea
   - Arrhythmias, such as premature ventricular contractions (PVCs) or ventricular tachycardia (VT)
   - Abnormal hemodynamic profile:
     Elevated PAS and PAD pressures
     Elevated PCW pressure
     Increased SVR
3. Increased atrial pressure
   - S_4 may develop as the atria attempt to eject blood into rigid ventricles
   - Atrial arrhythmias may occur (e.g., PAC, AF) due to the increase in atrial pressure
   - Palpitations
   - Elevated A wave on PCW waveform
   - Elevated RA pressure
4. Left outflow tract obstruction
   - Systolic murmur as blood flows through a narrowed outflow tract due to septal hypertrophy; heard at apex

Restrictive Cardiomyopathy

Signs and symptoms of restrictive cardiomyopathy and pericarditis are similar. Diagnosis can usually be made after an echocardiogram.

1. Inability to maintain adequate cardiac output
   - Activity intolerance
   - Weakness
   - Sinus tachycardia
   - Arrhythmias
   - Decreased CO/CI
2. Increased left ventricular filling pressures
   - Dyspnea
   - Jugular vein distention
   - S_3
   - Narrowed pulse pressure
   - Systolic murmur with mitral valve insufficiency
   - Abnormal hemodynamic profile:
     Elevated PAS, PAD, and PCW pressures
     Elevated SVR
     Elevated V wave on PCW waveform with mitral valve insufficiency
3. Increased right ventricular pressures
   - Peripheral edema
   - Hepatomegaly
   - Jaundice
   - Jugular vein distention
   - Systolic murmur with tricuspid valve insufficiency
   - Kussmaul's sign (increased neck vein distention with inspiration)
   - Elevated V wave on the RA waveform if tricuspid valve insufficiency
4. Increased atrial pressures
   - Palpitations
   - S_4 may develop as the atria attempt to eject blood into rigid ventricles
   - Atrial arrhythmias may occur (e.g., PAC, AF) due to the increase in atrial pressure
   - Elevated A wave on PCW waveform
   - Elevated RA pressure
   - Elevated A wave on the RA waveform

Diagnostic Tests

Dilated Cardiomyopathy

- *Chest x-ray:* Left ventricular dilation with potential enlargement and dilatation of all four cardiac chambers.
- *12-Lead ECG:* ST-segment and T-wave changes; left axis deviation; and left ventricular hypertrophy.
- *Echocardiography:* Dilated left ventricle with an increase in chamber size (other chambers may be enlarged also); diminished ventricular contractility; decreased septal movement; elevated ventricular volumes and decreased ejection fraction.
- *Endomyocardial biopsy:* Not usually done.

Hypertrophic Cardiomyopathy

- *Chest x-ray:* Normal or left atrial and ventricular dilatation (potential enlargement of right heart chambers).
- *12-Lead ECG:* ST-segment and T-wave changes; septal Q waves due to septal hypertrophy; left ventricular hypertrophy.
- *Echocardiography:* Thickened ventricular walls with a decrease in chamber size; left ventricular obstruction created by thickened ventricular septum and motion of mitral valve leaflet.
- *Endomyocardial biopsy:* Abnormal myocardial fibers that are in disarray.

Restrictive Cardiomyopathy

- *Chest x-ray:* Normal or slight enlargement of left atria and ventricle.
- *12-Lead ECG:* ST-segment and T-wave changes; low QRS amplitude.
- *Echocardiography:* Thickened ventricular walls; enlarged atria; diminished ventricular contractility; decreased ventricular volumes; elevated ventricular end-diastolic pressures.
- *Endomyocardial biopsy:* Not usually done.

Patient Needs and Principles of Management

The primary objectives in the management of cardiomyopathy are to treat the underlying cause (if known), maximize cardiac function, assist the patient and family members to cope with a debilitating, chronic disease, and prevent complications associated with cardiomyopathy.

▶ Improvement of Cardiac Function

Dilated Cardiomyopathy

1. Improve myocardial oxygenation. As ventricular dilatation occurs, ventricular wall tension increases,

increasing the myocardial workload and oxygen consumption. Oxygen therapy should be initiated as necessary to increase oxygenation saturation. Pulse oximetry, mixed venous oxygenation saturation (SvO_2), and arterial blood gases are helpful in guiding sufficient oxygen therapy.

2. Increase myocardial contractility. Inotropic agents (e.g., digoxin, dobutamine) will strengthen myocardial contractions; phosphodiesterase inhibitors (e.g., amrinone, milrinone) cause vasodilation and produce a positive inotropic effect, decreasing the workload of the failing ventricle.

3. Decrease preload and afterload. Diuretics decrease excess fluid and ventricular end-diastolic volumes; fluid and sodium restrictions also may be necessary. Vasodilators (e.g., nitroprusside, hydralazine) dilate arterial and venous vessels, decreasing venous return and resistance to ventricular systolic ejection.

4. Mechanical cardiac assist devices (e.g., intraaortic balloon therapy, hemopump therapy, ventricular assist device therapy) may be instituted to assist with the augmentation of adequate cardiac output/cardiac index.

5. Dynamic cardiomyoplasty. This is a relatively new surgical procedure which has grown in popularity since 1985. During surgery the latissimus dorsi muscle is dissected and wrapped around the cardiac muscle. The muscle is electrically stimulated to contract in harmony with ventricular systole to strengthen myocardial contraction and improve cardiac output.

6. Cardiac transplant may be necessary if medical therapy does not relieve patient symptoms.

Hypertrophic Cardiomyopathy

The management of the patient with hypertrophic cardiomyopathy focuses on promoting myocardial relaxation and decreasing left ventricular obstruction.

1. Decrease myocardial contractility. Use beta blockers and/or calcium channel blockers to decrease heart rate, contractility, and myocardial oxygen consumption. One or both types of medications may be given in an effort to increase ventricular compliance, decrease ventricular outflow obstruction, and improve left ventricular function.

2. The following medications are usually contraindicated in patients with hypertrophic cardiomyopathy:
   - Diuretics, since a decrease in fluid volume decreases ventricle filling pressures and decreases cardiac output.
   - Inotropes (e.g., digoxin, dobutamine), since an increase in contractility will contribute to an increase in the left ventricular outflow obstruction.
   - Vasodilators (e.g., nitroglycerin, nitroprusside), since they decrease end-diastolic volume, leading to an increase in left ventricular outflow obstruction.

3. Reduce physical and psychological stress. Patients with hypertrophic cardiomyopathy are at an increased risk for sudden cardiac death, which may occur during stressful periods. It is important that strenuous physical activity be limited. In addition, sudden changes in position should be avoided, since the heart cannot respond to fluid shifts created by sudden position changes. Valsalva's maneuver should also be avoided. Psychological stress should also be decreased. Teach patients strategies to use to enhance self-relaxation. Relaxation therapy may include rhythmic breathing, biofeedback, and/or imagery.

4. Cardiac surgery. Myectomy may be indicated for individuals who do not respond to medical management and have severe left ventricular outflow obstruction. Myectomy involves removal of a portion of the enlarged intraventricular septum in an attempt to decrease left ventricular outflow obstruction and improve myocardial functioning.

Restrictive Cardiomyopathy

1. Increase myocardial contractility. Inotropic agents (e.g., digoxin, dobutamine) strengthen myocardial contractility.

2. Decrease preload. Diuretics, sodium and fluid restrictions, and vasodilators will decrease ventricular end-diastolic volumes. The rigid ventricle is very sensitive to small fluid changes, significantly increasing ventricular end-diastolic pressure.

3. Cardiac surgery. Fibrotic cardiac tissue can be selectively excised in an effort to increase ventricular compliance and cardiac output.

▶ Facilitate Coping

For most patients, cardiomyopathy is a chronic, potentially life-threatening disease. Patients and their families often face an uncertain long-term prognosis. Emotions may vacillate as the family unit struggles to cope with the implications of the disease and its effect on lifestyle. Emphasis is placed on assisting the patient to remain active and to cope with a progressive disease. Involvement of the family unit in symptom management is also important. Relaxation therapy can benefit not only the patient, but also the family.

AT THE BEDSIDE

Andrea to her nurse: "I have to make it through this. You have to help me. I want my baby to make it also. I know the risks—they're scary, but I'm going to walk out of this hospital with my baby. I know I will!"

Although Andrea's nurse provided Andrea with support and encouragement, she was scared also. She knew that Andrea was critically ill. She was very worried that Andrea might not make it to delivery. She also wondered, even if Andrea did make it to delivery, how her dysfunctional heart would handle the stress and massive fluid shifts which would occur during labor and after delivery. Although she too wanted Andrea to leave the hospital with her baby, she was not as certain that it would happen.

▶ Prevention and Management of Complications

1. *Arrhythmias:* Continuous ECG monitoring; daily 12-lead ECGs; observe for potential side effects of cardiac medications; encourage family to learn CPR.
2. *Hemodynamic instability:* Pulmonary artery pressure monitoring; manage patient based on trends in hemodynamic parameters (i.e., RA, PAS, PAD, and PCW pressures; CO; CI; SVR; and PVR).
3. *Thromboembolic event:* Anticoagulation is necessary for patients with severely compromised left ventricular function and for patients experiencing atrial fibrillation. In both circumstances, thrombi may develop due to increased fluid volume and stasis.
4. *Endocarditis:* Antibiotic prophylaxis is recommended for patients with valve involvement. Prophylaxis should be given prior to dental work, surgery, or other invasive procedures.

Valvular Disease

Valvular disorders result from both congenital and acquired causes. Valves on the left side of the heart are more commonly affected because they are constantly exposed to higher pressures. Normally, when a valve opens, there are no pressure gradients, or differences, between the structures (chamber or vessel) above and below the valve. As valve disease progresses, pressure gradients between the two structures develop.

Valvular disorders are commonly classified as valve stenosis or valve insufficiency. A stenotic valve has a narrowed opening, permitting less blood to flow forward through it. An insufficient valve does not close properly, thus permitting some blood to flow backward instead of forward. Valve insufficiency is also referred to as valve regurgitation. Valve dysfunction may affect one or more valves.

The development of valve disease is usually a gradual process. As the case study illustrates, Mrs. Smith's valvular problems began with a bacterial endocarditis 15 years prior to the onset of her symptoms of mitral valve insufficiency.

Etiology and Pathophysiology

Valve disorders are caused by either congenital or acquired diseases (Table 22–2). Congenital valve disorders may affect any of the four valves and result in valve stenosis or

AT THE BEDSIDE
▶ *Valvular Disorder*

Mrs. Smith, a 48-year-old woman, was admitted to the coronary care unit with increasing shortness of breath and fatigue. She had bacterial endocarditis 15 years ago, which resulted in mitral valve insufficiency. On admission, she was in normal sinus rhythm with frequent premature atrial contractions, with a blood pressure of 150/94. Chest auscultation revealed rales in the left lower area. Hemodynamic parameters included:

RAP:	12 mm Hg
PAP:	35/25 mm Hg
PCWP:	24 mm Hg
CO:	4.8 L/minute
CI:	1.9 L/minute/m^2
SVR:	2100 dynes/second/cm^5

insufficiency. An example of a congenital valve disorder is an aortic valve with only one, instead of three, cusps. The unicusp valve causes an increase in turbulence as blood flows through the narrowed orifice. The individual may be

TABLE 22-2. ETIOLOGY OF VALVULAR DISORDERS

Mitral Stenosis
Rheumatic disease
Endocarditis
Degenerative process

Mitral Insufficiency
Rheumatic disease
Congenital
Endocarditis
Mitral valve prolapse
Papillary muscle dysfunction
Chordae tendineae dysfunction

Aortic Stenosis
Rheumatic disease
Congenital
Degenerative process

Aortic Insufficiency
Rheumatic disease
Congenital
Hypertension
Endocarditis
Marfan syndrome

Tricuspid Stenosis
Rheumatic disease
Congenital
Endocarditis

Tricuspid Insufficiency
Rheumatic disease
Marfan syndrome
Endocarditis
Ebstein's anomaly
Congenital
Secondary to left-sided valve disease
IV drug use

Pulmonic Stenosis
Rheumatic disease
Congenital
Endocarditis

Pulmonic Insufficiency
Primary pulmonary artery hypertension
Secondary to left-sided valve disease
Marfan syndrome
Endocarditis

asymptomatic until later in life when fibrotic tissue and calcium deposits form on the abnormal valve, leading to stenosis.

There are three types of acquired valve disorders: degenerative disease, rheumatic disease, or infective endocarditis. Degenerative disease may occur as the valve is damaged over time due to constant mechanical stress. This may occur with aging, or may be aggravated by conditions such as hypertension. Hypertension places significant pressure on the aortic valve, often causing insufficiency.

Individuals who develop rheumatic fever often experience valvular disease years later. Rheumatic disease contributes to gradual fibrotic changes of the valve, in addition to calcification of the valve cusps. Shortening of the chordae tendineae also may occur. Rheumatic fever commonly affects the mitral valve.

Infective endocarditis may occur as a primary or secondary infection. The valve tissue is destroyed by the infectious organism. Refer to Table 22–2 for a listing of other conditions which cause valve disease.

Pathophysiology of Mitral Stenosis

Several processes occur which together cause stenosis or narrowing of the mitral valve orifice (Figure 22–2). Gradual fusion of the commissures (the valve leaflet edges) and fibrosis of the valve leaflets are common. In addition, calcium deposits may invade the valve leaflets, further impeding their movement. As the mitral valve becomes increasingly stenotic, the left atrium has to generate significant amounts of pressure to propel blood forward through the mitral valve and into the left ventricle. Left atrial pressures are commonly increased, with left atrial dilatation occurring as the stenosis worsens. Increased left atrial pressures may lead to increased pulmonary vascular pressures as fluid backs up into the pulmonary system, resulting in right-sided heart failure.

Pathophysiology of Mitral Insufficiency

Adequate closure of the mitral valve is important so that blood is ejected forward, not backward, during ventricular systole. Damage to the mitral valve can affect the valve's ability to close properly (Figure 22–3). During ventricular systole, as blood is ejected forward into the aorta, blood is also ejected backward through the insufficient mitral valve. This abnormal blood flow contributes to an increase in left atrial volume, pressure, and eventually dilatation. Increased left atrial pressures may lead to increased pulmonary vascular pressures and right-sided heart failure. The left ventricle usually dilates and hypertrophies over time as end-diastolic volumes increase and cardiac output decreases.

Acute mitral insufficiency may occur due to dysfunction of the papillary muscles. Papillary muscle contraction is an important component of adequate mitral valve leaflet closure. Papillary muscles may rupture during an acute myocardial infarction if blood supply is diminished or eliminated by coronary artery disease. Loss of a papillary muscle causes sudden, severe insufficiency of the mitral valve, resulting in rapid increase in both left ventricular and atrial volumes and pressures. The pulmonary vascular system is quickly affected by the high left-sided pressures, with pulmonary edema developing acutely. In acute mitral insufficiency, there is no time for the heart to compensate for the sudden increases in volume and pressure, as there is with long-standing mitral insufficiency.

Pathophysiology of Aortic Stenosis

A similar process occurs in aortic stenosis as occurs in mitral stenosis (Figure 22–4). Fusion of the commissures, fibrosis of the valve leaflets, and calcium deposits may

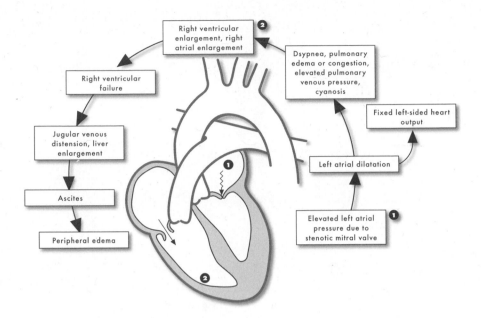

Figure 22–2. Cardiovascular effects of mitral stenosis.

occur on the aortic valve leaflets, impeding their movement. In aortic stenosis, the left ventricle has to generate a significant amount of pressure to propel blood forward through the aortic valve into the aorta. Left ventricular pressure increases lead to left ventricular dilatation and hypertrophy, as well as decreases in cardiac output. Left atrial volume and pressure may increase as pressure backs up from the left ventricle. Left atrial dilatation may eventually occur, and fluid may continue to back up into the pulmonary vascular system and to the right side of the heart, eventually causing right-sided heart failure.

Pathophysiology of Aortic Insufficiency
A similar process also occurs in aortic insufficiency as occurs with mitral insufficiency (Figure 22–5). Adequate

closure of the aortic valve is even more important than adequate closure of the mitral valve. If the aortic valve is not closed properly, blood flows backward from the aorta into the left ventricle during diastole. This can seriously affect forward blood flow into the aorta, and thus cardiac output. This causes significant increases in the volumes and pressures of the left ventricle, with the gradual development of left ventricular dilatation and hypertrophy. As with other left-sided valve dysfunctions, pulmonary vascular system dysfunction and right-sided failure can also occur.

Pathophysiology of Tricuspid Stenosis
Fused commissures or fibrosis of the valve leaflets may also narrow the tricuspid valve orifice. Right atrial pressures increase as the right atrium attempts to propel blood for-

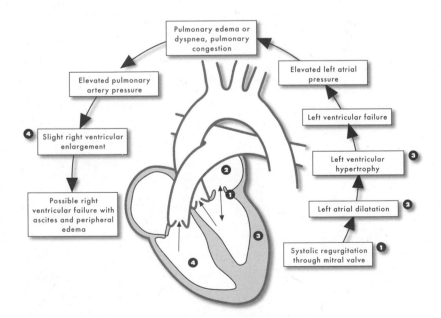

Figure 22–3. Cardiovascular effects of mitral insufficiency.

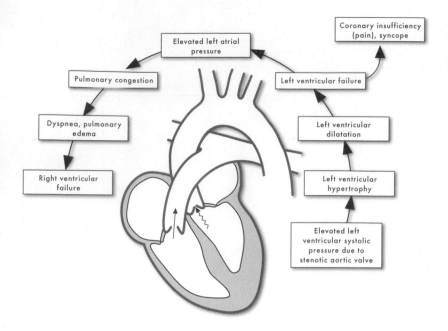

Figure 22–4. Cardiovascular effects of aortic stenosis.

ward into the right ventricle. Eventually, right atrial dilatation occurs and fluid may back up into the venous system.

Pathophysiology of Tricuspid Insufficiency

Damage to the tricuspid valve that prevents complete closure during ventricular systole causes the abnormal ejection of blood through the tricuspid valve into the right atrium. Right atrial volumes and pressures increase, leading eventually to dilatation and possible decreases in cardiac output.

Pathophysiology of Pulmonic Stenosis

Pulmonic stenosis develops as the pulmonic valve orifice becomes narrowed. Right ventricular pressures increase as the right ventricle attempts to eject blood forward into the pulmonary artery. Over time, right ventricular dilatation may occur, with decreases in right-sided cardiac output. The increased pressure may back up into the right atrium, causing an increase in volume and pressure, and eventually leading to dilatation. This can lead to volume and pressure increases in the venous system.

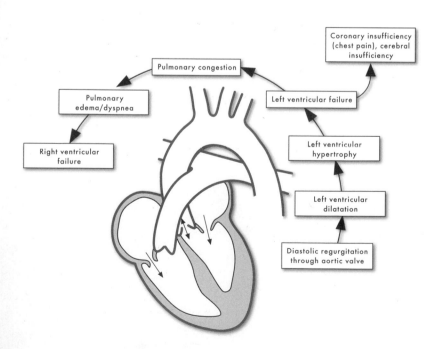

Figure 22–5. Cardiovascular effects of aortic insufficiency.

Pathophysiology of Pulmonic Insufficiency

Closure of the pulmonic valve prevents blood from backing up from the pulmonary artery into the right ventricle during diastole. An insufficient pulmonic valve will permit blood to flow backward into the right ventricle during diastole. Right-sided cardiac output decreases as blood flows backward instead of forward. An increase in right ventricular volume and pressure occurs, which may eventually lead to dilatation. The backflow of pressure may continue to the right atrium and then to the venous system.

Clinical Presentation

Mitral and Aortic Disease

The following signs and symptoms are found in all of the valvular disorders of the left side of the heart:

- Dyspnea
- Fatigue
- Increased pulmonary artery pressures (PAS, PAD, PCW)
- Decreased cardiac output

MITRAL STENOSIS
- Palpitations
- Hemoptysis
- Hoarseness
- Dysphagia
- Jugular vein distention (JVD)
- Orthopnea
- Cough
- Diastolic murmur
- Atrial arrhythmias (PAC, AF)
- Elevated A wave on PCW pressure waveform

MITRAL INSUFFICIENCY
- Paroxysmal nocturnal dyspnea
- Orthopnea
- Palpitations
- S_3 and/or S_4
- Rales
- Systolic murmur
- Atrial arrhythmias
- Elevated V wave on PCW pressure waveform

AORTIC STENOSIS
- Angina
- Syncope
- Decreased SVR
- S_3 and/or S_4
- Systolic murmur
- Narrowed pulse pressure

AORTIC INSUFFICIENCY
- Angina
- S_3
- Diastolic murmur
- Widened pulse pressure
- de Musset's sign (nodding of the head)

Tricuspid and Pulmonary Valve Disease

The following signs and symptoms are found in all of the valvular disorders of the right side of the heart:

- Dyspnea
- Fatigue
- Increased right atrial pressures
- Peripheral edema
- Hepatomegaly
- JVD

TRICUSPID STENOSIS
- Atrial arrhythmias
- Diastolic murmur
- Decreased CO
- Elevated A wave on RA pressure waveform

TRICUSPID INSUFFICIENCY
- Conduction delays
- Supraventricular tachycardia
- Systolic murmur
- Elevated V wave on RA pressure waveform

PULMONIC STENOSIS
- Cyanosis
- Systolic murmur
- Elevated A wave on RA pressure waveform

PULMONIC INSUFFICIENCY
- Diastolic murmur
- Elevated A wave on RA pressure waveform

Diagnostic Tests

- *Chest x-ray:* Shows specific cardiac chamber enlargement, pulmonary congestion, presence of valve calcification.
- *12-Lead ECG:* Useful in the diagnosis of right ventricular, left ventricular, and left atrial hypertrophy.
- *Echocardiogram:* Demonstrates the size of the four cardiac chambers, presence of hypertrophy, specific valve dysfunction, ejection fraction, and amount of regurgitant flow, if present.
- *Radionuclide studies:* Identify abnormal ejection fraction during inactivity and activity.
- *Cardiac catheterization:* Determines cardiac chamber pressures, ejection fraction, regurgitation, and pressure gradients, if present.

Patient Needs and Principles of Management

The primary objectives in the management of valvular disorders are to maximize cardiac function, reduce anxiety, and prevent complications associated with valve disease.

► Maximize Cardiac Function

Medical Management

1. Improve myocardial oxygenation. As ventricular dilatation occurs, there is an increase in ventricular wall tension, myocardial workload, and oxygen consumption. Oxygen therapy should be initiated, as necessary, to increase oxygen saturation. Pulse oximetry, mixed venous oxygenation saturation (SvO_2), and arterial blood gases are helpful in guiding sufficient oxygen therapy.
2. Decrease preload. Diuretics will decrease excess fluid and ventricular end-diastolic volumes. Fluid and sodium restrictions also may be necessary. (Exception: Preload usually is not decreased in patients with aortic insufficiency, since decreased left ventricular end-diastolic volumes may accentuate decreases in cardiac output.)
3. Decrease afterload. Afterload reduction may be indicated for patients with increased systemic vascular resistance and impaired left ventricular function (e.g., aortic stenosis or mitral insufficiency).
4. Improve contractility. Inotropic agents (e.g., digoxin, dobutamine) strengthen myocardial contractions and improve cardiac output.
5. Modify activity. Activity limitation will help to decrease myocardial oxygen consumption. Teach patients the importance of rest between activities.
6. Balloon valvuloplasty may be an option for stenotic mitral or aortic valves. A percutaneous catheter is inserted via the femoral artery under fluoroscopy and the balloon is inflated at the stenotic lesion in an effort to force open the fused commissures and improve valve leaflet mobility.

Surgical Management

Cardiac surgery is indicated when medical management doesn't alleviate patient symptoms. Patients may have better surgical outcomes if surgery is done prior to left ventricular dysfunction.

1. Valve repair. An increasing trend today is to have dysfunctional valves repaired instead of replaced. The hemodynamic function of the inherent valve is superior to any prosthetic valve. In addition, the risks associated with valve replacement are avoided. An open commissurotomy may be performed to relieve stenosis of any of the four heart valves. During open commissurotomy, the fused commissures are incised, thus mobilizing the valve leaflets. Valve leaflet reconstruction also may be done to patch tears in valve leaflets using pericardial patches for the repair. Chordae tendineae reconstruction may be performed to elongate fibrotic tendineae or to shorten excessively stretched tendineae. An annuloplasty ring may also be inserted to correct dilatation of the valve annulus.
2. Prosthetic valve replacement. Replacement of the native valve with a prosthetic, or artificial, valve is done for severely damaged valves or when repair is not possible. The entire native valve is removed and replaced with a mechanical or biological (porcine, bovine, or allograft) prosthetic valve.
3. Postoperative management after cardiac surgery is similar to coronary artery bypass surgery management (see Chapter 12, Cardiovascular System). Special considerations for patients having valve repair or replacement include the following:
   - Maintain adequate preload. Patients with valvular disease usually are accustomed to increased end-diastolic volumes. Although the valve is repaired, the heart will need time to adjust to the hemodynamic changes. Most patients will do better in the postoperative phase if fluids are adjusted based on presurgical RA and PCW pressures.
   - Monitor for conduction disturbances. The mitral, tricuspid, and aortic valves lie in close proximity to conduction pathways. Conduction disorders may be treated by temporary or permanent cardiac pacing.
   - Initiate anticoagulation therapy. Anticoagulation therapy is usually initiated for patients having valve replacement after the epicardial pacing wires are removed. This may be as early as the first postoperative day.

► Reducing Anxiety

Decrease anxiety. Teach the patient relaxation techniques. Deep breathing or imagery may help alleviate anxiety especially when symptoms of valve dysfunction occur.

► Prevention and Management of Complications

1. Arrhythmias: Continuous ECG monitoring; daily 12-lead ECG; observe for side effects of specific cardiac medications.

Patient Needs and Principles of Management, Cont.

2. *Hemodynamic instability:* PAP monitoring, manage patient based on trends in hemodynamic monitoring.

3. *Thromboembolic event:* Anticoagulation is necessary for patients with severely compromised left ventricular function or AF, and after valve surgery. Lifelong anticoagulation therapy is indicated for patients after mechanical valve replacement. Short-term anticoagulation therapy is usually initiated for patients having a biological valve replacement.

4. *Endocarditis:* Antibiotic prophylaxis is recommended for patients with valve disorders and for patients with prosthetic valves. Prophylaxis should be given prior to dental work, surgery, or other invasive procedures. Prior to discharge, teach the patient and family the importance of prophylaxis.

5. *Prosthetic valve dysfunction:* Biological valve dysfunction usually develops slowly with gradual signs and symptoms (e.g., presence of a new murmur, dyspnea, syncope). Mechanical valve dysfunction may occur slowly or suddenly. Rapid valve dysfunction requires emergency intervention as the patient presents with signs and symptoms of acute cardiac failure (hypotension, tachycardia, low cardiac output/cardiac index, congestive heart failure, cardiac arrest).

Pericarditis

Pericarditis is a chronic or acute inflammation of the pericardial lining of the heart. Acute pericarditis usually occurs secondary to another disease process and usually resolves within 6 weeks. Chronic pericarditis, however, may last for months.

Pericarditis may lead to pericardial effusion and/or cardiac tamponade. Pericardial effusion occurs as fluid builds up within the pericardial sac. Cardiac tamponade can occur as the pericardial fluid compresses the heart, restricts ventricular end-diastolic filling, and compromises cardiac function.

The case study is an example of the importance of accurate diagnosis of patients with chest pain. The pain of pericarditis may be similar to anginal pain, but the treatment is very different.

AT THE BEDSIDE
▶ *Pericarditis*

Mrs. Reb had an acute anterior myocardial infarction 5 days ago. She was readmitted to the CCU with dull, substernal chest pain, shortness of breath, and ST-segment elevations in the precordial leads and in leads I and II. The chest pain was unrelieved with nitroglycerin. Her pain was decreased after receiving 4 mg of morphine IV. Her pain was completely relieved when her nurse had her sit up and lean forward so that he could auscultate posterior breath sounds.

Etiology and Pathophysiology

A number of different conditions and situations can cause pericarditis (Table 22–3). Common causes include myocardial infarction, infections, neoplasm, radiation therapy, and uremia.

Normally the pericardial sac contains a small amount of clear serous fluid, typically less than 50 ml. This fluid lies between the visceral and parietal pleura and contributes to the ease with which the heart expands and contracts. An inflammation of the pericardium causes friction between the visceral and parietal pleura.

Inflammation of the pericardium causes an increase in pericardial fluid production, with increases of up to 1 L or more. A gradual build up of fluid may have little compromising effect on the heart as the pericardium expands and hemodynamic functioning is not altered. A sudden increase in pericardial fluid, however, will have dramatic effects on hemodynamic functioning.

TABLE 22–3. ETIOLOGY OF PERICARDITIS

Idiopathic
Infections (viral/bacterial)
Myocardial infarction
Cardiac surgery
Neoplasm
Radiation therapy
Rheumatic disease
Lupus erythematosus
Scleroderma
Uremia
Medication-induced

Chronic pericarditis causes fibrotic changes within the pericardial lining. The visceral and parietal pleura eventually adhere to each other, restricting the filling of the heart. This condition may be referred to as constrictive pericarditis. The pressure created by the constricted pericardium affects the heart's ability to distend properly, causing decreases in end-diastolic volume and cardiac output. These changes may contribute to increases in atrial pressures, leading to increases in pulmonary vascular and venous system pressures.

Clinical Presentation

Acute Pericarditis

- Sharp, stabbing, burning, dull, or aching pain in the substernal or precordial area, which increases with movement, inspiration, or coughing, or when the patient is in a recumbent position
- Pericardial friction rub
- Fever
- Sinus tachycardia
- Dyspnea, orthopnea
- Cough
- Fatigue
- Narrowed pulse pressure
- Hypotension
- Arrhythmias
- Elevated cardiac pressures (PA, PCW, RA)
- Decreased cardiac output
- Peripheral edema
- JVD

Chronic Pericarditis

- Dyspnea
- Anorexia
- Fatigue
- Abdominal discomfort
- Weight gain
- Activity intolerance
- JVD
- Peripheral edema
- Hepatomegaly
- Kussmaul's sign (increase in RA pressure during inspiration)

Diagnostic Tests

- *Chest x-ray:* Normal or enlarged heart; chronic pericarditis may reveal a decrease in heart size.
- *ECG:* ST-segment elevation in precordial leads (V leads) and leads I, II, or III; T-wave inversion after ST-segment returns to isoelectric line; decrease in QRS voltage.
- *Echocardiogram:* Presence of increased fluid in pericardial sac; chronic, constrictive pericarditis may demonstrate a thickened pericardium and diminished ventricular contractility.
- *Laboratory:* Elevated sedimentation rate and elevated WBC; causative organisms may be identified from blood cultures.
- *CT/MRI Scan:* Detects a thickened pericardium for patients with chronic pericarditis.

Patient Needs and Principles of Management

The primary principles of management of pericarditis are to correct the underlying cause, relieve pain and promote comfort, relieve pericardial effusion, and prevent and manage complications associated with pericarditis.

▶ Promoting Comfort and Relieving Pain

1. Decrease pain. Teach the patient that chest pain may be decreased or relieved by sitting up and/or leaning forward. Analgesics (e.g., aspirin) and narcotics (e.g., meperidine, morphine) administered around the clock will assist in pain relief.
2. Promote relaxation. Teach the patient relaxation techniques such as progressive muscle relaxation and visualization. This may assist the patient to cope. Relaxation techniques which include deep breathing should be avoided because pericardial pain usually increases with deep inspiration.
3. Limit activity. This is especially important during the acute period of inflammation. Activity can be gradually increased as fever and chest pain decrease. Assist patients to find a position of comfort. Patients often are more comfortable sitting up and leaning slightly forward.

▶ Correcting the Underlying Cause

1. Decrease pericardial inflammation. Nonsteroidal antiinflammatory agents (e.g., indomethacin, ibuprofen) will assist to decrease inflammation of the peri-

Patient Needs and Principles of Management, Cont.

cardium and the associated pain. Chronic, recurrent pericarditis may require corticosteroid therapy.
2. Eliminate infection. If the cause of the pericarditis is an infectious process, appropriate medications, including antibiotic therapy, are necessary.

▶ Relieving Pericardial Effusion

1. Pericardiocentesis. A needle is placed within the pericardial sac and fluid is withdrawn via the needle or is attached to a catheter and drained into a bottle. This procedure is performed to decrease fluid in the pericardium, in an effort to improve myocardial function. Culture specimens of the drained fluid should be obtained and sent to the laboratory for analysis.
2. Pericardiotomy/pericardial window. This is a surgical procedure in which a section of the pericardium is removed in an effort to decrease pericardial pressure on the heart and to allow pericardial fluid to drain more readily. It may be performed for recurrent pericardial effusions.
3. Pericardiectomy. This involves surgically removing the entire pericardium. This may be necessary for

chronic pericarditis that is refractory to other interventions.

▶ Prevention and Management of Complications

1. Monitor for signs and symptoms of acute heart failure. These include hypotension, tachycardia, increased respiration, extreme dyspnea, pink frothy sputum, decreased oxygen saturation, decreased peripheral pulses, and decreased urinary output. Oxygen therapy and inotropic agents will assist in improvement of myocardial contractility. Assessment of the need for surgical intervention for pericarditis may be indicated.
2. Cardiac tamponade. Monitor for signs and symptoms of cardiac tamponade. These include hypotension, tachycardia, tachypnea, dyspnea, pulsus paradoxus, narrowed pulse pressure, muffled heart sounds, and distended neck veins. Emergency pericardiocentesis is necessary in order to prevent further hemodynamic compromise.

Aortic Aneurysm

An aortic aneurysm is an area of aortic wall dilatation. Aneurysms are most prevalent in men, commonly occurring during their early 50s to late 60s. Without treatment, mortality from aneurysms is high.

AT THE BEDSIDE
▶ *Aortic Aneurysm*

Mr. Smith, 62 years old, was admitted to the ICU with substernal chest pain. The chest pain was unrelieved by nitroglycerin. The pain decreased in intensity after 8 mg of morphine sulfate. His admitting ECG was normal. His chest x-ray revealed a widened mediastinum, and an aortogram demonstrated a thoracic aneurysm. He has nitroprusside infusing at 1.0 µg/kg/minute to maintain his systolic blood pressure below 100 mm Hg. Suddenly, Mr. Smith yells out, "The pain, the pain . . .

it's back . . . it's even worse than before." A rapid assessment reveals the following:

BP:	190/100 mm Hg
HR:	110 beats/minute
RR:	30 breaths/minute
Color:	Gray
Skin:	Moist and cool
Pain:	Rated 10 on a 0 to 10 scale, described as tearing in the middle of his chest and between his shoulder blades

Aneurysms frequently are classified by types (Figure 22–6). A fusiform aneurysm is characterized by distention of the entire circumference of the affected portion of the aorta. A saccular aneurysm is characterized by distention of one side of the aorta. The distention of a saccular aneurysm resembles a bulging sac. Aneurysms may also be classified according to their location (Figure 22–7):

- Ascending: between the aortic valve and the innominate artery

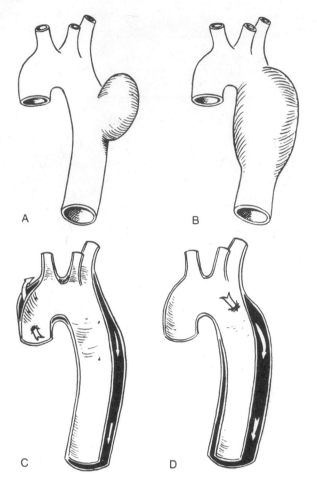

Figure 22–6. Diagram of different types of aortic aneurysms. (A) Fusiform aneurysm. (B) Saccular aneurysm. (C,D) Two aortic dissections. *(From: Underhill SL, Woods SL, Sivarajan ES, Halpenny CJ: Cardiac nursing, 1st ed. Philadelphia: JB Lippincott, 1982, p. 680.)*

- Transverse: between the innominate artery and the left subclavian artery
- Descending: from the left subclavian artery to the diaphragm
- Thoracoabdominal: from the diaphragm to the aortic bifurcation

Aneurysms have the potential to dissect or rupture. A dissection occurs when the intimal aortic wall is disrupted and blood extends into the aortic vessel layers (Figure 22–6C and 22–6D). Rupture occurs when all three layers of the aorta are disrupted and massive hemorrhage occurs. Both dissection and rupture are life-threatening events. The case study demonstrates the sudden onset of signs and symptoms associated with aortic rupture and the emergent need for life-saving interventions.

Etiology and Pathophysiology

Aortic aneurysms are caused by a variety of conditions, including atherosclerosis, cystic medial necrosis, genetic

link, congenital abnormality, hypertension, Marfan syndrome, and trauma to the chest.

The aorta is composed of three layers: the intima, media, and tunica adventitia. Aneurysm development is initiated by degeneration of smooth muscle cells and elastic tissue in the medial layer of the aorta. This weakens the vessel wall, potentially leading to dilatation of all layers of the aorta. The aortic wall may be further weakened with age, as well as from hypertension.

As the aortic aneurysm gradually expands, there is an increase in the risk for aortic dissection. Dissection is caused by a tear in the intima. Blood leaves the central aorta via the intimal tear and flows through the medial layer of the aorta (Figure 22–6C and 22–6D). This creates a false lumen. As the amount of blood increases in the medial layer, the pressure in the false lumen increases, compressing the central aorta (Figure 22–6D). This compression may decrease or totally obstruct blood flow through the aorta and/or its arterial branches. Dissections are classified as acute if they have occurred less than 2 weeks since the

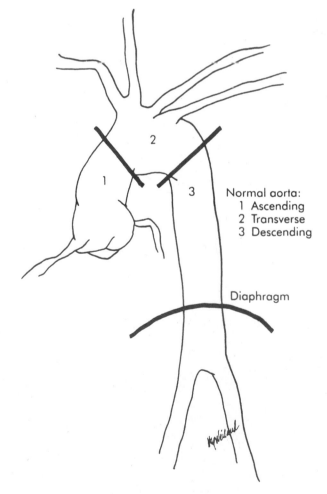

Figure 22–7. Classification of aortic aneurysms according to location. *(From: Seifert PC: Cardiac surgery. St. Louis, MO: CV Mosby, 1994, p. 321.)*

onset of symptoms. They are classified as chronic if they occurred more than 2 weeks since the onset of symptoms.

Two additional classifications exist for identifying the location of aortic dissections (Figure 22–8). The first classifies the dissection as Type A, involving the ascending aorta, or Type B, involving the descending aorta (distal to the left subclavian artery). Another classification system for aortic dissection has three categories for the dissection: Type I: the original intimal tear begins in the ascending aorta and the dissection extends to the descending aorta; Type II: the original intimal tear begins and is contained in the ascending aorta; and Type III: the original intimal tear begins and is contained in the descending aorta.

Clinical Presentation

Patients rarely demonstrate early signs of an aortic aneurysm. Diagnosis is commonly made during a routine physical exam or chest x-ray. Signs and symptoms of an aortic aneurysm occur as the aneurysm enlarges and compresses adjacent organs, structures, and/or nerve pathways.

Thoracic Aneurysm

- Ripping, tearing, or splitting pain, located at the anterior chest or posterior chest between the scapula, of an intense or excruciating nature
- Dysphagia
- Hoarseness, cough
- Dyspnea

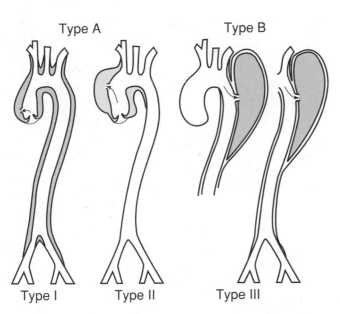

Figure 22–8. Classification for the location of aortic dissections. The Stanford system classifies aortic dissections based on involvement (Type A) of the ascending aorta or noninvolvement (Type B). The DeBakey system classifies dissections into Types I, II, or III. *(From DeBakey ME, et al.: Surgical management of dissecting aneurysms of the aorta. Journal of Thoracic Cardiovascular Surgery. 1965;49:131; adapted by Seifert PC: Cardiac surgery. St. Louis, MO: CV Mosby, 1994, p. 321.)*

AT THE BEDSIDE
▶ *Aortic Aneurysm*

Mr. Smith: "The pain I had in my chest prior to surgery was horrific! It felt like a sharp object was being pushed into my chest and out my back. I was really frightened."

- Different blood pressures when comparing right and left arms
- Different pulses when comparing right and left peripheral pulses

Abdominal Aneurysm

- Dull, constant abdominal or low back or lumbar pain
- Abdominal mass
- Pulsations in the abdomen
- Reduced lower extremity pulses
- Nausea and/or vomiting

Aortic Dissection

- Sudden intense pain in chest or back (or sudden increase in the intensity of pain)
- Dyspnea
- Syncope
- Abdominal discomfort or bloating
- Extremity weakness
- Oliguria or hematuria
- Hemiparesis, hemiplegia, or paraplegia
- Speech or visual disturbances
- Decreased hemoglobin and hematocrit

Aortic Rupture

- Sudden cessation of pain
- Reoccurrence of pain
- Signs and symptoms of shock, with the exception of BP (high in rupture); including tachycardia, increased RR, pallor, moist skin, and restlessness

Diagnostic Tests

- *Chest x-ray:* Shows the dilated aorta, widening of the mediastinum, and mediastinal mass.
- *Aortography:* Determines the origin, size, and location of the aneurysm and involvement of additional arterial branches.
- *CT/MRI scan:* Determines the size of the aorta, size of the aneurysm, extent of a dissection, involvement of additional arterial branches, lumen diameter, and wall thickness.

Patient Needs and Principles of Management

The primary objectives in the management of aortic aneurysm are relieving pain and anxiety, decreasing stress on the aneurysm, surgical repair, patient teaching, and prevention of complications.

► Relieving Pain and Anxiety

Administer narcotics (e.g., morphine, Demerol) as necessary. Unrelieved pain is likely to increase anxiety, tachycardia, and hypertension, all of which may aggravate the condition. Relaxation therapy, with deep breathing exercises or imagery, may be extremely helpful.

► Decreasing Stress on Aneurysm Wall

1. Decrease afterload. Vasodilators (e.g., nitroprusside) or ganglionic blocking agents (e.g., trimethaphan camsylate [Arfonad]) may be prescribed to lower blood pressure and thus pressure on the aneurysm. Blood pressures should be maintained as low as possible (systolic BP 90 to 120 mm Hg), without compromising perfusion to vital organs.
2. Decrease preload. Limit oral and IV fluids, decrease sodium intake, and administer diuretics as indicated. A decrease in preload will decrease the circulating blood volume, thus decreasing pressure on the aneurysm.
3. Decrease myocardial contractility with beta blockers (e.g., propranolol, esmolol, labetalol). A decrease in the strength of each cardiac contraction will decrease the pulsatile pressure on the aneurysm.

► Patient Teaching

1. If the patient will be medically managed, follow-up chest x-rays, CT scans, MRI scans, and/or ultrasounds will be needed at 6-month intervals to assess the status of the aneurysm. The importance of these studies should be stressed.
2. Diet modification. Teach the patient and family the importance of following a low-sodium diet. Consult a nutritionist for recipes and tips for food preparation.
3. Smoking cessation. Assist patient with programs available to assist with smoking cessation.
4. Physical/psychological stress modification. Teach the patient and family the hazardous effects of stress and the importance for modification. Discuss activity limitations and relaxation therapy.
5. Medications. Teach the patient and family the importance of compliance with the medication regimen. Stress that the medications are essential even though the patient may be asymptomatic.

► Surgical Management

Surgery is indicated for acute aneurysm rupture, aortic dissection in the ascending aorta, aortic dissection refractory to medical therapy, and asymptomatic patients with a fusiform aneurysm 6 or more cm in diameter (normal diameter is 2.5 to 3 cm).

1. During surgery the aortic aneurysm is resected and a prosthetic graft is sutured in place. The original aortic wall may be wrapped around the prosthetic graft for additional support.
2. If an acute dissection or rupture occurs and the patient is waiting for the operating room team to arrive:
   - Administer narcotics for pain.
   - Titrate vasodilators to maintain the patient's BP as low as possible (90 to 120 mm Hg if tolerated). This will decrease the pressure on the aneurysm.
   - Administer fluids to prevent hypovolemia.
   - Administer blood replacement products to maintain adequate hemoglobin and hematocrit levels.
3. Postoperative management:
   - Same interventions as previously described to relieve pain and anxiety and decrease stress on the aorta wall. It is important to decrease pressure on the repaired aorta so that suture lines can heal and bleeding will be kept to a minimum.
   - Continuous ECG and hemodynamic monitoring.
   - Complete assessment every 1 to 2 hours.
   - Gradual rewarming of the patient is important. Prevent postoperative shivering, which will increase blood pressure and place additional stress on suture lines.
   - Ventilator management to maximize oxygenation.
   - Keep the head of the bed less than 45 degrees the first 2 postoperative days to avoid additional tension on the prosthetic graft. Activity may be progressed more rapidly depending on institution standards and surgeon preference.
   - Initiate anticoagulation. Anticoagulation therapy is initiated for patients receiving prosthetic valves.

► Prevention and Management of Complications

1. Hemorrhage. Hourly assessment of vital signs and hemodynamic parameters. Daily hemoglobin and hematocrit.

Patient Needs and Principles of Management, Cont.

2. Arrhythmias. Continuous ECG monitoring; daily 12-lead ECGs.
3. Hemodynamic instability. Arterial and pulmonary artery pressure monitoring; manage hemodynamic parameters based on trends.
4. Altered perfusion. Arteries originating from the aorta may be compromised, leading to myocardial infarction, cerebral insufficiency/CVA, bowel necrosis, renal failure, paraplegia, and limb ischemia. Assess and monitor the patient for these conditions.
5. Aortic insufficiency. Aortic insufficiency may develop if the aneurysm is located in the ascending aorta. Enlargement or dissection of the aneurysm may dilate or damage the aortic valve, causing signs of acute congestive heart failure and pulmonary edema.

Cardiac Transplantation

From the early work of Dr. Christian Barnard in 1967, cardiac transplantation has evolved over 3 decades to a standard modality for the treatment of end-stage cardiac disease. When medical, surgical, or pharmacologic interventions have failed to improve quality of life and functional capacity, cardiac transplantation offers patients improved survival. The international 1-year survival rate is 80% to 90% and 72% at 10 years. The primary indications for cardiac transplantation include cardiomyopathies or ischemic heart disease. Other indications include cardiac valvular disease, congenital heart disease, and myocarditis.

Candidate Selection

Patients usually have a less than 1-year survival without cardiac transplant and are in New York Heart Association (NYHA) functional class III or IV. Due to the shortage of available organs, the patient must pass an extensive screening process to ascertain that he or she is appropriate for the candidate list (Table 22–4). Patients must be emotionally stable and free of alcohol or drug addictions. They must demonstrate a commitment to the rigors of being a candidate and eventual recipient through compliance with their medical regimens.

The period of waiting for an available donor can be extremely stressful for the patients and their family. It is important to explore their perceptions of the transplant process, what outcomes they are anticipating, and what methods they have utilized to cope in the past. Support group participation or meetings with a psychiatric clinical nurse specialist or nurse practitioner may be beneficial. Fear of death and critical illness may heighten the patient's anxiety. Family members may need proximity to the patient, and this may assist in alleviating anxiety. Incorporating their involvement in direct patient care may enhance their coping abilities.

AT THE BEDSIDE
▶ *Cardiac Transplant*

Robert T., a 54-year-old, white, married, unemployed man is admitted to the surgical ICU for idiopathic cardiomyopathy after an orthotopic heart transplant (OHT). He is orally intubated with a mediastinal chest tube draining 60ml sanguinous fluid per hour. Atrial and ventricular epicardial wires, a left radial arterial line, and a right subclavian Swan-Ganz catheter are in place.

Temperature:	35.8°C
BP:	140/82 mm Hg
Heart rate:	90/minute NSR without ectopy; remnant P wave present
Respiratory rate:	18/minute
Ventilator settings:	0.50 FiO_2
	TV of 700 ml
	Assist control mode, rate of 14/minute
	PEEP 5 cm H_2O
CO:	3.80 L/minute
Urine:	60 ml/hour
CI:	2.0 L/minute/m²
Mediastinal tube:	60 ml/hour
SVR:	1800 dyne/second/cm⁵
SVO_2	58%
SPO_2	96%
Neurology:	Moves all extremities on command; neurologically intact

Pretransplant Process

The greatest delay for cardiac transplantation occurs because of the shortage of donors. When a brain-dead

TABLE 22–4. RECIPIENT SELECTION CRITERIA

End-stage cardiac disease
Condition that can no longer be managed by conventional medical or surgical therapy
Placement in NYHA functional class III or IV
Life expectancy of less than 1 year
Age under 65 years
Absence of other conditions that limit survival:
    Fixed pulmonary vascular resistance of greater than 6 to 8 Wood units
    Systemic infection
    Irreversible renal insufficiency
    Irreversible pulmonary insufficiency
    Recent pulmonary embolus
    Active peptic ulcer
    Malignancy
Absence of smoking or alcohol and drug abuse
Compliant, well-motivated patient

From: Dressler DK: The patient undergoing cardiac transplant surgery. In Guzzetta CE, Dossey BM: Cardiovascular nursing holistic practice. St. Louis, MO: Mosby-Year Book, 1992.

donor is identified, he or she must be carefully managed to maintain cardiovascular stability and avoid electrolyte and renal complications. UNOS (United Network for Organ Sharing) coordinates the allocation of organs based on a nationwide waiting list. The donor must be of a compatible ABO blood type to the recipient and of similar body size and weight. The recipient is tested for relative immunologic compatability with the donor to avoid hyperacute rejection. Panel-reactive antibody (PRA) screening is performed using the recipient's serum with a random pool of lymphocytes. If no lymphocyte destruction occurs, the crossmatch is negative and the transplant may proceed. The donor's cardiac function must be normal as assessed by an echocardiogram, nuclear studies, or cardiac catheterization. The donor should have stable hemodynamic profiles on minimal inotropic support.

This process may take several hours, and it is imperative that the patient and family be frequently updated and made aware of the clinical plan of care. Pretransplant teaching should be reviewed to clarify misconceptions and correct knowledge deficits. If cardiac output is compromised, decreased cerebral perfusion may compromise the attention span. During this time, the recipient needs close monitoring to maintain cardiovascular stability. The recipient may require antiarrhythmic therapy, inotropes, diuretics, or afterload reduction agents to achieve major organ perfusion adequate for cellular function. Anticoagulation therapy may be instituted to decrease risk of embolization secondary to atrial fibrillation, reduced left ventricular function, or peripheral venous stasis.

The most unstable patient may be maintained on a cardiac assist device such as the IABP (intraaortic balloon pump) or VAD (ventricular assist device) to promote stabilization or to "bridge" him or her to transplantation.

Transplant Surgical Techniques

Two surgical options exist for cardiac transplantation. The majority, 95%, are orthotopic transplants in which the recipient's heart is removed and replaced by the donor heart in the normal anatomic position (Figure 22–9). The surgical approach is a median sternotomy; the recipient's heart is

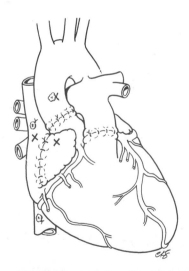

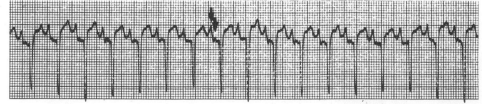

Figure 22–9. Orthotopic method of transplantation. Both the donor and the recipient SA nodes are intact (x). This results in an ECG tracing as shown. Note the double P wave, at independent rates. *(From: Weber BL: Cardiac surgery and heart transplantation. In Hudak CM, Gallo BM: Critical care nursing: A holistic approach. Philadelphia: JB Lippincott, 1994.)*

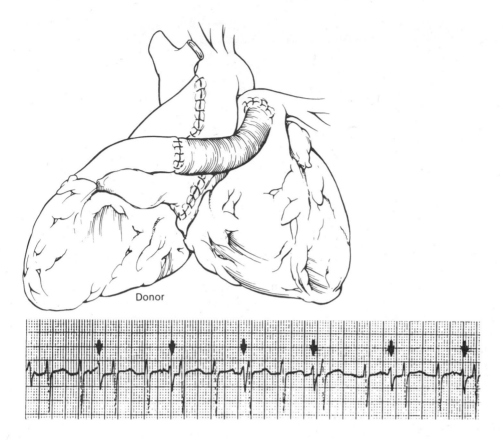

Donor

Figure 22–10. Heterotopic method of transplantation. The donor heart is anastomosed with a Dacron graft to the recipient's heart. This results in an ECG tracing as shown. Note the "extra" QRS at an independent rate. *(From: Weber BL: Cardiac surgery and heart transplantation. In Hudak CM, Gallo BM:* Critical care nursing: A holistic approach. *Philadelphia: JB Lippincott, 1994.)*

incised in the left and right atria, pulmonary artery, and aorta. The atrial septum and the posterior and lateral walls of the recipient's atria are left intact, including the SA node. The inferior and superior vena cavae to the right atrium and the pulmonary veins to the left atrium are left intact. In the pericardial cavity the donor heart is placed and aligned with interatrial septum and atrial wall remnants. Finally, the donor and recipient's aortas and pulmonary arteries are aligned and anastomosed. The fact that the donor's heart is denervated results in no sympathetic or parasympathetic influence, so the donor heart must rely on noncardiac mediators to increase cardiac output. There will be a remnant P wave on the ECG, but this does not depolarize the atria or cross the surgical suture line.

The other surgical option is a heterotopic approach, used in about 5% of cardiac transplants and also known as a "piggyback" approach. The donor heart is placed to the right side of the pleural cavity and performs as an auxillary pump for the native heart (Figure 22–10). This may be an option in a size mismatch between donor and recipient or for moderate to severe pulmonary hypertension. Synthetic tube grafts may be utilized between the two hearts' atria, aortas, and pulmonary arteries to complete parallel anastomoses. Several limitations exist with this technique, including limited space in the thoracic cavity and thromboembolism from the native heart, requiring anticoagulation. Long-term problems may arise from progressive ischemia to arrhythmias in the native heart.

Patient Needs and Principles of Management

The postsurgical care will be similar to care following conventional open heart surgery (see Chapter 12, Cardiovascular System). The primary objectives in the early postoperative period include stabilizing cardiovascular function, monitoring altered immune response and graft protection, and providing posttransplant psychological adjustment.

Patient Needs and Principles of Management, Cont.

▶ Stabilizing Cardiovascular Function

1. Cardiac denervation. The effect of the remnant atrial tissue with an intact sinus node in the recipient, along with the SA node of the donor, creates an electrocardiographic second, or "remnant," P wave. The recipient's remnant sinus node wave of depolarization does not cross the atrial suture line. Instead, the donor's SA node initiates the depolarization of the donor heart and elicits a QRS complex. The two sets of atria may be in separate rhythms as the donor heart is denervated and the recipient's is still under autonomic nervous system influence. Postoperatively there is loss of vagal influence, and the patient usually has a higher resting heart rate than normal.

   • The posttransplant patient requires more stabilization prior to exercise or position changes to avoid orthostasis due to these effects from denervation. With loss of vagal tone, should the sinus rate decrease, there is a stronger potential for junctional rhythms to result.

   • With heterotopic heart transplant patients, two separate telemetries are used to differentiate each heart. Right chest wall leads correspond to the donor heart and left chest wall leads correspond to the native heart.

   • Surgical manipulation and postoperative edema may decrease donor SA node automaticity, and therefore the patient may require temporary pacing or Isuprel to increase the heart rate.

   • Should arrhythmias such as SVT occur, the denervated heart will not respond to digitalis, Valsalva's maneuver, or carotid sinus pressure. Beta blockers or calcium channel blockers are used to decrease heart rate in these circumstances. It is important to assess the patient for response to Isuprel, as the drug can increase myocardial oxygen consumption.

   • Denervation creates a more long-term concern in these patients as the patient will no longer experience angina if the myocardium becomes ischemic. Pain impulses are not transmitted to the brain, so patients must be taught to report other signs of declining cardiac function (i.e., decreased exercise tolerance). This is seen in chronic rejection where even with diffuse coronary artery disease, the patient does not experience angina. The patient transplanted for ischemic cardiac disease may find this difficult to comprehend.

2. Ventricular failure. Any element of pulmonary hypertension can result in right ventricular dysfunction and eventually compromise left ventricular function also. Inotropic and vasodilating agents may be required to enhance cardiac function. It is essential to rule out any cardiac injury during harvesting and implantation which may have an impact on cardiac function. In reviewing the operative procedure, rule out reperfusion injuries or postbypass problems.

3. Bleeding. Risk factors include cardiopulmonary bypass (CPB), altered coagulation factors if right ventricular (RV) failure compromised hepatic function, and preoperative anticoagulation therapy. The recipient's pericardium may be enlarged from pretransplant cardiomegaly. With a smaller donor heart there is more room for blood accumulation without early detection. If there is greater than 100 to 200 ml/hour of bleeding for 2 hours, the patient may need to be reexplored. All medications should be reviewed for potential effect on platelet function and coagulation factors.

▶ Monitoring Altered Immune Response and Graft Protection

After cardiac transplantation, the patient is pharmacologically managed with immunosuppressive treatment for graft protection, with titrating for the best graft function with the least adverse effects. By virtue of these agents, patient survival has been tremendously enhanced, with a decrease in the need for retransplantation.

1. Immunosuppression. Most patients are maintained on triple-therapy immunosuppression: cyclosporine, azathioprine, and corticosteroids.

   • Cyclosporine creates a "selective immunosuppression" by selectively inhibiting T cells. T cells dependent on humoral immunity continue intact and no bone marrow suppression occurs. T-cell lymphocytes become unresponsive to IL-1, ultimately preventing maturation of helper and cytotoxic T cells. Adverse effects include hypertension, nephrotoxicity, hepatotoxicity, hirsutism, tremors, and gum hyperplasia. When the first intravenous (IV) dose is administered, it is important to assess the patient closely for potential histamine-type reactions with cardiovascular collapse. This is related to the IV solution preparation and is not seen with the oral preparation. A daily trough level is measured to assess therapeutic dosage and avoid toxicity.

   • Azathioprine (Imuran) is an antimetabolite that interferes with DNA synthesis. Rejection is prevented by decreasing the body's ability to generate helper and cytoxic killer T cells. It is administered to prevent rejection and is given in 1 mg/kg doses. Major adverse effects include bone marrow suppression, hepatic injury, pancreatitis,

Patient Needs and Principles of Management, Cont.

myopathy, and sepsis. The major bone marrow effects include thrombocytopenia, leukopenia, and macrocytic anemia. It is imperative to check WBC and platelet counts daily before administering Imuran. If the WBC's are less than 5000/mm^3 discuss either holding the drug or dosage reduction with the physician.

- Corticosteroids are administered to both prevent and treat rejection. They are able to decrease antibody production and inhibit antigen-antibody production, as well as interfere with production of mediators IL-1 and IL-2. Both their antiinflammatory and immunosuppressive properties offer the patient benefits. Immediately postoperatively, they are administered in high doses, and then tapered over 6 days to a maintenance dose. In situations of acute or chronic rejection the patient may be "pulsed" with steroids. These doses are 500 to 1000 mg IV every day for 3 days, during which other steroids are discontinued. The patient then resumes another tapering wean to maintenance dose steroids. Complications from steroid treatment are numerous and include infection, hyperlipidemia, diabetes, hypertension, osteoporosis, sodium and water retention, metabolic alkalosis, peptic ulceration, pancreatitis, increased appetite, adrenopituitary suppression, lymphocytopenia, opportunistic infections, and aseptic necrosis of femoral and humoral heads. The patient often receives ulcer prophylaxsis with a histamine blocker or antacids. Strict fluid and electrolyte balance must be maintained, and close assessment must be maintained for glucose intolerance. The antiinflammatory response may mask an infection; therefore, identification of malaise, anorexia, myalgias, change in wound appearance, cough, or sore throat must be reported. With all these immunosuppressive agents, the patient has an intrinsic risk for malignancies and needs comprehensive teaching regarding this and all preventive therapies to follow.

- Newer therapies offer further improvement in transplant outcomes. OKT3 (Orthoclone), a monoclonal antibody, may be given to reverse acute rejection. Antibodies that react with T$_3$ cells' surface antigens are produced, interfering with T-cell antigen recognition and making it more difficult for active T cells to recognize the target organ. OKT3 is administered for a 10- to 14-day course of therapy as a daily bolus dose of 5 to 10 mg IV. There is a danger of flash pulmonary edema; therefore the patient is premedicated with steroids, acetaminophen, and diphenhydramine.

Vital signs are monitored every 15 minutes for 1 hour after the dose is given with emergency intubation and resuscitative equipment available. While receiving the treatment of OKT3, cyclosporine is usually held and then titrated back up during the last 3 days of treatment. CD3 levels are monitored in the laboratory on the fourth and tenth day of therapy to assess effectiveness. Some centers utilize a monoclonal or polyclonal antibody for induction therapy in the immediate postoperative period. Others reserve medications such as OKT3 for rescue therapy.

2. Infection risk. The immunosuppressive drugs decrease the normal immune response, increasing the risk for nosocomial or suprainfections (Table 22–5). In the immediate posttransplant period, when steroid doses are highest, the patient is more vulnerable to these infections. Infections are a major cause of morbidity and mortality, and prevention and early detection are crucial.

TABLE 22–5. COMMON INFECTIONS IN CARDIAC RECIPIENTS

Bacterial Infections
Early
   Escherichia coli
   Enterococci
   Klebsiella organisms
   Pseudomonas organisms
   Serratia organisms
   Staphylococcus organisms
   Streptococcus organisms
Late
   Legionella organisms
   Listeria organisms
   Mycobacterium organisms
   Nocardia organisms
   Salmonella organisms

Viral Infections
CMV
Herpes simplex
Epstein-Barr virus
Varicella-zoster virus

Fungal Infections
Aspergillus organisms
Cryptococcus organisms
Histoplasmosis
Coccidiodomycosis
Blastomycosis
Candida organisms

Parasitic Infections
Pneumocystis organisms
Toxoplasmosis

From: Dressler DK: The patient undergoing cardiac transplant surgery. In Guzzetta CE, Dossey BM: Cardiovascular nursing holistic practice, St. Louis, Mo: Mosby-Year Book, 1992.

- The most challenging aspect of determining an infection is the clinical presentation, which is often masked by immunosuppression therapy. The patient's temperature may not elevate as high as in nonimmunosuppressed patients and the WBC may not elevate as rapidly. It is imperative to assess the individual trend in each patient and have a strong suspicion if patients appear more fatigued, complain of sore throats, develop a new cough, or run low-grade temperatures. Bacterial, fungal, viral, and protozoal infections may compromise the posttransplant recipient.

- Aggressive skin care to decrease dermal injuries, adequate nutrition and hydration, removing all invasive devices as soon as possible, and limiting unnecessary procedures may assist in reducing risks for sepsis. Patients and families should receive thorough education regarding transmission of infections. Antimicrobial therapy is instituted postoperatively while invasive devices are in place but should be utilized appropriately to avoid growth of antibiotic-resistant organisms. Thorough skin and oral assessments should be incorporated into daily assessment to rule out viral or fungal infections.

3. Assessing for rejection. Routinely, the patient will undergo a posttransplant endomyocardial biopsy to rule out rejection (Figure 22–11). Under fluoroscopy, utilizing a cardiac bioptome via the right internal jugular vein into the right ventricle, multiple (three to five) samples are taken of the myocardium to rule out rejection. The patient is then treated with the appropriate protocol (pulsed steroids or monoclonal antibodies). These biopsies are performed serially posttransplant during clinic visits to monitor for rejection. Other diagnostic procedures such as transesophageal echocardiogram and chest x-ray every 6 months may be performed. Cyclosporine levels are measured monthly. These data provide further guidance for earlier detection of rejection.

▶ Providing Posttransplant Psychological Adjustment

Many emotions impact on the posttransplant patient. Often the patient and family have altered their roles and responsibilities during the illness. The posttransplant goal is to encourage role readjustment and resumption of preillness activities of daily living. The return to independence may frighten them after the "security" of the hospital environment.

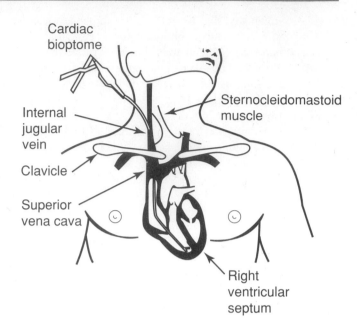

Figure 22–11. Endomyocardial biopsy technique. *(From: Macdonald SN: Heart transplantation. In Smith SL: Tissue and organ transplantation: implications for professional nursing practice. St. Louis, Mo: Mosby-Year Book, 1990.)*

1. They must be supported and assisted toward their return to home and with the plan of care.

2. Involvement in a transplant support group may benefit the patient and family, reduce anxieties, and clarify misconceptions. Meeting other recipients may validate their feelings and enhance the patient's adjustments.

3. Some recipients experience body image concerns related to hirsutism and increased weight. Reviewing cosmetic methods for dealing with these changes may decrease their concerns.

4. Weight loss may be enhanced through dietary counseling and participation in cardiac rehabilitation activities.

5. Quality-of-life issues should be explored with patients to heighten the positive side of transplantation and the future that awaits them.

6. Steroids may cause periods of mood swings from episodes of depression to euphoria. Counseling with the patient and family may reduce confusion over the cause of personality changes. During pulsed steroid therapy it is very important to assess for steroid psychosis. Closer monitoring and reassurance during this therapy may assist in diminishing this side effect.

Intraaortic Balloon Pump Therapy

The intraaortic balloon pump (IABP) provides cardiac assistance by improving myocardial oxygen supply and reducing cardiac workload. The IABP catheter is inserted percutaneously or via a surgical incision into the femoral artery. It is advanced into the aorta and, when correctly positioned, lies below the subclavian artery and above the renal arteries.

The IABP works on the principle of counterpulsation. Gas (helium or CO_2) moves back and forth from the IABP console to the IABP catheter, causing the balloon to inflate and deflate (Figure 22–12). The balloon inflates during ventricular diastole, increasing intraaortic pressure and blood flow to the coronary arteries. The balloon deflates just prior to ventricular systole, decreasing intraaortic pressure. This pressure decrease reduces the resistance to left ventricular ejection, or afterload.

Indications and Contraindications

Common indications for intraaortic balloon pump therapy include angina that is refractory to medical therapy, left ventricular failure, cardiogenic shock, and failure to wean from cardiopulmonary bypass after cardiac surgery. Patient symptoms necessitating the need for IABP therapy include symptoms of cardiogenic shock (tachycardia, systolic BP < 90 mm Hg, mean arterial pressure < 70 mm Hg, cardiac index < 2.2 to 2.5 L/minute/m^2, PCW pressure > 18 mm Hg), decreased oxygenation, unstable angina, inadequate peripheral perfusion, and decreased urine output. Contraindications to IABP therapy include moderate to severe aortic insufficiency and aortic aneurysms.

IABP Timing

Balloon inflation and deflation are synchronized to left ventricular (LV) systole and diastole from the ECG signal and arterial pressure waveform. Accurate timing of the IABP is essential to avoid obstructing LV ejection and severely compromising cardiac function. An ECG lead should be selected that optimizes the R wave. This is important since the IABP is usually set to deflate when it sees the R wave, which represents the beginning of ventricular depolarization just prior to ventricular systole. Inflation of the balloon is timed by observing the arterial pressure waveform for the dicrotic notch, an indicator of aortic valve closure at the beginning of diastole. Proper timing of IABP requires extensive knowledge and skill development, which is beyond the scope of this book. Refer to specific IABP manufacturers' recommendations for timing guidelines. A general overview of the process, however, is described in the following section.

Prior to assessing IABP timing, set the IABP frequency to 1:2 (Figure 22–13). In this mode the IABP will assist every other beat.

Inflation

- Identify the dicrotic notch of the assisted systolic waveform.
- Adjust inflation slightly after the dicrotic notch of the unassisted systolic waveform.
- Adjust inflation to occur just before the dicrotic notch and a sharp V wave is formed. The dicrotic notch will no longer be visible.
- The diastolic augmentation should be equal to or greater than the unassisted systole.

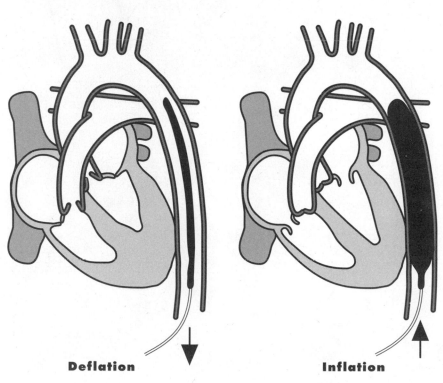

Deflation   **Inflation**

Figure 22–12. Counterpulsation. Intraaortic balloon pump inflation and deflation within the aorta.

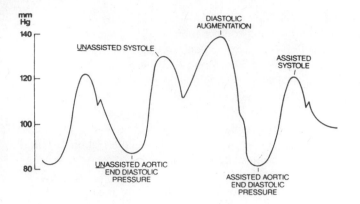

Figure 22–13. Intraaortic balloon pump frequency of 1:2. *(Datascope Corporation: Mechanics of intraaortic balloon counterpulsation. Montvale, NJ: Datascope, 1989.)*

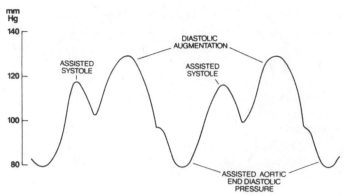

Figure 22–14. Intraaortic balloon pump frequency of 1:1. *(Datascope Corporation: Mechanics of intraaortic balloon counterpulsation. Montvale, NJ: Datascope, 1989.)*

Deflation

- Set the balloon to deflate so that the balloon-assisted aortic end-diastolic pressure is as low as possible, while maintaining optimal diastolic augmentation and not impeding on the next systole.
- Resume 1:1 pumping and observe the arterial waveform for characteristics of proper timing (Figure 22–14). Many of the IABP consoles perform automatic timing. Even if this mode is used, hourly assessment of the accuracy of timing is essential.

Inaccurate IABP Timing

Inaccurate timing of the IABP will decrease, instead of increase, myocardial performance. Common IABP timing errors include early and late inflation, as well as early and late deflation.

Early Inflation

Early inflation occurs when the IABP inflates too soon, thus impeding systolic ejection or the unassisted systolic pressure (Figure 22–15A). This timing error can lead to aortic

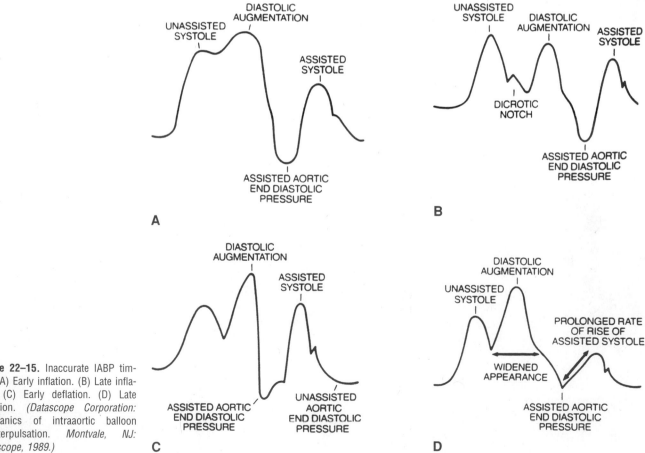

Figure 22–15. Inaccurate IABP timing. (A) Early inflation. (B) Late inflation. (C) Early deflation. (D) Late deflation. *(Datascope Corporation: Mechanics of intraaortic balloon counterpulsation. Montvale, NJ: Datascope, 1989.)*

regurgitation, premature closure of the aortic valve, and an increase in left ventricular end-diastolic volume.

Late Inflation

If the IABP inflates too late, the diastolic augmentation effect of the IABP is diminished (Figure 22–15B). This will decrease the amount of perfusion to the coronary arteries.

Early Deflation

Early deflation occurs when the IABP does not remain inflated long enough, resulting in reduced diastolic augmentation (Figure 22–15C). This may result in an increase, instead of a decrease, in the assisted systolic pressure. Early deflation will also decrease coronary artery perfusion and inhibit optimal afterload reduction.

Late Deflation

Late deflation occurs when the IABP remains inflated too long, thus impeding the patient's next systolic ejection or the assisted systolic pressure (Figure 22–15D). This results in a decrease in left ventricular ejection and an increase in afterload.

IABP Weaning

Weaning can be done by gradually decreasing the frequency of the IABP ratio (1:1 to 1:8, depending on the balloon console) or by decreasing the IABP volume. Patients are ready to wean from the IABP when:

- Heart rate and rhythm are normal
- Mean arterial pressure is greater than 70 mm Hg with minimal vasopressor support
- Cardiac index is greater than 2.2 to 2.5 L/minute/m^2
- Pulmonary wedge pressure is less than 18 mm Hg
- Oxygenation saturation is adequate
- Urine output is adequate

Patient Needs and Principles of Management

▶ IABP Maintenance

1. Monitor hemodynamic parameters to evaluate the effectiveness of IABP therapy and to identify the need to adjust prescribed vasoactive agents.
2. Frequently (every 1 hour) monitor neurologic status and circulation to the extremity distal to the balloon catheter.
3. Limit activity to maintain proper catheter position.
   - Maintain bedrest.
   - Immobilize the affected leg so that the IABP catheter does not become dislodged or kinked.
   - Maintain HOB less than 45 degrees to avoid catheter kinking.
   - Log roll every 2 hours and perform range of motion for the affected extremity.
4. Check the insertion site every 2 hours for bleeding or hematoma formation.
5. Change the insertion site dressing daily using aseptic technique.

▶ IABP Removal

1. Discontinue anticoagulant therapy 4 to 6 hours prior to IABP removal.
2. Turn the IABP off just prior to removal.
3. Assist the physician with removal of the balloon.
4. Ensure that hemostasis is obtained after pressure is maintained on the insertion site for 30 to 45 minutes after balloon catheter removal.

5. Apply a pressure dressing to the insertion site for 2 to 4 hours.
6. Monitor vital signs and hemodynamic parameters every 15 minutes for 1 hour every 30 minutes for 1 hour, and then every hour.
7. Assess peripheral perfusion to the affected extremity after catheter removal every 1 hour for 2 hours, and then every 2 hours.
8. Restrict activity of the decannulated extremity and maintain bedrest with the patient's HOB no greater than 45 degrees for 24 hours.

▶ Prevention and Management of Complications

1. IABP catheter misalignment. If the IABP catheter is advanced too far, the brachial artery may become occluded; thus left arm (brachial, radial) pulses will be diminished or absent and signs of limb ischemia will be present. If the catheter is not in far enough, the mesenteric and/or renal arteries may be occluded. Signs of this include decreased or absent bowel sounds, increased abdominal girth or firmness, and decreased urine output.
2. Thromboemboli. Anticoagulation is recommended to decrease the development of thromboemboli related to the indwelling IABP catheter. Fast flushing and withdrawing blood samples should be avoided from the central aortic lumen of the IAB

catheter. If this must be done, ensure that the IABP is on standby and that extreme care is taken to ensure that air bubbles are not introduced into the system. If the patient experiences asystole, turn the IABP console to the internal mode. In this mode, the catheter will flutter within the aorta so that thrombi formation is prevented. Refer to specific IABP manufacturer recommendations.

3. Hemorrhage. Monitor the central aortic pressure via the IABP catheter. This should be connected to a transducer, a pressured flush system, and an alarm system. Accidental disconnection of the central aortic lumen could cause rapid exsanguination.

4. Intraaortic balloon rupture. Signs of rupture include:
   - Loss of balloon augmentation.
   - Obvious blood or brown particles in the IAB catheter tubing.
   - Depending on the model of the IABP console, "a catheter problem" alarm may be activated.
   - Sudden hemodynamic instability.

If the intraaortic balloon ruptures, turn the IABP console off, clamp the IABP catheter, notify the physician, and prepare for IABP removal/replacement. Observe your patient's hemodynamic status and adjust vasoactive medications accordingly.

Ventricular Assist Devices

Patients with cardiogenic shock following a myocardial infarction (MI), coming off cardiopulmonary bypass (CPB), or with cardiomyopathies may require additional assistance when cardiac output remains low despite maximal medical therapy. IABP support offers 8% to 12% augmentation to the patient's cardiac output, but this may be inadequate, requiring placement of a ventricular assist device (VAD). Greater support for the failing ventricle(s) can be provided with a VAD. The goals of utilizing a VAD are to reduce myocardial ischemia and workload, limit permanent cardiac damage, and restore adequate organ perfusion.

Indications

Appropriate candidates for VAD include those patients with end-stage cardiac disease, cardiomyopathies, post-CPB, and acute MI with cardiogenic shock. Another indication for insertion is to "bridge" the patient prior to cardiac transplantation until a suitable donor is located. Post-MI a patient may be "bridged" in the hope of myocardial recovery and eventual weaning from the device.

The appropriate selection of a candidate for these devices is based on hemodynamic criteria. If preload has been maximized, afterload reduced, and drug therapy instituted to maximal levels, and yet the patient is still cardiovascularly compromised, a VAD may be critical to achieve survival. Appropriate parameters to consider for VAD placement are:

- Cardiac index < 2 L/minute/m^2
- Systemic vascular resistance > 2100 dyne/second/cm^5

- Mean arterial pressure < 60 mm Hg
- Left or right atrial pressure > 20 mm Hg
- Urine output < 30 ml/hour
- Pulmonary wedge pressure > 15 to 20 mm Hg

The exclusion criteria for use of a VAD include the following:

- Shock > 12 to 18 hours where reversibility is unlikely
- Acute cerebral vascular damage
- Cancer with metastasis
- Renal failure (unrelated to cardiac failure)
- Severe hepatic disease
- Coagulopathy
- Severe systemic sepsis, resistant to therapy
- Severe pulmonary disease
- Severe peripheral vascular disease
- Psychological instability
- Alcohol or drug addiction

General Description of VAD Principles

The VAD "unloads" the native ventricle or ventricles by way of artificial ventricles or a blood pump. Cardiac output is enhanced by blood circulating at a physiologic rate and by augmenting systemic and coronary circulation.

VAD support is predominately utilized for the left ventricle. However, if the right ventricle is compromised, support can be provided to both ventricles. This would necessitate separate VADs, yet the systems would function in tandem.

VADs are comprised of nonpulsatile pumps (roller and centrifugal) or pulsatile pumps (pneumatically driven or implantable electromagnetically driven). Nonpulsatile pumps are inserted in the operating room (Figure 22–16). Atrial cannulation is via the right superior pulmonary vein or into the upper portion of the left atria at the junction with the right superior pulmonary vein. Aortic cannulation is placed low in the ascending aorta. Blood flow is diverted via the atrial cannulation and is returned via the aortic cannulation.

Roller pumps deliver blood flow by compressing blood and moving it forward. Flow is continuous, but nonpulsatile. Generally this is chosen for resuscitative purposes. Centrifugal pumps are vortex pumps with two magnetic cones rotating to create a "tornado effect." Blood flow is adjusted by liter per minute based on revolutions per minute. These pumps are nonthrombogenic acrylic cones and flow is designed to reduce turbulence, thus reducing hemolysis.

Pulsatile pumps include internal or external pneumatic pumps and electric pumps. Pulsatile flow is believed to reduce microcirculatory shunting and edema formation and yield more physiologically acceptable assistance. There is superior flow assistance with pulsatile systems as they can assume flow for the assisted ventricle even during ventricular tachycardia or fibrillation.

The external pneumatic pump contains inflow and outflow valves that keep blood moving forward. The pumping chambers rest close to the thorax and are connected by transcutaneous cannula to the inflow and outflow sites. The inflow cannula is surgically placed in either the left atrium (LA) or left ventricle (LV). Atrial cannulation is associated with less bleeding and less trauma to the ventricle. However, if the patient is a transplant candidate, it is more important to use LV cannulation. This affords LA protection which will be anastomosed to the donor heart. The outflow exits the chest below the costal margin and connects to the pneumatic pump, returning to the aorta.

The inflow conduit of the internal pneumatic pump is inserted into the LV cavity after excising a core of the LV apex. The outflow conduit is anastamosed to the ascending aorta. Blood flows from the LV into the inflow to the pump and is ejected into the ascending aorta.

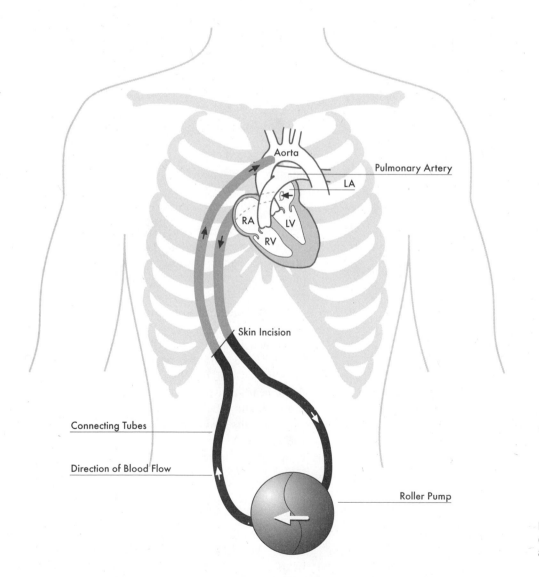

Figure 22–16. Left ventricular assist device cannula inserted into the left atria and the aorta.

The electric pump consists of an abdominally placed, battery-powered titanium blood pump. The inflow conduit is inserted into the LV cavity and the outflow conduit is placed into the aorta. A percutaneous electric line connects the blood pump to the portable system controller, which clips to a belt or waistband. The pump can generate a cardiac output up to 10 L/minute. The patients can wear either a shoulder holster or a belt bag with 5 to 8 hours battery life to increase mobility, even permitting them to go home and await transplantation.

The hemopump is a temporary cardiac assist device that employs an axial flow pump to augment LV output. The catheter is inserted through the femoral artery, advanced into the aorta, through the aortic valve, and is placed into the LV. Power is transmitted to the pump via a flexible drive shaft from an external motor and rotating magnet, which connects to an external power source. The hemopump does not require LV synchronization and can generate 3.5 L/minute of nonpulsatile blood flow.

Weaning and Recovery

The plan for weaning should revolve around hemodynamic stability and the patient's other physiologic systems' response. Neurologic, pulmonary, renal, and hematologic systems must be recovered from multiorgan insults. Assessment of CO, CI, SVR, PCW pressure, MAP, and SVO$_2$ will guide decisions for initiating weaning. Pharmacologic support should be at a stable level with good major organ perfusion.

The arterial line waveform is assessed for the dicrotic notch appearance, evidence that there is adequate LV pressure for aortic opening. A MUGA scan may be done with the VAD off for 4 minutes and if EF is > 30% with the VAD off, then weaning can start. The VAD will be turned down at small increments to assess tolerance throughout the weaning process. Heparin must be initiated before weaning and the device never set at less than 2 L/minute flow to avoid clot formation. At completion of weaning, the patient returns to the operating room for surgical removal.

Patient Needs and Principles of Management

The primary objectives in managing the patient with a VAD are to optimize cardiac output, maximize coping, and prevent complications.

▶ Optimize Cardiac Output

1. Initially, the risk of biventricular failure still is paramount after the device's insertion and the patient must be closely evaluated. Cardiovascular profiles should be measured every 2 to 4 hours and changes in cardiac output (CO) and cardiac index (CI) reported to the physician. Pharmacologic support should be titrated to achieve the most stable mean arterial pressure (MAP) and adequate Svo$_2$.
2. The VAD should be assessed for proper function to achieve an improved cardiovascular profile. The amount the VAD is delivering should be considered when measuring CO to assess for the natural heart's intrinsic CO. As myocardial recovery occurs, more support occurs from the heart and less from the VAD. The patient can then support CO without as much mechanical support.

▶ Maximize Coping

The patient and family may be overwhelmed by the suddenness of the disease, the ICU environment, the equipment related to the VAD, and the threat of loss of life. Transplantation, if discussed, may significantly increase their stress. They may require intense information sharing and clarification of misconceptions.

1. Promote emotional and psychological adaptation and assess for nonverbal clues of fear or anxiety. Frequent updates regarding goals for the day and present plan of care need to be provided in an interdisciplinary manner. The advanced practice nurse and the patient's primary nurse may coordinate this process.
2. Realistic information related to prognosis needs to be addressed with the patient and family. Often, 20% to 40% of patients on VAD die awaiting a donor heart, and families need support to cope with this possibility. Early involvement with social work and chaplains also may assist patients and families. Closely assess for other situational stressors and review prior coping strategies the patient or family found helpful.

▶ Prevent Complications

1. Thromboembolism. Anticoagulation therapy may include heparin, dextran, aspirin, or dipyridamole in order to reduce the risk for thromboembolism.

Patient Needs and Principles of Management, Cont.

Peripheral vascular impairment may occur secondary to vascular catheters. Frequent neurovascular checks should be performed and any change reported immediately. Assess for the 5 Ps of vascular complications:

- Pallor
- Pain
- Parasthesia
- Paralysis
- Pulselessness

2. Bleeding. Monitor hemoglobin, hematocrit, and coagulation factors frequently. Assess all catheter sites and wounds for oozing. The patient needs to be evaluated for spontaneous oozing or occult bleeding. The patient needs close monitoring of therapy so he or she is safely anticoagulated but not in a dangerous range should a sudden match for a transplantation heart occur. Ideally the partial thromboplastin time (PTT) should be 1.5 times normal. The anticoagulation therapy may increase the propensity for cardiac tamponade to occur. This is a surgical emergency and may require reoperation for stabilization. Clues to this complication include the following:

- Elevated atrial pressures
- Reduced CO as pump cannot fill properly
- Elevated pulmonary pressures
- Diastolic equalization
- Reduced MAP
- Declining MvO_2

3. Arrhythmias. Possible treatment with medications or electrical cardioversion may be required. Biventricular support may maintain nearly normal hemodynamics during arrhythmias. Assess the effect of arrhythmias on cardiac output and augment the VAD accordingly. Treat all electrolyte abnormalities aggressively to enhance contractility. Validate with physicians whether CPR may be performed for asystole, depending on the specific VAD.

4. Decreased renal function. Possible etiologies in the VAD patient for reduced renal function include hypoperfusion before VAD insertion, prolonged CPB time, massive transfusions, and hemolysis with release of hemoglobin. Assess daily BUN and creatinine values for further decline in renal function. It is imperative that all medications be assessed for nephrotoxicity and doses be based on creatinine clearance. Adequate vasopressor therapy in the dopaminergic range is beneficial to enhance renal perfusion. Maintain adequate fluid balance so

preload is within normal limits. Monitor urinalysis for potential abnormalities, and avoid any period of hypotension which could further insult the kidneys.

5. Infection. The large cannulas exiting the skin create great portals of entry for pathological organisms. Patients on VAD support are so metabolically stressed that they are more prone to infections, and strict precautions need to be followed. It is imperative they not become colonized, especially if they are pretransplant, as sepsis could preclude their receiving a heart. The best plan of action is prevention and includes:

- Strict hand washing before and after all patient care activities
- Strict aseptic technique
- Pan-culture for temperature >101°F
- Monitor wounds for erythema, exudate, or edema
- Assess for shift to the left on differential count

6. Immobility. Dermal injury may arise from the degree of immobility during the patient's critical phase of illness. Meticulous skin care and frequent position changes assist in reducing problems. Aggressive nutritional support will assist in decreasing the degree of catabolism. Immobility may result in significant muscle mass loss and negative nitrogen balance. Bedside physical therapy is crucial until the patient is more stable and can begin ambulating. Foot splints may be applied to diminish the risk of foot drop.

7. Poor device performance. Dangers related to VAD mechanical problems include thrombus formation, in-flow obstructions, or device failures. Frequent device evaluation is needed, particularly with any change in the patient's clinical status. Device failure may result in inadequate or no systemic perfusion, so emergency measures must be implemented rapidly (Table 22–6).

TABLE 22–6. EMERGENCY MEASURES FOR VAD FAILURE OR CARDIAC ARREST

- Back-up VAD in place and ready for operation if mechanical failure occurs.
- Discuss with surgeons if CPR can be performed.
- Assess availability of blood products should emergency transfusions be necessary.
- Have vascular clamps available for cannula disconnections.
- Educate all team members regarding emergency measures if problem with VAD occurs.
- Patients can be safely cardioverted and defibrillated with VAD in place.
- Connect to emergency power outlets in case of an electrical outage.

AT THE BEDSIDE
■ *Thinking Critically*

You are caring for a patient who just returned to the SICU from cardiac surgery. He was admitted to the hospital with mitral insufficiency and today he had a St. Jude mechanical valve inserted into the mitral position. Your assessment includes:

Temperature:	36.2°C
HR:	Temporarily atrial-paced at 80 beats/minute
BP:	86/60 mm Hg
RR:	Assist control of 12 via the Bear ventilator
PAS:	15 mm Hg
PAD:	8 mm Hg
PCW:	4 mm Hg
RA:	3 mm Hg
CO:	4.9 L/minute
CI:	1.9 L/minute/m^2
SVR:	2200 dynes/second/cm^5

What is the probable reason for his hypotension and low cardiac output/cardiac index? What interventions should be immediately initiated to improve his cardiac status?

SELECTED BIBLIOGRAPHY

Cardiomyopathy—General

Bohachick P: Psychosocial adjustment of patients and spouses to severe cardiomyopathy. *Research in Nursing and Health.* 1990; 13(6):385–92.

Casey PE: Pathophysiology of dilated cardiomyopathy: Nursing implications. *Journal of Cardiovascular Nursing.* 1987;2(1): 1–12.

Courtney-Jenkins A: The patient with hypertrophic cardiomyopathy. *Journal of Cardiovascular Nursing.* 1987;2(1):33–47.

Elkayam U: Pregnancy and cardiovascular disease. In Braunwald E (ed.): *Heart disease: A textbook of cardiovascular medicine,* 4th ed. Philadelphia: WB Saunders, 1992.

Finkelmeier BA (ed.): *Cardiothoracic surgical nursing.* Philadelphia: JB Lippincott, 1995.

Guzzetta CE, Dossey BM (eds.): *Cardiovascular nursing holistic practice.* St. Louis, MO: CV Mosby, 1992.

Pettrey LJ, Leflar-DiLeva KM: Preparing for cardiomyoplasty: A new horizon in cardiac surgery. *Dimensions of Critical Care Nursing.* 1994;13(5):226–237.

Seifert PC (ed.): *Cardiac surgery.* St. Louis, MO: CV Mosby, 1994.

Wenger NK, Abelmann WH, Roberts WC: Cardiomyopathy and specific heart muscle disease. In Hurst JW, Schlant RC, Rackley CE, et al. (eds.): *The heart,* 7th ed. New York: McGraw-Hill, 1990.

Woods SL, Froelicher ESS, Halpenny CJ, Motzer SU (eds.): *Cardiac nursing,* 3rd ed. Philadelphia: JB Lippincott, 1995.

Wynne J, Braunwald E: The cardiomyopathies and myocarditis: Toxic, chemical, and physical damage to the heart. In Braunwald E (ed.): *Heart disease: A textbook of cardiovascular medicine,* 4th ed. Philadelphia: WB Saunders, 1992.

Cardiomyopathy—Critical Care Management

Abou-Awadi NL, Joseph KA: Hemopump left ventricular support in the peripartum cardiomyopathy patient. *Journal of Cardiovascular Nursing.* 1994;8(2):36–44.

Alspach G (ed.): *AACN core curriculum for critical care nursing,* 4th ed. Philadelphia: WB Saunders, 1991.

Canobbio MM (ed.): *Cardiovascular disorders.* St. Louis, MO: CV Mosby, 1990.

Pettrey LJ, Leflar-DiLeva KM: Preventing complications in the dynamic cardiomyoplasty patient. *Dimensions of Critical Care Nursing.* 1994;13(5):238–240.

Purcell JA: Advances in the treatment of dilated cardiomyopathy. *AACN Clinical Issues in Critical Care Nursing.* 1990;1(1): 31–45.

Vargo R, Dimengo JM: Surgical alternatives for patients with heart failure. *AACN Clinical Issues in Critical Care Nursing.* 1993;4(2):244–259.

Wingate S: Dilated cardiomyopathy. Part I. *Focus on Critical Care.* 1984;11(4):49–56.

Valvular Disorders

Abramczyk EL, Brown MM: Valvular heart disease. In Kinney MR: *Comprehensive cardiac care,* 7th ed. St. Louis, MO: CV Mosby, 1991.

Alspach G (ed.): *AACN core curriculum for critical care nursing,* 4th ed. Philadelphia: WB Saunders, 1991.

Blaisdell MW, Good L, Gentzler RD: Percutaneous transluminal valvuloplasty. *Critical Care Nurse.* 1989;9(3):62–68.

Braunwald E: Valvular heart disease. In Braunwald E (ed.): *Heart disease: A textbook of cardiovascular medicine,* 4th ed. Philadelphia: WB Saunders, 1992.

Canobbio MM (ed.): *Cardiovascular disorders.* St. Louis, MO: CV Mosby, 1990.

Cavallo GAO: The person with valvular heart disease. In Guzzetta CE, Dossey BM (eds.): *Cardiovascular nursing holistic practice.* St. Louis, MO: CV Mosby, 1992.

Finkelmeier BA (ed.): *Cardiothoracic surgical nursing.* Philadelphia: JB Lippincott, 1995.

Finkelmeier BA, Hartz RS, Fisher EB, Michaelis LL: Implications of prosthetic valve implantation: An 8-year follow-up of patients with procine bioprosthesis. *Heart and Lung.* 1989;18(6):565–574.

Guzzetta CE, Dossey BM (eds.): *Cardiovascular nursing holistic practice.* St. Louis, MO: CV Mosby, 1992.

Hurst JW, Schlant RC, Rackley CE, et al. (eds.): *The heart,* 7th ed. New York: McGraw-Hill, 1990.

Kinney MR, Craft MS: The person undergoing cardiac surgery. In Dossey BM, Guzzetta CE (eds.): *Cardiovascular nursing holistic practice.* St. Louis, MO: CV Mosby, 1992.

Kirklin JW, Barratt-Boyes BG (eds.): *Cardiac surgery,* 2nd ed. New York: Churchill Livingstone, 1993.

Seifert PC (ed.): *Cardiac surgery.* St. Louis, MO: CV Mosby, 1994.

Woods SL, Froelicher ESS, Halpenny CJ, Motzer SU (eds.): *Cardiac nursing,* 3rd ed. Philadelphia: JB Lippincott, 1995.

Pericarditis—General

Lorell BH, Braunwald E: Pericardial disease. In Braunwald E (ed.): *Heart disease: A textbook of cardiovascular medicine,* 4th ed. Philadelphia: WB Saunders, 1992.

Finkelmeier BA (ed.): *Cardiothoracic surgical nursing.* Philadelphia: JB Lippincott, 1995.

Guzzetta CE, Dossey BM (eds.): *Cardiovascular nursing holistic practice.* St. Louis, MO: CV Mosby, 1992.

Shabetai R: Pericardial disease. In Hurst JW, Schlant RC, Rackley CE, et al. (eds.): The heart, 7th ed. New York: McGraw-Hill, 1990.

Kirklin JW, Barratt-Boyes BG (eds.): *Cardiac surgery,* 2nd ed. New York: Churchill Livingstone, 1993.

Muirhead J: Constrictive pericarditis: A review. *Progress in Cardiovascular Nursing.* 1988;3(4):122–127.

Seifert PC (ed.): *Cardiac surgery.* St. Louis, MO: CV Mosby, 1994.

Woods SL, Froelicher ESS, Halpenny CJ, Motzer SU (eds.): *Cardiac nursing,* 3rd ed. Philadelphia: JB Lippincott, 1995.

Pericarditis—Critical Care Management

Alspach G (ed.): *AACN core curriculum for critical care nursing,* 4th ed. Philadelphia: WB Saunders, 1991.

Bennett SJ: Pericarditis: Nursing care makes the difference. *Advancing Clinical Care.* 1990;5(6):42–43.

Bressler MJ: Acute pericarditis and myocarditis. *Emergency Medicine.* 1992;24(8):34–42.

Canobbio MM (ed.): *Cardiovascular disorders.* St. Louis, MO: CV Mosby, 1990.

Conner RP: Acute pericarditis and the electrocardiogram. *Critical Care Nurse.* 1983;3(5):40–42.

Diamond T: The ST segment axis: A distinguishing feature between acute pericarditis and acute myocardial infarction. *Heart and Lung.* 1985;14(6):629–631.

Spodick DH: Acute pericardial disease. *Heart and Lung.* 1985;14(6):599–604.

Abdominal Aneurysm—General

Cooley DA: *Surgical treatment of aortic aneurysms.* Philadelphia: WB Saunders, 1986.

DeBakey ME, et al.: Surgical management of dissecting aneurysms of the aorta. *Journal of Cardiovascular Surgery.* 1965;49:130.

Eagle KA, DeSanctis RW: Diseases of the aorta. In Braunwald E (ed.): *Heart disease: A textbook of cardiovascular medicine,* 4th ed. Philadelphia: WB Saunders, 1992.

Finkelmeier BA (ed.): *Cardiothoracic surgical nursing.* Philadelphia: JB Lippincott, 1995.

Guzzetta CE, Dossey BM (eds.): *Cardiovascular nursing holistic practice.* St. Louis, MO: CV Mosby, 1992.

Kirklin JW, Barratt-Boyes BG (eds.): *Cardiac surgery,* 2nd ed. New York: Churchill Livingstone, 1993.

Phipps WJ, Long BC, Woods NF: *Shaffer's medical-surgical nursing,* 7th ed. St. Louis, MO: CV Mosby, 1980.

Seifert PC (ed.): *Cardiac surgery.* St. Louis, MO: CV Mosby, 1994.

Underhill SL, Woods SL, Froelicher ESS, Halpenny CJ, Motzer SU (eds.): *Cardiac nursing,* 1st ed. Philadelphia: JB Lippincott, 1982.

Waldhausen JA, Pierce WS: *Johnson's surgery of the chest,* 5th ed. St. Louis, MO: CV Mosby, 1985.

Woods SL, Froelicher ESS, Halpenny CJ, Motzer SU (eds.): *Cardiac nursing,* 3rd ed. Philadelphia: JB Lippincott, 1995.

Abdominal Aneurysm—Critical Care Management

Alspach G (ed.): *AACN core curriculum for critical care nursing,* 4th ed. Philadelphia: WB Saunders, 1991.

Barringer TP: Ascending aortic arch aneurysms and dissections: Discussion and nursing management. *Progress in Cardiovascular Nursing.* 1991;6(1):13–20.

Canobbio MM (ed.): *Cardiovascular disorders.* St. Louis, MO: CV Mosby, 1990.

Cisar NS: Traumatic descending thoracic aneurysms: Discussion and nursing care. *Progress in Cardiovascular Nursing.* 1990;5(1):13–20.

Hotter AN: Preventing cardiovascular complications following AAA surgery. *Dimensions of Critical Care Nursing.* 1987;6(1):10–19.

Weiland AP: Thoracic aneurysms. *Critical Care Quarterly.* 1986;9(3):20–31.

Wheat MW: Acute dissecting aneurysms of the aorta. In Goldberger E (ed.): *Treatment of cardiac emergencies.* St. Louis, MO: CV Mosby, 1990.

IABP Therapy

Ardire L, Boswell J: Intraaortic balloon pump timing in the patient with hypotension. *Focus on Critical Care.* 1992;19(2):146–149.

Daily EK, Tilkian AG: Intraaortic balloon pumping. In Tilkian AG, Daily EK (eds.): *Cardiovascular procedures: Diagnostic techniques and therapeutic procedures.* St. Louis, MO: CV Mosby, 1986.

Datascope Corporation: *Mechanics of intraaortic balloon counterpulsation.* Montvale, NJ: Datascope, 1989.

Goran S: Vascular complications of the patient undergoing intraaortic balloon pumping. *Critical Care Clinics of North America.* 1989;1(3):459–467.

Lynn-McHale DJ, McGrory J: Intraaortic balloon pump management. In Boggs RL, Wooldridge-King M (eds.): *AACN procedure manual,* 3rd ed. Philadelphia: WB Saunders, 1993.

Patacky MG, Garvin BJ, Schwirin PM: Intraaortic balloon pumping and stress in the coronary care unit. *Heart and Lung.* 1985;14:142–148.

Quall SJ: *Comprehensive intraaortic balloon pumping.* St. Louis, MO: CV Mosby, 1984.

Schott KE: Intra-aortic balloon counterpulsation as a therapy for shock. *Critical Care Nursing Clinics of North America.* 1990; 2(2):187–193.

Shinn AE, Joseph D: Concepts of intraaortic balloon counterpulsation. *Journal of Cardiovascular Nursing.* 1994;8(2): 45–60.

Shoulders-Odom B: Managing the challenge of IABP therapy. *Critical Care Nurse.* 1991;11(2):60–62.

Whitman G: Intraaortic balloon pumping and cardiac mechanics: A programmed lesson. *Heart and Lung.* 1978;7: 1034–1050.

Wojner AW: Assessing the five points of the intra-aortic balloon pump waveform. *Critical Care Nurse.* 1994;14(3):48–52.

Ventricular Assist Devices (VAD)

Abou-Awadi NL, Joseph KA: Hemopump left ventricular support in the peripartum cardiomyopathy patient. *Journal of Cardiovascular Nursing.* 1994;8(2):36–44.

Benning CR, Smith A: Psychosocial needs of family members of liver transplant patients. *Clinical Nurse Specialist.* 1994;8(5): 280–88.

Dressler DK: The patient undergoing cardiac transplant surgery. In Guzzetta CE, Dossey BM (eds.) *Cardiovascular nursing holistic practice.* St. Louis, MO: Mosby-Year Book, 1992.

Finkelmeier BA: Mechanical assist devices. *Cardiothoracic surgical nursing.* Philadelphia: JP Lippincott, 1995.

Frazier OH: First use of an utethered, vented electric left ventricular assist device for long-term support. *Circulation.* 1994; 89(6):2908–2914.

Hooks MA: Immunosuppressive agents used in transplantation. In Smith SL: *Tissue and organ transplantation: Implications for professional nursing practice.* St. Louis, MO: Mosby-Year Book, 1990.

Lewandowski AV: The bridge to cardiac transplantation: Ventricular assist device. *Dimensions of Critical Care Nursing.* 1995;14(1):17–25.

McCarthy P, Sabik JF: Implantable circulatory support devices as a bridge to heart transplantation. *Seminars in Thoracic and Cardiovascular Surgery.* 1994;6(3):174–180.

McCauley MF: Pulmonary artery balloon counterpulsation as a treatment for right ventricular failure. *Journal of Cardiovascular Nursing.* 1994;8(2):61–68.

Moroney DA, Reedy JE: Understanding ventricular assist devices: A self-study guide. *Journal of Cardiovascular Nursing.* 1994;8(2):1–15.

Quaal SJ: Cardiac assist devices. *AACN Clinical Issues in Critical Care Nursing.* 1991;2(3):475–476.

Quaal SJ: The person with heart failure and cardiogenic shock. In Guzzetta CE, Dossey BM (eds.): *Cardiovascular Nursing Holistic Practice.* St. Louis, MO: Mosby-Year Book, 1992.

Seifert PC: Ventricular and other circulatory assist devices. In Seifert PC (ed.): *Cardiac surgery.* St. Louis, MO: Mosby-Year Book, 1994.

Shinn JA: Management modalities: Cardiovascular system. In Hudak CM, Gallo BM: *Critical care nursing: A holistic approach.* Philadelphia: JB Lippincott, 1994.

Weber BL: Cardiac surgery and heart transplantation. In Hudak CM, Gallo BM: *Critical care nursing: A holistic approach.* Philadelphia: JB Lippincott, 1994.

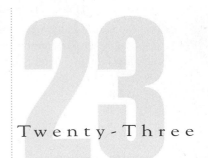

Advanced Respiratory Concepts

---

1. Discuss the definition, selection, application, pressure-controlled/inverse ratio, and assessment of pressure support, volume-assured pressure support, volume support, and high-frequency ventilation in critically ill patients.

2. Describe the use of minimum minute volume and flow-by as ventilator options for use in critically ill patients.

3. Identify factors important to the promotion of positive weaning outcomes in the long-term mechanically ventilated patient.

4. Describe the use of weaning predictors in the long-term mechanically ventilated patient.

5. Discuss weaning mode selection and weaning planning for the long-term mechanically ventilated patient.

6. Describe the use of Svo_2 monitoring in the critically ill patient.

■ *What Heals: Imagery and Ventilator Weaning*

Critical Care Nurse: "Mr. S. was a long-term patient in the critical care unit following his cardiac surgery because of respiratory complications and an inability to wean him from the ventilator. With the help of physical therapy and a lot of encouragement, we finally were able to mobilize him to the chair with assistance. We again tried to wean him. He managed to do well, and each day, he was weaned from one less ventilator-assisted breath. His most difficult time, however, was at night. He would become tense, could not relax, and would end up losing all ground. We would then have to increase the rate on the ventilator again.

"As I spoke with his wife one evening, she mentioned that he enjoyed golfing and had played for many years. I realized that I might be able to use this imagery to help him relax. I approached him with the plan and he agreed. I turned down the lights and closed the door. I suctioned him, made sure he was lying in a comfortable position, and began guiding him to slow his breathing by counting, ". . . in 2,3 . . . out 2,3 . . . ." His respirations at that time were 36, he was slightly diaphoretic, and his blood pressure was elevated. Holding his hand and gently wiping his brow, I began a guided imagery of what I knew about golfing.

"I continued to coach him with his breathing and asked if he could imagine his favorite golf course on a beautiful warm day, with a slight breeze rustling the tree tops. Not knowing too much about golf, I asked him to imagine the things around him on the golf course, noting what he saw and what he could feel and hear. I encouraged him to relax his body and continue his slow, diaphragmatic breathing as he started to play golf on the first hole.

"As he continued his imaging, I noticed his blood pressure had come down considerably and his respirations had decreased. I stayed with him a few minutes longer, encouraging him to continue this image. Then I slowly withdrew my hand and slipped out of the room, telling him I would check on him soon. I found him sleeping a few minutes later.

"We did not have to increase the ventilator rate that night. We had broken the cycle by a golf game. He continued to be weaned successfully."

CED & BMD

Adapted from: Tierney K: Relaxing with the ventilator. In Dossey BM, Guzzetta CE, Kenner CV: Critical care nursing: Body-mind-spirit, *3rd ed. Philadelphia: JB Lippincott, 1992, p. 215.*

ADVANCED MODES OF MECHANICAL VENTILATION

Pressure Modes of Ventilation: Concepts

Volume ventilation, for the last 20 years the most popular form of ventilation, is rapidly being replaced with new and complex pressure modes of ventilation. Although the basic concepts related to volume and pressure ventilation have not changed, new forms of pressure ventilation have resulted in characteristics that make widespread clinical application attractive.

Volume ventilation delivers the prescribed volume at a set flow rate regardless of the pressure required (Chapter 6, Airway and Ventilatory Management). Pressure ventilation, on the other hand, limits the pressure. Therefore, volume varies with each breath and is affected by airway resistance, compliance of the lung and chest wall, and the pressure level selected. Given the critical nature of many patients requiring mechanical ventilation and the fact that a changing volume can result in adverse blood gas changes, it is easy to see why volume ventilation has been such a popular option.

Pressure Support Ventilation (PSV)

Pressure support ventilation, first described in the early 1980s as a form of ventilation for the stable, spontaneously breathing patient during weaning, is now a popular mode of ventilation in most critical care units. The clinical success of pressure support has resulted in many other pressure modes of ventilation being used clinically. An understanding of how pressure support works will serve as a basis for understanding these new, more complex modes of pressure ventilation.

Pressure support ventilation requires that a pressure level be selected by the clinician. When the patient initiates a breath, the ventilator senses the negative pressure

(the sensitivity is usually set at −1 to −2 cm H_2O) and delivers a high flow of gas to the patient until the selected pressure level is reached early in inspiration. This pressure level is then maintained throughout the inspiratory phase. The ventilator cycles off and exhalation begins when flow decreases to approximately one-quarter of the original flow (the cycle-off mechanism varies with different ventilators). This occurs as the lungs fill toward the end of the inspiration. The characteristic decelerating flow pattern associated with PSV (Figure 23–1A) has been credited with one of the major positive outcomes associated with pressure support ventilation: improved gas distribution. In contrast, volume ventilation provides a steady gas flow throughout inspiration. This is referred to as a square flow pattern (Figure 23–1B).

Flow patterns are important because they affect lung filling in different ways. Gas moving down the airways always takes the path of least resistance and tends to preferentially fill alveoli that are open and compliant. Closed or partially open alveoli are less compliant and do not fill easily. With volume ventilation, gas flow is turbulent and distribution of gas is uneven; closed alveoli stay closed, while compliant alveoli receive most of the fresh gases. With pressure ventilation, flow is high initially but slow towards the end of the breath; gas is distributed more evenly. It is thought that this is because the slower end-inspiratory flow rate results in less turbulent gas flow (called laminar flow), decreased resistance, and better alveolar filling.

Another important characteristic of pressure support ventilation, in addition to improved gas distribution, is that it enables patients to determine inspiratory time, volume, and respiratory rate. This characteristic is thought to explain why pressure support is seen as a "comfortable" mode for spontaneously breathing patients. Guidelines for patient selection for, use of, and complications of pressure support ventilation are delineated in Table 23–1.

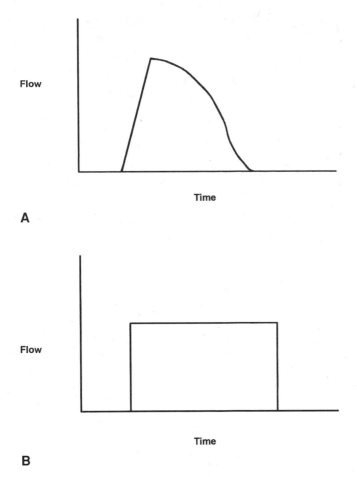

Flow

Time

A

Flow

Time

B

Figure 23–1. (A) Decelerating flow pattern seen with pressure support ventilation. (B) Square flow pattern seen with volume ventilation.

Pressure Controlled/Inverse Ratio Ventilation (PC/IRV)

One of the most dreaded complications associated with adult respiratory distress syndrome (ARDS) is barotrauma (Chapter 6, Airway and Ventilatory Management). Investigators have linked this serious complication to the very high airway pressures required to ventilate the noncompliant lungs of patients with ARDS. With ARDS, the lungs are stiff, and a severe V/Q mismatch exists. Many of the lung units are collapsed and therefore contribute little to blood oxygenation (shunt). Other lung units overfill (dead-space) but cannot make up the difference in oxygenation. The achievement of acceptable PaO_2 and $PaCO_2$ levels requires a high minute ventilation rate.

PC/IRV is actually two modes of ventilation in combination designed to ventilate patients with ARDS. The pressure control option allows the clinician to control (or limit) the pressure during inspiration to a level that is less likely to result in barotrauma (< 35 cm H_2O). The inverse ratio option is employed to overcome the tidal volume decrease that occurs when pressure is limited. Inspiration, which is normally shorter than expiration (normal inspiratory to

TABLE 23–1. PRESSURE SUPPORT VENTILATION (PSV)

Definition

Pressure support ventilation (PSV) is a form of ventilation used to augment spontaneous respirations with a selected amount of positive airway pressure. This mode can be thought of as an "inspiratory splint." There are two applications of PSV: (1) stand-alone mode and (2) mixed mode where a back-up rate is set. As with any pressure mode of ventilation, *changes in compliance or resistance can result in changes in tidal volume.*

Patient Selection

1. Patients who are stable, ready to wean, and with a dependable ventilatory drive.
2. PSV helps overcome resistance associated with circuits and airways.

Application

1. Adjust PSV level to obtain a tidal volume of 10 to 12 ml/kg (called PSV max). This level may also be used as the "resting level."
2. Decrease PSV level as tolerated. The speed of PSV decrease varies between patients (from hours to days). Aim for a tidal volume of 5 to 10 ml/kg during wean trials and a respiratory rate ≤ 25 breaths/minute. Monitor both parameters hourly.

Assessment

1. *Comfort:* The patient controls inspiratory and expiratory time, rate, and volume. The patient should be comfortable and without dyspnea (RR ≤ 25 breaths/minute, eupneic respiratory pattern). Generally, the tidal volume should be 10 ml/kg when "resting" (called PSV max) and 5 to 10 ml/kg during wean trials.
2. *Secretions* can increase resistance and decrease tidal volume. Ensure airway patency with adequate humidification and suctioning as needed. If secretions are copious, pressure support may be contraindicated.
3. *Compliance changes:* Any change in lung status (i.e., pulmonary edema) will result in a decreased tidal volume.
4. *Conditioning:* PSV is good for promoting endurance of the respiratory muscles by gradually increasing workload over time. For example, when the PSV level is set at a higher level, little effort (work) is required. The work is increased as the PSV level is gradually lowered. It is important to remember that when other activities are taking place (i.e., sitting up in a chair, physical therapies) or when there are physical impediments to breathing (i.e., ascites, obesity, distention), the PSV level may need to be increased. Use respiratory rate and tidal volume to determine optimal level of support.

Complications

1. Caution when chest tube leaks and cuff leaks are present: Patients with large air leaks from chest tubes and/or endotracheal tube cuffs should not be placed on PSV. When a leak is present, the patient will not be able to control the parameters of inspiratory time, rate, or volume.
2. PSV should be used *very* cautiously in patients with asthma or in patients with rapidly changing physical status (i.e., with acute bronchospasm, airway resistance increases and tidal volume will decrease).

expiratory ratio is 1:2 or 1:3), is lengthened to as long as expiration (1:1) or longer (2:1, 3:1, 4:1). This lengthened expiration results in more time to attain the desired tidal volume. Since noncompliant lungs collapse (empty) readily, a short expiration does not present a problem. Furthermore, by making inspiration longer, the lungs are not allowed to collapse completely, thereby making ventilation easier during subsequent breaths. This concept of incomplete exhalation time is referred to as auto-PEEP and is a desirable goal of PC/IRV.

AT THE BEDSIDE
► *Complex Ventilator Modes: PC/IRV*

Mrs. X. was admitted to the RICU in respiratory distress. Her history included a flulike illness that progressively got worse, necessitating a trip to the ER. Mrs. X.'s chest radiograph showed bilateral diffuse infiltrates in a honeycomb pattern consistent with ARDS. Once intubated she was placed on assist-control at a rate of 20/minute. Her airway pressures were very high (65 cm H_2O) and she required an FiO_2 of 1.0 and 10 cm H_2O of PEEP. ABGs on these settings were pH = 7.23, $PaCO_2$ = 38 mm Hg, and PaO_2 = 52 mm Hg. Mrs. X. was agitated, thrashing, and asynchronous with the ventilator, despite a sensitivity setting of –1 cm H_2O, a short inspiratory time, and a high ventilator rate.

The decision was made to sedate and paralyze Mrs. X. and place her on the PC/IRV mode. Settings were:

PC level: 35 cm H_2O
Rate: 20/minute
I:E ratio: 2:1
FiO_2:   0.6
PEEP: 10 cm H_2O (auto-PEEP on these settings was 5 cm H_2O, providing a total PEEP level of 15 cm H_2O)

ABGs after 30 minutes were pH = 7.34, $PaCO_2$ = 35 mm Hg, and PaO_2 = 66 mm Hg.

The team felt that the positive results were reflective of the improved gas distribution associated with the decelerating pressure waveform associated with PC/IRV. Further, they felt that by decreasing (controlling) the high inspiratory pressures, the risk of barotrauma was lessened.

AT THE BEDSIDE

Nurse: "I could see Mrs. X was really struggling to breathe. She was diaphoretic, tachypneic, and just wild. Sedation didn't help much, and I knew that given her acidosis and hypoxemia, we had to act quickly or she would code. I gave her fentanyl and Ativan for her discomfort and agitation, but it wasn't until we paralyzed her and switched to PC/IRV that things started turning around."

The obvious benefits of PC/IRV, such as controlled pressure and prolonged inspiration, are only some of the positive implications of this mode. As noted previously, pressure ventilation allows for a decelerating flow pattern (Figure 23–1A) that tends to optimize gas distribution. In the ARDS patient, the decelerating flow pattern allows for improved gas distribution and ultimately lower minute ventilation requirements. The unique flow pattern of pressure ventilation combined with a prolonged inspiration appears to result in superior ventilation, with improved oxygenation often the result.

Despite the theoretical advantages of PC/IRV, the negative outcomes associated with ARDS (mortality, barotrauma) have not decreased with the use of PC/IRV. Since this mode option currently tends to be used in the "worse-case scenarios," it will be difficult to make comparisons with conventional (volume) ventilation. Furthermore, barotrauma may not be the result of high peak inspiratory pressures (and associated shear forces), but instead may be due to high mean airway pressures. Since PC/IRV requires that pressure, though lower, be maintained for a longer period, the mean airway pressure is often higher than with conventional ventilation. Studies will need to be done that elucidate the pathophysiology associated with barotrauma. Guidelines for patient selection for, use of, and complications of PC/IRV are summarized in Table 23–2.

TABLE 23–2. PRESSURE CONTROLLED/INVERSE RATIO VENTILATION (PC/IRV)

Definition
PC/IRV is actually two modes of ventilation used in combination to lower peak airway pressure and improve gas distribution (and oxygenation).

Patient Selection
Patients with ARDS with PaO_2 ≤ 60 mm Hg and peak inspiratory pressures ≥ 60 mm H_2O in whom the risk of barotrauma is present.

Application
1. Select the pressure level. Generally this is around 35 cm H_2O.
2. Select inspiratory/expiratory ratio (1:1, 2:1, 3:1, 4:1).
3. Select respiratory rate (this is usually high—in most cases *above* 20).
4. Set PEEP (the amount dialed in) may stay the same initially. However, with the prolonged inspiratory time secondary to inverse ratios, auto-PEEP may occur. Auto-PEEP may be a desirable outcome!
5. FiO_2 is initially high but can be decreased as oxygenation improves.
6. Patients placed on PC/IRV require sedation, and often, paralytic agents. This is because the inverse ratio is not physiologic and patient/ventilator asynchrony will result in inadequate ventilation.

Assessment
1. Arterial blood gases, end-tidal CO_2, and pulse oximetry to monitor adequacy of oxygenation and ventilation.
2. With changing compliance or resistance (agitation, secretions, pneumothorax, bronchospasm, abdominal distention, fluid overload, etc.), tidal volume will be affected. Monitor tidal volume hourly and with *any* position change.
3. Patient comfort/synchrony. If paralytic agents are used, the appropriate use of sedatives and analgesics should be ensured.

Complications
1. A high index of suspicion for barotrauma. Acute changes in oxygenation, ventilation, tidal volume, and vital signs may herald a pneumothorax.
2. Acute changes in lung compliance and resistance affect tidal volume.

Volume-Guaranteed Pressure Modes of Ventilation

As noted earlier in the discussion on pressure ventilation, a major drawback to the use of pressure ventilation is the inability to ensure a consistent volume delivery. Delivered volume is dependent on compliance, resistance, and pressure level. In severely ill patients, such as the patient with ARDS, changes in compliance can result in changes in volume delivery and ultimately lead to blood gas abnormalities. Ventilator manufacturers, responding to this concern with pressure ventilation, designed mode options that guarantee a prescribed tidal volume while delivering the volume as a pressure breath (decelerating flow pattern, etc.). The technology associated with these new mode options is sophisticated and characteristics vary between manufacturers. However, the inherent concepts are similar and can be applied in the clinical setting. Two different examples of volume-guaranteed pressure modes of ventilation are described below.

Volume-Assured Pressure Support Ventilation (VAPS) (Bear 1000, Bear Medical Systems, Riverside, CA)

This mode option allows the clinician to select the desired tidal volume with a pressure option (called pressure augmentation). This means that the ventilator will deliver the breaths as pressure breaths unless it is determined, by measuring compliance and flow, that the prescribed tidal volume will not be attained. Then, the ventilator automatically delivers the rest of the breath as a volume breath. The pressure waveforms may vary and will change as the clinician adjusts the pressure level (Figure 23–2). In nonspontaneously breathing patients a rate is also set.

Volume Support (VS) and Pressure-Regulated Volume Control (PRVC) (Siemens Medical, Iselin, NJ)

These mode options are similar to VAPS in that the breaths are delivered as pressure breaths and volume is ensured. The difference between them, however, is in the delivery manner of the breaths. With VS, the pressure level for the breaths is adjusted on a breath-to-breath basis to maintain the desired volume. The pressure waveforms (Figure 23–3) show stepwise changes in pressure levels as needed in the spontaneously breathing patient. In the nonspontaneously breathing patient, the same mechanism is in place to ensure the desired tidal volume, but a mandatory rate and inspiratory time also are selected for the breaths. This mode option is called PRVC. Table 23–3 summarizes the selection criteria for, use of, and complications associated with volume-guaranteed pressure modes (VAPS, VS, PRVC, etc.) of ventilation.

Alternative Ventilator Options

It is clear that pressure modes of ventilation appear promising and that they likely will assume a dominant role in the future of mechanical ventilation. Despite the popularity of

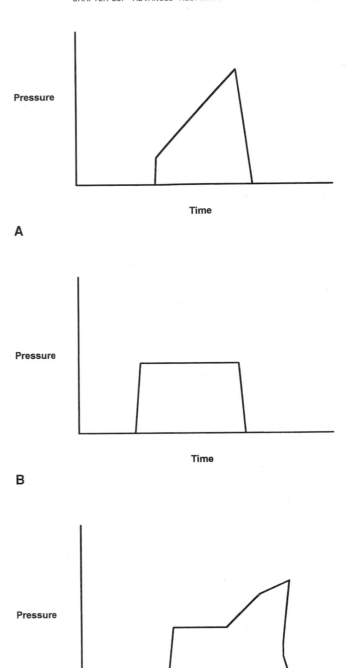

Figure 23–2. (A) Accelerating pressure waveform seen with volume ventilation. (B) Square pressure waveform associated with pressure ventilation. (C) Volume-assured pressure support breath begins as pressure breath (square waveform), but when the ventilator senses that desired volume will not be reached, the rest of the breath is delivered as a volume breath (accelerating waveform).

pressure ventilation, however, other mode options will continue to be explored for use in selected clinical situations. Examples include high-frequency ventilation, the minimum minute volume option, and flow-by.

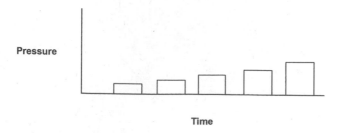

Figure 23–3. VS Pressure waveforms (square) adjusted on breath-to-breath basis. Note how the level of pressure support changes to deliver the desired tidal volume. These changes are made in a gradual stepwise fashion.

High-Frequency Ventilation (HFV)

HFV, once considered an extreme but promising mode of ventilation, has only gained true widespread acceptance in neonatal critical care. It is likely that use in adult ventilation will continue to be explored for use in selected cases. Given the superiority of the new pressure modes and our lack of knowledge of HFV, it is unlikely to emerge as a popular clinical mode option.

HFV is defined as mechanical ventilation using higher than normal breathing rates. Generally, this means greater than 100 breaths/minute in the adult. The volumes delivered with HFV are very small (dead-space ventilation), with peak airway pressures less than with conventional ventilation. HFV may be used in adults at high risk for barotrauma complications or when improved gas distribution is necessary. How gases actually move through the lungs with HFV has not been clearly elucidated but is sometimes referred to as augmented dispersion. This mechanism is quite different than with conventional ventilation where gases are delivered by bulk flow and includes phenomenon such as Taylor dispersion (how the gases in front of the bulk flow move through the lungs), molecular diffusion (the traditional concept of how gases mix in the alveoli secondary to diffusion), and the Pendelluft phenomenon (intraunit gas mixing).

Although a few studies have been done that support the proposed benefits of high-frequency ventilation in adults, there is little evidence that the use of this mode results in improved survival. Furthermore, the complications associated with HFV, in addition to the difficulty of becoming proficient in its use, limit applicability. The indications for, uses of, and complications associated with HFV are summarized in Table 23–4.

Minimum Minute Volume (MMV)

This mode option is only available on a few ventilators (e.g., Bear 1000, Bear Medical Systems, Riverside, CA; Hamilton Veolar, Hamilton Medical, Reno, NV). MMV ensures that spontaneously breathing patients on CPAP, SIMV, PSV, or other spontaneous ventilatory modes receive a minimum minute volume. In order to do this, tidal volume, rate, and minimum minute volume are set by

TABLE 23–3. VOLUME-GUARANTEED PRESSURE MODES (VAPS, VS, PRVC)

Definition

Volume-guaranteed pressure modes provide spontaneous and controlled pressure ventilation mode options while ensuring that a predetermined tidal volume is delivered. The volume-guarantee characteristic is provided in one of two ways. Either the pressure level is automatically adjusted by the ventilator to attain the predetermined volume, or the breath starts as a pressure breath but is completed as a volume breath. The decelerating flow pattern characterized by pressure ventilation is a desired outcome of these modes.

Patient Selection

1. Acutely ill patients: This mode can be selected so that volume is guaranteed while providing pressure ventilation.
2. Chronically ill patients: This option may be used as a "safety" in spontaneously breathing patients in whom pressure ventilation is desired. May be especially helpful for night use (when respiratory rates and volumes normally decrease) and in patients in whom secretions are a problem. (For example, as secretions build, resistance increases and tidal volume goes down. This mode option will prevent the decreased tidal volume and potential atelectasis.)

Application Please note: Application varies with specific ventilators.

1. Volume desired is selected and mode selection (pressure augmentation, volume support, etc.) is activated.
2. Pressure level is adjusted (i.e., in VAPS) to attain acceptable tidal volume while delivering it as a pressure breath (this is automatically done with VS).
3. Respiratory rate is selected for controlled modes and as a back-up.
4. Airway pressure monitoring is necessary with these modes to accurately apply and assess the mode options.

Assessment

1. Arterial blood gases, end-tidal CO_2, and pulse oximetry.
2. Monitor pressure waveforms to determine the need for pressure/volume adjustment (alarms will also indicate when pressure limits are exceeded, indicating compliance changes).

Complications

1. Barotrauma is a potential complication of all mechanical ventilation.
2. These modes, if not understood, will be hard to assess. An understanding of the specific ventilator mode characteristics and the ability to interpret airway pressure waveforms are essential to prevent errors in mode application.

the clinician. As long as the patient meets the minimum minute volume requirement, the ventilator does not provide additional support. However, should the minimum minute volume not be attained, additional "back-up" breaths are delivered to achieve the MMV level. A negative aspect of this mode option is that since minute volume is determined by respiratory rate and tidal volume, the potential exists for the patient to meet the minute volume requirement by breathing rapidly and shallowly. To prevent this, safeguards such as high rate alarms are activated to alert the clinician to undesirable respiratory rates and patterns.

Flow-by

Available only on some ventilators, this option provides for a high flow of gas past the patient's airway opening (patient

TABLE 23–4. HIGH-FREQUENCY VENTILATION (HFV)

Definition

Adult high-frequency ventilation is mechanical ventilation using respiratory rates higher than 100 breaths/minute. The rationale for using HFV is to reduce airway pressure swings associated with barotrauma and to improve the efficiency of ventilation. Two systems commonly are employed to deliver gas at high frequencies: jets and oscillators.

Patient Selection

1. Patients with large pulmonary air leaks (i.e., bronchopleural fistulas) in whom a decreased pressure and improved gas distribution are desired (and in whom conventional modes have failed).
2. In lithotripsy when a quiet thoracoabdominal wall is indicated.
3. Airway surgical procedures.

Jets

With high-frequency jet ventilation (HFJV) a small tube is placed in the circuit or airway (generally as far down the airway as possible), and a high-velocity "jet" of gas is injected at desired frequencies. Exhalation is passive and additional fresh gases are entrained from a bias (or cross) flow of source gas. Tidal volume is difficult to assess and is the product of rate, frequency, and the entrained gases. Jet ventilation is associated with frequencies between 100 to 600 breaths/minute.

Application

Rate, inspiratory time, jet pressure, and PEEP are all set by monitoring pressure, chest movement, and arterial blood gases. Auto-PEEP is frequently present.

Oscillators

High-frequency oscillators (HFO) move in a back-and-forth motion (piston-generated) and so have "inspiratory" and "expiratory" phases. Fresh gas is supplied by a bias flow. Tidal volume is dependent on the oscillator displacement volume and the magnitude and location of the bias flow.

Application

Rate, amplitude, inspiratory time, and bias flow pressure are all adjusted using visual inspection of chest motion, arterial blood gases, and pressure measurements. As with jet ventilation, auto-PEEP is common.

Assessment

1. Arterial blood gases, pulse oximetry, and end-tidal CO_2 monitoring.
2. Chest movement: Generally the chest is seen to "vibrate." With adequate gas exchange, the patient may not initiate spontaneous breaths. Return of spontaneous effort may be indicative of increased $Paco_2$.
3. Auto-PEEP is a common and often desirable outcome of these modes, but may be excessive and result in barotrauma and decreased cardiac output.

Complications

1. Adequate humidification is often difficult to attain, and airway obstruction is possible.
2. Tracheobronchitis (especially with jet ventilation).
3. Excessive auto-PEEP and barotrauma.

wye) during spontaneous breathing (e.g., SIMV). Spontaneous inspirations are "flow triggered." With this option, flow is always present in the system and triggering occurs when the ventilator senses a flow difference (between flow entering and exiting the system) indicating the beginning of inspiration. The flow-triggering sensitivity is adjusted by the clinician. This method differs from traditional pressure-triggered systems which require that a negative pressure be sensed within the ventilator before a breath is delivered. Research has demonstrated that the flow-by method of gas

flow delivery can result in less work of breathing for the patient; thus, many believe it is a superior method. It is likely that many new ventilators will provide this option in the future.

WEANING PATIENTS FROM LONG-TERM MECHANICAL VENTILATION

"Weaning" refers to the gradual withdrawal of ventilatory support as the patient assumes a greater portion of spontaneous ventilation. In some patients, this process is rapid and is termed short-term mechanical ventilation ($\leq$ 3 days). In others, this process takes longer than 3 days, sometimes requiring weeks or even months to accomplish. In these long-term mechanically ventilated patients, the weaning

AT THE BEDSIDE
▶ *Weaning*

Mr. H. was a 75-year-old admitted to the ER in respiratory distress. He was intubated and placed on the ventilator secondary to profound hypercarbia and acidosis and then transferred to the MICU for management of his respiratory failure and right upper lobe pneumonia.

After 2 days of treatment with mechanical ventilation (AC of 14/minute), antibiotics, fluid and nutritional replacement, and bronchodilators, the care team assessed Mr. H.'s wean potential. Major impediments to weaning included factors such as:

- Poor nutritional status (albumin = 1.8 g/dl)
- Anxiety and agitation
- Immobility
- Persistent upper lobe infiltrate
- Copious secretions
- NIP = −15 cm H_2O
- Minute ventilation = 15 L/minute with a $Paco_2$ of 50 mm Hg

The team recognized that these factors contributed to Mr. H.'s high work of breathing (secretions, respiratory rate, minute ventilation) and his overall weak and debilitated state (nutrition, immobility, NIP). They acknowledged that these factors must be addressed before active weaning could successfully occur. It was likely that prolonged ventilation would be necessary. A ventilatory mode was selected that would allow for gradual respiratory muscle conditioning while overall improvement in physical status occurred. An IMV of 8/minute plus a PSV of 15 cm H_2O was selected for daytime use. At night the IMV was increased to a rate of 12, or that level required to obliterate spontaneous effort.

One week later, Mr. H. was sitting in a chair at the bedside and beginning to ambulate with the help of the nurse and physical therapist. Serial BWAP assessments demonstrated improvement (47% to 62%), and the team felt it was time to progress Mr. H.'s wean. The plan was designed so that Mr. H. was placed on PSV alone during the day and continued to rest at night on IMV plus PSV. The plan called for a stepwise decrease in the daytime PSV level with a starting level of 20 cm H_2O (this was PSV max, Vt = 500 ml, RR = 25/minute). The level was decreased by 5 cm H_2O once Mr. H. could tolerate 12 hours without signs of fatigue. With any signs of intolerance, the level was increased until Mr. H. was comfortable and Vt and RR were within target ranges. A tracheostomy was placed during week 3 of hospitalization.

It took Mr. H. 6 weeks to finally reach a PSV of 5 (the lowest level of the plan), and it was at that time that the team initiated tracheostomy collar trials. Night rest was continued until Mr. H. could tolerate 12 hours without signs of intolerance. He was decannulated and sent home with his family 1 week later.

process varies and consists of three phases: (1) the prewean phase (that period of time when the patient is still suffering from the underlying disease or condition); (2) the wean phase (the time when trials of decreased ventilatory support are attempted but progress varies); and (3) the outcome phase (extubation, terminal weaning, or partial ventilatory support) (see Chapter 6, Figure 6–16).

Although many attempts have been made to discover the physiologic variables most important to weaning and the modes of ventilation most conducive to rapid and suc-

TABLE 23–5. TRADITIONAL WEAN CRITERIA (PULMONARY SPECIFIC)

*Negative inspiratory pressure (NIP) ≤ -20 cm H_2O
 Positive expiratory pressure (PEP) $\geq +30$ cm H_2O
*Spontaneous tidal volume (STV) ≥ 5 ml/kg
 Vital capacity (VC) ≥ 10 to 15 ml/kg
*Fraction of inspired oxygen (Fio_2) $\leq 50\%$
*Minute ventilation (MV) ≤ 10 L/minute

*These criteria are considered the most reliable because they are *not* effort dependent.

cessful wean trials, answers are unavailable. Regardless, research in the area of weaning offers guidance to clinicians working with these patients. The following discussion of weaning consists of wean assessment, wean planning, and weaning modes and methods.

Wean Assessment

Long-term mechanical ventilation is associated with high costs, numerous iatrogenic complications, and ethical concerns related to prolonged ventilation of the elderly and those with terminal diseases. It is no wonder that investigators continue to test methods for assessing weaning potential. Commonly referred to as weaning predictors, parameters, indices, or criteria, these tools include traditional pulmonary measurements of strength, endurance, and gas exchange (Table 23–5). Newer integrated clinical weaning indices combine numerous factors, both pulmonary and nonpulmonary, in an attempt to improve weaning assessment and prediction (Table 23–6).

Assessment of weaning potential starts with an evaluation of the underlying reason for mechanical ventilation (sepsis, pneumonia, trauma, etc.). Resolution of the underlying cause is necessary before gains in weaning can be expected. However, it is important to remember that reso-

TABLE 23–6. CLINICAL INTEGRATED WEANING INDICES

Index	Components	Clinical Application
Burns Wean Assessment Program (BWAP) (Comprehensive) (Burns et al., 1994)	• 26 factors important to weaning: 12 general and 14 pulmonary	• Tested as prewean index and throughout wean process • Useful as prewean checklist • Active, progressive wean trials indicated with scores of $\geq 65\%$
Wean index (WI) (Pulmonary specific) (Jabour et al., 1991)	• Strength, endurance, gas exchange combined in single index	• Tested at end of wean process (extubation) • Useful to evaluate components and as extubation criteria • WI threshold ≤ 4 associated with success
Index of rapid shallow breathing or frequency/tidal volume (f/VT) (Pulmonary specific) (Yang and Tobin, 1991)	• Respiratory rate and tidal volume	• Tested at end of wean process (extubation) • Pattern of rapid shallow breathing may precede respiratory muscle fatigue and failure • f/VT ≤ 105 associated with success
Compliance, rate, oxygenation, and pressure index (CROP) (Pulmonary specific) (Yang and Tobin, 1991)	• Combined compliance, respiratory rate, oxygenation (a/A ratio), and pressure (NIP) in a single index	• Tested at end of wean process (extubation) • CROP > 13 associated with success

TABLE 23-7. BURNS' WEAN ASSESSMENT PROGRAM (BWAP)

Patient Name _____ Patient History

I. General Assessment

Yes	No	Not Assessed	
____	____	____	1. Hemodynamically stable (pulse rate, cardiac output)?
____	____	____	2. Free from factors that increase or decrease metabolic rate (seizures, temperature, sepsis, bacteremia, hypo/hyperthyroid)?
____	____	____	3. Hematocrit > 25% (or baseline)?
____	____	____	4. Systemically hydrated (weight at or near baseline, balanced intake and output)?
____	____	____	5. Nourished (albumin > 2.5, parenteral/enteral feedings maximized)? *If albumin is low and anasarca or third spacing is present, score for hydration should be "no."
____	____	____	6. Electrolytes within normal limits (including Ca^{++}, Mg^+, PO_4)? *Correct Ca^{++} for albumin level.
____	____	____	7. Pain controlled (subjective determination)?
____	____	____	8. Adequate sleep/rest (subjective determination)?
____	____	____	9. Appropriate level of anxiety and nervousness (subjective determination)?
____	____	____	10. Absence of bowel problems (diarrhea, constipation, ileus)?
____	____	____	11. Improved general body strength/endurance (i.e., out of bed in chair, progressive activity program)?
____	____	____	12. Chest x-ray improving?

II. Respiratory Assessment

Yes	No	Not Assessed	
Gas Flow and Work of Breathing			
____	____	____	13. Eupnic respiratory rate and pattern (spontaneous RR <25, without dyspnea, absence of accessory muscle use)? *This is assessed *off* the ventilator while measuring #20–23.
____	____	____	14. Absence of adventitious breath sounds (rhonchi, rales, wheezing)?
____	____	____	15. Secretions thin and minimal?
____	____	____	16. Absence of neuromuscular disease/deformity?
____	____	____	17. Absence of abdominal distention/obesity/ascites?
____	____	____	18. Oral ETT > #7.5 or trach > #7.5?
Airway Clearance			
____	____	____	19. Cough and swallow reflexes adequate?
Strength			
____	____	____	20. NIP <–20 (negative inspiratory pressure)?
____	____	____	21. PEP > +30 (positive expiratory pressure)?
Endurance			
____	____	____	22. STV > 5 ml/kg (spontaneous tidal volume)?
____	____	____	23. VC > 10-15 ml/kg (vital capacity)?
ABGs			
____	____	____	24. pH 7.30–7.45?
____	____	____	25. $PaCo_2$ ~ 40 mm/Hg (or baseline) with MV <10 L/minute? *This is evaluated while on ventilator.
____	____	____	26. Pao_2 >60 on Fio_2 <40%?

*If unsure how to obtain information refer to tutorial menu for help.

lution of the underlying cause of ventilation is frequently not sufficient to ensure successful weaning. Patients who require prolonged ventilation, sometimes referred to as the "chronically, critically ill," often suffer from a myriad of factors that impede weaning. Even with resolution of the disease or condition which necessitated mechanical ventilation, overall status is often below baseline (weak, malnourished, etc.). Therefore, a systematic, comprehensive approach to weaning assessment is important. One example of a tool that encourages such an approach is the Burns Wean Assessment Program (BWAP). The factors important to weaning are listed in the BWAP bedside checklist (Table 23–7).

In addition to factors listed in the BWAP, it is important to assess the effect neurologic status may have on weaning. Although alertness is important for successful extubation (i.e., ability to protect the airway), it may not be essential for resumption of spontaneous breathing. Therefore, the difference between weaning and extubation must be recognized so that care planning is effective.

Weaning predictors are numerous and they provide information related to the components important to weaning, but their ability to predict weaning outcome reliably has proved disappointing. These predictors generally have been tested at the end of the weaning process (extubation) so clinical application of the scores during the weaning process is difficult. Regardless, they provide useful information related to the components important to weaning.

Wean Planning

Once impediments to weaning are identified, plans that focus on improving the factors are made in conjunction with a multidisciplinary team. A collaborative approach to assessment and planning greatly enhances outcomes in the long-term mechanically ventilated patient. However, if care planning is to be successful, it must also be systematic. Since the wean process is dynamic, regular reassessment and adjustment of plans are necessary. Tools like the BWAP, the Wean Index (WI), and f/VT can be used as serial measurements to assess and track wean progress. Other methods to systematically track and adjust weaning plans include care delivery models such as care maps, computer applications, and collaborative weaning teams. Although proponents of each will champion the virtues of specific methods, it is likely that any systematic, collaborative approach that is comprehensive will be equally successful.

Weaning Trials, Modes, and Methods

A wide variety of weaning modes and methods are available and include IMV, SIMV, CPAP, T-piece (Chapter 6, Airway and Ventilatory Management), and PSV, discussed earlier in this chapter. To date no data support the superiority of any mode for weaning; however, some general concepts related to the application of the different modes apply to each. One such concept relates to the work required by the different modes. The goal of all wean trials is to condition the muscles without unduly fatiguing them.

Respiratory Muscle Conditioning and Fatigue

Work in the area of weaning has clearly demonstrated that respiratory muscles fatigue, and that, once fatigued, require from 12 to 24 hours of rest to recover. In order for the respiratory muscles to rest, the inspiratory workload must be diminished. Generally, this means complete cessation of spontaneous effort, but in the case of PSV, a high level of PSV may accomplish the necessary "unloading." Respiratory muscle conditioning requires that workload be increased over time and that muscles are rested adequately between trials. Signs of fatigue include dyspnea, tachypnea, chest-abdominal asynchrony, and elevated $PaCO_2$ (a late sign). These signs indicate a need for increased ventilatory support and rest. Prolonging trials once the patient is fatigued serves no useful purpose and may be extremely detrimental physiologically and psychologically.

Weaning Trials

Weaning trials generally provide for progressively lower levels of support for increasing time intervals. A popular and common sense approach to wean trial progression is to wean during the daytime and allow the patient to rest at night until the lowest level of support identified in the wean plan is reached and tolerated for a specified amount of time. It is useful to adopt general weaning guidelines that the multidis-

AT THE BEDSIDE

Nurse: "Mr. H. had been in the chair for only 20 minutes when he began to complain of shortness of breath and asked to go back to bed. I knew he was weak and any physical effort wore him out. I also knew he got discouraged easily when he was short of breath. I noted his increased respiratory rate of 32/minute and also that his tidal volume had decreased from the target volume of 400 ml to 250 ml. His PSV level was at its lowest level, 5 cm H_2O. After suctioning Mr. H. to see if secretions were the reason for the decreased Vt and increased RR (they weren't), I increased the PSV level to 10 and finally to 15 cm H_2O. Finally, he said he felt better and I could see why—his RR was 22 and his Vt was 470 ml—a big improvement! Mr. H. decided to stay in the chair for another hour."

ciplinary team all agree on. These guidelines should specify when weaning should occur and how to promote sleep and rest (Table 23–8). Wean plans need to be communicated clearly to all members of the health care team (especially the patient!) so that outcomes are optimal. It may well be that the most important aspect of weaning is not the mode of ventilation, but the presence of a plan of care that provides for the dynamic nature of the wean process.

Wean Mode Selection

Wean mode selection is often determined by clinician preference and experience with the modes. For the progression of trials on any mode to be successful, however, the concepts related to conditioning and fatigue must be incorporated into the plan. For example, with PSV, the level of PSV should not be arbitrarily determined, but rather assessed by decreasing the level of support to attain the target tidal volume and spontaneous respiratory rate. When sustained increases in respiratory rate and decreases in tidal volume occur during trials, the level of support should be increased and the patient rested (Table 23–1). Do not progress below that level of ventilatory support until the patient is able to maintain the level without signs of fatigue.

In the volume modes, such as IMV/SIMV and AC, the inspiratory time is set by the respiratory therapist, physician, or nurse. When a volume mode (IMV/SIMV) is used for weaning, the inspiratory time adjustment must be made carefully since inspiratory time determines how fast the patient can take a breath. In a patient who is dyspneic, this parameter can significantly affect comfort. In addition, work of breathing will increase since the patient will work during the breath to get more flow (to get the breath faster). We often refer to this phenomenon as "out-of-phase," or patient-ventilator asynchrony. This asynchrony can result in respiratory muscle fatigue and is to be avoided. When the

TABLE 23–8. GENERAL WEANING GUIDELINES

Active Weaning Should Occur:
1. When patient is stable and reason for mechanical ventilation is resolved or improving.
2. When the wean score indices (BWAP, etc.) are improving. A temporary hold and even an increase in support will be necessary when setbacks occur.
3. During the daytime (patient's ventilatory muscles should rest at night).

Considerations for Temporary Hold
1. When wean score drops (investigate factors and intervene as necessary).
2. During procedures that require that the patient be flat or in the Trendelenburg position (i.e., during line insertion).
3. During "road trips" (increased ventilatory support will protect the patient while off the unit).
4. If suctioning is excessive (every half hour).
5. When febrile, bacteremic, septic, or with *Clostridium difficile* disease.
6. During acute events (bronchospasm, hypotension).

Rest and Sleep
Rest is important for psychological and physiologic reasons. Complete rest in the mechanically ventilated patient is defined as that level of ventilatory support that does *not* require muscular work (cessation of spontaneous activity). Decisions about *when* rest is important include the following:
1. When an acute event has occurred (i.e., hypercarbic respiratory failure, pulmonary embolus, pulmonary edema) and for the first 24 hours following admission.
2. A reasonable approach for the chronic or nonacute patient is to work on active weaning trials during the day with rest at night until most of the daytime wean is accomplished (10 hours or more). Then, night wean trials can be accomplished fairly rapidly. At night, the patient should be allowed to sleep—if work of breathing is high, sleep will not be possible. Ventilator rate should be high enough to allow for relaxation and optimal resting. Night sleeping aids should be given early in the night to enhance sleep and ventilatory synchronization *and* so that the drugs can be metabolized before the daytime trials begin.
3. Whenever possible, the patient should be rested the night before extubation and extubated early in the day.

patient's spontaneous respiratory rate is high, the ventilator response may not be rapid enough. Further complicating this situation is the fact that the ventilator sensitivity must also be set. If it is not sensitive enough, or in the presence of auto-PEEP, the patient may have to generate an excessive amount of pressure to get a breath. This ultimately results in fatigue and unsuccessful wean trials. It is this potential problem that has lead to the development and application of the flow-by option described earlier in this chapter and also to the combined use of SIMV and PSV. Since PSV allows the patient to set his or her own inspiratory time and rate, some clinicians believe that mixing the modes prevents the problems associated with IMV alone. Generally, the PSV level is set to obtain the desired tidal volume for the spontaneous breaths. Then, IMV is weaned followed by PSV.

Spontaneous breathing options such as T-piece trials and/or continuous positive airway pressure (CPAP) continue to be popular wean trial choices (see Chapter 6, Airway and Ventilatory Management). Trials using these options are gradually lengthened until rest with positive pressure modes is no longer required. Again, the key to successful use of these options is to provide adequate respiratory muscle rest between trials.

CONTINUOUS MIXED VENOUS OXYGEN MONITORING (Sᵥo₂)

Sᵥo₂ Monitoring Principles

The pulmonary artery catheter allows clinicians many monitoring capabilities that help guide therapeutic interventions in the critically ill (Chapter 5, Hemodynamic Monitoring). One such option is the continuous monitoring of mixed venous oxygenation. S_vO_2 catheters are different from other pulmonary artery catheters in that they have two special fiberoptic bundles within the catheter that determine the oxygen saturation of hemoglobin by measuring the wavelength (color) of reflected light. Light is transmitted down one bundle and is reflected off the oxygen-saturated hemoglobin, returning up the other bundle. This information is quantified by the bedside computer and numerically displayed as the percentage of saturation of the mixed venous blood.

S_vO_2 monitoring is used to continuously monitor how well the body's demand for oxygen is being met under different clinical conditions. To understand this concept, an understanding of how the tissues are supplied with oxygen is necessary.

Blood leaves the left heart 100% saturated with oxygen and is transported to the tissues for cellular use based on the amount of perfusion (cardiac output). Under normal conditions, only about 25% of the oxygen available on the hemoglobin is extracted by the tissues, with blood returning to the right heart with approximately 75% of the hemoglobin saturated with oxygen. Normal values for oxygen saturation are 70% to 80%.

In situations where tissue demand for oxygen increases, however, oxygen saturation of blood returning to the right heart will be lower than 70%. Clinical situations of increased tissue demand for oxygen include fever, pain, anxiety, sepsis, seizures, and some "routine" nursing activities like turning and suctioning. In contrast, hypothermia dramatically decreases oxygen consumption by the tissues. Interventions, then, are directed at decreasing or increasing the oxygen requirements as needed.

This concept of oxygen utilization is often referred to as supply and demand (or more accurately consumption) and is the essential concept inherent in S_vO_2 monitoring. Since tissue oxygenation is dependent on hemoglobin level, saturation of hemoglobin, oxygen consumption, and cardiac output, the saturation of blood returning to the pulmonary artery tells us much about the interaction of these four variables. Indications for the use of continuous S_vO_2 monitoring are found in Table 23–9.

AT THE BEDSIDE
▶ Svo_2

Mrs. R., a 35-year-old with pancreatitis and ARDS, was experiencing a progressively worsening oxygenation status. The care team decided to replace Mrs. R.'s pulmonary artery catheter with an Svo_2 catheter to better monitor and manage Mrs. R. Once the Svo_2 catheter was in place and calibrated, it was noted that Mrs. R.'s Svo_2 was only 60%. A quick assessment of oxygen supply variables yielded the following:

Hct: 23%
Cardiac output: 6 L/minute
PCW: 18 mm Hg
Sao_2:   91% on an Fio_2 of 0.6, PEEP of 15 cm H_2O

Given the high level of ventilatory support already in place, the team felt that augmentation of oxygen-carrying capacity with transfusions of packed red blood cells (PRBC) would provide the greatest boost to oxygenation. Following the infusion of 2 units of PRBC, the Svo_2 increased to 75%. Over the course of the next few days, ventilatory support was gradually decreased by monitoring the effect of ventilatory changes on Svo_2 in conjunction with other supply-side variables.

On day 6 of Mrs. R's hospitalization, she became increasingly agitated and her Svo_2 once again decreased to 60%. She was febrile and her sputum was noted to be purulent appearing. Sputum cultures were obtained and other reasons for Mrs. R.'s agitation were also considered. A STAT chest radiograph was obtained to rule out pneumothorax (it was ruled out), and a blood gas test was obtained. ABG results were pH = 7.32, $Paco_2$ = 45 mm Hg, and Pao_2 = 55 mm Hg. Her ventilator settings were IMV = 12/minute, Fio_2 = 0.45, PEEP = 5 cm H_2O, Hct = 29%, and cardiac output = 6 L/minute.

The team recognized that both supply and demand needed to be addressed to optimize oxygenation in Mrs. R. Thus, ventilatory settings were increased as follows:

Fio_2:   0.55
PEEP: 10 cm H_2O
IMV: 15/minute

Since Mrs. R.'s CO and Hct were considered adequate, the team then considered Mrs. R.'s demand requirements. Their assessment indicated that agitation and fever were both increasing demand, so both sedatives and antipyretics were ordered in conjunction with fluids and antibiotics. Mrs. R.'s Svo_2 increased to 75% following these interventions.

TABLE 23–9. INDICATIONS FOR CONTINUOUS Svo_2 Measurement

The Svo_2 catheter can be used to monitor alterations in hemodynamic and pulmonary status and manage:

- Titration of vasoactive drugs
- Volume loading and blood replacement
- Ventilatory and oxygenation changes
- Routine care interventions such as turning and suctioning

The Svo_2 catheter may reduce the need for frequent ABGs and COs.

Selected Examples of Clinical Applications

Svo_2 and Low Cardiac Output

In low "output" states, hemoglobin is moved more slowly through the body, so there is a decrease in oxygen delivery (supply). There also is more time for oxygen extraction at the tissue level. Svo_2 levels in someone with cardiogenic shock are typically low (below 70%) due to slow perfusion and high tissue extraction of oxygen. The addition of an inotropic agent such as dobutamine may increase the cardiac output and thus increase the Svo_2. Conversely, decreases in Svo_2 may be observed as inotropic agents are weaned, indicating decreases in cardiac output.

AT THE BEDSIDE

Nurse: "Mrs. R.'s Svo_2 had been hovering around 67% all night. I knew that her Sao_2 and Svo_2 had decreased with turning, suctioning, and almost any intervention, and yet I also knew that she needed these therapies to prevent complications. I discussed the situation with the respiratory therapist and we planned to increase the ventilator Fio_2, as well as provide sedation and pain relief, prior to activities. We worked together all night and were successful in keeping Mrs. R.'s Svo_2 around 70%. It was a great feeling to know that our plans prevented complications and resulted in a good night's sleep for Mrs. R.!"

Svo_2 and High Output States

In sepsis, cardiac output is often very high (> 10 L/minute). In this hypermetabolic output state, blood moves very quickly past the tissues and extraction is less than optimal. Svo_2 levels are frequently above normal (> 80%), indicating that extraction of oxygen at the tissue level is low. Despite the availability of oxygen, tissue hypoxia exists and is confirmed with lactic acid measurements.

A related concept that has recently been described is that of "supply-dependent consumption." This condition is observed in sepsis and is described as the inability of the tissues to extract oxygen normally. Essentially, more "supply" is required before consumption can increase. Although this concept seems quite strange, it means that oxygen sup-

TABLE 23–10. SUPPLY AND CONSUMPTION CALCULATION

A. Arterial side (supply) =
[(Hbg × arterial oxygen saturation × 1.34*) × cardiac output] × 10**

B. Venous side (return) =
[(Hbg × venous oxygen saturation × 1.34) × cardiac output] × 10**

C. Consumption = A – B***   Normal = 250 ml/minute

*A constant reflecting the amount of oxygen in milliliters that the hemoglobin can hold.
**A constant to convert the unit of measurement to milliliters.
***Simplified calculation omitting the negligible contribution of oxygen dissolved in plasma.

ply must be increased so that oxygen utilization can occur. The three ways oxygen supply is increased include increasing cardiac output (fluids followed by inotropes), increasing saturation (FiO_2 level, PEEP, etc.), and increasing hemoglobin (transfusion of red cells). The SvO_2 catheter then allows for rapid calculation and assessment of supply and consumption (Table 23–10) and can be used to improve outcomes in sepsis.

SvO_2 and Blood Loss

In acute blood loss, hemoglobin is decreased and the body extracts more from the available hemoglobin. SvO_2 levels will decrease and are an early indication of acute blood loss. Transfusions (providing they are adequate in number and rate) result in an increase in SvO_2.

Troubleshooting

The instructions for calibration of the SvO_2 catheter must be followed if readings are to be accurate. It is also important that measurements be compared periodically with co-oximeter measurements of SvO_2 drawn slowly from the distal port of the pulmonary artery. The SvO_2 monitor can be recalibrated if saturations vary. This is referred to as an in vivo calibration.

It is also important that the catheters be free floating in the PA and not have fibrin or clots attached to the end which might affect the fiberoptic measurement of saturation. A guide for this is called "light intensity" and refers to the amount of transmitted light required to obtain a suitable reflected signal back to the monitor. Guidelines for the levels of light intensity help the clinician assess the accuracy of the SvO_2 readings. The size and position of the light intensity signal help the nurse detect such complications as a catheter in wedge position or clot formation.

SvO_2 catheters can be helpful in the assessment of oxygenation in the critically ill. An additional benefit may be a reduction in the need for frequent cardiac output measurements, arterial blood gas parameters, and hemoglobin levels. However, as with any tool, the successful applica-

tion of SvO_2 monitoring is dependent on user familiarity and a comprehensive understanding of essential concepts.

SELECTED BIBLIOGRAPHY

Advanced Modes of Ventilation

Anderson JB: *Improved care for the critically ill: Introducing pressure regulated volume control (PRVC) and volume support (VS)*. Sweden: Siemens-Elema AB, Life Support Systems Division, 1992.

Bear Medical Systems: *Bear 1000 operations manual*. Riverside, CA: Bear, 1992.

Tobin MJ (ed.): *Principles and practice of mechanical ventilation*. New York: McGraw-Hill, 1994.

Weaning from Long-Term Mechanical Ventilation

Burns SM, Barton D, Fahey S, Slack D: Weaning from mechanical ventilation: A method for assessment and planning. *AACN Clinical Issues in Critical Care Nursing*. 1991;2(3):372–387.

Burns SM, Burns JE, Truwit JD: Comparison of five clinical weaning indices. *American Journal of Critical Care*. 1994;3(5):342–352.

Burns SM, Clochesy JM, Goodnough-Hanneman SK, Ingersoll GL, Knebel AR, Shekleton ME: Weaning from long-term mechanical ventilation. *American Journal of Critical Care*. 1995;4(1):4–22.

Daly BJ, Rudy EB, Thompson KS, Happ MB: Development of a special care unit for chronically critically ill patients. *Heart and Lung*. 1991;20:45–52.

Goodnough-Hanneman SK, Ingersoll GL, Knebel AR, Shekleton ME, Burns SM, Clochesy JM: Weaning from short-term mechanical ventilation: A review. *American Journal of Critical Care*. 1994;3:421–443.

Jabour ER, Rabil DM, Truwit JD, Rochester DF: Evaluation of a new weaning index based on ventilatory endurance and the efficiency of gas exchange. *American Review of Respiratory Disease*. 1991;144:531–537.

Knebel AR, Shekleton ME, Burns SM, Clochesy JM, Goodnough-Hanneman SK, Ingersoll GL: Weaning from mechanical ventilation: Concept development. *American Journal of Critical Care*. 1994;3:416–420.

Yang KL, Tobin MJ: A prospective study of indexes predicting the outcome of trials of weaning from mechanical ventilation. *New England Journal of Medicine*. 1991;324:1445–50.

SvO_2 Monitoring

Cilley RE, Sharenberg AM, Bongiorno PF, Guire KE, Bartlett RH: Low oxygen delivery produced by anemia, hypoxia, and low cardiac output. *Journal of Surgical Research*. 1991;51:425–433.

Kupeli I, Satwicz PR: Mixed venous oximetry. *International Anesthesiology Clinics*. 1989;27:176–183.

Shoemaker WC, Appel PL, Kram HB, Bishop M, Abraham E: Hemodynamic and oxygen transport monitoring to titrate therapy in septic shock. *New Horizons*. 1993;1:145–159.

Advanced Neurologic Concepts

> ## ► Knowledge Competencies
>
> 1. Describe the etiology, pathophysiology, clinical presentation, patient needs, and principles of management of increased intracranial pressure (ICP).
> 2. Compare and contrast the pathophysiology, clinical presentation, patient needs, and management approaches for the following conditions:
>
> - Aneurysm
> - Head injury
> - Acute spinal cord injury
> - Space-occupying lesions

■ *What Heals: Unrestricted Visiting Policies*

The raging debate over unrestricted visiting policies in critical care continues. It is a debate because most critical care units continue visiting restrictions. Even if all units across the United States were to change to unrestricted visiting tomorrow, it would be doomed to fail.

Why would it fail? Because critical care nurses are the gatekeepers of the ICU doors. It is known, for example, that regardless of whether there is a liberal or restrictive visiting policy in place, sometimes we allow family members open visiting and sometimes we enforce strict visiting policies. We are the ones who individually regulate the frequency and length of the visits. We are the ones who either enforce or disregard the policy.

Unrestricted visiting is believed to produce havoc and confusion and interfere with patient care because additional time must be spent explaining things to families, thereby leaving less time for the patient. In short, families get in the way. As long as we continue to view and treat families as outsiders who get in the way, they will remain so. It is time for a fresh approach. What would happen if we made families a part of team and put them to work? What if we contracted with them not only on visitation times but also on what they could do to help? What if we contracted with them by discussing the psychophysiologic care needs of the patient and negotiated their role and which aspects of care they might feel comfortable in providing? What if we made families a part of the team—with an important role to play and important tasks to perform?

What is being suggested here is nothing new. Besides opening the labor and delivery door to husbands, we have let parents into pediatric hospitals for unrestricted visiting to play an extended patient care role with their children. Why not also incorporate families of critically ill patients into the health care team? The advantages to families are clear. Because they are taking these sick patients home earlier and earlier to become their sole caretakers, families could be given the teaching, experience, and practice they need before the patient goes home. Also, the therapeutic benefits for the family of knowing that they are actually doing something that is important in the care of their loved one could be powerful.

We would need to assess each situation carefully because some families will be unsuitable, unable, or unwilling to take on this responsibility. We would have to monitor and evaluate the care being rendered by the family. However, most families would do well with the proper contracting, teaching, and help. If we

changed our view of the family from being an outsider to a part of the health care team, our attitudes and beliefs about visiting would change. So too would our behaviors regarding visiting.

CEG & BMD

Adapted from: Guzzetta CE. Comments. Capsules and Comments in Critical Care Nursing. 1994;1:64–65.

PATHOLOGICAL CONDITIONS

Intracranial Pressure

Cerebral Hemodynamics

Intracranial pressure (ICP) is the pressure exerted by the cerebral spinal fluid (CSF) within the ventricles of the brain. ICP is normally less than 10 mm Hg. The Monro-Kellie hypothesis states that in the adult, the cranial vault or skull is nondistensible and the three components of the vault (brain tissue, intravascular blood, and CSF) have limited compressibility. An increase in volume of one component necessitates a reciprocal decrease in volume in either or both of the other components. If the reciprocal decrease does not occur, there is a rise in ICP.

Although the skull is considered a closed cavity, compensatory mechanisms allow for some adaptation to an increase in volume. The ability of the brain to adjust to volume changes is called compliance. A person with good compliance has intact compensatory mechanisms for adapting to changes in volume. Compensation occurs through four mechanisms:

- Displacement of some CSF to the dural sac
- Compression of the low-pressure venous system
- Decreased production of CSF
- Cerebral vasoconstriction

As these mechanisms are saturated, compliance is decreased, resulting in poor compliance. With decreased compliance, a small increase in volume will result in a large increase in ICP. Patients with decreased compliance may maintain increased ICP even when volume returns to previous levels. Cerebral compliance is evaluated by interpreting the ICP pulse waveform.

Cerebral Perfusion Pressure

Cerebral perfusion pressure (CPP) is the pressure at which the cells are perfused, or the blood pressure gradient across the brain. It is calculated as the difference between the mean arterial pressure (MAP) and the mean ICP:

$$CPP = MAP - ICP$$

CPP provides an estimate of cerebral blood flow (CBF). Decreases in CPP reduce CBF. CBF is maintained at a rate that meets the metabolic needs of the brain. If metabolic needs are high, cerebral vasodilation occurs with a subsequent increase in CBF. Conversely, when metabolic needs are low, there is decreased CBF.

The normal range for CPP is 70 to 100 mm Hg. A CPP of at least 50 to 60 mm Hg is necessary for adequate cerebral perfusion. CPP below 30 mm Hg results in irreversible neuronal hypoxia, leading to brain death.

CBF is constant in healthy adults with MAP ranging from 60 to 160 mm Hg. As CPP decreases, cerebral vessels dilate to maintain CBF within a normal range. When CPP increases, cerebral vasoconstriction occurs to maintain CBF within a normal range. With MAP less than 60 or greater than 160 mm Hg, or a CPP less than 50 or greater than 150 mm Hg, this autoregulation may stop functioning, and CBF becomes dependent on systemic arterial pressure. If this occurs, an increase in MAP will increase CBF and increase ICP. A drop in MAP to less than 60 mm Hg will decrease CBF, resulting in neuronal hypoxia and eventually brain death. Factors that increase CBF include:

- Increased CO_2 concentration. P_{CO_2} greater than 45 mm Hg results in cerebral vasodilation and increased CBF.

- Decreased O_2 concentration. Arterial P_{O_2} less than 50 mm Hg results in cerebral vasodilation and increased CBF.
- Cerebral vasodilating drugs, such as anesthetic agents (halothane, nitrous oxide), some antihypertensive agents (Nipride), and some histamines.
- Activity (e.g., seizures, fever, pain, and cerebral trauma).

CPP is usually calculated hourly along with the documentation of ICP. Examining ICP alone is of little value. An ICP in the normal range of 0 to 15 mm Hg may be high enough to prevent adequate perfusion of cells, depending on a patient's mean arterial pressure. Patients in hypotensive states, such as trauma patients, are at risk for impaired cerebral perfusion even with a normal ICP.

Increased ICP

Many factors are associated with increased ICP and intracranial hypertension (intracranial hypertension is defined as a sustained elevated ICP of 15 to 20 mm Hg or higher). These factors are grouped below by their effects on brain volume, blood volume, CSF volume, and activities.

- *Increased brain volume.* Mass lesions (e.g., hematomas, abscesses, tumors, aneurysms) or cerebral edema (e.g., head injury, Reye's syndrome, ischemia).
- *Increased blood volume.* Venous outflow obstruction from compression of jugular veins (neck flexion, hyperextension, rotation); increased intrathoracic pressure or increased intraabdominal pressure from Trendelenburg position, prone position, extreme hip flexion, Valsalva maneuver, coughing, PEEP, endotracheal suctioning; or cerebral vasodilation (hypoxia, hypercapnia, increased metabolic demands, drug effects).
- *Increased CSF volume.* Obstruction of CSF flow, decreased reabsorption of CSF (e.g., subarachnoid hemorrhage), or increased production of CSF.
- *Activities.* Isometric muscle contractions, emotional upset, noxious stimuli (pain, invasive procedures), seizures, or clustering of activities (e.g., bathing, turning, weighing).

Cerebral Edema

Cerebral edema is defined as an abnormal accumulation of water or fluid in the intracellular space and/or extracellular space, resulting in increased brain volume. Cerebral edema can be life-threatening because it may increase ICP, cause neurological deficits, and produce herniation. Two types of cerebral edema are vasogenic edema and cytotoxic edema.

Vasogenic edema occurs as a result of increased capillary permeability of the arterial walls, allowing plasma and protein to leak into the extracellular space. It is seen with intracranial tumors, cerebral trauma, cerebral ischemia, or hemorrhage.

Cytotoxic edema is associated with a hypoxic or anoxic event, such as cardiac arrest, where intracellular fluid and sodium increases and extracellular fluid volume decreases.

Clinical Presentation of Increasing ICP

- Deterioration in level of consciousness (LOC)
  Early: confusion, restlessness, lethargy
  Late: stuporous and comatose
- Pupillary dysfunction
  Early: gradual dilation, sluggish reaction to light
  Late: ipsilateral pupil dilation, nonreactive to light, papilledema (edema of the optic nerve from compression)
  Terminal: bilateral pupil dilation, nonreactive to light
- Visual abnormalities
  Early: blurred vision, diplopia
  Late: more pronounced blurred vision, diplopia
- Motor weakness
  Early: hemiparesis, monoparesis
  Late: hemiplegia, decortication, decerebration
- Headache
  Slight or vague
- Vomiting
- Altered blood pressure and heart rate
  Early: no change
  Late: increasing systolic pressure, widening pulse pressure, bradycardia (Cushing's response)
  Very late: decreased blood pressure, tachycardia
- Altered respiratory pattern
  Dependent on level of brain dysfunction

ICP Monitoring

ICP monitoring is considered in patients who have evidence of, or are at significant risk for, increased ICP. ICP can be measured in the cerebral ventricles, subarachnoid space, epidural space, subdural space, or brain parenchyma (Figure 24–1). A variety of different types of ICP monitoring systems are available (Table 24–1). ICP values depend on the site selected for monitoring.

The monitoring system has three parts—a sensor, a transducer, and a recording instrument. In one system the sensor is a fluid-filled catheter, cannula, or bolt that communicates between the intracranial space being monitored and the transducer. The transducer converts the pressure signal into an electrical signal for recording. The recorder is usually a bedside monitor with a digital readout and a waveform display.

The ICP monitoring system is a closed system with no continuous flush system. The transducer must be level with the inferred anatomical reference point of the foramen of Monro. This reference point may be the top of the ear, the external auditory meatus, or the point lateral to outer canthus of the eye. Whichever point is used, consistency is essential. Any change in the height of the patient's

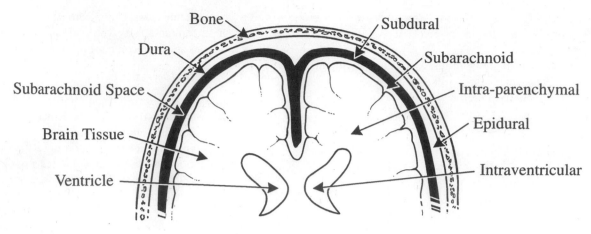

Figure 24–1. Locations for intracranial pressure (ICP) monitoring systems.

head requires the transducer to be leveled to the anatomical reference point and ideally rezeroed to atmospheric pressure prior to obtaining readings to ensure the highest accuracy.

The fiberoptic transducer-tipped catheter (FTC) is also available for ICP monitoring. The FTC contains a miniature transducer at the tip, so leveling to an anatomical point is not required. Just before insertion the catheter is zero-balanced to atmospheric pressure. The FTC can be inserted into the ventricle, subarachnoid space, epidural space, subdural space, or brain parenchyma. It has its own monitor so a patient can be transported while accurate ICP readings are obtained.

ICP Waveforms

With continuous ICP monitoring, there are fluctuations in waveforms that correlate with specific physiological events. Examination of these waveforms can be helpful in evaluating changes in the patient's condition.

The ICP pulse waveform is a continuous, real-time pressure display that corresponds to each heartbeat (Figure 24–2). The normal pulse wave has three or more defined peaks (Figure 24–3):

P1 Percussion wave: sharp peak, consistent in amplitude
P2 Tidal wave: variable in shape and magnitude
P3 Dicrotic wave: occurs after dicrotic notch

TABLE 24–1. TYPES OF ICP MONITORING DEVICES

Type	Advantages	Disadvantages
Intraventricular catheter (fluid-filled or fiberoptic)	Provides highly accurate and reliable readings Able to drain CSF to reduce ICP Able to collect CSF specimens for analysis Able to evaluate cerebral compliance by injection of fluid	Increased risk of infection Catheter may become plugged with blood or cerebral tissue CSF leakage may occur around insertion site Insertion may be difficult if ventricles small
Subarachnoid screw/bolt (fluid-filled or fiberoptic)	Easy to insert at bedside Able to collect CSF specimens for analysis Provides accurate readings Decreased CSF drainage around insertion site	Bolt may become plugged with blood or cerebral tissue Less accurate at high ICP pressures Tendency for dampened waveforms Increased risk of infection
Epidural catheter or sensor (fiberoptic)	Easy to insert Brain or subarachnoid space not penetrated, so decreased risk of infection	Indirect measurement of ICP so readings not as accurate Unable to collect CSF specimens
Subdural catheter or sensor (fluid-filled or fiberoptic)	Low risk of bleeding Direct measure of pressure	Unable to collect CSF specimens Accuracy and reliability poor over time as they are often placed during surgical closure of skull
Intraparenchymal (fiberoptic)	Easy to insert Provides accurate readings May eventually replace epidural, subdural, and subarachnoid monitors. Useful when unable to obtain ventricular access	Expensive Fiberoptic can be broken if cable is kinked or stretched Requires separate monitor

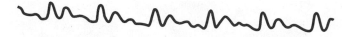

Figure 24–2. Intracranial pressure (ICP) pulse waveform.

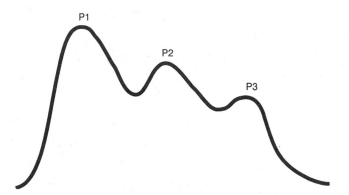

Figure 24–3. Components of a normal intracranial pressure (ICP) pulse waveform.

The pulse waveform at low pressures is a descending sawtoothed pattern with a distinct P_1. As mean ICP rises, a progressive elevation of P_2 occurs, causing the pulse waveform to appear more rounded. When P_2 is equal to or higher than P_1, decreased compliance exists (Figure 24–4).

Trend recordings compress continuous ICP recording data into time periods to reflect general trends in ICP over longer time periods (minutes to hours). Three distinct pressure waves have been identified (Figure 24–5). A waves (plateau waves) are sudden increases in pressure lasting 5 to 20 minutes. They begin from a baseline of an already elevated ICP (greater than 20 mm Hg) and reflect cerebral ischemia. B waves are sharp, rhythmic oscillations of pressure (up to 50 mm Hg) occurring every 0.5 to 2 minutes. They are seen in relationship to fluctuations in the respiratory cycle, such as Cheyne-Stokes respirations. They are not clinically significant, but may progress to A waves. C waves are small rhythmic waves with pressures up to 20 mm Hg occurring four to eight times per minute. They relate to normal changes in systemic arterial pressure, and their clinical significance is unknown.

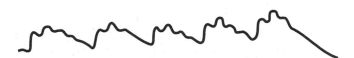

Figure 24–4. Intracranial pressure (ICP) pulse waveform demonstrating poor compliance.

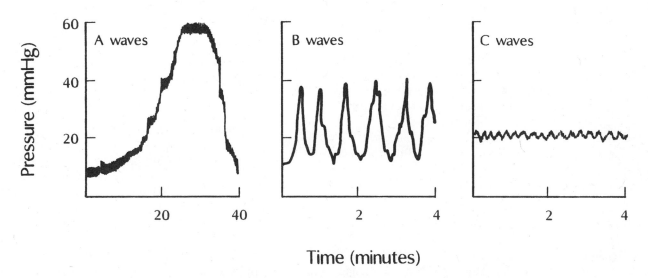

Figure 24–5. Intracranial pressure waveforms.

Patient Needs and Principles of Management

Increased intracranial pressure must be aggressively treated to prevent permanent neurological damage. The goals of management include monitoring for neurological changes, maintaining adequate oxygenation and ventilation, and managing factors which increase ICP.

► Monitoring for Changes in Neurological Status

1. Assess baseline neurological signs; then reassess periodically and compare to previous findings. Include level of consciousness, Glasgow Coma Scale score, pupillary size and reaction to light, eye movement, and motor/sensory function.
2. Assess vital signs and compare with previous findings to identify trends.

► Maintaining Adequate Oxygenation and Ventilation

1. Assess rate, depth, and pattern of respirations. Auscultate chest for normal breath sounds.
2. Administer O_2 as ordered.
3. Monitor ABGs for abnormalities. Hypercarbia and hypoxia can result in cerebral vasodilation and increased ICP.
4. In the patient with intracranial hypertension, hyperventilating the patient will rapidly reduce the Pco_2 level and ICP by constricting cerebral blood vessels and decreasing CBF. This decreased blood flow can cause ischemia in injured brain tissue, and therefore is no longer routinely used to decrease ICP.
5. Hyperventilate lungs with 100% oxygen for at least 20 to 30 seconds prior to suctioning and limit the duration of suctioning to less than 10 seconds. Attempt to reduce coughing with endotracheal suctioning when possible. Endotracheal suctioning produces a transient but significant increase in ICP. Hyperventilating provides adequate oxygenation so that an increase in CO_2 will not exacerbate increased ICP.
6. Secure the endotracheal tube noncircumferentially with tape. Circumferential ties around the patient's neck may obstruct venous return.
7. Turn patients every 2 hours to enhance ventilation.

► Managing Factors Which Increase ICP

1. Drug therapy to decrease cerebral edema.
   - Osmotic diuretics reduce cerebral edema and enhance circulating blood volume by pulling extracellular fluid from brain tissue into the blood vessels. Mannitol is the most commonly used agent. The dosage and frequency are related to the ICP, CPP, and serum osmolality. Therapy is directed at keeping the serum osmolality between 300 and 315 mOsm/L. Serum osmolality, glucose, and electrolytes must be closely monitored during osmotic diuretic therapy.
   - Corticosteroids may also be used to decrease cerebral edema, depending on the cause of the intracranial hypertension. Steroids appear to be effective in the management of vasogenic edema associated with intracranial tumors; however, steroid use in head injuries is controversial. The drug of choice is dexamethasone (Decadron). Patients on steroids must be monitored for gastric irritation, stress ulcer, gastric hemorrhage, and hyperglycemia. Stools should be monitored for the presence of occult blood. An antacid or H_2 receptor may be administered to prevent gastric irritation. Cortiosteroids are tapered gradually to avoid the risk of adrenal insufficiency.
2. Blood pressure management. Management of blood pressure is determined by the level of ICP and CPP. The goal is to maintain a CPP of approximately 60 to 70 mm Hg. If the patient is hypotensive, fluids are infused to ensure euvolemia. Fluid management is guided by CVP and/or PCWP. Vasopressors, such as phenylephrine hydrochloride (Neo-Synephrine) may be titrated to achieve an optimal CPP with minimal effect on ICP. Antihypertensives may be indicated if the systolic pressure exceeds 160 mm Hg or when CPP exceeds 85 to 100 mm Hg. Intravenous beta blockers, such as labetalol, are the drugs of choice.
3. Seizure control. Seizure activity increases CBF and ICP. Phenytoin (Dilantin) is used to prevent and control seizure activity. Phenobarbital may be used if the patient has a drug reaction or allergy to Dilantin. Blood levels are monitored to ensure therapeutic levels are maintained for control of potential seizure activity.
4. Elimination of high intrathoracic pressure. Neuromuscular paralysis may be used to prevent increases in intrathoracic and venous pressure that occur with coughing, "bucking" of the ventilator, or patient-ventilator asychrony. Pancuronium bromide (Pavulon) and vecuronium bromide (Norcuron) are commonly used agents. Sedation, with benzodiazepines and/or barbiturates, is always used in conjunction with neuromuscular paralysis.

Patient Needs and Principles of Management, Cont.

5. Management of uncontrolled intracranial hypertension. Barbiturate coma therapy may be indicated for the management of uncontrolled intracranial hypertension that does not respond to other therapies. Barbiturate coma therapy decreases cerebral metabolism, decreases CBF, and decreases ICP. Drugs commonly used are pentobarbital (Nembutal) and thiopental (Pentothal). Once the barbiturate coma is induced, the usual parameters of neurological assessment, such as pupillary, gag, and swallowing reflexes, are lost. However, asymmetrical or dilated pupils may occur in response to brain stem compression, and therefore pupillary assessment should continue. Invasive monitoring devices, such as the ICP monitor, pulmonary artery catheter, arterial blood pressure monitor, and cardiac monitor are necessary. The patient is maintained on a ventilator via an endotracheal tube or tracheostomy tube. Complications associated with barbiturate coma include hypotension, dehydration, hypothermia, and cardiac depression.

6. Maintain normal body temperature. Elevated temperature, shivering, and other activities that increase oxygen consumption exacerbate increased ICP. Initiate treatment for temperature elevations and avoid shivering.

7. Positioning and moving patients. Increased intrathoracic pressure, intraabdominal pressure, and neck flexion impairs venous drainage from the brain.
   - Elevate head of bed 30 to 45 degrees. Avoid the Trendelenburg or prone position and extreme hip flexion greater than 90 degrees.
   - Maintain the head in a neutral position, avoiding extreme flexion or hyperextension of the neck or rotation of the head.
   - Assist the patient in moving up in bed. Do not ask the patient to push with his or her heels or arms. If the patient is able to follow simple directions, instruct the patient to exhale upon turning or moving. The Valsalva maneuver and isometric exercises are avoided as they may increase ICP.

8. Minimize environmental stimuli.
   - Avoid clustering patient care activities together (suctioning, bathing, turning).
   - Maintain a calm, quiet environment. Control the environment for noise, odors, temperature, and other noxious stimuli. Avoid unnecessary conversation regarding the patient's condition at the bedside.
   - Provide soft, soothing stimuli, such as soft music, therapeutic touch, and the voice of loved ones on a tape recorder, for short periods of time throughout the day.

9. Bowel management. Prevent constipation to avoid straining at stool through the administration of stool softeners.

10. CSF drainage. Drainage of CSF through a catheter inserted in the lateral ventricle (ventriculostomy) is a temporary measure used to reduce ICP rapidly (Figure 24–6). It is the treatment of choice when increased ICP is due to hydrocephalus. The catheter is inserted through a burr hole made into the skull and connected to an external collecting and measuring system.
    - CSF drainage is controlled by adjusting the height of the drainage system relative to a reference point on the patient, usually at the level of the foramen of Monro, at the top of the ear, or at the outer canthus of the eye. The height of the fluid column of the drainage system above the reference point creates hydrostatic pressure that opposes ICP. If the drainage system is raised, CSF drainage will decrease; when the drainage system is lowered,

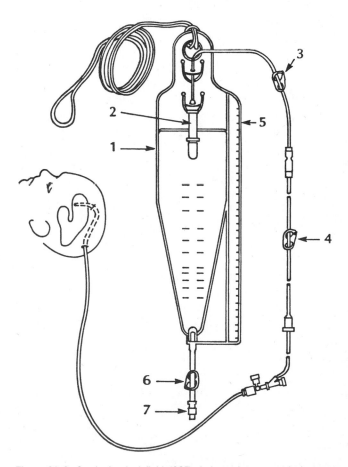

Figure 24–6. Cerebral spinal fluid (CSF) drainage into a ventriculostomy bag for control of intracranial pressure (ICP). (1) Collection bag. (2) Drip chamber. (3) Distal tube clamp. (4) Proximal tube clamp. (5) Height scale. (6) Tube clamp. (7) Withdrawal site.

Patient Needs and Principles of Management, Cont.

CSF drainage will increase. Rapid drainage of CSF can result in ventricular collapse; therefore, CSF is drained in a controlled manner based on a predetermined ICP. This is accomplished by maintaining the drainage system at a specific height, such as 10 cm above the top of the ear.

- CSF drainage is also monitored for the amount and color. Bright red blood indicates new hemorrhage and warrants physician notification.

- To decrease the risk of infection, preassembled closed drainage systems are available. Sterile technique is essential whenever the system is entered for CSF samples. CSF samples are usually sent daily for culture and sensitivity testing, glucose and protein evaluation, and for cell counts to monitor the patient for signs of infection.

Aneurysm

Etiology, Risk Factors, and Pathophysiology

A cerebral aneurysm is a saccular outpouching of a cerebral artery. Intracranial aneurysms may be congenital, degenerative, or traumatic in origin. Most aneurysms are congenital in origin and are located near the circle of Willis. Aneurysms may also be found on the internal carotid artery, anterior cerebral artery, middle cerebral artery, or the basilar arteries. Rupture of a cerebral aneurysm usually results in a subarachnoid hemorrhage. Rupture occurs more frequently in females than males, most often between the ages of 30 and 60 years.

Cerebral aneurysms have a variety of sizes (Table 24–2) and shapes (Table 24–3). When the aneurysm ruptures, blood under high pressure is forced into the subarachnoid space, increasing ICP and decreasing CPP. Fibrin, platelets, and fluid seal off the site of bleeding, resulting in a clot that may occlude blood flow into the area

TABLE 24–2. ANEURYSMS CLASSIFIED BY SIZE

Designation	Size
Small	< 15 mm
Large	15 to 25 mm
Giant	25 to 50 mm
Super-giant	> 50 mm

or interfere with CSF absorption. The released blood is an irritant to the brain tissue, causing an inflammatory response that increases cerebral edema and spasm.

Clinical Presentation

Before Rupture

Most patients are completely asymptomatic until the time of bleeding, however, there may be "warning signs," often called prodromal signs, that are either ignored or attributed to other causes. These include:

- Dilated pupil
- Ptosis
- Pain above and behind the eye
- Localized headache
- Neck pain
- Upper back pain
- Nausea and vomiting

AT THE BEDSIDE
▶ Aneurysm

B.D. is a 34-year-old loan officer at a bank who experienced the sudden onset of a severe headache while at work. She was taken to the emergency department of a local hospital where she described her headache as the "worst headache of my life." She had been having headaches with some nausea over the past several weeks. She now reports slight nausea and blurred vision. She keeps asking, "What is wrong with me?"

TABLE 24–3. ANEURYSMS CLASSIFIED BY SHAPE

Designation	Shape
Berry	Berry-shaped with a neck or stem
Fusiform	Outpouching of an arterial wall with tapering at either end
Dissecting	Intimal layer pulled away from medial layer and blood is forced between the layers

After Rupture

As blood is forced into the subarachnoid space, the patient experiences a violent headache, often described by the patient as the "worst headache of my life." Immediate loss of consciousness may occur, or a decrease in the level of consciousness. Vomiting is common. Other signs and symptoms include:

- Deficits in cranial nerves III, IV, and VI
- Those related to meningeal irritation (nausea, vomiting, stiff neck, pain in the neck and back, blurred vision)
- Those related to stroke syndrome (hemiparesis, hemiplegia, aphasia, cognitive deficits)
- Those related to increased ICP and cerebral edema (seizures, hypertension, bradycardia, widening pulse pressure)
- Those related to pituitary dysfunction secondary to the location of the gland to the aneurysm (diabetes insipidus and hyponatremia)

Diagnostic Tests

- *CT scan:* Identifies aneurysm location, and individuals at high risk for developing vasospasm.
- *Angiography:* Performed immediately if there is evidence of intracerebral hematoma or a possible arteriovenous malformation. Angiography is delayed if subarachnoid hemorrhage (SAH) from aneurysmal bleed is well established by CT scan. Angiography is performed immediately before surgery to identify specific location, size, and shape of the aneurysm, to identify any vascular anomalies, and to determine the presence of vasospasm.
- *Lumbar puncture:* Performed when CT scan is not available or if CT scan fails to demonstrate blood in CSF in a patient with a history characteristic of SAH without increased ICP.

Patient Needs and Principles of Management

The patient who survives the initial rupture of a cerebral aneurysm is at risk to develop complications that increase morbidity and mortality. The best management is surgery; however, until a decision is made about surgery, the goal is to prevent a rebleed.

► General Principles of Management

1. Institute aneurysm precautions to prevent elevations in blood pressure that may lead to rebleeding (Table 24–4).
2. Maintain complete bedrest. Apply elastic stockings and/or a sequential compression device to prevent deep vein thrombosis and pulmonary embolus from immobility.
3. Control hypertension. In the early hours and days after rupture, blood pressure is usually elevated, reflecting the body's response to an increased ICP. As ICP decreases, the blood pressure also decreases. If the blood pressure continues to be elevated from cerebral edema or a hematoma, mannitol may be administered. Mannitol will decrease cerebral edema, decrease neurological deficits, and improve cerebral blood flow. Systolic blood pressure is maintained at 150 mm Hg. Systolic pressures above 150 mm Hg may be treated with nitroprusside, propranolol, or hydralazine.
4. Administer drug therapy (anticonvulsants, stool softeners, steroids, analgesics, sedatives) as indicated.
5. Reduce anxiety. Be alert for cues that indicate areas of concern. Provide explanations and support, and allow patient choices whenever possible.

TABLE 24–4. TYPICAL ANEURYSM PRECAUTIONS

Purpose:
To provide the patient with a quiet environment that controls and minimizes physiological and psychological stress and promotes rest and relaxation.

Interventions:
Provide a quiet single room to minimize environmental stimuli.
Remove telephone.
Control natural and artificial light.
Provide television, radio, and reading materials if they do not upset or overstimulate the patient.
Maintain bedrest with head of bed at 30 to 45 degrees.
Limit visitors to immediate family and significant others.
Instruct visitors to avoid discussions or topics that may upset patient.
Place "Aneurysm Precaution" sign on patient's door.
Discourage and control any activity that results in a Valsalva's maneuver (e.g., coughing, straining at stool, pushing up in bed with elbows, turning with the mouth closed).

Patient Needs and Principles of Management, Cont.

▶ Prevention and Management of Complications

The major complications of an aneurysm rupture or bleeding are rebleeding, cerebral vasospasm, and hydrocephalus.

Rebleeding occurs most frequently in the first 2 weeks after initial hemorrhage.

1. Frequently assess for signs and symptoms of rebleeding (sudden, severe headache; nausea and vomiting; decrease in or loss of consciousness; and/or new neurological deficits).
2. Institute aneurysm precautions and interventions described above to prevent elevations in blood pressure that may lead to rebleeding (Table 24–4).

Cerebral vasospasm is the narrowing of a cerebral blood vessel, which may cause decreased perfusion, ischemia, and/or infarction of cerebral tissue. Vasospasm develops 4 to 14 days after initial hemorrhage, peaking at 7 days.

1. Frequently assess for signs and symptoms of vasospasm [gradual neurological deterioration (e.g., paresis/paralysis of a limb or side of the body, cranial nerve deficits, aphasia), decreased level of consciousness, presence of high risk factors (hyponatremia, decreased fluid volume)].
2. Maintain normal fluid volume to avoid dehydration, which may increase the incidence of vasospasm.

Cerebral perfusion may be increased by increasing fluid volume with crystalloids or colloids. Fluid restriction, steroids, and mannitol may be used if cerebral edema is present.

3. Increase CPP by increasing blood pressure with crystalloids, colloids, or vasopressors (dopamine, phenylephrine) if necessary.
4. Drug management for vasospasm utilizes calcium channel blockers (nicardipine, nimodipine).

Hydrocephalus develops as a result of blood in the CSF interfering with the reabsorption of CSF. Diagnosis is based on a CT scan that reveals dilated ventricles containing blood. Hydrocephalus is classified as acute, subacute, or delayed.

- *Acute.* Occurs within 24 hours after intraventricular hemorrhage. Characterized by the abrupt onset of stupor or persistent coma. CSF drainage with a ventriculostomy is the treatment of choice.
- *Subacute.* Occurs within first few days to 7 days after aneurysm hemorrhage. Characterized by gradual or abrupt drowsiness. CSF drainage with a ventriculostomy or lumbar puncture is the treatment of choice.
- *Delayed.* Occurs 10 or more days after aneurysm hemorrhage. Characterized by gradual onset of symptoms (dull, quiet personality and gait difficulty) after surgery and/or failure to progress in recovery. Surgical placement of ventriculoperitoneal shunt is the treatment of choice.

Head Injury

Etiology, Risk Factors, and Pathophysiology

Head injury refers to injury of the skull or brain, or both, that is severe enough to interfere with normal function and to require treatment. Major causes of head injury are motor vehicle accidents (MVAs), falls, and assaults. Most MVAs occur in the summer, on weekends, and during normal weather conditions. Falls are more common in the elderly, and assaults are more prevalent in urban areas. The incidence of head injury is higher in males than females and higher in people 15 to 24 years of age.

Head injuries result when excessive forces are applied to the head. Injuries may occur from blunt trauma (a direct blow to the head) or from penetrating trauma (missile or impalement). Injuries result from stress, force, and/or strain (effect of stress). Strain is classified into three components: compression (pushing of tissue together), tension (pulling of tissue apart, traction), and shearing (sliding of parts of tissue over other parts). Classifications of head injuries by mechanism of injury are summarized in Table 24–5.

Head injury is divided into two components: primary head injury and secondary head injury. Primary head injury refers to the biomechanical effects of trauma on the brain and skull as a direct result of the initial insult. Secondary head injury refers to the complications that result in additional pathophysiological changes and dysfunction of the brain tissue. Causes of secondary head injury include

AT THE BEDSIDE
▶ *Head Injury*

K.S. is a 30-year-old construction worker who was involved in a single-vehicle, high-speed, rollover accident in which he was ejected. He was cyanotic at the scene, with fixed pupils of 6 mm, and a Glasgow Coma Scale score of 3. He was unresponsive, with no movement of the left side of his body and decerebration on the right side of his body. He was immediately transported to a trauma center where he was diagnosed with severe blunt head trauma with a left subdural hematoma (SDH) and a midline shift. An ICP monitor was placed, with an opening ICP of 37 mm Hg. A craniotomy with burr holes and hematoma evacuation was performed in the operating room. Other injuries included a left femur fracture, left clavicular fracture, left acetabular fracture, and a significant splenic injury.

hypoxemia, hypotension, increased ICP, respiratory complications, infection, and electrolyte imbalances. These problems compromise the oxygen and nutrient supply necessary for adequate cerebral cell metabolism and contribute to a poor patient outcome, including death.

The major pathophysiological changes associated with head injury include loss of autoregulatory mechanisms, cerebral edema, and increased ICP.

Loss of Autoregulatory Mechanisms
As discussed earlier, autoregulatory mechanisms maintain constant CBF over a wide range of CPP (between 50 and 150 mm Hg) and within a wide range of blood pressures and ICPs. When CPP decreases, cerebral vasodilation occurs to maintain CBF by increasing cerebral blood volume. When CPP increases, cerebral vasoconstriction occurs, maintaining CBF with a lower cerebral blood volume.

TABLE 24–5. CLASSIFICATION OF MECHANISMS OF HEAD INJURY

Type	Description	Result
Deformation	Distortion of skull either inward or outward	Injury to the skull without injury to the brain Injury to the skull causing injury to the brain
Acceleration-deceleration	Rapid changes in velocity of the brain within the skull along a straight line	Injury to the brain without injury to the skull
Rotation	Acceleration-deceleration of the brain in directions other than a straight line (side-to-side and twisting)	Injury to the brain without injury to the skull

The injured brain may not be able to compensate for an increase in intracranial volume or direct injury to the brain, resulting in significant elevations of ICP. Cerebral blood flow becomes dependent on changes in blood pressure and CPP. This loss of autoregulation is seen clinically when ICP rises with increases in systemic blood pressure. The extent of this autoregulatory loss varies in head injury patients.

Cerebral Edema
With direct focal injury there is a simultaneous localized loss of autoregulation of the arterioles, resulting in a local increase in CBF. These changes increase the pressure in the capillaries and venules and alter the blood-brain barrier, resulting in the movement of fluid, plasma proteins, and electrolytes into the cerebral extracellular space, which in turn, causes vasogenic edema.

Although these vascular changes provide increased perfusion to selected areas of the brain, other areas do not receive adequate blood supply, especially as cerebral edema develops. Hypercapnia from inadequately perfused areas contributes to local acidosis, vasodilation, and sodium and water accumulation (cytotoxic edema), increasing cerebral edema. Maximal edema occurs 3 to 5 days after injury.

The resulting cerebral edema can be localized or global and often exaggerates the amount and severity of neurological deficits. As decompensation develops, ICP increases, and herniation syndromes can develop rapidly.

Increased ICP
The major sources of increased ICP in head injuries are cerebral edema and expanding lesions, such as hematomas. Compression of any blood vessels can result in ischemia and infarction of specific areas. Neuronal necrosis can be caused by direct injury or hypoxia precipitated by the combined forces that cause the cerebral edema.

ICP increases when the normal compensatory mechanisms discussed earlier are exhausted. An increased ICP negatively effects CBF and the viability of neurons. CPP is used to evaluate CBF. A CPP less than 60 mm Hg results in cerebral ischemia as blood flow is compromised. When CPP is sustained at a low level, irreversible neuronal changes occur and death results.

Types of Head Injuries
Injuries to the head are caused by a variety of situations, including skull fractures, focal brain injuries and diffuse brain damage.

Skull Fractures
Skull fractures are classified as linear, comminuted, depressed, or basilar.

1. Linear skull fractures, also known as simple fractures, resemble a line or single crack in the skull. Generally, they are not displaced and require no

treatment. If the fracture extends into an orbit or paranasal sinus or crosses a major vascular channel, observation for secondary injuries may be warranted.

2. Comminuted skull fractures refer to fragmentation of the bone into many pieces.

3. Depressed skull fractures are characterized by an inward depression of bone fragments to at least the thickness of the skull. The dura may or may not be torn. Depressed skull fractures are classified as open or compound in the presence of a communicating scalp laceration. When depressed skull fractures are open, asepsis is used to care for the scalp laceration because of the potential for infection from hair, dirt, and pieces of the impacting object. Surgery to elevate the depressed bone is accomplished within 24 hours. Fracture fragments are removed from grossly contaminated wounds. If they cannot be replaced in the wound, a plate cranioplasty (plate made of acrylic or metal) may be placed; however, placement may be delayed due to cerebral edema and to prevent local infection. A course of antibiotics may be given if removal of fragments is not possible or if more than 24 hours elapse before debridement.

4. Basilar skull fractures involve the base of the skull, including the anterior, middle, or posterior fossa. These fractures are difficult to confirm with x-rays, and therefore diagnosis is based on clinical presentation of the patient. Clinical manifestations of a basilar skull fracture include periorbital ecchymosis (raccoon's eyes), mastoid ecchymosis (Battle's sign), rhinorrhea (CSF or blood leaking from the nose), otorrhea (CSF or blood leaking from the ears), hemotympanum (CSF or blood behind the tympanic membrane), and conjunctival hemorrhage without evidence of direct trauma. The presence of otorrhea or rhinorrhea indicates a dural tear with increased risk of meningitis. Although most CSF leaks stop simultaneously, those which persist after 7 to 14 days may require dural repair. Management includes bedrest, antibiotics, head-up position, and occasionally, lumbar subarachnoid drainage of CSF for 3 to 4 days.

Focal Injuries

Focal injuries, also known as expanding mass lesions, account for most head injuries. They are produced by an object striking the head or acceleration-deceleration forces. These lesions may cause local brain damage at the site of injury, taking up space, increasing ICP, and causing brain shift and herniation. Focal injuries include cerebral contusions and hematomas (epidural, subdural, and intracerebral).

1. Cerebral contusions and lacerations involve cortical bruising and laceration of vessels and brain tissues with subsequent tissue necrosis. They may be classified as coup (occurring at the site of impact) or contrecoup (occurring opposite the site of impact). The primary sites of injury are the frontal and temporal lobes. The size and severity of the contusion depend upon the area of contact and degree of acceleration. Clinical presentation depends on the site and extent of brain injury. Isolated contusions do not generally produce immediate loss of consciousness. Coma is usually the result of a concussion or diffuse injury. Frontal injuries result in personality, behavior, motor, and speech deficits. Temporal lobe contusions result in language, memory, and intellectual ability deficits and are monitored closely because of their proximity to the tentorium and midbrain, increasing the potential for herniation. Management focuses on monitoring for signs of increased ICP and neurological changes.

2. Epidural hematoma is a blood clot located between the dura and the skull and most commonly is found in the temporal region. Epidural hematomas are associated with temporal or parietal skull fractures that lacerate an underlying artery or vein. The accumulated bleeding forms the hematoma. They are potentially fatal because of rapid expansion with resulting brain displacement and herniation. Clinical presentation depends on the source and rapidity of the bleeding. The classic triad of symptoms include an immediate loss of consciousness at the time of injury, a lucid interval lasting a few minutes to a few hours, and then a lapse into unconsciousness again. Other symptoms include increasingly severe headache, seizures, vomiting, hemiparesis, and pupillary dilation. Management consists of emergency surgery to evacuate the hematoma.

3. Subdural hematoma (SDH) refers to bleeding within the subdural space between the dura mater and arachnoid layer of the meninges. Since the arachnoid layer adheres closely to the brain, bleeding into the subdural space creates immediate direct pressure on the brain. Bleeding results from rupture of the bridging veins between the brain and dura, bleeding from contused or lacerated brain tissue, or extension from an intracerebral hematoma.

   • *Acute SDH* occurs within 48 hours after injury and is associated with major cerebral trauma with contusion. Patients present with progressive decreased level of consciousness, headache, agitation, and confusion. Motor deficits, pupillary abnormalities, and cranial nerve dysfunction may be seen, reflecting extensive bleeding, primary brain injury, and compressive effects. Treatment consists of craniotomy with a burr hole with evacuation of the hematoma and coagulation of actively bleeding vessels.

- *Subacute SDH* can develop 2 to 14 days following injury. It is strongly suspected in a patient who fails to regain consciousness.
- *Chronic SDH* can occur up to several months following the initial injury. The hematoma develops slowly, presenting with the same signs as a space-occupying lesion. Symptoms include an increasingly severe headache, confusion, and drowsiness. Treatment of subacute and chronic SDH includes burr holes and evacuation.

4. Intracerebral hematoma (ICH) is a well-defined blood clot that is deep within the brain tissue. The most frequent sites are the frontal and temporal lobes. ICH occurs as a result of closed head injuries and/or depressed skull fractures. Small, deep hematomas occur from shear forces and indicate diffuse axonal injury (DAI). Clinical presentation is similar to that of contusions with the course and outcome dependent on the size and location of the hematoma. ICH is complicated by progressive focal edema and mass effect, resulting in neurological deterioration that can occur soon after injury or as long as 7 to 10 days after injury. Delayed hemorrhage may occur in areas that were injured at the time of impact but appeared normal on the initial CT scan. Clot formation and neurological deterioration occur within a few days of the original injury. Delayed hemorrhage is associated with poor outcome and a high incidence of intracranial hypertension. Patients with disseminated intravascular coagulation, hypoxia, hypotension, or alcohol abuse have an increased incidence of delayed hemorrhage.

Diffuse Brain Injuries

These insults produce widespread damage that is scattered throughout the brain. Diffuse brain injuries involve microscopic damage to cells deep in the white matter and may be impossible to visualize on CT scan. They occur as lateral head motion produces angular movement of the brain within the skull causing shearing or stretching of axonal nerve fibers. Damage is variable and dependent on the amount of accelerative force transmitted to the brain. Diffuse brain injuries include concussion with little or no brain dysfunction and diffuse axonal injuries (DAI) that produce disabling deficits.

1. Cerebral concussion is a transient, temporary neurogenic dysfunction caused by rapid acceleration-deceleration or by a sudden blow to the head. It is suspected that this temporary change in function results from transient ischemia or neuronal depolarization after a sudden release of acetylcholine. Mild concussion is the most common brain injury. It generally does not require hospitalization. Symptoms include confusion, disorientation, and sometimes amnesia. Symptoms last only a few minutes. Classic concussion involves temporary loss of consciousness, amnesia, and sometimes mild neurological impairment. Unconsciousness usually lasts less than 5 minutes and no longer than 6 hours. The duration of amnesia is often a predictor of the severity of the injury. Patients often are admitted to a hospital for a short observational period to monitor for delayed intracranial bleeding.

2. Diffuse axonal injury (DAI) is the most severe form of brain injury. It also has been called a shearing injury. The hallmark of DAI is immediate and prolonged coma (more than 6 hours). The coma is the result of severe, widespread damage to the white matter, disconnecting the cerebral hemispheres from the brain stem reticular activating system. Since DAI is microscopic in nature, the severity of injury is determined by the patient's clinical characteristics and duration of coma. Clinical findings of DAI include deep and prolonged coma, initial decortication (flexion) or decerebration (extension), increased ICP, hypertension, excessive sweating, and an elevated temperature. The clinical course and outcome are dependent upon the severity of axonal injury. The patient may be comatose for up to 3 months and may never regain full consciousness. Survivors of DAI have major residual disabilities including deficits in cognition, memory, speech, motor function, and personality.

Clinical Presentation

Assessment of the head trauma patient includes evaluation of the level of consciousness, pupillary response, cranial nerve response, vital signs, and motor and sensory function.

Level of Consciousness

The level of consciousness is the most sensitive indicator of neurological function. A Glasgow Coma Scale (GCS) score of 13 to 15 indicates mild head injury; 9 to 12 indicates moderate head injury; and a score of 8 or less indicates severe head injury or coma. A decreasing GCS indicates neurological deterioration and warrants notification of the physician.

Pupillary Response and Shape

Pupillary changes in size, shape, or reactivity indicate neurological deterioration and warrant physician notification. Pupillary asymmetry of 1 mm or greater, an irregularly shaped or oval pupil, and sluggishly reacting pupils are all significant.

Cranial Nerve Changes

Other brain stem reflexes that can be assessed include corneal, gag, oculocephalic, and oculovestibular reflexes. Absent reflexes indicate a poor prognosis.

Vital Signs

Blood pressure and heart rate are assessed to ensure adequate perfusion to the brain. ICP and CPP are monitored for changes. CPP falls when there is arterial hypotension or increased ICP. As ICP rises and CBF falls, the systemic arterial blood pressure rises to maintain adequate cerebral perfusion. This is part of the Cushing's reflex (increased systolic blood pressure, widening pulse pressure, and bradycardia). When autoregulation is lost following severe head injury, a rise in arterial blood pressure may accompany a rise in ICP, leading to decreased CPP. A change in blood pressure and heart rate without an accompanying change in the level of consciousness indicates nonneurologic causes.

Cardiac rate, rhythm, and conduction changes occur with many intracranial injuries. Progressive bradycardia, junctional escape rhythms, and idioventricular rhythms occur with cerebral hemorrhage and increased ICP. Acute subdural hematoma is associated with atrial and ventricular ectopy and conduction defects. ST and T-wave changes follow cerebral ischemia and increased ICP. Neurogenic T waves, inverted T waves with increased amplitude and duration, may be seen.

Changes in respiratory pattern are associated with the level of intracranial injury or the degree of pressure exerted on the brain stem. Centers controlling the regulation of respirations are scattered throughout the brain with each center responsible for a unique respiratory pattern. Changes in respirations assist in identifying the area of injury and indicate neurologic deterioration.

Motor and Sensory Function

Alterations in sensory and motor function may be present (Chapter 15, Neurologic System). Responses on both sides of the body should be evaluated and compared.

Diagnostic Tests

- *Skull films:* Locates skull fractures.
- *CT Scan:* Identifies space-occupying lesions, contusions, and hemorrhagic or edematous areas in the brain.
- *MRI:* Differentiates between gray and white matter; detects small hemorrhages in DAI.
- *Evoked potential studies:* Reflects brain response to specific sensory stimuli (visual, auditory, somatosensory) to locate lesions and clarify prognosis.

Patient Needs and Principles of Management

The goals in the management of the head-injured patient are to minimize secondary brain injury in order to optimize functional recovery, relieve anxiety, and prevent and manage complications.

▶ Minimize Secondary Brain Injury

1. Maintenance of patient airway, oxygenation, and ventilation.

   - The severely head-injured patient is intubated and placed on a ventilator to maintain an airway and monitored to prevent hypoxia and hypercapnia.
   - Provide sufficient levels of oxygen to ensure adequate cerebral oxygenation. The ability to maintain adequate oxygenation may be compromised by pulmonary contusion, atelectasis, or pneumonia. Shunting of blood to the lungs secondary to a sympathetic discharge can result in neurogenic pulmonary edema (see the section on complications).

   - Hyperventilation, although not routinely used to decrease CO_2 and ICP, may be particularly harmful in head-injured patients. The ability of the cerebral blood vessels to react to changes in CO_2 and O_2 is reduced and limits the effectiveness of hyperventilation. Hyperventilation may also reduce the seizure threshold in head-injured patients.

2. Management of factors which increase ICP. Refer to strategies previously discussed for increased ICP.

▶ Relieve Patient and Family Anxiety

Families and significant others may experience fear, helplessness, and loss of control. The family can participate in the patient's care to the extent with which they are comfortable. The family is encouraged to talk about current events and about the patient's past to facilitate communication with a semicomatose or comatose patient.

AT THE BEDSIDE
▶ *Making Families a Part of the Health Care Team*

Families can become an integral part of the health care team with an important role to play and important tasks to perform. Nurses can contract with families to be involved in the care of their loved one, depending on the condition of the patient and the involvement of the family. The following are some suggestions for activities with which families might get involved:

Orientation, Distraction, and Socialization Techniques

- Updating the patient on family, local, social, and national news
- Reading books and newspapers
- Bringing in the patient's favorite music tapes to be played at the bedside
- Praying with the patient
- Guiding the patient in deep breathing and relaxation exercises

Daily Hygiene Tasks

- Tooth brushing
- Bathing
- Hair combing
- Toileting
- Back rubs
- Foot and skin care

Procedures and Therapies

- Cooking
- Feeding
- Providing nasogastric feedings
- Assisting with range-of-motion exercises
- Giving medications
- Doing dressing changes
- Doing catheter care
- Suctioning the patient

▶ Prevent and Manage Complications

1. Neurogenic pulmonary edema. Neurogenic pulmonary edema may occur in massive head injury or abrupt elevations in ICP. The process occurs in two steps. First, there is a shift of blood from the systemic to the pulmonary circulation due to a massive sympathetic discharge occurring at the time of injury. A generalized vasoconstriction results in a shift of blood from the high-resistance systemic circulation to the low-resistance pulmonary circulation. Pulmonary edema occurs because of an increase in pulmonary capillary pressure and hydrostatic pressure. Second, the pulmonary hypervolemia damages the pulmonary capillary membranes, allowing the shift of fluid into the alveolar spaces. Even after normal cardiac and hemodynamic function have been reestablished, fluid remains in the alveolar spaces, causing a defect in O_2 exchange and systemic hypoxemia. The clinical presentation of neurogenic pulmonary edema is the same as that of acute pulmonary edema—dyspnea, restlessness, anxiety, confusion, diaphoresis, cyanosis, rapid and shallow respirations, rales and rhonchi, rapid heart rate, elevated blood pressure, and distended neck veins. Management includes elevating the head of the bed and administering oxygen, diuretics, and PEEP to keep the alveoli from collapsing.

2. Herniation. Cerebral herniation is the distortion and displacement of the brain from one compartment to another within the intracranial cavity. Herniation is a life-threatening event that occurs with expanding mass lesions or hematomas and rapidly increasing ICP. The standard neurological assessment is intended to detect early signs of herniation. The classic signs of herniation are:

   - Deterioration in the level of consciousness
   - Pupillary abnormality (ipsilateral fixed and dilated pupil)
   - Motor abnormality (contralateral hemiparesis, abnormal flexion or decortication, abnormal extension or decerebration)
   - Brain stem dysfunction (cranial nerve displacement and compression)
   - Alteration in vital signs (Cushing's triad, altered respiratory pattern)

AT THE BEDSIDE
▶ *Acute Spinal Cord Injury*

D.J. was a 19-year-old college student returning home from a party late one night when he struck another vehicle head-on. He felt intense pain throughout his neck and body that was soon replaced with the sensation of a tight band squeezing his chest. His arms and legs became lifeless. He struggled to take each breath as paramedics worked rapidly to free him from the wreckage and transport him to the hospital. At the hospital, his respirations were shallow at a rate of 40 breaths/minute. He was intubated and placed on mechanical ventilation. A CT scan and cervical spine x-rays revealed a C4-5 subluxation with cord compression. His eyes expressed fear and panic.

Acute Spinal Cord Injury

Etiology, Risk Factors, and Pathophysiology

Spinal cord injury (SCI) may result from motor vehicle accidents, falls, acts of violence, or sports-related injuries. Most SCIs occur in males under the age of 40 years, with 50% occurring between the ages of 15 and 25 years. SCI can result in permanent paralysis and total loss of sensation below the level of injury. The ability to breathe may be diminished or destroyed. Bowel, bladder, and sexual function may be affected. Significant psychologic, social, and economic ramifications are also related to SCI.

SCI results from concussion, contusion, laceration, transection, hemorrhage, or damage to the blood vessels that supply the spinal cord. Concussion is a jarring of the spinal cord that causes temporary loss of function lasting 24 to 48 hours. Contusion is a bruising of the spinal cord that includes bleeding into the spinal cord, subsequent edema, and possible necrosis from compression by the edema or damage to the tissue. The extent of neurological deficits depends on the severity of the contusion and the presence of necrosis. Laceration is an actual tear in the spinal cord that results in permanent injury. Contusion, edema, and cord compression are seen with a laceration. Transection is a severing of the spinal cord that can be complete or incomplete. Hemorrhage is bleeding in and around the spinal cord, acting as an irritant which results in edema and neurological deficits. Damage to the blood vessels that supply the spinal cord results in ischemia and possible necrosis and neurological deficits.

The major mechanisms of SCI are flexion, flexion-rotation, hyperextension, and compression.

SCI can be classified by the level and/or degree (complete or incomplete) of injury. Spinal levels include cervical, thoracic, and lumbar. Cervical and lumbar injuries occur more frequently because these areas have the greatest flexibility and movement. A cervical injury may result in paralysis of all four extremities, or quadriplegia. Injuries of the thoracic and lumbar areas result in paraplegia.

The degree of involvement may be complete or incomplete. Complete SCI results in total loss of sensory and motor function due to complete interruption of motor and sensory pathways below the level of injury. Incomplete SCI results in mixed loss of motor and sensory function because some spinal tracts remain intact. Incomplete SCI is divided into five syndromes (Table 24–6).

The pathophysiology of SCI is multiphasic, involving cellular damage to the spinal cord, hemorrhage, vascular damage, structural changes in the gray and white matter, and subsequent biochemical responses. Blood flow to the spinal cord is decreased significantly during the acute phase of injury, resulting in changes in metabolic function and the release of free radicals from ischemic areas. Free-radical

TABLE 24–6. INCOMPLETE SCI SYNDROMES

Type	Mechanism of Injury	Motor Deficits	Sensory Deficits
Central cord syndrome	Hyperextension	Weakness/paralysis of upper extremities greater than lower extremities	Same as motor distribution Varying bowel and bladder dysfunction
Anterior cord syndrome	Hyperflexion	Paralysis below injury level	Loss of temperature and pain sensation below injury level
Posterior cord syndrome	Blunt or penetrating trauma	None	Loss of touch, position, and vibration sensation below injury level
Brown-Séquard's syndrome (lateral cord syndrome)	Penetrating trauma	Ipsilateral motor paralysis below injury level	Contralateral loss of pain and temperature sensation below injury level Ipsilateral loss of touch, pressure, and vibration sensation below injury level
Horner's syndrome	Incomplete cord transection of cervical sympathetic neurons	Ipsilateral eyelid ptosis Ipsilateral eye recession into orbit Ipsilateral pupil smaller than contralateral pupil	Ipsilateral loss of facial sweating

release increases ischemia, vasospasm, and hypoxia. The spinal cord may also suffer concussion or contusion, further compounding damage.

Sudden, complete transection of the spinal cord results in the temporary suppression of reflexes controlled by segments below the level of injury, also known as spinal shock. After a period of hours to months, usually 7 to 10 days, the spinal neurons gradually regain their excitability with the return of motor, sensory, and reflex function below the level of injury, or the spinal neurons will develop their own reflex activity with the development of muscle spasticity.

Neurogenic shock occurs following cervical and upper thoracic cord injury. Neurogenic shock results from the loss of control of the sympathetic nervous system which normally increases heart rate, contractility, and vasoconstricts the blood vessel walls. Loss of sympathetic outflow results in hypotension, bradycardia, and vasodilatation.

Clinical Presentation
Specific functional losses from spinal cord injury are summarized in Table 24–7.

Spinal Shock

- Complete loss of motor, sensory, and reflex function below the level of injury (flaccid paralysis)
- Loss of spinal reflexes
- Loss of pain, proprioception, temperature, and pressure sensation below the level of injury
- Bowel and bladder dysfunction
- Loss of the ability to perspire below the level of injury

Neurogenic Shock

- Hypotension (from peripheral vasodilation)
- Bradycardia (from dominance of the parasympathetic nervous system)
- Inability to increase heart rate
- Inability to sweat below the level of injury
- Hypothermia or poikilothermia (from disruption of the transmission between the hypothalamus and sympathetic nervous system)

TABLE 24–7. FUNCTIONAL LOSSES FROM SCI

Level of Injury	Motor Function	Sensory Function	Respiratory Function	Bowel and Bladder
C1-C4	Quadriplegia Loss of all motor function from neck down	Loss of all sensory functions in the neck and below	Loss of involuntary (phrenic) and voluntary (intercostals) respiratory function Ventilatory support and tracheostomy necessary	No bowel or bladder control
C5	Quadriplegia Loss of all function below upper shoulders Can control head	Loss of sensation below clavicle and in most portions of arms, hands, chest, abdomen, and legs	Phrenic nerve intact but not intercostal muscles	No bowel or bladder control
C6	Quadriplegia Loss of all function below shoulders and upper arms	Loss of everything listed for C5 but greater arm and thumb sensation	Phrenic nerve intact but not intercostal muscles	No bowel or bladder control
C7	Quadriplegia Loss of motor control to portion of arms and hands	Loss of sensation below clavicle and portion of arms and hands	Phrenic nerve intact but not intercostal muscles	No bowel or bladder control
C8	Quadriplegia Loss of motor control to portion of arms and hands	Loss of sensation below chest and in portion of hands	Phrenic nerve intact but not intercostal muscles	No bowel or bladder control
T1-T6	Paraplegia Loss of everything below midchest area	Loss of sensation below midchest area	Phrenic nerve intact Some intercostal muscle impairment	No bowel or bladder control
T6-T12	Paraplegia Loss of motor control below the waist	Loss of sensation below the waist	No interference with respiratory function	No bowel or bladder control
L1-L3	Paraplegia Loss of most control of legs and pelvis	Loss of sensation to the lower abdomen and legs	No interference with respiratory function	No bowel or bladder control
L3-L4	Paraplegia Loss of motor control to portion of lower legs, ankles, and feet	Loss of sensation to portion of lower legs, feet, and ankles	No interference with respiratory function	No bowel or bladder control
L4-S5	Paraplegia Degree varies Segmental motor control of legs, ankles, and feet	Degree varies Loss of sensation to portion of legs, ankles, and feet	No interference with respiratory function	Bowel and bladder control may or may not be impaired

Diagnostic Tests
- *X-rays:* Cervical, thoracic, and lumbar spine x-rays identify presence of injury. Immobilization of the spinal column must be maintained to prevent additional trauma.

- *Myelogram:* Determines sources of pressure on the spinal cord.
- *CT Scan:* Defines and delineates bone injury and cord compression.
- *MRI:* Detects soft tissue involvement.

Patient Needs and Principles of Management

Management of the SCI patient focuses on stabilization of the spinal cord; maintenance of adequate oxygenation and ventilation; recognizing and managing neurogenic shock; maintaining bladder and bowel function; prevention of secondary neuronal injury; and prevention and treatment of complications.

▶ Stabilization of the Spinal Cord

1. All trauma patients are treated as if they have a SCI until proven otherwise. This includes spinal immobilization with a hard cervical collar and spinal board in the prehospital setting and a cervical collar and bedrest in the ICU until injury is ruled out or confirmed clinically and radiographically.
2. Traction is used in unstable cervical fractures and/or when subluxation has occurred. If surgical intervention cannot be performed due to patient instability, severe bleeding, or edema at and around the site of injury, traction will maintain alignment, prevent movement of unstable bones and bone fragments, and reduce fractures and dislocations. Traction devices include Gardner-Wells tongs and a halo device (see manufacturer's literature for more information). Traction devices are rarely used in thoracic, lumbar, or sacral injuries. Bedrest is the most often used therapy.
3. Early surgical intervention to stabilize the spine is dependent on the type of injury and the patient's hemodynamic status. Compression unrelieved by traction, a burst fracture, or progressive neurological deficit from edema or intrathecal hemorrhage usually requires rapid surgical intervention. Early surgery may preserve, improve, or restore spinal cord function.
4. Drug therapy. Methylprednisolone administration has been shown to maintain spinal cord blood flow. It must be initiated within 8 hours of injury, with a loading dose of 30 mg/kg IV over 15 minutes, followed 45 minutes later with a maintenance dose of 5.4 mg/kg/hour IV for 23 hours.

▶ Maintenance of Adequate Oxygenation and Ventilation

Altered respiratory function is a major problem for patients with high thoracic or cervical SCI. Injuries at or above C4 result in ventilatory dependency because of the inability to breathe spontaneously. This occurs due to loss of phrenic nerve function (C3-5) that innervates the diaphragm and paralysis of the intercostal muscles (innervated by T1-11). The abdominal muscles are innervated by T6-L1. In addition, paralysis of intercostal and abdominal muscles results in ineffective coughing and retention of secretions. Pneumonia and aspiration are common complications in patients with SCI. Management includes:

1. Prophylactic intubation in patients with high thoracic or cervical SCI. Intubation in a patient with a lower lesion may be indicated if the patient is breathing spontaneously at a rate of greater than 30 breaths/minute, aspiration is a risk, and/or the vital capacity is less than 500 ml.
2. Aggressive pulmonary care. Chest physiotherapy every 4 hours, assisted coughing ("quad" coughing), incentive spirometry, and suctioning are all indicated. Bronchoscopy may be performed if these interventions do not successfully clear secretions. Vigorous suctioning may stimulate the vagus nerve, leading to profound bradycardia.
3. Perform physical assessment of the chest. Inspection, palpation, percussion, and auscultation are performed along with vital signs during the first 72 hours following injury. Chest expansion and abdominal movement are assessed to determine accessory muscle use.
4. Monitor pulmonary function. Tidal volume, minute ventilation, and vital capacity are assessed on a periodic basis. A progressive decline in serial vital capacity measurements indicates the need for intubation and mechanical ventilation.
5. Monitor ABGs and pulse oximetry. Initially, the PaO_2 is maintained above 80 mm Hg to avoid

Patient Needs and Principles of Management, Cont.

hypoxemia which may accentuate the SCI. $PaCO_2$ is also monitored to evaluate for hypoventilation.

6. Ensure adequate force of expiration. Abdominal tone is lost in SCI, preventing the active force of expiration. SCI patients expire more effectively lying flat than sitting up. An elastic abdominal binder will assist expiration through constant abdominal pressure when the patient is sitting up.

▶ Management of Neurogenic Shock

Neurogenic shock causes significant hemodynamic alterations.

1. Differentiating neurogenic shock from other types of shock. Hypotension in neurogenic shock reflects fluid displacement into the vasodilated periphery, not a true lack of fluid volume. Overhydration will not correct hypotension and may lead to pulmonary edema or congestive heart failure.
2. Inotropic drug therapy to treat hypotension. Dopamine hydrochloride and/or dobutamine hydrochloride in low doses are used to maintain MAP at 80 to 90 mm Hg.
3. Monitoring of ECG and blood pressure. A pulmonary artery catheter may be indicated to monitor the hemodynamic status of the patient.
4. Monitoring for bradycardia. Suctioning or turning the patient may cause a vasovagal response, with the heart rate falling below 40 beats/minute, that is best treated with atropine sulfate.
5. Monitor body temperature. The goal is to achieve and maintain normothermia. The hypothermic patient may be warmed with warm blankets, a heat lamp, and warmed IV fluids. The hyperthermic patient may be cooled with a fan, lightweight clothing, and the light spraying of water on the skin that will act as perspiration to promote heat loss through evaporation.

▶ Maintenance of Skin Integrity

The patient with SCI is at high risk for skin breakdown due to decreased blood flow to the skin and decreased cutaneous response to focal pressure as a result of the SCI. Management is focused on prevention, including manual turning every 2 hours; use of a rotation, kinetic therapy, or low air-loss bed; and continuous monitoring for pressure areas and open sores.

▶ Maintenance of Urinary Function

Areflexia caused by spinal shock leads to urinary retention. An indwelling catheter is placed on admission and maintained until hemodynamic stability. Scheduled intermittent catheterizations are then initiated to decrease the incidence of infection associated with indwelling catheters.

▶ Maintenance of Maximum Mobility

During spinal shock, there is a total loss of motor function below the level of injury. Flaccid paralysis progresses to spastic paralysis. Management to prevent further injury and maintain range of motion to all joints includes:

1. Continuous assessment of motor function during the acute phase. All major muscle groups are graded for strength every 4 hours. Decreased motor function may be seen with swelling at the injury site, loss of vertebral alignment, or intrathecal hematoma formation. Significant changes warrant physician notification.
2. Maintain immobilization. Immobilization is maintained with tongs. Spinal stability is facilitated with mechanical beds including kinetic therapy treatment tables or Stryker frames. A halo device may also be used to maintain vertebral stability.
3. Perform passive range of motion. Passive range of motion is performed every 4 hours to prevent contractures. Joints are positioned in the neutral position whenever possible. Adjunctive devices, such as antirotation boots, antidrop foot splints, trochanter rolls, and wrist splints are useful in maintaining the correct position.

▶ Relief of Patient and Family Anxiety

Fear, uncertainty, and anxiety are common emotions in the ICU following SCI. The psychological and emotional trauma of SCI can be overwhelming. Sudden paralysis does not allow patients or family to prepare for this major insult. Fear focuses on the injury and life-and-death issues. Anxiety results from the ICU environment, feelings of total dependence, sensory deprivation, helplessness, and an unknown future.

A trusting relationship must be established between the patient and the ICU staff. Use of verbal communication, touch, eye contact, and patience, honesty, and consistency are reassuring to the patient. Encouraging self-care within the patient's abilities will decrease feelings of complete dependence. Contracting with the patient may be helpful in setting limits for some patients. The family and significant others should be incorporated into the plan of care, increasing the patient's sense of autonomy.

The patient, family, and significant others should be informed by the physician about the degree of injury, the diagnosis, and the prognosis as soon as possible after the injury. This information will allow them to understand the reality of the situation and begin to deal with the fear.

▶ Prevention and Management of Complications

The SCI patient is at risk for developing deep vein thrombosis (DVT), gastrointestinal problems, and autonomic dysreflexia.

Deep Vein Thrombosis

The SCI patient has significant risk factors for DVT including fractures, immobilization, edema, and surgery. Prevention and early detection are crucial and include:

1. Measure midcalf and midthigh circumference of the legs daily. Assess these areas for edema and warmth.
2. Promote venous return. Provide antiembolism hose or alternating pneumatic pressure devices on the legs. Perform range-of-motion exercises every 4 hours. Kinetic treatment tables, which can rotate the patient continuously, also promote circulation in the patient with SCI.
3. Provide heparin (5000 units subcutaneously twice daily) or low-molecular-weight heparin (3500 anti-Xa units subcutaneously once daily).

Gastrointestinal Problems

Gastrointestinal (GI) complications following SCI include gastric dilatation, paralytic ileus, and stress ulcers. The location and degree of SCI determines the degree of alteration in bowel elimination. GI complications occur as a result of disturbances in autonomic reflexes and atonia, and may last for up to 72 hours after SCI.

1. A nasogastric tube is used initially for gastric decompression.
2. Once peristalsis returns, nasogastric feedings are started and a daily bowel program instituted. This includes daily stool softeners, glycerine suppositories, bisacodyl suppository laxatives, and/or digital

stimulation. The use of a bowel regimen makes it possible to establish bowel continence.

3. Stress ulcers are managed prophylactically with H_2 receptor blocking agents (ranitidine, cimetadine), antacids, or a pepsin inhibitor (Carafate). Gastric pH is monitored, and stools are monitored for the presence of blood.

Autonomic Dysreflexia

Autonomic dysreflexia (AD) is a life-threatening complication that occurs when there is an uninhibited response to the sympathetic nervous system. This massive sympathetic response occurs primarily with injuries above T6. Although it usually appears in the first year following injury, it can occur anytime after spinal shock has subsided. AD may result from a variety of stimuli, including overdistended bladder (most common), full rectum, infection, skin stimulation, pressure sores, pain, and sudden changes in environmental temperature. The stimulus causes massive vasoconstriction that clinically presents with a severe headache, hypertension (may result in cerebral hemorrhage or myocardial infarction), tachycardia, diaphoresis, nasal stuffiness, bradycardia, flushing above the level of injury, and pallor and coolness below the level of injury.

1. Move the patient into a sitting position immediately. Treatment is then focused on relieving the stimulus. Physician notification is especially important at this time.
2. Identify and treat the underlying cause (e.g., impaction, bladder distention).
3. Monitor blood pressure and pulse closely. Pharmacological therapies may be indicated if symptoms continue after removal of the cause. Nitropaste, nifedipine, and hydralazine will dilate blood vessels and help reduce blood pressure. Prevention is the best way to treat AD in SCI patients, and a good bowel and bladder program and skin care will help in prevention.

Space-Occupying Lesions

Etiology, Risk Factors, and Pathophysiology

Patients with space-occupying lesions or intracranial or brain tumors are cared for in critical care units when they are postoperative or when they present with acute symp-

toms. Intracranial tumors are found in people of all ages; however, there is a decline in their incidence after age 60. This may be a reflection of neural and endocrine activity. The incidence of intracranial tumors is slightly higher in men than in women.

AT THE BEDSIDE
▶ *Space-Occupying Lesions*

V. L. was a 46-year-old engineer whose wife began noticing a change in his behavior. V. L., who enjoyed building model airplanes, was having difficulty concentrating and was becoming frustrated and easily angered. Concerned, she scheduled an appointment with their physician. A complete neurological exam, in which V. L. admitted to having severe headaches over the past month, raised suspicion of a space-occupying lesion. A CT scan and MRI confirmed the presence of a frontal lobe lesion. A needle biopsy revealed a glioblastoma. V. L. and his wife were devastated with the diagnosis and anxious about V. L.'s impending surgery for resection of the tumor.

Classification

Intracranial tumors are classified by distinguishing criteria:

- *Primary and secondary tumors.* Primary intracranial tumors originate from the cells and structures in the brain. Secondary or metastatic intracranial tumors originate from structures outside the brain, such as primary tumors of the breast, lungs, and gastrointestinal tract.
- *Histological origins.* During the early stage of embryonic development two types of undifferentiated cells are found—the neuroblasts and the glioblasts. The neuroblasts become neurons, the basic unit of structure in the nervous system. The glioblasts form a variety of cells that support, insulate, and metabolically assist the neurons. The glioblasts are collectively referred to as glial cells and are subdivided into astrocytes (star-shaped cells), oligodendrocytes, and ependymal cells (which line the ventricles). This is the basis of a broad category of intracranial tumors called gliomas. Gliomas are subdivided into astrocytomas, oligodendrogliomas, and ependymomas. Gliomas are graded based on histological criteria related to the degree of differentiation from the parent cell. The higher the grade, the more malignant the tumor. The reader is referred to the neurological literature for a more detailed description of the specific types of intracranial tumors.
- *Anatomical location.* This refers to the actual site of the tumor, such as the frontal lobe, temporal lobe, pons, or cerebellum. Knowing the location of the tumor helps in predicting deficits based on the normal functions of that anatomical area. Anatomical location may also refer to the location of the tumor in reference to the tentorium. Supratentorial refers to tumors located above the tentorium (cerebral hemispheres), and infratentorial refers to tumors located below the tentorium (brain stem and cerebellum).
- *Benign and malignant intracranial tumors.* The distinction between benign and malignant intracranial tumors is based on histological examination. Cells that are well differentiated tend to indicate a much better prognosis than poorly differentiated cells. However, a histologically benign tumor may be surgically inaccessible. This "benign" tumor will continue to grow and ultimately contribute to the individual's death. These "benign" tumors may convert to more histologically malignant types as they develop.

Pathophysiology

Intracerebral tumors occupy space and, because the brain has a limited degree of compressibility, can increase ICP. The brain has limited compensatory mechanisms with which to maintain normal ICP. Normal ICP is maintained by decreasing the volume of brain tissue, CSF, and/or cerebral blood flow.

- *Brain volume.* In a slow-growing tumor the brain tissue has a limited degree of compressibility. In fast-growing tumors, the brain is essentially not compressible.
- *Displacement of CSF.* Some CSF can be displaced into the dural sac, resulting in decreased CSF volume within the ventricles and subarachnoid space. When the limits of this displacement are surpassed, pressure within the ventricle and subarachnoid space increases, causing a rise in ICP.
- *Cerebral blood volume.* Compression of the venules in the tissue surrounding an intracranial tumor results in an elevation of capillary pressure and the development of vasogenic edema. The increased venous pressure decreases CSF absorption and results in an increased CSF volume and pressure. Cerebral venous stasis will also cause vasodilation, increasing intracranial cerebral blood volume. Once the limits of compensation are reached, ICP rises.

Clinical Presentation

There is no classic clinical presentation seen in patients with intracranial tumors. The clinical presentation is dependent on compression or infiltration of specific brain tissue (location) and the development of increased ICP (Table 24–8).

The most common initial signs and symptoms of intracranial tumors are alterations in consciousness and/or

TABLE 24–8. CLINICAL PRESENTATION OF BRAIN TUMORS RELATED TO LOCATION

Location	Clinical Presentation
Frontal lobe	Inappropriate behavior
	Inattentiveness
	Inability to concentrate
	Emotionally labile
	Quiet but flat affect
	Expressive aphasia
	Seizures
	Headache
	Impaired memory
Parietal lobe	Hyperesthesia
	Paresthesia
	Astereognosis (inability to recognize an object by feeling it)
	Autotopagnosia (inability to locate or recognize parts of the body)
	Loss of left-right discrimination
	Agraphia (inability to write)
	Acalculia (difficulty in calculating numbers)
Temporal lobe	Psychomotor seizures
Occipital lobe	Visual loss in half of the visual field
	Seizures
Pituitary and hypothalamus region	Visual deficits
	Headache
	Hormonal dysfunction of the pituitary gland
	Water imbalance and sleep alterations in tumors of the hypothalamus
Ventricles	Symptoms of increased ICP associated with obstruction of CSF flow
Cerebellum	Ataxia
	Incoordination
	Symptoms of increased ICP associated with obstruction of CSF flow

cognition, headache, seizures, and vomiting. The clinical presentation of increased ICP has been discussed previously. Many patients with intracranial tumors develop papilledema as a result of increased pressure on the optic nerve.

Diagnostic Tests

- *CT Scan and MRI:* Identify the presence of space-occupying lesion.

To further evaluate an intracranial tumor and to determine the best treatment, other diagnostic studies may be performed, including cerebral angiography, visual field and funduscopic examination, audiometric studies, chest films, and endocrine studies.

Patient Needs and Principles of Management

There are three general approaches to the management of intracranial tumors: drug therapy, including chemotherapy; radiation therapy; and surgery. These modalities may be used alone or in any combination. Variables considered in selecting appropriate treatment include the type of tumor, its location and size, related symptoms, and the general condition of the patient.

► Drug Therapy

1. Dexamethasone (Decadron) is administered to decrease cerebral edema. It usually is started when the tumor is diagnosed and the presence of cerebral edema and increased ICP is confirmed. Significant improvements in neurological status are seen soon after initiation of therapy. If surgery is recommended, dexamethasone is administered preoperatively, continued postoperatively, after hospital discharge, and during chemotherapy and radiation therapy. Other medications administered include H₂ blockers, such as cimetidine (Tagamet), and antacids to reduce gastric irritation, phenytoin (Dilantin) to prevent seizures, acetaminophen (Tylenol) to relieve mild headaches, and docusate sodium (Colace) to prevent straining at stool.

2. Chemotherapy is the use of drugs or chemicals that act as cellular poisons to destroy tumors. Unfortu-

nately, chemotherapeutic agents affect normal tissue as well as tumor cells. Chemotherapy is offered to patients with low-grade astrocytomas/glioblastomas who have already received surgery and irradiation and continue to have significant regrowth of the tumor or no improvement in their condition.

▶ Radiation Therapy

The objective of radiation therapy is to destroy tumor cells without injuring normal cells. A course of radiation therapy can increase survival rates after surgery. The treatment dose depends on the histological type, radioresponsiveness, location of the tumor, and the level of patient tolerance.

▶ Surgery

Surgery is often the last step in positive diagnosis of an intracranial tumor through histological examination of a tissue biopsy. Some tumors, although histologically benign, cannot be completely removed. A partial resection of the tumor mass will temporarily relieve symptoms of compression, and increased ICP may be relieved. Obstruction of CSF flow may require a shunting procedure to relieve CSF pressure. Laser surgery may be used to dissect or shrink tumors without injuring surrounding tissue. Areas of the brain formerly inaccessible to the neurosurgeon may be accessible by laser surgery.

▶ Postoperative Management

Most patients undergo elective operations for intracranial tumors. They are relatively stable on admission to the critical care unit with no or limited neurological deficit. Postoperative management includes monitoring neurological and respiratory status, controlling pain, providing wound care, and reducing anxiety.

1. Neurological assessment. Neurological assessment is performed frequently to determine the presence and extent of increased ICP. In the immediate postoperative period, neurologic assessment may be performed as frequently as every 15 to 30 minutes for the first 8 to 12 hours and then every hour for the next 12 hours. As the patient stabilizes, the frequency of assessment may be reduced to every 1 to 2 hours. Current findings are compared with baseline findings to determine trends. Changes may be subtle or rapid. Increases in blood pressure or decreases in heart rate may indicate increasing ICP. Most patients will not have an ICP monitor in place unless the patient had evidence of cerebral edema during surgery. Small changes in vital signs and/or level of consciousness may be the first clue that cerebral edema due to surgical manipulation or retraction is developing. Although slight increases in blood pressure may be due to pain, anxiety, or nausea and vomiting, the suspicion of intracranial hypertension must always be present. Serum electrolytes and osmolality testing are performed routinely to detect electrolyte imbalance. A decreased sodium and chloride level can result in weakness, lethargy, and coma. A decreased potassium level may result in confusion. Both may affect neurological signs and create confusion about the etiology of a change in condition.

2. Monitoring ventilatory status. The majority of patients admitted to a critical care unit after intracranial tumor removal are conscious and extubated. The following strategies are performed to ensure adequate ventilation:
   - Monitor respirations for signs of hypoventilation and respiratory depression. Hypoxia and hypercapnia increase CBF and ICP. Sedation is used carefully to avoid respiratory depression.
   - Monitor oxygen saturation via pulse oximetry.
   - Monitor ABG results.
   - Elevate HOB 30 degrees following supratentorial surgery. The HOB may be flat if the patient has undergone infratentorial surgery.
   - Maintain the patient's neck in a neutral position.

3. Pain management. Increasing headache in an awake patient is a significant indicator of increasing ICP and warrants physician notification. Sedation is used carefully to avoid masking the presence of an increasing headache. Pain is managed with acetaminophen (Tylenol), Tylenol with codeine, or morphine sulfate. Morphine sulfate is used in small doses in the critical care unit because it can be reversed easily. If the patient is not completely awake postoperatively, pain is monitored by assessing for restlessness, pulling on the head dressing, or a change in vital signs.

4. Wound care. In the adult, most intracranial tumors are located in the supratentorial region or above the cerebral hemispheres. The scalp incision is made within the boundary of the hairline directly over the area to be explored. After surgery, a turban-style dressing is applied initially and removed after 24 hours. The dressing is monitored for evidence of blood or CSF drainage. The incision is monitored for redness, drainage, or signs of wound infection.

5. Reducing anxiety. The diagnosis of an intracranial tumor causes anxiety, uncertainty, fear, and hope for the patient and family. For the patient who is con-

scious and oriented, the prospect of cranial surgery accentuates fears—fear of loss of life, permanent disability, loss of independence, and loss of mental ability. In addition, the patient's head may be entirely shaved in the operating room. The family usually experiences many of the same feelings. An individualized teaching plan initiated preoperatively and used postoperatively in the critical care unit will provide information about what is happening and what can be expected, and will help decrease anxiety.

▶ Prevention and Management of Complications

The major complications in the postoperative period are related to increasing ICP from cerebral edema and intracranial hemorrhage and hematoma. In addition, other potential complications include infection, thrombophlebitis, and diabetes insipidus.

1. Cerebral edema. Postoperative cerebral edema may occur due to the long surgical procedure and/or the retraction of brain tissue to expose the operative area. Elevating the head of the bed 30 degrees facilitates drainage of blood from the brain. Corticosteroids (Decadron) are administered to reduce cerebral edema. Cerebral edema is suspected if the patient presents postoperatively with greater neurological deficits than were present preoperatively. A CT scan is obtained and compared to the preoperative CT scan for significant changes in cerebral edema or shift. If the change is significant, an ICP monitor may be placed and appropriate therapy initiated based on the ICP reading (see the previous discussion on the management of increased ICP).

2. Intracranial hemorrhage and hematoma. Bleeding may occur from the epidural space at the edges of the craniotomy or from the tumor itself, especially if total removal of the tumor was not possible. Bleeding within the skull is characterized by signs and symptoms of increasing ICP. Clinical signs include increasing headache, decreasing level of consciousness, and the development of new focal neurological signs (e.g., weakness of an arm or leg). If an intracranial bleed is suspected, mannitol is administered, a CT scan is obtained, and the patient is returned to the OR for surgical removal of the hemorrhage and management of the bleeding points. Postoperative management is directed toward controlling ICP.

3. Infection. Microorganisms responsible for infection, and more specifically meningitis, can enter the meninges from contamination during surgery or a CSF or wound infection. Presence of a dural tear is indicated by clear drainage on the head dressing or from the ear or nose. The drainage on the dressing appears as a "halo sign" with the center bloody or serous and the outer circle clear or yellowish. CSF drainage from the ear or nose is confirmed by testing the drainage with a Dextrostix. If the drainage is CSF, the fluid will test positive for glucose. The patient must not be suctioned nasally or allowed to blow the nose. The physician is notified immediately. To prevent the development of infection, strict aseptic technique is followed in the management of the surgical site. A wet head dressing is reinforced immediately and the physician notified.

4. Thrombophlebitis. The neurosurgical patient is prone to the development of thrombophlebitis due to the induction of hypothermia during surgery and the projected operative time of 3 to 16 hours with the patient in one position. Thigh-high elastic stockings and sequential compression air devices are initiated during surgery and maintained postoperatively to prevent stasis of blood in the lower legs and to enhance venous return to the heart. Postoperatively, the patient's legs are assessed for redness, swelling, and pain.

5. Diabetes insipidus. Supratentorial surgery can lead to transient diabetes insipidus (DI). DI is caused by a disturbance in the posterior lobe of the pituitary gland, which produces antidiuretic hormone (ADH). If ADH is not secreted in sufficient amounts, the patient will produce large volumes of dilute urine with a low specific gravity. Significant fluid and electrolyte imbalances with dehydration may result. Management includes IV therapy that correlates with urine output followed by administration of aqueous vasopressin (Pitressin) or desmopressin acetate (DDAVP). The patient's hydration status, electrolytes, and serum osmolarity are monitored closely.

SELECTED BIBLIOGRAPHY

What Heals: Unrestricted Visiting Policies

Henneman EA, Cardin S, Papillo J: Open visiting hours in the critical care setting—Effect on nursing staff. *Heart and Lung.* 1989;18:291–292.

Hickey M, Lewandowski L: Critical care nurses' role with families. A descriptive study. *Heart and Lung.* 1988;17:670–676.

Neurological Critical Care Management

Cardona VD, Hurn PD, Mason PJB, Scanlon AM, Veise-Berry SW: *Trauma nursing from resuscitation through rehabilitation,* 2nd ed. Philadelphia: WB Saunders, 1994.

Clochesy JM, Breu C, Cardin S, Rudy EB, Whittaker AA (eds.): *Critical care nursing.* Philadelphia: WB Saunders, 1993.

Hickey JV: *The clinical practice of neurological and neurosurgical nursing,* 3rd ed. Philadelphia: JB Lippincott, 1992.

Marshall SB, Marshall LF, Vos HR, Chestnut RM: *Neuroscience critical care: Pathophysiology and patient management.* Philadelphia: WB Saunders, 1990.

Techniques to Reduce Anxiety

Amato CA: Malignant glioma: Coping with a devastating illness. *Journal of Neurosurgical Nursing.* 1991;23:212–223.

Muss-Clum N, Ryan M: Brain injury and the family. *Journal of Neurosurgical Nursing.* 1981;13:165–169.

Rogers PM, Kreutzer JS: Family crisis following head injury: A network intervention strategy. *Journal of Neurosurgical Nursing.* 1984;16:343–346.

Sisson R: Effects of auditory stimuli on comatose patients with head injury. *Heart and Lung.* 1990;19:373–378.

Sullivan J: Individual and family responses to acute spinal cord injury. *Critical Care Nursing Clinic of North America.* 1990; 2:407–414.

Key Reference Information

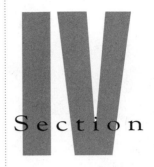

Section IV

Normal Values Table

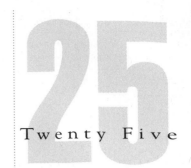

Twenty Five

Abbreviation	Definition	Normal Value	Formula
BSA	Body surface area	Meters squared (m^2)	Value obtained from a nomogram based on height and weight
MAP	Mean systemic arterial pressure	85–90 mm Hg	MAP estimate = diastolic pressure + 1/3 pulse pressure
CVP	Central venous pressure	5–12 cm H_2O	
PA	Mean pulmonary artery pressure	10–17 mm Hg	
PCWP	Mean pulmonary capillary wedge pressure	5–12 mm Hg	
CO	Cardiac output	5–6 L/minute	
CI	Cardiac index	2.5–3.5 L/minute/m^2	$CI\ (L/minute/m^2) = \dfrac{cardiac\ output\ (L/minute)}{body\ surface\ area\ (m^2)}$
SVR	Systemic vascular resistance	900–1200 dynes/second/cm^5	$SVR\ (TPR)\ (dynes/second/cm^5) = \dfrac{(MAP\ [mm\ Hg] - CVP\ [mm\ Hg]) \times 79.9}{cardiac\ output\ (L/minute)}$
PVR	Pulmonary vascular resistance	120–200 dynes/second/cm^5	$PVR\ (dynes/second/cm^5) = \dfrac{(PA\ [mm\ Hg] - PCWP\ [mm\ Hg]) \times 79.9}{cardiac\ output\ (L/minute)}$
HR	Heart rate	60–90 beats/minute	
SV	Stroke volume	50–100 ml/beat	$SV\ (ml/beat) = \dfrac{cardiac\ output\ (ml)}{heart\ rate}$
SI	Stroke index	35–50 mL/m^2	$SI\ (ml/minute/m^2) = \dfrac{stroke\ volume}{body\ surface\ area}$
RVSW	Right ventricular stroke work	51–61 g/m/m^2	$RVSW = SI \times MPAP \times 0.0144$
LVSW	Left ventricular stroke work	8–10 g/m/m^2	$LVSW = SI \times MAP \times 0.0144$
EF	Ejection fraction	70%	$Ejection\ fraction = \dfrac{SV}{EDV}$
EDV	End-diastolic volume	50–90 ml	
dp/dt	First time derivative of left ventricular pressure	13–14 seconds	
P_{AO_2}	Mean partial pressure of oxygen in alveolus	104 mm Hg	
P_{ACO_2}	Partial pressure of carbon dioxide in alveolus	40 mm Hg	
Pa_{O_2}	Partial pressure of oxygen in arterial blood	Will vary with patient's age and the FiO_2. On room air: 80–95 mm Hg. On 100% O_2: 640 mm Hg	
Pa_{CO_2}	Partial pressure of carbon dioxide in arterial blood	35–45 mm Hg	
Pv_{O_2}	Partial pressure of oxygen in mixed venous blood	Will vary with the FiO_2, cardiac output, and oxygen consumption from 35–40 mm Hg	
Pv_{CO_2}	Partial pressure of carbon dioxide in mixed venous blood	41–51 mm Hg	
$P(A-a)_{O_2}$	Alveolar-arterial oxygen gradient	25–65 mm Hg at $FiO_2 = 1.0$	$P(A-a)_{O_2}\ (mm\ Hg) = P_{AO_2} - Pa_{O_2}$
Sa_{O_2}	Percentage of oxyhemoglobin saturation of arterial blood	97% (air)	

continued

Abbreviation	Definition	Normal Value	Formula
$S_{V}O_2$	Percentage of oxyhemoglobin saturation of mixed venous blood	75% (air)	
$C_{a}O_2$	Arterial oxygen content	Will vary with hemoglobin concentration and $P_{a}O_2$ on air from 19–20 ml/100 ml	$C_{a}O_2$ (ml O_2/100 ml blood or vol %) = $(Hb \times 1.39) S_{a}O_2 + (P_{a}O_2 \times 0.0031)$
$C_{V}O_2$	Mixed venous oxygen content	Will vary with $C_{a}O_2$, cardiac output, and O_2 consumption from 14–15 ml/100 ml	
$C(a–v)O_2$	Arteriovenous oxygen content difference	4–6 ml/100 ml	$C(a–v)O_2$ (ml/100 ml or vol %) = $C_{a}O_2 - C_{V}O_2$
O_2 avail	Oxygen availability	550–650 ml/minute/m^2	O_2 avail (ml/minute/m^2) = $CI \times C_{a}O_2 \times 10$
O_2 ext ratio	Oxygen extraction ratio	0.25	O_2 ext ratio = $\dfrac{C(a–v)O_2}{C_{a}O_2}$
P_B	Barometric pressure		
V_{O_2}	Oxygen consumption	115–165 ml/minute/m^2	O_2 ext ratio = $\dfrac{C(a–v)O_2}{C_{a}O_2}$
V_{CO_2}	Carbon dioxide production	192 ml/minute	
R or RQ	Respiratory quotient	0.8	RQ = $\dfrac{V_{CO_2}}{V_{O_2}}$
FRC	Functional residual capacity	2400 ml	
VC	Vital capacity	65–75 ml/kg	
IF	Inspiratory force	75–100 cm H_2O	
EDC	Effective dynamic compliance	35–45 ml/cm H_2O females 40–50 ml/cm H_2O males	EDC (ml/cm H_2O) = $\dfrac{\text{tidal volume (ml)}}{\text{peak airway pressure (cm } H_2O)}$
V_D	Dead space	150 ml	$V_D/V_T = \dfrac{P_{a}CO_2 - P_{E}CO_2}{P_{a}CO_2}$
V_T	Tidal volume	500 ml	
V_D/V_T	Dead space to tidal volume ratio	0.25–0.40	
Q_S/Q_T	Right-to-left shunt (percentage of cardiac output flowing past nonventilated alveoli or the equivalent)	5–8%	$Q_S/Q_T(\%) = \dfrac{0.0031 \times P(A–a)O_2}{C(a–v)O_2 + (0.0031 \times P[A–a]O_2)} \times 100$ Valid only when arterial blood is 100% saturated

Adapted from: Hall J, Schmidt G, Wood L: Principles of critical care. New York: McGraw Hill, 1993, cover tables I–IV.

Pharmacology Tables

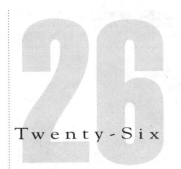

Twenty-Six

TABLE 26–1. INTRAVENOUS MEDICATION ADMINISTRATION GUIDELINES

Drug	Usual IV Dose Range*	Standard Dilution	Infusion Times/Comments/Drug Interactions
Acetazolamide	5 mg/kg/24h or 250 mg qd-qid	Undiluted	Infuse at 500 mg/minute
Acyclovir	5 mg/kg q8h	D5W 100 ml	Infuse over at least 60 minutes
Adenosine	6 mg initially, then 12 mg × 2 doses	Undiluted	Inject over 1–2 seconds Drug interactions: theophylline (1); persantine (2)
Amikacin			
Standard dose	7.5 mg/kg q12h	D5W 50 ml	Infuse over 30 minutes
Single daily dose	20 mg/kg q24h	D5W 50 ml	Drug interactions: neuromuscular blocking agents (3) Therapeutic levels: Peak: 20–40 mg/L; trough: <8 mg/L Single daily dose: trough level at 24 hours = 0 mg/L; peak levels unnecessary
Aminophylline			
Loading dose	6 mg/kg	D5W 50 ml	Infuse loading dose over 30 minutes Maximum loading infusion rate 25 mg/minute Aminophylline = 80% theophylline Drug interactions: cimetidine, ciprofloxacin, erythromycin, clarithromycin (4)
Infusion dose		500 mg in D5W 500 ml	Therapeutic levels: 10–20 mg/L
CHF	0.3 mg/kg/hour		
Normal	0.6 mg/kg/hour		
Smoker	0.9 mg/kg/hour		
Ammonium chloride	mEq Cl = Cl deficit (in mEq/L) × 0.2 × wt (kg)	100 mEq in NS 500 ml	Maximum infusion rate is 5 ml/minute of a 0.2-mEq/ml solution; correct 1/3 to 1/2 of Cl deficit while monitoring pH and Cl; administer remainder as needed
Amphotericin B	0.5–1.5 mg/kg q24h	D5W 250 ml	Infuse over 2–6 hours Do not mix in electrolyte solutions (e.g., saline, Ringer's lactate)
Ampicillin	0.5–3 g q4–6h	NS 100 ml	Infuse over 15–30 minutes
Ampicillin/sulbactam	1.5–3 g q6h	NS 100 ml	Infuse over 15–30 minutes
Amrinone			
Loading dose	0.75–3 mg/kg	Undiluted	Inject over 1–2 minutes Do not mix in dextrose-containing solutions; may be injected into running dextrose infusions through a Y-connector or directly into tubing
Infusion dose	5–20 µg/kg/minute	300 mg in NS 120 ml	
Anistreplase (APSAC)	30 U IV	SW 5 ml	Infuse over 5 minutes, give with aspirin 325 mg PO immediately Preparation should be discarded if not used within 6 hours
Atenolol	5 mg IV over 5 minutes, 5 mg IV 10 minutes later	Undiluted	Inject 1 mg/minute
Atracurium			
Intubating dose	0.4–0.5 mg/kg	Undiluted	Inject over 60 seconds to prevent histamine release
Maintenance dose	0.08–0.1 mg/kg	Undiluted	Inject over 60 seconds to prevent histamine release
Infusion dose	5–9 µg/kg/minute	1000 mg in D5W 150 ml	Continuous infusion. Final volume = 250 ml, conc = 4 mg/ml Drug interactions: aminoglycosides (3); anticonvulsants (5)

*Usual dose ranges are listed; refer to appropriate disease state for specific dose.
Abbreviations: IVP, IV push; IVPB, IV piggy back; D5W, dextrose-5%-water; NS, normal saline; SW, sterile water.
Drug interactions: (1) antagonizes adenosine effect; (2) potentiates adenosine effect; (3) potentiates effect of neuromuscular blocking agents; (4) inhibits theophylline metabolism; (5) antagonizes effect of neuromuscular blocking agents: (6) metabolism inhibited by cimetidine; (7) metabolism inhibited by ciprofloxacin; (8) increased digoxin concentrations; (9) metabolism inhibited by erythromycin; (10) increased nephrotoxicity; (11) increased heparin requirements.

continued

TABLE 26–1. INTRAVENOUS MEDICATION ADMINISTRATION GUIDELINES (continued)

Drug	Usual IV Dose Range*	Standard Dilution	Infusion Times/Comments/Drug Interactions
Aztreonam	0.5–2 g q6–12h	D5W 100 ml	Infuse over 15–30 minutes
Bretylium			
Bolus dose	5–10 mg/kg	Undiluted	Infuse over 5–10 seconds
Infusion dose	1–5 mg/minute	2 g in D5W 500 ml	Continuous infusion
Bumetanide			
Bolus dose	0.5–1 mg	Undiluted	Maximum injection rate: 1 mg/minute
Infusion dose	0.08–0.3 mg/hour	2.4 mg in NS 100 ml	Continuous infusion
Calcium (elemental)	100–200 mg of elemental calcium IV over 15 minutes followed by 100 mg/hour	1000 mg in NS 1000 ml	Ca chloride 1 g = 272 mg (13.6 mEq) of elemental calcium Ca gluconate 1 g = 90 mg (4.65 mEq) of elemental calcium
Cefamandole	0.5–2 g q4–8h	D5W 50 ml	Infuse over 15–30 minutes
Cefazolin	0.5–1 g q6–8h	D5W 50 ml	Infuse over 15–30 minutes
Cefmetazole	2 g q6–12h	D5W 50 ml	Infuse over 15–30 minutes
Cefonicid	1–2 g q24h	D5W 50 ml	Infuse over 15–30 minutes
Cefoperazone	1–2 g q12h	D5W 50 ml	Infuse over 15–30 minutes
Cefotaxime	1–2 g q4–6h	D5W 50 ml	Infuse over 15–30 minutes
Cefotetan	1–2 g q12h	D5W 50 ml	Infuse over 15–30 minutes
Cefoxitin	1–2 g q4–6h	D5W 50 ml	Infuse over 15–30 minutes
Ceftazidime	0.5–2 g q8–12h	D5W 50 ml	Infuse over 15–30 minutes
Ceftizoxime	1–2 g q8–12h	D5W 50 ml	Infuse over 15–30 minutes
Ceftriaxone	0.5–2 g q12–24h	D5W 50 ml	Infuse over 15–30 minutes
Cefuroxime	0.75–1.5 g q8h	D5W 50 ml	Infuse over 15–30 minutes
Chlorothiazide	0.5–1 g qd-bid	SW 18 ml	Inject over 3–5 minutes
Chlorpromazine	10–50 mg q4–6h	Dilute with NS to a final concentration of 1 mg/ml	Inject at 1 mg/minute
Cimetidine			
IVPB	300 mg q6–8h	D5W 50 ml	Infuse over 15–30 minutes IVP dose may be injected over at least 5 minutes
Infusion dose	37.5 mg/hour	D5W 250 ml	Continuous infusion Drug interactions: theophylline, warfarin, phenytoin, lidocaine, benzodiazepines (6)
Ciprofloxacin	200–400 mg q12h	Premix solution 2 mg/ml	Infuse over 60 minutes Drug interactions: theophylline, warfarin (7)
Clindamycin	150–900 mg q8h	D5W 100 ml	Infuse over 30–60 minutes
Conjugated estrogens	0.6 mg/kg/d × 5 days	NS 50 ml	Infuse over 15–30 minutes
Cosyntropin	0.25 mg IV	Undiluted	Inject over 60 seconds
Cyclosporine	5–6 mg/kg q24h	D5W 100 ml	Infuse over 2–6 hours Drug interactions: digoxin (8); erythromycin (9); amphotericin, NSAID (10) IV dose = 1/3 PO dose Therapeutic levels: trough: 50–150 ng/ml (whole blood-HPLC)
Dantrolene			
Bolus dose	1–2 mg/kg	SW 60 ml	Administer as rapidly as possible
Maximum dose	10 mg/kg		Do not dilute in dextrose or electrolyte-containing solutions
Maintenance dose	2.5 mg/kg q4h × 24h	SW 60 ml	Infuse over 60 minutes
Desmopressin	0.3 mg/kg	NS 50 ml	Infuse over 15–30 minutes
Dexamethasone	0.5–20 mg	NS 50 ml	May give doses ≤ 10 mg undiluted IVP over 60 seconds
Diazepam	2.5–5 mg q2–4h	Undiluted	Inject 2–5 mg/minute Active metabolites contribute to activity
Diazoxide	50–150 mg q5–15min	Undiluted	Inject over 30 seconds Maximum 150 mg/dose
Digoxin			
Digitalizing dose	0.25mg q4-6h up to 1 mg	Undiluted	Inject over 3–5 minutes
Maintenance dose	0.125–0.25 mg q24h		Drug interactions: amiodarone, cyclosporine, quinidine, verapamil (8) Therapeutic levels: 0.5–2.0 ng/ml

TABLE 26–1. INTRAVENOUS MEDICATION ADMINISTRATION GUIDELINES (continued)

Drug	Usual IV Dose Range*	Standard Dilution	Infusion Times/Comments/Drug Interactions
Diltiazem			
Bolus dose	0.25–0.35 mg/kg	Undiluted	Inject over 2 minutes
Infusion dose	5–15 mg/hour	125 mg in D5W 100 ml	Continuous infusion (final concentration = 1 mg/ml)
Diphenhydramine	25–100 mg IV q 2–4 h	Undiluted	Inject over 3–5 minutes
			Competitive histamine antagonist, doses > 1000 mg/24 h may be required in some instances
Dobutamine	2.5–20 µg/kg/minute	500 mg in D5W 250 ml	Continuous infusion
Dopamine			
Renal dose	< 5 µg/kg/minute	400 mg in D5W 250 ml	Continuous infusion
Inotrope	5–10 µg/kg/minute	400 mg in D5W 250 ml	Continuous infusion
Pressor	> 10 µg/kg/minute	400 mg in D5W 250 ml	Continuous infusion
Doxacurium			
Intubating dose	0.025–0.08 mg/kg	Undiluted	Inject over 5–10 seconds
Maintenance dose	0.005–0.01 mg/kg	Undiluted	Inject over 5–10 seconds
Infusion dose	0.25 µg/kg/minute	25 mg in D5W 50 ml	Continuous infusion
			Dose based on lean body weight
			Drug interactions: aminoglycosides (3); anticonvulsants (5)
Doxycycline	100–200 mg q12–24h	D5W 250 ml	Infuse over 60 minutes
Droperidol	0.625–10 mg q1–4h	Undiluted	Inject over 3–5 minutes
Enalaprilat	1.25–5 mg q6h	Undiluted	Inject over 5 minutes
			Initial dose for patients on diuretics is 0.625 mg
Epinephrine	1–4 µg/minute	1 mg in D5W 250 ml	Continuous infusion
Erythromycin	0.5–1 g q6h	NS 250 ml	Infuse over 60 minutes
			Drug interactions: theophylline (4); cyclosporine (9)
Erythropoietin	12.5–525 U/kg 3 × per week	Undiluted	Inject over 3–5 minutes
Esmolol			
Bolus dose	500 µg/kg	Undiluted	Inject over 60 seconds
Infusion dose	50–400 µg/kg/minute	5 g in D5W 500 ml	Continuous infusion
Ethacrynic acid	50 mg	D5W 50 ml	Inject over 3–5 minutes
	May repeat × 1		Maximum single dose 100 mg
Etidronate	7.5mg/kg qd × 3d	NS or D5W 500 ml	Infuse over at least 2 hours
Famotidine	20 mg q12h	D5W 100 ml	Infuse over 15–30 minutes
Fentanyl			
Bolus dose	25–75 µg q1–2h	Undiluted	Inject over 5–10 seconds
Infusion dose	50–100 µg/hr	Undiluted	Continuous infusion
Filgastrim	1–20 µg/kg × 2–4 weeks	D5W	Preferred route of administration is subcutaneous
Fluconazole	100–800 mg q24h	Premix solution 2 mg/ml	Maximum infusion rate 200 mg/hour (IV rate is 15–30 minutes)
Flumazenil			
Reversal of conscious sedation	0.2 mg initially, then 0.2 mg q 60 seconds to a total of 1 mg	Undiluted	Inject over 15 seconds
			Maximum dose of 3 mg in any 1-hour period
Benzodiazepine overdose	0.2 mg initially, then 0.3 mg × 1 dose, then 0.5 mg q30 seconds up to a total of 3 mg	Undiluted	Inject over 30 seconds
			Maximum dose of 3 mg in any 1-hour period
Continuous infusion	0.1–0.5 mg/h	5 mg in D5W 1000 ml	Continuous infusion
Foscarnet			
Induction dose	60 mg/kg q8h	Undiluted	Infuse over 1 hour
Maintenance dose	90–120 mg/kg q24h	Undiluted	Infuse over 2 hours
Furosemide			
Bolus dose	20–40 mg q1–2h	Undiluted	Maximum injection rate 40 mg/minute
Infusion dose	3–15 mg/hour	100 mg in NS 100 ml	Continuous infusion
Gallium nitrate	100–200 mg/m² qd × 5d	D5W 1000 ml	Infuse over 24 hours
Ganciclovir	2.5 mg/kg q12h	D5W 100 ml	Infuse over 1 hour

continued

TABLE 26–1. INTRAVENOUS MEDICATION ADMINISTRATION GUIDELINES (continued)

Drug	Usual IV Dose Range*	Standard Dilution	Infusion Times/Comments/Drug Interactions
Gentamicin			
Loading dose	2–3 mg/kg	D5W 50 ml	Infuse over 30 minutes
Maintenance dose	1.5–2.5 mg/kg q8–24h	D5W 50 ml	Infuse over 30 minutes
Single daily dose	5–7 mg/kg q24h	D5W 50 ml	Infuse over 30 minutes
			Critically ill patients have an increased volume of distribution requiring increased doses
			Drug interactions: neuromuscular blocking agents
			Therapeutic levels:
			Peak: 4–10 mg/L
			Trough: < 2 mg/L
			Single daily dose: trough level at 24 hours = 0 mg/L; peak levels unnecessary
Glycopyrrolate	5–15 µg/kg	Undiluted	Inject over 60 seconds
Granisetron	10 µg/kg	D5W 50 ml	Infuse over 15 minutes
Haloperidol (lactate)			
Bolus dose	1–10 mg q2–4h	Undiluted	Inject over 3–5 minutes
Infusion dose	10 mg/h	100 mg in D5W 100 ml	Continuous infusion
			In urgent situations the dose may be doubled every 20–30 minutes until an effect is obtained
			Decanoate salt is only for IM administration
Heparin	10–25 U/kg/hour	25,000 units in D5W 500 ml	Drug interactions: nitroglycerin (11)
Hydralazine	5–20 mg q4–6h	Undiluted	Inject over 3–5 minutes; doses every 30 minutes may be required for eclampsia
Hydrochloric acid	mEq = (0.5×BW × (103-serum Cl))	100 mEq in SW 1000 ml	Maximum infusion rate = 0.2 mEq/kg/hour
Hydrocortisone	12.5–100 mg q6–12h	Undiluted	Inject over 60 seconds
Hydromorphone	1–4 mg q4–6h	Undiluted	Inject over 60 seconds
			Dilaudid-HP available as 10 mg/ml
Imipenem	0.5–1 g q6–8h	D5W 100 ml	Infuse over 30–60 minutes
Isoproterenol	1–10 µg/minute	2 mg in D5W 500 ml	Continuous infusion
Ketamine			
Bolus dose	1–4.5 mg/kg	Undiluted	Inject over 60 seconds
Infusion dose	5–45 µg/kg/minute	200 mg in D5W 500 ml	Continuous infusion
Labetalol			
Bolus dose	20 mg q15min	Undiluted	Inject over 2 minutes
Infusion dose	1–4 mg/minute	200 mg in D5W 160 ml	Continuous infusion
Levothyroxine	25–200 mg q24h	Undiluted	Inject over 5–10 seconds
			IV dose = 75% of PO dose
Lidocaine			
Bolus dose	1 mg/kg	Undiluted	Inject over 60 seconds
Infusion dose	1–4 mg/minute	2 g in D5W 500 ml	Continuous infusion
			Drug interactions: cimetidine (6)
			Therapeutic levels: 1.5–5.0 mg/L
Lorazepam			
Bolus dose	0.5–2 mg q1–4h	Dilute 1:1 with NS before administration	Inject 2 mg/minute
Infusion dose	0.06 mg/kg/hour	20 mg in D5W 250 ml	Monitor for lorazepam precipitate in solution
			Use in-line filter during continuous infusion to avoid infusing precipitate into patient
Magnesium (elemental)			Magnesium 1 g = 8 mEq
Magnesium deficiency	25 mEq over 24 hours followed by 6 mEq over the next 12 hours	25 mEq in D5W 1000 ml	Continuous infusion
Acute myocardial infarction	15–45 mEq over 24–48 hours followed by 12.5 mEq/day for 3 days	25 mEq in D5W 1000 ml	Continuous infusion
Ventricular arrhythmias	16 mEq over 1 hour followed by 40 mEq over 6 hours	40 mEq in D5W 1000 ml	16 mEq (2 g) may be diluted in 100 ml D5W and infused over 1 hour

TABLE 26–1. INTRAVENOUS MEDICATION ADMINISTRATION GUIDELINES (continued)

Drug	Usual IV Dose Range*	Standard Dilution	Infusion Times/Comments/Drug Interactions
Mannitol			
Diuretic	12.5–100 g over 1–2 hours	Undiluted	Inject over 3–5 minutes
Cerebral edema	1.5–2 g/kg over 30–60 minutes	Undiluted	Inject over 3–5 minutes
Meperidine	25–100 mg q2–4h	Undiluted	Inject over 60 seconds Avoid in renal failure
Metaraminol			
Bolus dose	0.5–5 mg	Undiluted	Inject over 60 seconds
Continuous infusion	20–500 µg/min	100 mg in NS 500 ml	Continuous infusion
Methadone	5–20 mg qd	Undiluted	Inject over 3–5 minutes Accumulation with repetitive dosing
Methyldopate	0.25–1 g q6h	D5W 100 ml	Infuse over 30–60 minutes
Methylprednisolone	10–500 mg q6h	Undiluted	Inject over 60 seconds
Metoclopramide			
Small intestine intubation	10 mg × 1	Undiluted	Inject over 3–5 minutes
Antiemetic	2 mg/kg before chemo, then 2 mg/kg q2h × 2, then q3h × 3	D5W 50 ml	Infuse over 15–30 minutes
Metoprolol	5 mg q2min × 3	Undiluted	Inject over 3–5 minutes
Metronidazole	500 mg q6h	Premix solution 5 mg/ml	Infuse over 30 minutes
Mezlocillin	3 g q4h	D5W 100 ml	Infuse over 15–30 minutes
Midazolam			
Bolus dose	0.025–0.35 mg/kg q1–2h	Undiluted	Inject 0.5 mg/minute
Infusion dose	0.5–5 µg/kg/minute	50 mg in D5W 100 ml	Continuous infusion Unpredictable clearance in critically ill patients Drug interactions: cimetidine (6)
Milrinone			
Loading dose	50 µg/kg	1 mg/ml	Infuse over 10 minutes Available in 5-ml syringe
Maintenance dose	0.375–0.75 µg/kg/minute	50 mg in D5W 250 ml	Continuous infusion
Mivacurium			
Intubating dose	0.25 mg/kg	Undiluted	Inject over 60 seconds
Maintenance dose	0.1 mg/kg	Undiluted	Inject over 60 seconds
Infusion dose	9–10 µg/kg/minute	50 mg in D5W 100 ml	Continuous infusion Drug interactions: aminoglycosides (3); anticonvulsants (5)
Morphine			
Bolus dose	2–10 mg	Undiluted	Inject over 60 seconds
Infusion dose	2–5 mg/h	100 mg in D5W 100 ml	Continuous infusion
Nafcillin	0.5–2 g q4–6h	D5W 100 ml	Infuse over 30–60 minutes
Naloxone			
Bolus dose	0.4–2 mg Max 10 mg	Undiluted	Inject over 60 seconds
Infusion dose	3–5 µg/kg/h	2 mg in D5W 250 ml	Continuous infusion
Neostigmine	25–75 µg/kg	Undiluted	Inject over 60 seconds
Nitroglycerin	10–200 µg/minute	50 mg in D5W 250 ml	Continuous infusion Drug interactions: heparin (11)
Nitroprusside	0.5–10 µg/kg/minute	50 mg in D5W 250 ml	Continuous infusion Maintain thiocyanate < 10 mg/dl
Norepinephrine	4–10 µg/minute	4 mg in D5W 250 ml	Continuous infusion
Ofloxacin	200–400 mg q12h	D5W 100 ml	Infuse over 60 minutes
Ondansetron			
Chemotherapy-induced nausea and vomiting	32 mg 30 minutes before chemotherapy	D5W 50 ml	Infuse over 15–30 minutes
Postoperative nausea and vomiting	4 mg × 1 dose	Undilated	Inject over 2–5 minutes

continued

TABLE 26–1. INTRAVENOUS MEDICATION ADMINISTRATION GUIDELINES (continued)

Drug	Usual IV Dose Range*	Standard Dilution	Infusion Times/Comments/Drug Interactions
Oxacillin	0.5–2 g q4–6h	D5W 100 ml	Infuse over 30 minutes
Pamidronate	60–90 mg × 1 dose	D5W 1000 ml	Infuse over 24 hours
Pancuronium			
Intubating dose	0.06–0.1 mg/kg	Undiluted	Inject over 60 seconds
Maintenance dose	0.01–0.015 mg/kg	Undiluted	Inject over 60 seconds
Infusion dose	1 μg/kg/minute	50 mg in D5W 250 ml	Continuous infusion
			Metabolite contributes to activity
			Drug interactions: aminoglycosides (3); anticonvulsants (5)
Penicillin G	8–24 MU divided q4h	D5W 100 ml	Infuse over 15–30 minutes
Pentamidine	4 mg/kg q24h	D5W 50 ml	Infuse over 60 minutes
Pentobarbital			
Bolus dose	20 mg/kg	NS 100 ml	Infuse over 2 hours
Infusion dose	1 mg/kg/hour initially, then	NS 250 ml	Continuous infusion
	0.5–3.5 mg/kg/hour	2g in NS 250 ml	Therapeutic levels: 20–50 mg/L
Phenobarbital			
Status epilepticus	20 mg/kg	Undiluted	Inject over 3–5 minutes
			Therapeutic levels: 15–40 mg/L
Phentolamine			
Bolus dose	2.5–10 mg prn	Undiluted	Inject over 3–5 minutes
Continuous infusion	1–5 mg/minute	50 mg in D5W 100 ml	Continuous infusion
Phenylephrine	20–30 μg/minute	15 mg in D5W 250 ml	Continuous infusion; 0.5mg over 20–30 seconds
Phenytoin	15 mg/kg	Undiluted	Maximum infusion rate: 25 to 50 mg/minute
Status epilepticus			Drug interactions: cimetidine (6); neuromuscular blocking agents (5)
			Therapeutic levels: 10–20 mg/L
Phosphate (potassium)	0.08–0.24 mmol/kg	Function of K^+ concentration	Infuse over 6–8h
			1 mmol of PO_4 = P 31 mg
			Solution should be made no more concentrated than 0.4 mEq/ml of K^+
Piperacillin	2–4 g q4–6h	D5W 100 ml	Infuse over 15–30 minutes
Piperacillin/tazobactam	3.375g IV q6h	D5W 100 ml	Infuse over 30 minutes
			Each 2.25-g vial contains 2 g piperacillin and 0.25 g tazobactam
Plicamycin	15–25 μg/kg qd × 3–4 d	NS 1000 ml	Infuse over 4 to 6 hours
Potassium chloride	5–40 mEq/hour	40 mEq in 1000 ml (NS, D5W, etc)	Cardiac monitoring should be used with infusion rates > 20 mEq/hour
Prednisolone	4–60 mg q24h	Undiluted	Inject over 60 seconds
Procainamide			
Loading dose	15 mg/kg	D5W 50 ml	Maximum infusion rate 25–50 mg/minute
Infusion dose	1–4 mg/minute	2g in D5W 500 ml	Continuous infusion
			Therapeutic levels:
			Procainamide: 4–10 mg/L
			NAPA: 10–20 mg/L
Propofol			
Bolus dose	0.25–0.5 mg/kg	Undiluted	Infuse over 1–2 minutes
Infusion dose	5–50 μg/kg/minute	Undiluted	Continuous infusion
Propranolol			
Bolus dose	0.5–1 mg q5–15 min	Undiluted	Infuse over 60 seconds
Infusion dose	1–4 mg/hour	50 mg in D5W 500 ml	Continuous infusion
Protamine	<30 minutes: 1–1.5 mg/100 U; 30–60 minutes: 0.5–0.75 mg/100 U; > 120 minutes: 0.25–0.375 mg/100 U	50 mg in SW 5 ml	Inject over 3–5 minutes; do not exceed 50 mg in 10 minutes
Pyridostigmine	100–300 μg/kg	Undiluted	Use to reverse long-acting neuromuscular blocking agents
			Inject over 60 seconds
Quinidine gluconate	600 mg initially, then 400 mg q2h, maintenance 200–300 mg q6h	800 mg in D5W 50 ml	Infusion rate 1 mg/minute; use cardiac monitor
			Therapeutic levels: 1.5–5 mg/L

TABLE 26–1. INTRAVENOUS MEDICATION ADMINISTRATION GUIDELINES (continued)

Drug	Usual IV Dose Range*	Standard Dilution	Infusion Times/Comments/Drug Interactions
Ranitidine			
IVPB	50 mg q6–8h	D5W 50 ml	Infuse over 15–30 minutes
			IVP dose should be injected over at least 5 minutes
Infusion dose	6.25 mg/hour	150 mg in D5W 150 ml	Continuous infusion
Rocuronium			
Intubating dose	0.45–1.2 mg/kg	Undiluted	Inject over 60 seconds
Maintenance dose	0.075–0.15 mg/kg	Undiluted	Inject over 60 seconds
Infusion dose	10–14 µg/kg/minute	50 mg in D5W 100 ml	Continuous infusion
Streptokinase			
Acute myocardial infarction	1.5 MU	D5W 45 ml	Infuse over 30 minutes
Deep venous thrombosis, pulmonary embolism	250,000 U over 30 minutes, then 100,000 U/hour over 24–72 hours	D5W 90 ml	Continuous infusion
Succinylcholine	0.6–2 mg/kg	Undiluted	Infuse over 60 seconds
t-PA	100 mg	100 mg in D5W 100 ml	Infuse 60 mg/hour during first hr, then 20 mg/hour for 2 hours
Thiamine	100 mg qd × 3	D5W 50 ml	Infuse over 15–30 minutes
Thiopental	3–4 mg/kg	Undiluted	Inject over 3–5 minutes
Ticarcillin	3 g q3–6h	D5W 100 ml	Infuse over 15–30 minutes
Ticarcillin/clavulanate	3.1 g q4–6h	D5W 100 ml	Infuse over 15–30 minutes
Tobramycin			
Loading dose	2–3 mg/kg	D5W 50 ml	Infuse over 30 minutes
Maintenance dose	1.5–2.5 mg/kg q8–24h	D5W 50 ml	Infuse over 30 minutes
			Critically ill patients have an increased volume of distribution requiring increased doses
			Drug interactions: neuromuscular blocking agents (3)
			Therapeutic levels:
			Peak: 4–10 mg/L
			Trough: < 2 mg/L
Torsemide	5–20 mg qd	Undiluted	Inject over 60 seconds
Trimethaphan	0.3–5 mg/minute	500 mg in D5W 500 ml	Continuous infusion
Trimethaprim-sulfamethoxazole			
Common infections	4–5 mg/kg q12h	TMP 16 mg-SMX 80 mg per D5W 25 ml	Infuse over 60 minutes
PCP	5 mg/kg q6h	TMP 16 mg-SMX 80 mg per D5W 25 ml	Infuse over 60 minutes
			Therapeutic levels: 100–150 mg/L
Urokinase Pulmonary embolism	4,400 U/kg over 10 minutes, then 4,400 U/h over 12 hours	D5W 195 ml	Continuous infusion
Vancomycin	1 g q12h	D5W 250 ml	Infuse over at least 1 hour to avoid "red-man" syndrome
			Therapeutic levels:
			Peak: 20–40 mg/L
			Trough: <10 mg/L
Vasopressin	0.2–0.4 U/minute	100 units in D5W 250 ml	Maximum infusion rate 0.9 U/minute
Vecuronium			
Intubating dose	0.1–0.28 mg/kg	Undiluted	Inject over 60 seconds
Maintenance dose	0.01–0.015 mg/kg	Undiluted	Inject over 60 seconds
Infusion dose	1 µg/kg/minute	20 mg in D5W 100 ml	Continuous infusion
			Metabolite contributes to activity
			Drug interactions: aminoglycosides (3); anticonvulsants (5)
Verapamil			
Bolus dose	0.075–0.15 mg/kg	Undiluted	Inject over 1–2 minutes
			Continuous infusion
			Drug interactions: digoxin (8)

TABLE 26–2. NEUROMUSCULAR BLOCKING AGENTS

Agent	Dose	Onset/Duration	Comments
Depolarizing Agents			
Succinylcholine	Intubating dose: 1–2 mg/kg	Onset: 1 minute Duration: 10 minutes	Prolonged paralysis in pseudocholinesterase deficiencies Contraindications: Family history of malignant hyperthermia, neuromuscular disease, hyperkalemia, open eye injury, major tissue injury (burns, trauma, crush), increased intracranial pressure Side effects: bradycardia (especially in children), tachycardia, increased serum potassium concentration
Nondepolarizing Agents ***Short-Acting***			
Mivacurium	Intubating dose: 0.25 mg/kg Maintenance dose: 0.1 mg/kg Continuous infusion: 9.0–10.0 µg/kg/minute	Onset: 5 minutes Duration: 15–20 minutes Duration: 15 minutes	Metabolized by pseudocholinesterase Intubating dose: initial 0.15 mg/kg followed in 30 seconds by 0.1 mg/kg
Intermediate-Acting			
Atracurium	Intubating dose: 0.5 mg/kg Maintenance dose: 0.08–0.10 mg/kg Continuous infusion: 5–9 µg/kg/minute	Onset: 2 minutes Duration: 30–40 minutes Duration: 15–25 minutes	Histamine release with bolus doses > 0.6 mg/kg and may precipitate asthma or hypotension Elimination independent of renal or hepatic function Metabolized in the plasma by Hofmann elimination and ester hydrolysis Duration not prolonged by renal or liver failure Used when succinylcholine is contraindicated or not preferred
Rocuronium	Intubating dose: 0.45–1.2 mg/kg Maintenance dose: 0.075–0.15 mg/kg Continuous infusion: 10–14 µg/kg/minute	Onset: 0.7–1.3 minutes Duration: 22 67 minutes Duration: 12–17 minutes	Not associated with histamine release Used when succinylcholine is contraindicated or not preferred Metabolized by liver; duration not significantly prolonged by renal failure, but prolonged in patients with liver disease No adverse cardiovascular effects
Vecuronium	Intubating dose: 0.1–0.15 mg/kg Maintenance dose: 0.01–0.15 mg/kg Continuous infusion: 1 µg/kg/minute	Onset: 2 minutes Duration: 30–40 minutes Duration: 15–25 minutes	Not associated with histamine release Bile is the main route of elimination Metabolized by liver; minimal reliance on renal function, although active metabolite accumulates in renal failure Used when succinylcholine is contraindicated or not preferred No adverse cardiovascular effects
Long-Acting			
Doxacurium	Intubating dose: 0.025–0.8 mg/kg Maintenance dose: 0.005–0.01 mg/kg Continuous infusion: 0.25 µg/kg/minute (not generally recommended)	Onset: 4–5 minutes Duration: 55–160 minutes Duration: 35–45 minutes	No adverse cardiovascular effects Predominantly renally eliminated; significant accumulation in renal failure
Pancuronium	Intubating dose: 0.06–0.1 mg/kg Maintenance dose: 0.01–0.015 mg/kg Continuous infusion: 1 µg/kg/minute (not generally recommended)	Onset: 2–3 minutes Duration: 60–100 minutes Duration: 25–60 minutes	Tachycardia (vagolytic effect) Metabolized by liver; minimal reliance on renal function, although active metabolite accumulates in renal failure

TABLE 26–3. VASOACTIVE AGENTS

Agent and Dose	Receptor Specificity									Pharmacologic Effects
	α	β₁	β₂	DM	SM	VD	VC	INT	CHT	*Comments*
Inotropes										
Dobutamine										Useful for acute management of low cardiac output states; in chronic CHF intermittent infusions palliate symptoms but do not prolong survival
2–10 µg/kg/minute	1+	3+	2+	—	—	1+	1+	3+	1+	
>10–20 µg/kg/minute	2+	4+	3+	—	—	2+	1+	4+	2+	
Isoproterenol	—	4+	3+	—	—	3+	—	4+	4+	Used primarily for temporizing treatment of life-threatening bradycardia
2–10 µg/kg/minute										
Amrinone										Useful for acute management of low cardiac output states; can be combined with dobutamine
Loading dose										
0.75 mg/kg										
Maintenance dose:										Associated with the development of thrombocytopenia
5–15 µg/kg/minute	—	—	—	—	2+	2+	—	3+	3+	
Milrinone										Useful for acute management of low cardiac output states; can be combined with dobutamine
Loading dose: 50 µg/kg over 10 minutes										
Maintenance dose:										
0.375–0.75 µg/kg/minute	—	—	—	—	2+	2+	—	3+	3+	
Mixed										
Dopamine										Doses above 20–30 µg/kg/minute usually produce no added response; 2 µg/kg/minute may protect kidneys when giving other vasopressors
2–5 µg/kg/minute	—	3+	—	4+	—	—	—	2+	1+	
5–10 µg/kg/minute	—	4+	2+	4+	—	—	—	4+	2+	
10–20 µg/kg/minute	3+	4+	1+	—	—	—	3+	3+	3+	
Epinephrine										Mixed vasoconstrictor/inotrope; stronger inotrope than norepinephrine; does not constrict coronary or cerebral vessels; give as needed to maintain BP
0.01–0.05 µg/kg/minute	1+	4+	2+	—	—	1+	1+	4+	2+	
>0.05 µg/kg/minute	4+	3+	1+	—	—	—	3+	3+	3+	
Vasopressors										
Norepinephrine										Mixed vasoconstrictor/inotrope; useful when dopamine inadequate; give as needed to maintain BP (usually ≤20 µg/minute)
2–20 µg/minute titrate to effect	4+	2+	—	—	—	—	4+	1+	2+	
Phenylephrine										Pure vasoconstrictor without direct cardiac effect; may cause reflex bradycardia; useful when other pressors cause tachyarrhythmias; give as much as needed to maintain BP
Start at 30 µg/minute IV and titrate	4+	—	—	—	—	—	4+	—	—	
Metaraminol										Predominant vasoconstrictor with mild inotropic effect; especially useful for shock associated with spinal anesthesia or CNS lesions
0.5–5 mg slow IV bolus, titrate to effect	2+ – 3+	0	1+	0	—	0	3+	1+	1+	
Vasodilators										
Nitroglycerin										Tachyphylaxis, headache
20–100 µg/minute	—	—	—	—	4+	4+ A<V	—	—	1+	
Nitroprusside										Monitor thiocyanate levels if infusion duration >48 hours; maintain thiocyanate level <10 mg/dl
0.5–10 µg/kg/minute	—	—	—	—	4+	4+ A=V	—	—	1+	

α₁: α₁-adrenergic; β₁: β₁-adrenergic; β₂: β₂-adrenergic; DM: dopaminergic; SM: smooth muscle; VD: vasodilator; VC: vasoconstrictor; INT: inotropic; CHT: chronotropic.
Vasoconstrictors usually are given by central vein and should be used only in conjunction with adequate volume repletion. All can precipitate myocardial ischemia. All except phenylephrine can cause tachyarrhythmias.
Modified from: Gonzalez ER, Meyers DG: Assessment and management of cardiogenic shock. In Oronato JC (ed.): Clinics in emergency medicine: Cardiovascular emergencies. *New York: Churchill Livingstone, 1986, p. 125, with permission.*

TABLE 26–4. ANTIARRHYTHMIC AGENTS

Agents	Indications	Dosage	Comments
Class IA			
Procainamide	Ventricular ectopy; conversion of atrial fibrillation and atrial flutter; WPW	Loading dose: (IV) 15 mg/kg at 25–50 mg/minute, (PO) 1 g Maintenance dose: (IV) 2–5 mg/minute; (PO): 500 mg q3h or SR 500–1500 mg q6h	N-acetyl procainamide is active metabolite; lupus-like syndrome; rash; agranulocytosis; QT prolongation Therapeutic range: PA 4–10 mg/L, NAPA 10–20 mg/L
Quinidine	Ventricular ectopy; conversion of atrial fibrillation and atrial flutter; WPW	Quinidine sulfate: 200–300 mg PO q6h Quinidine gluconate: 324–648 mg PO q8h	Diarrhea, nausea, headache dizziness; hypersensitivity reactions including thrombocytopenia; hemolysis; fever; hepatitis; rash; QT prolongation; increased digoxin level Dosage adjustment should be made when switching from one salt to another: Quinidine sulfate (83% quinidine), gluconate (62% quinidine), polygalacturonate (60% quinidine) Therapeutic range: 2.5–5 mg/L
Disopyramide	Ventricular ectopy; conversion of atrial fibrillation and atrial flutter; WPW	100–300 mg PO q6h; SR: 100–300 mg PO q12h	Anticholinergic effects; negative inotropy; QT prolongation Therapeutic range: 2–4 mg/L
Class IB			
Lidocaine	Malignant ventricular ectopy; WPW	1.5 mg/kg IV over 2 minutes, then 1–4 mg/minute	No benefit in atrial arrhythmias Seizures; paresthesias; delirium; levels increased by cimetidine; minimal hemodynamic effects Therapeutic range: 1.5–5 mg/L
Mexiletine	Malignant ventricular ectopy	150–300 mg PO q6–8h with food	No benefit in atrial arrhythmias Less effective than IA and IC agents Nausea; tremor; dizziness; delirium; levels increased by cimetidine Therapeutic range: 0.5–2 mg/L
Tocainide	Malignant ventricular ectopy	200–600 mg PO q8h with food	No benefit in atrial arrhythmias Less effective than IA and IC agents Nausea; tremor; dizziness; delirium; agranulocytosis; pneumonitis; minimal hemodynamic effects Therapeutic range: 4–10 mg/L
Class IC			
Flecainide	Life-threatening ventricular arrhythmias refractory to other agents Prevention of symptomatic, disabling, paroxysmal supraventricular arrhythmias, including atrial fibrillation or flutter and WPW in patients without structural heart disease	100–200 mg PO q12h	Proarrhythmic effects; moderate negative inotropy; dizziness; conduction abnormalities Therapeutic range: 0.2–1 mg/L
Propafenone	Life-threatening ventricular arrhythmias refractory to other agents SVT, WPW, and paroxysmal atrial fibrillation or flutter in patients without structural heart disease	150–300 mg PO q8h	Proarrhythmic effects; negative inotropy; dizziness; nausea; conduction abnormalities
Class IB/IC (hybrid electrophysiologic effects)			
Moricizine	Life-threatening ventricular arrhythmias refractory to other agents	100–300 mg PO q8h	Proarrhythmic effects; dizziness; nausea; headache

TABLE 26–4. ANTIARRHYTHMIC AGENTS (continued)

Agents	Indications	Dosage	Comments
Class II (beta-blocking agents)			
Propranolol	Slowing ventricular rate in atrial fibrillation, atrial flutter, and SVT; suppression of PVCs	Up to 0.5–1 mg IV, then 1–4 mg/hour (or 10–100 mg PO q6h)	Not cardioselective; hypotension; bronchospasm; negative inotropy
Esmolol	Slowing ventricular rate in atrial fibrillation, atrial flutter, SVT, and MAT	Loading dose: 500 µg/kg over 1 minute; Maintenance dose: 50 µg/kg/minute; rebolus and increase q5min by 50 µg/kg/minute to maximum of 400 µg/kg/minute	Cardioselective at low doses; hypotension; negative inotropy; very short half-life
Metoprolol	Slowing ventricular rate in atrial fibrillation, atrial flutter, SVT, and MAT	Initial IV dose: 5 mg q5min up to 15 mg, then 25–100 mg PO q8–12h	Cardioselective at low doses; hypotension; negative inotropy
Class III			
Amiodarone	Life-threatening ventricular arrhythmias, supraventricular arrhythmias, including WPW refractory to other agents	800–1600 mg PO qd for 1–3 weeks, then 600–800 mg PO qd for 4 weeks, then 100–400 mg PO qd	Half-life >50 days; pulmonary fibrosis; corneal microdeposits; hypo/hyperthyroidism; bluish skin; hepatitis; photosensitivity; conduction abnormalities; mild negative inotropy; increased effect of coumadin; increased digoxin level. Therapeutic range: 1–2.5 mg/L
Bretylium	Refractory ventricular tachycardia and ventricular fibrillation	5–10 mg/kg IV boluses q10min up to 30 mg/kg, then 0.5–2 mg/minute	Initial hypertension, then postural hypotension; nausea and vomiting; parotitis; catecholamine sensitivity
Sotalol	Life-threatening ventricular arrhythmias	80–160 mg PO q12h; may increase up to 160 mg PO q8h	Beta blocker with Class III properties; proarrhythmic effects; QT prolongation
Class IV (calcium channel antagonists)			
Verapamil	Conversion of SVT; slowing ventricular rate in atrial fibrillation, atrial flutter, and MAT	IV bolus: 5–10 mg over 2–3 minutes (repeat in 30 minutes prn), continuous infusion: 2.5–5 µg/kg/minute; PO: 40–160 mg PO q8h	Hypotension; negative inotropy; conduction disturbances; increased digoxin level; generally contraindicated in WPW
Diltiazem	Conversion of SVT; slowing ventricular rate in atrial fibrillation, atrial flutter, and MAT	IV bolus: 0.25 mg/kg over 2 minutes (repeat in 15 minutes prn with 0.35 mg/kg IV); Maintenance infusion: 5–15 mg/hour; PO: 30–90 mg PO q6h	Hypotension; less negative inotropy than verapamil; conduction disturbances; rare hepatic injury; generally contraindicated in WPW
Miscellaneous Agents			
Adenosine	Conversion of SVT, including WPW	6 mg rapid IV bolus; if ineffective, 12 mg rapid IV bolus 2 minutes later; follow bolus with fast flush; use smaller doses if giving through central venous line	Flushing; dyspnea; nodal blocking effect increased by dipyridamole and decreased by theophylline and caffeine; very short half-life ($\approx$ 10 seconds)
Atropine	Initial therapy for symptomatic bradycardia	0.5 mg IV bolus; repeat q5 min prn to total of 2 mg IV	May induce tachycardia and ischemia
Digitalis	Slowing AV conduction in atrial fibrillation and atrial flutter	Loading dose: 0.5 mg IV, then 0.25 mg IV q4–6h up to 1 mg; Maintenance dose: 0.125–0.375 mg PO/IV qd.	Heart block; arrhythmias; nausea; yellow vision; numerous drug interactions, generally contraindicated in WPW. Therapeutic range: 0.5–2.0 ng/ml

Abbreviations: MAT, multifocal atrial tachycardia; SR: Sustained Release; SVT, supraventricular tachycardia; WPW, Wolff-Parkinson-White.

TABLE 26–5. THERAPEUTIC DRUG MONITORING

Drug	Usual Therapeutic Range	Usual Sampling Time
Antibiotics		
Amikacin	Peak: 20–40 mg/L Trough: <10 mg/L Single daily dose: 0 mg/L at 24 h	Peak: 30–60 minutes after a 30-minute infusion Trough: just before next dose Single daily dose: trough level just before next dose
Chloramphenicol	Peak: 10–25 mg/L Trough: 5–10 mg/L	Peak: 30–90 minutes after a 30-minute infusion Trough: just before the next dose
Flucytosine	Peak: 50–100 mg/L Trough: <25 mg/L	Peak: 1–2 hours after an oral dose Trough: just before next dose
Gentamicin	Peak: 4–10 mg/L Trough: <2 mg/L Single daily dose: 0 mg/L at 24 h	Peak: 30–60 minutes after a 30-minute infusion Trough: just before next dose Single daily dose: trough level just before next dose
Tobramycin	Peak: 4–10 mg/L Trough: <2 mg/L	Peak: 30–60 minutes after a 30-minute infusion Trough: just before next dose
Netilmicin	Peak: 4–10 mg/L Trough: <2 mg/L Single daily dose: 0 mg/L at 24 h	Peak: 30–60 minutes after a 30-minute infusion Trough: just before next dose Single daily dose: trough level just before next dose
Vancomycin	Peak: 20–40 mg/L Trough: <10 mg/L	Peak: 1 hour after end of a 1-hour infusion Trough: just before next dose
Sulfonamides (sulfamethoxazole, sulfadiazine, cotrimoxazole)	Peak: 100–150 mg/L	Peak: 2 hours after 1-hour infusion Trough: not applicable
Antiarrhythmics		
Amiodarone	0.5–2 mg/L	Trough: just before next dose
Digoxin	0.5–2 µg/ml	Peak: 8–12 hours after administered dose Trough: just before next dose
Disopyramide	2–4 mg/L	Trough: just before next dose
Flecainide	0.2–1.0 mg/L	Trough: just before next dose
Lidocaine	1.5–5 mg/L	Anytime during a continuous infusion
Mexiletine	0.5–2 mg/L	Trough: just before next dose
Procainamide/NAPA	Procainamide: 4–10 mg/L NAPA: 10–20 mg/L	IV: immediately after IV loading dose, anytime during continuous infusion PO: trough: just before next dose
Quinidine	2.5–5 mg/L	Trough: just before next dose
Tocainide	4–10 mg/L	Trough: just before next dose
Anticonvulsants		
Carbamazepine	4–12 mg/L	Trough: just before next dose
Pentobarbital	20–50 µg/ml	IV: immediately after IV loading dose, anytime during continuous infusion
Phenobarbital	15–40 mg/L	Trough: just before next dose
Phenytoin	10–20 mg/L	IV: 2–4 hours after dose Trough: PO/IV: just before next dose Free phenytoin level: 1–2 mg/L
Valproic acid	50–100 mg/L	Trough: just before next dose
Bronchodilators		
Theophylline	10–20 mg/L	IV: prior to IV bolus dose, 30 minutes after end of bolus dose, anytime during continuous infusion PO: peak: 2 hours after rapid-release product, 4 hours after sustained-release product Trough: Just before next dose
Miscellaneous		
Cyclosporine	50–150 ng/ml (whole blood, HPLC)	Trough: IV, PO: just before next dose

Advanced Cardiac Life Support Algorithms

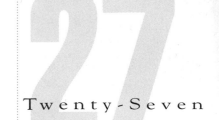

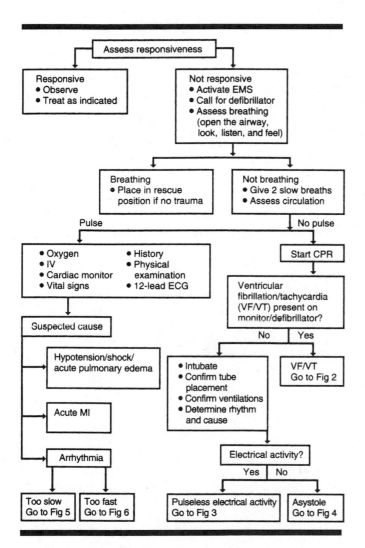

Figure 27–1. Universal Algorithm for Adult Emergency Cardiac Care (ECC).*

*All figures in this chapter from: Advanced cardiac life support: Part III. Journal of the American Medical Association. 1992;268:2216.

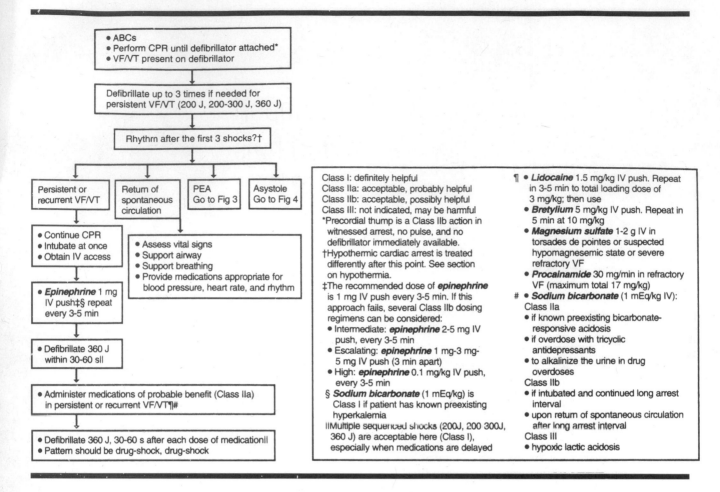

Figure 27–2. Algorithm for Ventricular Fibrillation and Pulseless Ventricular Tachycardia (VF/VT).

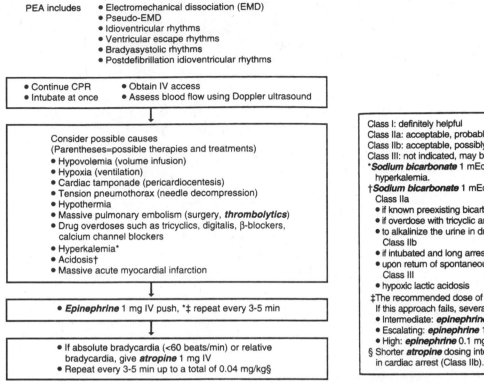

PEA includes
- Electromechanical dissociation (EMD)
- Pseudo-EMD
- Idioventricular rhythms
- Ventricular escape rhythms
- Bradyasystolic rhythms
- Postdefibrillation idioventricular rhythms

- Continue CPR
- Intubate at once
- Obtain IV access
- Assess blood flow using Doppler ultrasound

Consider possible causes
(Parentheses=possible therapies and treatments)
- Hypovolemia (volume infusion)
- Hypoxia (ventilation)
- Cardiac tamponade (pericardiocentesis)
- Tension pneumothorax (needle decompression)
- Hypothermia
- Massive pulmonary embolism (surgery, *thrombolytics*)
- Drug overdoses such as tricyclics, digitalis, β-blockers, calcium channel blockers
- Hyperkalemia*
- Acidosis†
- Massive acute myocardial infarction

- *Epinephrine* 1 mg IV push, *‡ repeat every 3-5 min

- If absolute bradycardia (<60 beats/min) or relative bradycardia, give *atropine* 1 mg IV
- Repeat every 3-5 min up to a total of 0.04 mg/kg§

Class I: definitely helpful
Class IIa: acceptable, probably helpful
Class IIb: acceptable, possibly helpful
Class III: not indicated, may be harmful
**Sodium bicarbonate* 1 mEq/kg is Class I if patient has known preexisting hyperkalemia.
†*Sodium bicarbonate* 1 mEq/kg:
   Class IIa
   - if known preexisting bicarbonate-responsive acidosis
   - if overdose with tricyclic antidepressants
   - to alkalinize the urine in drug overdoses
      Class IIb
   - if intubated and long arrest interval
   - upon return of spontaneous circulation after long arrest interval
      Class III
   - hypoxic lactic acidosis
‡The recommended dose of *epinephrine* is 1 mg IV push every 3-5 min. If this approach fails, several Class IIb dosing regimens can be considered.
   - Intermediate: *epinephrine* 2-5 mg IV push, every 3-5 min
   - Escalating: *epinephrine* 1 mg-3 mg-5 mg IV push (3 min apart)
   - High: *epinephrine* 0.1 mg/kg IV push, every 3-5 min
§ Shorter *atropine* dosing intervals are possibly helpful in cardiac arrest (Class IIb).

Figure 27-3. Algorithm for Pulseless Electrical Activity (PEA) (Electromechanical Dissociation [EMD]).

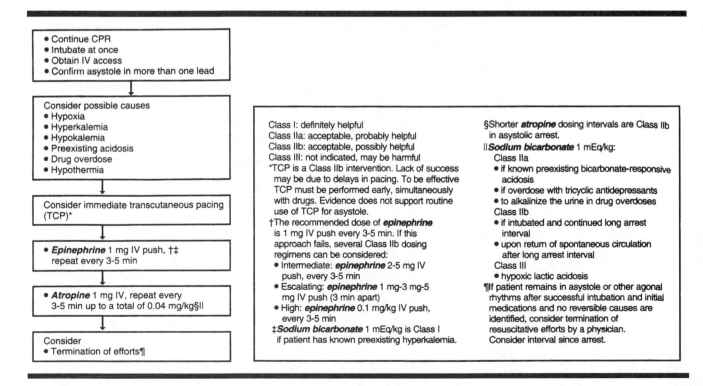

- Continue CPR
- Intubate at once
- Obtain IV access
- Confirm asystole in more than one lead

Consider possible causes
- Hypoxia
- Hyperkalemia
- Hypokalemia
- Preexisting acidosis
- Drug overdose
- Hypothermia

Consider immediate transcutaneous pacing (TCP)*

- *Epinephrine* 1 mg IV push, †‡ repeat every 3-5 min

- *Atropine* 1 mg IV, repeat every 3-5 min up to a total of 0.04 mg/kg§‖

Consider
- Termination of efforts¶

Class I: definitely helpful
Class IIa: acceptable, probably helpful
Class IIb: acceptable, possibly helpful
Class III: not indicated, may be harmful
*TCP is a Class IIb intervention. Lack of success may be due to delays in pacing. To be effective TCP must be performed early, simultaneously with drugs. Evidence does not support routine use of TCP for asystole.
†The recommended dose of *epinephrine* is 1 mg IV push every 3-5 min. If this approach fails, several Class IIb dosing regimens can be considered:
   - Intermediate: *epinephrine* 2-5 mg IV push, every 3-5 min
   - Escalating: *epinephrine* 1 mg-3 mg-5 mg IV push (3 min apart)
   - High: *epinephrine* 0.1 mg/kg IV push, every 3-5 min
‡*Sodium bicarbonate* 1 mEq/kg is Class I if patient has known preexisting hyperkalemia.

§Shorter *atropine* dosing intervals are Class IIb in asystolic arrest.
‖*Sodium bicarbonate* 1 mEq/kg:
   Class IIa
   - if known preexisting bicarbonate-responsive acidosis
   - if overdose with tricyclic antidepressants
   - to alkalinize the urine in drug overdoses
      Class IIb
   - if intubated and continued long arrest interval
   - upon return of spontaneous circulation after long arrest interval
      Class III
   - hypoxic lactic acidosis
¶If patient remains in asystole or other agonal rhythms after successful intubation and initial medications and no reversible causes are identified, consider termination of resuscitative efforts by a physician. Consider interval since arrest.

Figure 27-4. Asystole Treatment Algorithm.

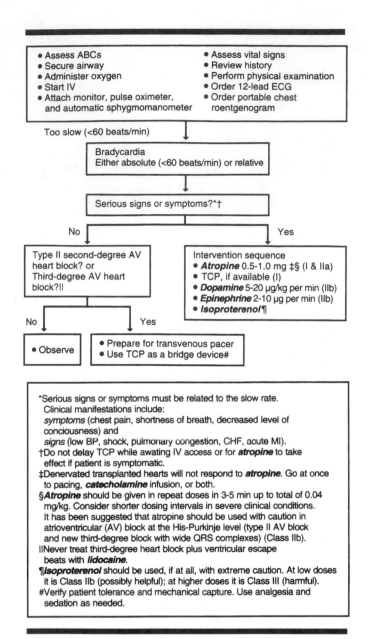

Figure 27–5. Bradycardia Algorithm (with the Patient Not in Cardiac Arrest).

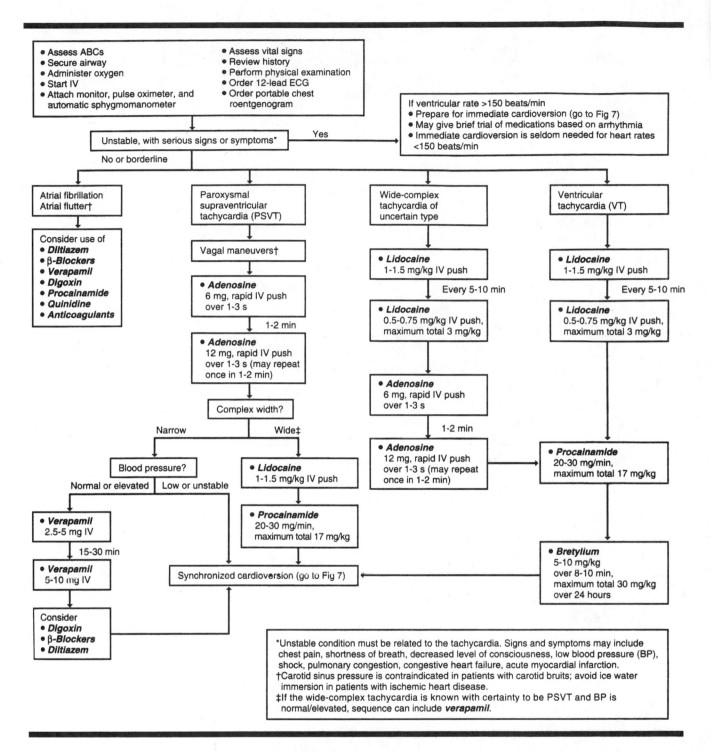

Figure 27–6. Tachycardia Algorithm.

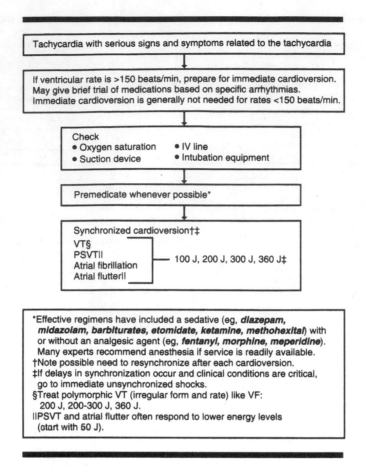

Tachycardia with serious signs and symptoms related to the tachycardia

If ventricular rate is >150 beats/min, prepare for immediate cardioversion.
May give brief trial of medications based on specific arrhythmias.
Immediate cardioversion is generally not needed for rates <150 beats/min.

Check
• Oxygen saturation   • IV line
• Suction device   • Intubation equipment

Premedicate whenever possible*

Synchronized cardioversion†‡
VT§
PSVT‖   100 J, 200 J, 300 J, 360 J‡
Atrial fibrillation
Atrial flutter‖

*Effective regimens have included a sedative (eg, *diazepam,
  midazolam, barbiturates, etomidate, ketamine, methohexital*) with
  or without an analgesic agent (eg, *fentanyl, morphine, meperidine*).
  Many experts recommend anesthesia if service is readily available.
†Note possible need to resynchronize after each cardioversion.
‡If delays in synchronization occur and clinical conditions are critical,
  go to immediate unsynchronized shocks.
§Treat polymorphic VT (irregular form and rate) like VF:
  200 J, 200-300 J, 360 J.
‖PSVT and atrial flutter often respond to lower energy levels
  (start with 50 J).

Figure 27–7. Electrical Cardioversion Algorithm (with the Patient Not in Cardiac Arrest).

Twenty-Eight

Alternative Therapies Table

BIOBEHAVIORAL COPING STRATEGIES

Relaxation Interventions

Relaxation is a psychophysiologic state characterized by a parasympathetic dominance involving multiple visceral and somatic systems and the absence of physical, mental, and emotional tension. Guide the patient in the use of one or several of the following interventions (Table 28-1).

Breathing Exercises

Teach breathing exercises in a simple manner, such as attend to the breath, inhale to the count of 4 and exhale to the count of 4; keep the upper chest still and allow the abdomen to fill with air; and on the exhale let the abdomen fall back to the spine.

Autogenics

Teach repetitions of self (auto)-generated (genic) suggestions, positive inner phrases, and dialogue that are said in the first person, present tense to create what is desired rather than what exists. Repeat this exercise for 10 minutes or longer. Pause for 15 seconds between phrases, and repeat each phrase three times. Start with a few relaxed abdominal breaths. The nurse says the words as the patient repeats silently:

"My right arm is warm and heavy."

"My right leg is warm and heavy."

"Heaviness and warmth are flowing through my body."

"My body breaths freely and easily."

"My heartbeat is calm and regular."

"My breathing is calm and relaxed."

"My mind is quiet and still."

"I am at peace."

Relaxation Response

Teach passive concentration on the slow repetition of a neutral word such as "one" that is repeated on the exhale.

Body Scanning

Focus on various parts of the body to detect areas of accumulated tension, such as accumulated tightness in the back and upper shoulders. With this awareness the patient then might use various breathing, relaxation, and imagery strategies to focus on the tense area to reverse or decrease the tension. Teach a system for scanning, such as a "head-to-toe" scan. The patient would start at the top of his or her head and go down the body to the feet. A systematic scan helps a patient learn deeper levels of inner awareness about where tension occurs in the body.

Prayer

Prayer is a fundamental, primordial, and important "language" humans speak. It is a way to connect to the spiritual core of healing, and may be directed or nondirected and said silently or aloud as a focusing device to evoke deep states of relaxation. Prayer helps us to enter a state where stress, crisis, and illness are experienced as a natural part of life, where acceptance transcends passivity.

General Relaxation Script

Introduction

Discuss the concept of relaxation with the patient. If the patient agrees to participate, proceed with the following:

1. Ask the patient to urinate, if necessary.
2. Dim the lights.
3. Close the drapes.
4. Ask the patient to remove eyeglasses or contact lenses.
5. Ask the patient to lie in a supine or semi-Fowler's position. It is sometimes helpful to place a small pillow under the knees to relieve lower back strain.

Give the patient the following instructions:

1. The purpose of the session is:
   - To relax in a wakeful state
   - To have a quiet, relaxing experience
2. First, I will guide you in a few breathing exercises to relax.
3. Then I will guide you in a head-to-toe relaxation session.
4. Then you will continue to relax for 20 minutes.
5. Now close your eyes (if you wish).
6. Find a comfortable position:
   - Hands at side of chest or on body—whatever is most comfortable
   - Legs uncrossed
7. At any time you may change positions, scratch, or swallow.
8. There may be noises around, but these will not be important if you concentrate on my voice.
9. Now think of relaxation:
   - Relax the body.
   - Relax the mind.
   - Allow yourself to let go of tension.
   - Allow relaxation to happen.
   - Do not strain for it, force it, or resist it.
10. I am going to guide you in relaxing.
11. To begin relaxing, take in three long, deep breaths. Breathe gently with your abdomen. This is the kind of relaxed breathing we do every night as we fall asleep. As you breathe in, let your stomach blow up like a balloon. As you exhale, let your stomach gently fall back to your spine.
12. Feel the relaxation coming over your body.
13. As you begin to relax, focus your attention on the top of your head. Let the muscles go; relax them and feel the relaxation moving in.
14. Let the relaxation flow to your forehead, temples, eyebrows, eyelids, and eyes—let go of the muscles; feel the relaxation and warmth.
15. Let the relaxation flow to your cheeks, lips, chin, and jaw:
    - Let your jaw drop down a little.
    - Let your lips part a little.
    - Let your tongue relax; just let it puddle in your mouth.
16. Relax these muscles; your whole face feels heavy, warm, and relaxed.
17. Let the relaxation flow down your throat, neck, shoulders, upper arms, elbows, lower arms, fingers, and fingertips:
    - Let these muscles hang heavy, loose, limp, and relaxed.
    - Notice how heavy and warm both arms feel; these are signs of relaxation. You might even

experience a slight tingling, which is also a sign of relaxation.
18. Focus your attention on your back, spine, waist, and buttocks:
    - Smooth out these muscles, and let go of any tension.
    - Feel the relaxation and heaviness and warmth. Allow yourself to feel the bed supporting you—just let go.
19. Let the relaxation flow around to the side of your chest, abdomen, and waist; relax the muscles, and feel the relaxation, warmth, and heaviness.
20. Concentrate on your thighs, knees, calves, ankles, feet, and toes; feel how heavy your legs are, how comfortably heavy, warm, and relaxed.
21. Feel the relaxation from the top of your head to your toes:
    - Be relaxed, peacefully calm.
    - Be very quiet, silent, and relaxed.
22. Feel this relaxation flowing through your body. If there are any places in your body that are still tense, move them a little bit, and relax them.
23. Now, as you continue to relax, select a word such as the word "one" or "relax." With each exhale say the word "one" silently to yourself. Focus all of your attention on your breathing and on the word "one."
24. If a distracting thought occurs, acknowledge the passing thought. Let it go and return your concentration on your breathing and the word "one."
25. Continue this exercise for the next 20 minutes and allow the experience to relax you even more than you already are now.
26. I will be leaving the room now and will quietly come back in 20 minutes.
27. At that time, I will guide you in counting back from 5 to 1. You will come back into the room easily and quietly. You will feel very relaxed, calm, and peaceful.
28. Now continue to relax your body and your mind.

Imagery Interventions

Imagery is information gained through sensory modes—visual, auditory, olfactory, gustatory, tactile, and kinesthetic—a bridge between conscious processing of information and physiologic change where a person chooses to create healing images (see Table 28-2 for imagery interventions). The following are various types of imagery:

- *Receptive:* "Bubbles up," as if one received images. Go inward: listen to body-mind.
- *Active:* Conscious formation of image. Direct image: body area or activity that requires attention.
- *Concrete:* Real life: under the microscope. Biologic correctness.

TABLE 28–1. IMPLEMENTATION AND EVALUATION OF RELAXATION INTERVENTIONS

Patient Outcomes	Implementation	Evaluation
The patient will demonstrate decreased anxiety, tension, and other manifestations of the stress response as a result of the relaxation intervention.	Guide the patient in the relaxation exercise. Evaluate for decrease in anxiety, tension, and other manifestations of the stress response as evidenced by heart rate within normal limits, decreased respiratory rate, return of blood pressure toward normal, resolution of anxious behaviors such as anxious facial expressions and mannerisms, repetitive talking or behavior, inability to sleep, or restlessness.	The patient exhibited decreased anxiety, tension, and other manifestations of the stress response as evidenced by normal vital signs; slow, deep breathing pattern; and decreased anxious behaviors.
The patient will demonstrate a stabilization or decrease in pain as a result of the relaxation intervention.	Evaluate for decrease in pain as evidenced by reduction or elimination of pain control medication and increase in activities or mobility.	The patient's intake of pain medication stabilized and then decreased with relaxation skills practice. The patient began to participate in activities previously limited by pain.
The patient will link breathing awareness to a commonly occurring cue and use this combination to reduce tension.	Teach awareness of breathing patterns and habitual linking of relaxing breathing to a cue in the environment.	The patient used turning in bed as a cue to take a slow, deep breath and to relax jaw muscles.

From: Dossey B, Keegan L, Guzzetta C, Kolkmeier L: Holistic nursing: A handbook for practice, *2nd ed. Gaithersburg, MD: Aspen, 1995.*

- *Symbolic:* Metamorphosis: personal energy of a person. Can't be forced.
- *Process:* Step-by-step goal to be achieved. Mechanics of biologic correct images.
- *End stage:* Image final healed state to follow process imagery.
- *General healing:* An event, healing light, forgiveness, inner guide/advisor.
- *Packaged:* Commercial tapes that have general images.
- *Customized:* Images that bubble up. Become personalized by a person.

General Breathing Imagery Script

1. Guide the patient in how to integrate breathing with imagery suggestions and to become aware of how images may involve one or more of the senses.
2. Image the body as hollow and allow each breath to fill the hollow body slowly with relaxation.
3. In the mind's eye, see the breath as a soft color and breathe that color into all parts of the body.
4. Breathe and feel relaxation move up one side of the body and down the other side; breathe and feel the relaxation move up the front of the body and down the back; breathe and feel the relaxation move up through the soles of the feet and relax the inside of the body; breathe and feel the relaxation move down from the top of the head, over the skin, and back into the feet.

General Imagery Variations

To vary the general imagery script, begin with a head-to-toe relaxation session and add on one of the following modifications:

1. Let your imagination choose a place that is safe and comfortable . . . a place where you can retreat at any time. This is a healthy technique for you to learn . . . this place will help you survive your daily stressors. This safe and special place is very important, particularly while you are in the hospital.
2. Form a clear image of a pleasant outdoor scene, using all of your senses. Smell . . . smell the fragrance of flowers or the breeze. Feel . . . feel the texture of the surface under your feet. Hear . . . hear all the sounds in nature, birds singing, wind blowing. See . . . see all the different sights around as you let yourself turn in a slow circle to get a full view of this special place. (Include taste if appropriate.)
3. Let a beam of light, such as the rays of the sun, shine on you for comfort and healing. Allow yourself to experience the warmth and relaxation.
4. Form an image of a meadow. Imagine that you are in the meadow. . . . The meadow is full of beautiful grass and flowers. In the meadow, see yourself sitting by a stream . . . watching the water . . . flowing by . . . slowly and gently.
5. Imagine a mountain scene. See yourself walking on a path toward the mountain. You hear the sound of your shoes on the path . . . smell the pine trees . . . feel the cool breeze as you approach your campsite in the mountain. You are now higher up the mountain. . . resting in your campsite. Look around at the beauty of this place.
6. Imagine yourself in a bamboo forest. . . . You are walking in a large bamboo forest. The bamboo is very tall. . . . You lean against a strong cluster of bamboo . . . hear the swaying . . . and hear the

TABLE 28–2. IMPLEMENTATION AND EVALUATION OF IMAGERY INTERVENTIONS

Patient Outcomes	Implementation	Evaluation
The patient will demonstrate skills in imagery.	Following an assessment, guide the patient in an imagery exercise.	The patient participated in the imagery exercise by choice.
	Assess the patient's levels of anxiety with this new process	The patient demonstrated no signs of anxiety with the imagery process.
	After the imagery process experience, assess effectiveness through patient dialogue.	The patient stated that the imagery experience was helpful.
	Encourage the patient to recognize daily self-talk and the images that lead to balance and inner peace.	
	Help the patient to create images of desired health habits, feelings, and desires for daily living.	The patient reported creating images of desired health habits, feelings, and desires for daily living.
	Teach the patient coping power over daily events and ability to move toward a healthy life style.	The patient reported increased coping with daily stressors.
	Teach the patient to recognize images leading to self-defeating lifestyle habits.	The patient reported recognition of negative images leading to self-defeating behavior; the patient created positive images.
The patient will participate in drawing, if appropriate.	Encourage the patient to draw images and symbols as a communication process with self.	The patient used drawing as a communication process with self.

From: Dossey B, Keegan L, Guzzetta C, Kolkmeier L: Holistic nursing: A handbook for practice, 2nd ed. Gaithersburg, MD: Aspen, 1995.

rustling of the bamboo leaves, gently moving in the wind.

7. Look into the sky of your mind . . . see the fluffy clouds. A cloud gently comes your way . . . and the cloud surrounds your body. You climb up on the cloud and lie down. Feel yourself begin to float off gently in a gentle breeze.

Music Therapy

Music therapy is the systematic use of music to produce relaxation and desired change in behaviors, emotions, and physiology. Let the patient choose music from an audiocassette library (see Chapter 8, Alternative Therapies). See Table 28-3 for music therapy interventions.

General Music Therapy Script

Introduction

Discuss the concept of relaxation and music therapy with the patient. If the patient agrees to participate, follow the General Relaxation Script (Steps 1 through 22) and then proceed with the following:

Music Tapes

1. Now, as you continue to relax, I will turn on the music.
2. Listen to the music:
   - Tell yourself that you would like to go wherever the music takes you.
   - Allow yourself to follow the music.
   - Let the music suggest to you what to think and what to feel.
   - Do not try to analyze the music.
   - If you find distracting thoughts occurring, simply let them go and return all of your concentration back to the music.
   - Allow the music to relax you even more than you are now.
3. The music will play for 20 minutes, and I will leave the room.
4. I will quietly come back into the room before the music is over.
5. When the music is over, I will guide you in counting back from 5 to 1. You will come back into the room easily and quietly. You will feel very relaxed, calm, and peaceful.
6. Now continue to relax your body and your mind; let the music help you.

Music Script Variations

To vary the general music therapy script, begin with a head-to-toe relaxation session and add on one of the following modifications:

1. Allow yourself to receive a music bath. Let yourself be immersed in the musical sounds as if you were in a warm tub of water or standing under the warm water in a shower.
2. Let the music take you to a peaceful place. Become aware of the images of this place, such as textures, colors, and fragrances.

TABLE 28–3. IMPLEMENTATION AND EVALUATION OF MUSIC THERAPY INTERVENTIONS

Patient Outcomes	Implementation	Evaluation
The patient will select the music of choice and will participate in music therapy sessions to achieve a relaxed response and facilitate healing.	Provide the patient with various taped musical selections to facilitate selecting the music of choice. Guide the patient in music therapy sessions and help the patient to establish the routine of listening to music once or twice a day.	The patient chose the music of choice for listening and reported enjoying the music. The patient participated in music therapy sessions twice a day to facilitate healing.
The patient will demonstrate positive physiologic outcomes in response to the music therapy session, such as decreased respiratory rate, heart rate, blood pressure, muscle tension, and fatigue.	Assess the patient's physiologic outcomes in response to music therapy before and immediately after the session. Evaluate the patient's respiratory rate, heart rate, blood pressure, muscle tension, and fatigue.	The patient demonstrated decreased respiratory rate, heart rate, blood pressure, muscle tension, and fatigue.
The patient will demonstrate positive psychologic outcomes in response to the music therapy session such as: • positive emotions and relaxed feeling • decreased restlessness and agitation • decreased anxiety/depression • increased motivation • increased nonverbal expression of feelings • increased positive imagery • decreased isolation	Assess the patient's psychologic outcomes in response to music therapy before and immediately after the session. Evaluate the patient's: • emotions and level of relaxation • level of restlessness and agitation • level of anxiety/depression • level of motivation • ability to express feelings nonverbally • types of imagery experienced • level of social isolation	The patient demonstrated: • positive emotions and more relaxed feeling • reduced restlessness and agitation • decreased levels of anxiety (or depression) • increased motivation • increased nonverbal expression of feelings • increased positive imagery • decreased feelings of social isolation

Dossey B, Keegan L, Guzzetta C, Kolkmeier L. Holistic nursing: A handbook for practice, *2nd ed. Gaithersburg, MD: Aspen, 1995.*

3. Permit your ears to be large channels that run from the side of your head all the way to your toes. Allow the sounds of the music to flow into every cell in your body-mind-spirit.

4. Use your own voice as music. Begin with a spontaneous audible groan that you might make when you take off a tight belt or tight shoes, such as "ohhh" or "ahhh." Allow this healing groan to go as deep as possible without forcing it and feel the voice vibra-

tions in your body. The voice will change frequencies until your body finds its right healing tone.

Touch Therapies

Touch is done to diagnose, monitor, or treat the symptoms or illness itself; touch may focus on the end result of curing, decreasing, or stabilizing symptoms or illness, or preventing further complications. See Table 28-4 for touch interventions.

TABLE 28–4. IMPLEMENTATION AND EVALUATION OF TOUCH INTERVENTIONS

Patient Outcomes	Implementation	Evaluation
The patient will exhibit relaxation following a touch therapy session.	Encourage the patient to receive touch therapy in order to evoke the relaxation response. During the touch therapy session, help the patient decrease anxiety and fear, decrease pulse and respiratory rate, recognize a feeling of body-mind relaxation, develop a sense of general well-being, increase effectiveness in individual coping skills, increase a sense of belonging and lessened loneliness, and feel less alone and express that feeling.	The patient exhibited decreased anxiety and fear, demonstrated a decrease in pulse and respiratory rate, reported muscle relaxation, exhibited a satisfied facial expression and expressed inner calmness, and reported greater satisfaction in individual coping patterns.
The patient will demonstrate improved circulation.	Provide the patient with information about how touch therapies improve circulation and tissue perfusion.	Patients with light skin had a reddened color in the area where the nurse had used effleurage and petrosauge massage strokes. Skin in the massage area was warmer than before the therapy.
The patient will request touch therapy to maintain and enhance health.	Encourage the patient to ask for touch therapy. Suggest that the patient seek out the nurse. Recommend that the patient accept touch when offered by the nurse.	The patient asked for touch therapy.

Dossey B, Keegan L, Guzzetta C, Kolkmeier L: Holistic nursing: A handbook for practice, *2nd ed. Gaithersburg, MD: Aspen, 1995.*

- *Acupressure:* The application of finger and/or thumb pressure to specific sites along the body's energy meridians for the purpose of relieving tension and reestablishing the flow of energy along the meridian lines.
- *Foot reflexology:* The application of pressure to points on the feet that correspond to other parts of the body.
- *Shiatzu:* The use of the thumb and/or heel of the hand for deep pressure work along the energy meridian lines.
- *Therapeutic massage:* The use of the hands to apply deep pressure and motion on the skin and underlying muscles of the recipient for the purposes of physical and psychologic relaxation, improvement of circulation, relief of sore muscles, and other therapeutic effects, such as in giving or receiving a therapeutic back rub.
- *Therapeutic touch:* A specific technique of centering intention used while the practitioner moves the hands through the recipient's energy field for the purposes of assessing and treating energy field imbalance.

EMOTIONAL COPING STRATEGIES

Humor

Encourage the patient to use the creative faculty of discovering, expressing, or appreciating wit and comedy; using funny movies, video and audiotapes, or books can lead to laughter.

Interaction With Others

Ask the patient to identify in his or her imagination people who can best help with coping, as well as those who do not. If certain individuals make the patient feel sick or depressed, limit contact. Have family, friends, or clergy visit during hospital visiting hours or by phone.

Journals and Letters

Have the patient record factual or subjective interpretations of events, thoughts, feelings, and plans. These provide patient insight about imagery and thought processes, and may help the patient to give up those things for which one has no control.

Frustration of Environmental Events/Stimuli

Help the patient identify events and stimuli that are frustrating. Offering simple clarification of equipment and routines can decrease the anxiety-apprehension situations and alleviate further anxiety. Incorporate rehearsal and imagery exercises for reducing these stressors and situations in the imagination.

Denial

Give the patient permission to deny or suppress the effects of illness and hospitalization with which the patient cannot cope. Tell the patient it is okay to ignore the things one can't handle at the time. Have patient rehearse this in the imagination. This adaptive denial can reduce feelings of anxiety in patients with severe illness.

Anger and Fear

Encourage adaptive displacement through healthy, verbal expression of emotions to staff, family members, or friends. Use these situations in imagery scripts to help patients focus on their strengths, spiritual beliefs, family, or interests. Help patients list problems and situations in the imagination from the most to the least urgent. Assist with the immediate solutions for the most urgent problems, help identify those that can wait or be delegated, and encourage letting go of those beyond the patient's control.

COGNITIVE COPING STRATEGIES

Reframing

Help the patient identify undesired behaviors and thoughts and replace them with pleasant thoughts, situations, or images directed towards positive outcomes that can simultaneously inhibit unpleasant realities. For example, help a surgical patient who says that he or she doesn't have time for surgery to see hospitalization as only 4 days within that person's year.

Redefinition

When a patient takes on a victim role, encourage the patient to become an actor and rehearse a situation with confidence and control (e.g., rehearse in the imagination and become an actor who signed the operative permit and who has contracted with a surgeon to perform an important operation). When patients assume responsibility, anxiety decreases because individuals experience the self as in control and making important decisions.

Self-Hypnosis and Self-Talk

Help the patient identify constant internal dialogue during anxiety. Often it is the negative images of self-talk or internal conversation that impede the healing process. For example, a patient may say, "All I think about is the pain: I can't stand this any longer." The nurse can help the patient to change the dialogue to "I can be with this pain. My relaxation and imagery will help me work with the pain medicine."

Contracts

Ask the patient to identify and image small steps as follows: What changes are most wanted at this time? What is the first step? By what time today should an event occur? What reward can be given? How will life be different? How can the nurse help?

Assertiveness

A patient might complain that the doctor, nurse, or family member is forcing them to do something against their will, thereby increasing anxiety. The nurse can encourage the patient to rehearse in the imagination being assertive and asking questions until the situation is better understood.

Limit Setting

Ask the patient to image placing limits on what is tolerable and what is not. This empowers the patient to be more capable of being active in the decision making and become more involved in self-care.

PHYSICAL COPING STRATEGIES

Exercise

Suggest mild to moderate exercise depending on patient's condition, such as a walk down the hall corridors and stretching exercises; if the patient is confined to bed, use modified upper body stretching with lower leg exercises.

Healthy Eating

Have the patient make healthy food and snack choices according to the prescribed diet.

Stimulants

Have the patient reduce caffeine intake; substitute with herbal teas, water, and juices.

Therapeutic Touch/Massage

Schedule therapeutic touch or massages one or twice a day.

Handicrafts

Suggest that the patient get involved in needlepoint, knitting, playing cards, or solving puzzles.

Self-care Activities

Have the patient take a warm bath or shower and practice rhythmic breathing while bathing. Reinforce when the patient takes an active role in self-care activities.

Guidelines for the Transfer of Critically Ill Patients*

TRANSFERS WITHIN THE HOSPITAL

Transport Personnel and Equipment Requirements

Personnel

- A minimum of two people should accompany the patient.
- One of the accompanying personnel should be the critical care nurse assigned to the patient or a specifically trained critical care transfer nurse. This critical care nurse should have completed a competency-based orientation and meet the described standards for critical care nurses.
- Additional personnel may include a respiratory therapist, registered nurse, critical care technician, or physician. A respiratory therapist should accompany all patients requiring mechanical ventilation.

Equipment

The following minimal equipment should be available:

- Cardiac monitor/defibrillator
- Airway management equipment and resuscitation bag of proper size and fit for the patient
- Oxygen source of ample volume to support the patient's needs for the projected time out of the ICU, with an additional 30-minute reserve
- Standard resuscitation drugs: epinephrine, lidocaine, atropine
- Blood pressure cuff (sphygmomanometer) and stethoscope
- Ample supply of the IV fluids and continuous drip medications (regulated by battery-operated infusion pumps) being administered to the patient

- Additional medications to provide the patient's scheduled intermittent medication doses and to meet anticipated needs (e.g., sedation) with appropriate orders to allow their administration if a physician is not present
- For patients receiving mechanical support of ventilation, a device capable of delivering the same volume, pressure, and PEEP and an FiO_2 equal to or greater than what the patient is receiving in the ICU. For practical reasons, in adults an FiO_2 of 1.0 is most feasible during transfer because this eliminates the need for an air tank and air-oxygen blender. During neonatal transfer, FiO_2 should be precisely controlled.
- Resuscitation cart and suction equipment need not accompany each patient being transferred, but such equipment should be stationed in areas used by critically ill patients and be readily available (within 4 minutes) by a predetermined mechanism for emergencies that may occur en route.

Monitoring During Transfer

- If technologically possible, patients being transported should receive the same physiological monitoring during transfer that they were receiving in the ICU.
- Minimally, all critically ill patients being transferred must have continuous monitoring of ECG and pulse oximetry and intermittent measurement and documentation of blood pressure, respiratory rate, and pulse rate.
- In addition, selected patients, based on clinical status, may benefit from monitoring by capnography; continuous measurement of blood pressure, PAP,

*From: American Association of Critical Care Nurses: AACN's guidelines for the transfer of critically ill patients. Aliso Viejo, CA: AACN, 1993.

and ICP; and intermittent measurement of CVP, Pao, and CO.

- Intubated patients receiving mechanical support of ventilation should have airway pressure monitored. If a transfer ventilator is used, it should have alarms to indicate disconnects or excessively high airway pressures.

Pretransfer Coordination and Communication

- Physician-to-physician and/or nurse-to-nurse communication regarding the patient's condition and treatment preceding and following the transfer should be documented in the medical record when the management of the patient will be assumed by a different team while the patient is away from the ICU.
- The area to which the patient is being transferred (X-ray, operating room, nuclear medicine, etc.) must confirm that it is ready to receive the patient and immediately begin the procedure or test for which the patient is being transferred.
- Ancillary services (e.g., security, respiratory therapy, escort) must be notified as to the timing of the transfer and the equipment and support needed.
- The responsible physician must be notified either to accompany the patient or to be aware that the patient is out of the ICU at this time and may have an acute event requiring the physician's response to provide emergency care in another area of the hospital.
- Documentation in the medical record must include the indication for transfer, the patient's status during transfer, and whether the patient is expected to return to the ICU.

TRANSFERS BETWEEN HOSPITALS

Transport Personnel, Medication, and Equipment Requirements

Personnel

- A minimum of two people, in addition to the vehicle operator, should accompany the patient.
- One of the accompanying personnel should be a registered nurse, physician or advanced EMT capable of providing advanced airway management, including endotracheal intubation, intravenous therapy, arrhythmia interpretation and treatment, and basic and advanced cardiac and trauma life support.
- When a physician does not accompany the patient, there should be a mechanism available to communi-

cate with a physician regarding the patient's condition. Standing orders should be authorized if direct communication is not possible.

Medication Requirements

Transfer medications include drugs for advanced cardiac resuscitation, the management of acute physiologic derangements, and the specific needs of that patient (e.g., sedatives, analgesics, antibiotics).

The following is a complete list of transfer medications:

Bristojets
(1) Dextrose 50%/50 ml
(1) calcium chloride 1 gm/10 ml
(2) atropine sulfate 1 mg/10 ml
(2) lidocaine 100 mg/10 ml
(1) lidocaine 2 gm/10 ml
(4) sodium bicarbonate 50 mEq/50 ml
(4) epinephrine 1:10,000/10 ml
(1) Cetacaine spray
(10) Dextrostix
(1) potassium chloride 20 mEq/10 ml
(2) verapamil hydrochloride 5 mg/2 ml (Calan, Isoptin)
(1) nitroglycerin tablets 0.4 mg/tablet
(1) nitroprusside 50 mg/vial (Nipride)
(1) heparin sodium 1000 units/ml
(2) dexamethasone 20 mg/ml, 5 ml vial (Decadron)
(1) diphenhydramine hydrochloride 50 mg/ml (Benadryl)
(1) phytonadione (AquaMEPHYTON) 10 mg/ml (vitamin K)
(1) digoxin .25 mg/ml (Lanoxin)
(2) propranolol 1 mg/ml (Inderal)
(2) naloxone hydrochloride 2.0 mg/2 ml vial (Narcan)
(1) procainamide 100 mg/ml—10 ml total (Pronestyl)
(3) epinephrine 1:1000 ampules
(2) bretylium tosylate 500 mg/10 ml (Bretylol)
(2) phenytoin sodium 250 mg/5 ml—20 ml total (Dilantin)
(1) furosemide 100 mg/10 ml (Lasix)
(1) mannitol 12.5 gm/50 ml, 50–100 gm/50 ml
(1) nitroglycerin vial 5 mg/ml
(1) aminophylline 500 mg/20 ml
(2) dopamine 200 mg/5 ml (Intropin)
(1) isoproterenol 1 mg/5 ml (Isuprel)
(1) normal saline 30 ml
(1) sterile water 10 ml
(2) adenosine 6 mg/2 ml (Adenocard)
narcotics, sedatives, neuromuscular paralyzing agents added, based on anticipated patient need

Equipment

The following *minimal* equipment should be available:

- Cardiac monitor/defibrillator
- Airway management equipment and resuscitation bag of proper size and fit for the patient
- Oxygen source of ample volume to support the patient's needs for the projected time out of the ICU, with an additional 30-minute reserve
- Standard resuscitation drugs: epinephrine, lidocaine, atropine
- Blood pressure cuff (sphygmomanometer) and stethoscope

- Materials for intravenous therapy including cannulas, solutions, tubing, needles and syringes, and devices for regulation of continuous intravenous infusions
- Spinal immobilization devices
- Communication equipment to allow contact between the transporting vehicle and the referring and receiving hospitals

Table 29–1 is a complete list of transfer equipment.

TABLE 29–1. TRANSFER EQUIPMENT

Airway Management—Adult and Pediatric

(1) adult bag—valve system with oxygen reservoir
(1) end tidal CO_2 monitor
(1) PEEP valve
(1) small pediatric mask
(1) medium pediatric mask
(1) large pediatric mask
(1) small adult mask
(1) medium adult mask
(1) large adult mask
(2) O_2 tubing
(1) 50-ml flex tube with patient adapter
(1) pediatric bag—valve system with oxygen reservoir
(1) pressure gauge with airway adapter tubing and test lung
(1) tonsil suction
(2) #T–63 5/6 French suction catheters
(2) #5 suction catheters
(2) #8 suction catheters
(2) #10 suction catheters
(2) #14 suction catheters
(1) nasal cannula

Arterial Line Tubing and Monitoring Equipment

(3) three-way pressure stopcocks
(1) 6-ft pressure tubing
(1) 1-ft pressure tubing
(1) flush system
(1) adaptor tubing
(1) mercury manometer
(1) roll 1/2" adhesive tape
(1) roll 2" adhesive tape
(1) roll 2" Elastoplast tape

Syringes

(6) 1 cc TB
(3) 3 cc with 20-gauge needle
(3) 3 cc with 22-gauge needle
(3) 5 cc
(3) 10 cc
(2) 60 cc

Alcohol Wipes

IV Catheters

(2) #14
(2) #16
(2) #18
(2) #20
(2) #22
(2) #24
(2) #22 (1 inch)
(2) #24 (1.6 cm)

Butterfly Needles

(2) #23
(2) #25

Intubation Kit

(1) #1 Macintosh blade
(1) #2 Macintosh blade
(1) #3 Macintosh blade
(1) #4 Macintosh blade
(1) #0 Miller blade
(1) #1 Miller blade
(1) #2 Miller blade
(1) pediatric laryngoscope handle
(1) pediatric ET stylet
(1) adult ET stylet
(1) roll 1" adhesive tape
(1) wrist restraints
(1) Heimlich valve
(1) pediatric Magil forceps

(1) adult Magil forceps
(2) 10-cc syringes
(1) booted hemostat
(1) #2.5 uncuffed ET tube
(1) #3.0 uncuffed ET tube
(1) #3.5 uncuffed ET tube
(1) #4.0 uncuffed ET tube
(1) #4.5 uncuffed ET tube
(1) #5.0 uncuffed ET tube
(1) pair disposable scissors
(4) water-soluble lubricant
(1) #26 nasopharyngeal airway
(1) #30 nasopharyngeal airway
(1) #0 oral airway
(1) #1 oral airway
(1) #2 oral airway
(1) #3 oral airway
(1) #4 oral airway
(1) #5.0 cuffed ET tube
(1) #5.5 cuffed ET tube
(1) #6.0 cuffed ET tube
(1) #6.5 cuffed ET tube
(1) #7.0 cuffed ET tube
(1) #7.5 cuffed ET tube
(1) #8.0 cuffed ET tube
(1) scalpel with blade for cricothyroidotomy
(1) infant medium concentration mask with tubing
(1) pediatric rebreather mask
(1) adult rebreather mask
(1) adult Venturi mask

Dressing Sponges

(4) surgical combines
(8) 2 × 2 sponges
(8) 4 × 4 sponges
(1) 3" Kling
(1) Kerlix

continued

TABLE 29–1. TRANSFER EQUIPMENT (cont.)

IV Administration Sets

(3) regular (macro) drip administration sets
(3) mini (pediatric) drip administration sets
(2) Y-blood tubing drip sets
(5) three-way stopcocks with extensions

IV Solutions

(2) 1,000 ml normal saline
(2) 1,000 ml Ringer's lactate
(2) 500 ml normal saline
(4) 250 ml D_5W
(4) 360 ml D_5 1/2NS
(4) 250 ml D_5 1/4NS

Arm Boards

(1) short arm board
(1) pediatric arm board

Nasogastric Tubes

(1) #10 NG Tube
(1) #14 NG Tube
(1) #18 NG Tube
(1) catheter tip (60-cc) irrigating syringe
(4) blood pump bags
(1) 250-ml bottle normal saline for irrigation
(1) set pediatric electrodes
(1) set adult electrodes
(1) tube electrode jelly
(1) neonatal BP cuff
(1) infant BP cuff
(1) child BP cuff
(1) adult BP cuff
(1) stethoscope
(1) pair trauma scissors
(1) rubber tourniquets
(1) tube Betadine ointment
(1) roll 1" adhesive tape
(1) Kelly clamp

Needles

(6) 19-gauge needles
(6) 20-gauge needles
(6) 22-gauge needles
(6) 25-gauge needles
(1) bone marrow needle

Equipment

external pacemaker
monitor/defibrillator
transport ventilator
suction apparatus
MAST—adult and pediatric
spinal immobilization device
pulse oximeter
infusion pumps
neonatal isolette (if appropriate for mission)

Monitoring During Transfer

- All critically ill patients being transferred should have continuous ECG monitoring as a minimal level of monitoring.
- Intermittent measurement of blood pressure, respiratory rate, and pulse rate should be done and documented.
- Continuous monitoring of pulse oximetry is strongly recommended.

- Selected patients, based on clinical status, may benefit from monitoring by capnography; continuous measurement of blood pressure, measurement of CVP, PAP, or ICP; and/or end tidal CO_2.
- Intubated patients receiving mechanical support of ventilation should have airway pressure monitored. If a transfer ventilator is used, it should have alarms to indicate disconnects or excessively high airway pressures.

Transfer Algorithm

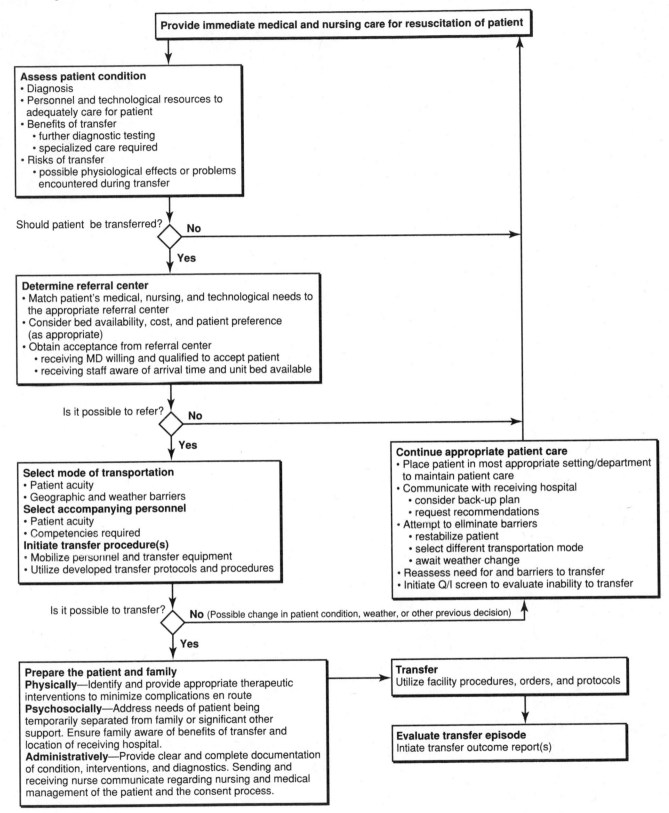

(From: American Association of Critical Care Nurses: AACN's guidelines for the transfer of critically ill patients. Aliso Viejo, CA: AACN, 1993.

Hemodynamic Monitoring Troubleshooting Guide

Thirty

30

TABLE 30-1. PROBLEMS ENCOUNTERED WITH ARTERIAL CATHETERS

Problem	Cause	Prevention	Treatment
Hematoma after withdrawal of needle	Bleeding or oozing at puncture site	Maintain firm pressure on site during withdrawal of catheter and for 5-15 minutes (as necessary) after withdrawal. Apply elastic tape (Elastoplast) firmly over puncture site. For femoral arterial puncture sites, leave a sandbag on site for 1-2 hours to prevent oozing. If patient is receiving heparin, discontinue 2 hours before catheter removal.	Continue to hold pressure to puncture site until oozing stops. Apply sandbag to femoral puncture site for 1-2 hours after removal of catheter.
Decreased or absent pulse distal to puncture site	Spasm of artery; Thrombosis of artery	Introduce arterial needle cleanly, nontraumatically. Use 1 U heparin/1 ml IV fluid.	Inject lidocaine locally at insertion site and 10 mg into arterial catheter. Arteriotomy and Fogarty catheterization both distally and proximally from the puncture site result in return of pulse in more than 90% of cases if brachial or femoral artery is used.
Bleedback into tubing, dome, or transducer	Insufficient pressure on IV bag	Maintain 300 mm Hg pressure on IV bag.	Replace transducer. "Fast flush" through system.
Hemorrhage	Loose connections; Loose connections	Use Luer-Lok stopcocks; tighten periodically. Keep all connecting sites visible. Observe connecting sites frequently. Use built-in alarm system. Use Luer-Lok stopcocks.	Tighten all connections. Tighten all connections.
Emboli	Clot from catheter tip into bloodstream	Always aspirate and discard before flushing. Use continuous flush device. Use 1 U heparin/1 ml IV fluid. Gently flush <2-4 ml.	Remove catheter.
Local infection	Forward movement of contaminated catheter; Break in sterile technique; Prolonged catheter use	Carefully suture catheter at insertion site. Always use aseptic technique. Remove catheter after 72-96 hours. Leave dressing in place until catheter is removed, changed, or dressing becomes damp, loosened, or soiled.	Remove catheter. Prescribe antibiotic.
Sepsis	Break in sterile technique; Prolonged catheter use; Bacterial growth in IV fluid	Use percutaneous insertion. Always use aseptic technique. Remove catheter after 72-96 hours. Change IV fluid bag, stopcocks, dome, and tubing no more frequently than at 72 hour intervals. Do not use IV fluid containing glucose. Use sterile dead-end caps on all ports of stopcocks. Carefully flush remaining blood from stopcocks after blood sampling.	Remove catheter. Prescribe antibiotic.

From: Daily E, Schroeder J: Techniques in bedside hemodynamic monitoring, *5th ed. St. Louis, MO: CV Mosby, 1994, pp. 165-166.*

TABLE 30–2. INACCURATE ARTERIAL PRESSURE MEASUREMENTS

Problem	Cause	Prevention	Treatment
Damped pressure tracing	Catheter tip against vessel wall	Usually cannot be avoided.	Pull back, rotate, or reposition catheter while observing pressure waveform.
	Partial occlusion of catheter tip by clot	Use continuous drip under pressure. Briefly "fast flush" after blood withdrawal (2-4 ml). Add 1 U heparin/1 ml IV fluid.	Aspirate clot with syringe and flush with heparinized saline (<2-4 ml).
	Clot in stopcock or transducer	Carefully flush catheter after blood withdrawal and reestablish IV drip. Use continuous flush device.	Flush stopcock and transducer; if no improvement, change stopcock and transducer.
	Air bubbles in transducer or connector tubing	Carefully flush transducer and tubing when setting up system and attaching to catheter.	Check system; flush rapidly; disconnect transducer and flush out air bubbles.
	Compliant tubing	Use stiff, short tubing.	Shorten tubing or replace softer tubing with stiffer tubing.
Abnormally high or low readings	Change in transducer air-reference level	Maintain air-reference port of transducer at midchest and/or catheter tip level for serial pressure measurements.	Recheck patient and transducer positions.
No pressure available	Transducer not open to catheter	Follow routine, systematic steps for setting up system and turning stopcocks.	Check system—stopcocks, monitor, and amplifier setup.
	Settings on monitor amplifiers incorrect—still on zero, cal, or off		
	Incorrect scale selection	Select scale appropriate to expected range of physiologic signal.	Select appropriate scale.

From: Daily E, Schroeder J: Techniques in bedside hemodynamic monitoring, 5th ed. St. Louis, MO: CV Mosby, 1994, p. 161.

TABLE 30–3. PROBLEMS ENCOUNTERED WITH PULMONARY ARTERY (PA) CATHETERS*

Problem	Cause	Prevention	Treatment
Phlebitis or local infection at insertion site	Mechanical irritation or contamination	Prepare skin properly before insertion. Use sterile technique during insertion and dressing change. Insert smoothly and rapidly. Use Teflon-coated introducer. Attach silver-impregnated cuff to introducer. Change dressings, stopcocks, and connecting tubing every 24-48 hours. Remove catheter or change insertion site every 4 days.	Remove catheter. Apply warm compresses. Give pain medication as necessary.
Ventricular irritability	Looping of excess catheter in right ventricle	Suture catheter at insertion site; check chest film.	Reposition catheter; remove loop.
	Migration of catheter from PA to RV	Position catheter tip in main right or left PA.	Inflate balloon to encourage catheter flotation out to PA. Advance rapidly out to PA.
	Irritation of the endocardium during catheter passage	Keep balloon inflated during advancement; advance gently.	
Apparent wedging of catheter with balloon deflated	Forward migration of catheter tip caused by blood flow, excessive loop in RV, or inadequate suturing of catheter at insertion site	Check catheter tip by fluoroscopy; position in main right or left PA. Check catheter position on x-ray film if fluoroscopy is not used. Suture catheter in place at insertion site.	Aspirate blood from catheter; if catheter is wedged, sample will be arterialized and obtained with difficulty. If wedged, slowly pull back catheter until PA waveform appears. If not wedged, gently aspirate and flush catheter with saline; catheter tip can partially clot, causing damping that resembles damped PAW waveform.
Pulmonary hemorrhage or infarction, or both	Distal migration of catheter tip	Check chest film immediately after insertion and 12-24 hrs later; remove any catheter loop in RA or RV.	
	Continuous or prolonged wedging of catheter	Leave balloon deflated. Suture catheter at skin to prevent inadvertent advancement. Position catheter in main right or left PA. Pull catheter back to pulmonary artery if it spontaneously wedges. Do not flush catheter when in wedge position.	Deflate balloon. Place patient on side (catheter tip down). Stop anticoagulation. Consider "wedge" angiogram.
	Overinflation of balloon while catheter is wedged	Inflate balloon slowly with only enough air to obtain a PAW waveform.	
	Failure of balloon to deflate	Do not inflate 7-Fr catheter with more than 1-1.5 ml air.	

Complication	Cause	Prevention	Treatment
"Overwedging" or damped PAW 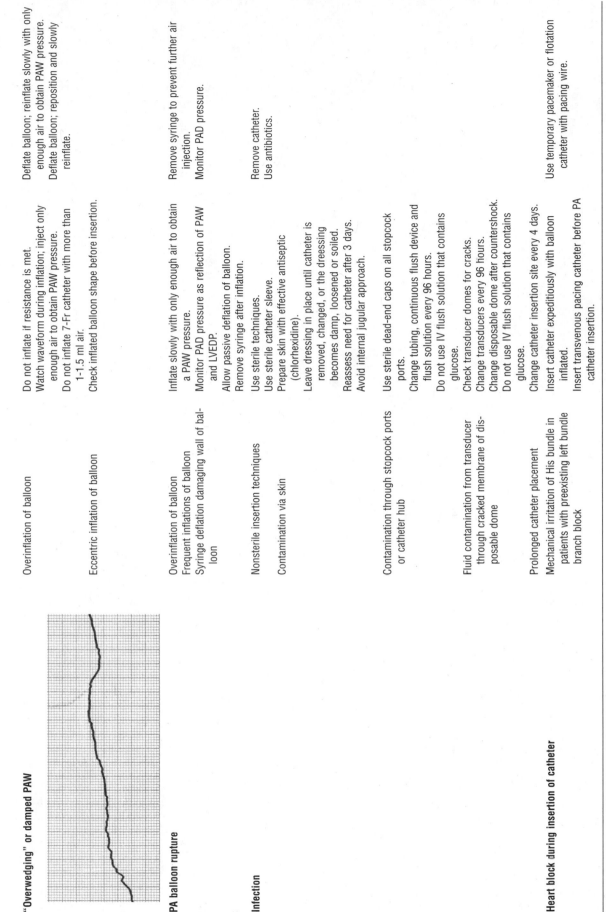	Overinflation of balloon	Do not inflate if resistance is met. Watch waveform during inflation; inject only enough air to obtain PAW pressure. Do not inflate 7-Fr catheter with more than 1-1.5 ml air.	Deflate balloon; reinflate slowly with only enough air to obtain PAW pressure.
	Eccentric inflation of balloon	Check inflated balloon shape before insertion.	Deflate balloon; reposition and slowly reinflate.
PA balloon rupture	Overinflation of balloon Frequent inflations of balloon Syringe deflation damaging wall of balloon	Inflate slowly with only enough air to obtain a PAW pressure. Monitor PAD pressure as reflection of PAW and LVEDP. Allow passive deflation of balloon. Remove syringe after inflation.	Remove syringe to prevent further air injection. Monitor PAD pressure.
Infection	Nonsterile insertion techniques Contamination via skin	Use sterile techniques. Use sterile catheter sleeve. Prepare skin with effective antiseptic (chlorhexidine). Leave dressing in place until catheter is removed, changed, or the dressing becomes damp, loosened or soiled. Reassess need for catheter after 3 days. Avoid internal jugular approach.	Remove catheter. Use antibiotics.
	Contamination through stopcock ports or catheter hub	Use sterile dead-end caps on all stopcock ports. Change tubing, continuous flush device and flush solution every 96 hours. Do not use IV flush solution that contains glucose.	
	Fluid contamination from transducer through cracked membrane of disposable dome	Check transducer domes for cracks. Change transducers every 96 hours. Change disposable dome after countershock. Do not use IV flush solution that contains glucose.	
	Prolonged catheter placement	Change catheter insertion site every 4 days.	
Heart block during insertion of catheter	Mechanical irritation of His bundle in patients with preexisting left bundle branch block	Insert catheter expeditiously with balloon inflated. Insert transvenous pacing catheter before PA catheter insertion.	Use temporary pacemaker or flotation catheter with pacing wire.

*PAW, pulmonary artery wedge; RV, right ventricle; PA, pulmonary artery.

From Daily E, Schroeder J: Techniques in bedside hemodynamic monitoring, 5th ed. S. Louis, MO: CV Mosby, 1994, pp. 134-136.

TABLE 30–4. INACCURATE PULMONARY ARTERY (PA) PRESSURE MEASUREMENTS*

Problem	Cause	Prevention	Treatment
Damped waveforms and inaccurate pressures 	Partial clotting at catheter tip	Use continuous drip with 1 U heparin/1 ml IV fluid. Hand flush occasionally. Flush with large volume after blood sampling. Use heparin-coated catheters.	Aspirate, then flush catheter with heparinized fluid (not in PAW position).
	Tip moving against wall	Obtain more stable catheter position.	Reposition catheter.
	Kinking of catheter	Restrict catheter movement at insertion site.	Reposition to straighten catheter. Replace catheter.
Abnormally low or negative pressures	Incorrect air-reference level (above midchest level)	Maintain transducer air-reference port at midchest level; rezero after patient position changes.	Remeasure level of transducer air-reference and reposition at midchest level; rezero.
	Incorrect zeroing and calibration of monitor	Zero and calibrate monitor properly.	Recheck zero and calibration of monitor.
	Loose connection	Use Luer-Lok stopcocks.	Check all connections.
Abnormally high pressure reading	Pressure trapped by improper sequence of stopcock operation	Turn stopcocks in proper sequence when two pressures are measured on one transducer.	Thoroughly flush transducers with IV solution; rezero and turn stopcocks in proper sequence.
	Incorrect air-reference level (below midchest level)	Maintain transducer air-reference port at midchest level; recheck and rezero after patient position changes.	Check air-reference level; reset at midchest and rezero.
Inappropriate pressure waveform	Migration of catheter tip (e.g., in RV or PAW instead of in PA)	Establish optimal position carefully when introducing catheter initially. Suture catheter at insertion site and tape catheter to patient's skin.	Review waveform; if RV, inflate balloon; if PAW, deflate balloon and withdraw catheter slightly. Check position under fluoroscope and/or x-ray after reposition.
No pressure available	Transducer not open to catheter Amplifiers still on cal, zero, or off	Follow routine, systematic steps for pressure measurement.	Check system, stopcocks.
Noise or fling in pressure waveform 	Excessive catheter movement, particularly in PA	Avoid excessive catheter length in ventricle.	Try different catheter tip position.
	Excessive tubing length	Use shortest tubing possible (<3 to 4 feet).	Eliminate excess tubing.
	Excessive stopcocks	Minimize number of stopcocks.	Eliminate excess stopcocks.

*PAW, pulmonary artery wedge; RV, right ventricle; PA, pulmonary artery.
*From Daily E, Schroeder J: Techniques in bedside hemodynamic monitoring, 5th ed. St. Louis, MO: CV Mosby, 1994, p. 137.

TABLE 30–5. TROUBLESHOOTING PROBLEMS WITH THERMODILUTION CARDIAC OUTPUT MEASUREMENTS*

Problem	Cause	Action
Cardiac output values lower than expected	Injectate volume greater than designated amount	Inject exact volume to correspond to computation constant used.
		Discontinue rapid infusion through proximal or distal port.
	Catheter tip in RV or RA	Verify PA waveform from distal lumen. Reposition catheter.
	Incorrect computation constant (CC)	Reset computation constant. Correct prior CO values:
		Incorrect CO value $\times \dfrac{\text{correct CC}}{\text{wrong CC}}$
	Left-to-right shunt (VSD)	Check RA and PA oxygen saturations.
		Use alternative CO measurement technique.
	Catheter kinked or thermistor partially obstructed with clot	Check for kinks at insertion site; straighten catheter; aspirate and flush catheter. Replace catheter.
	Faulty catheter (communication between proximal and distal lumens)	
Cardiac output values higher than expected	Injectate volume less than designated amount	Inject exact volume to correspond to computation constant.
		Carefully remove all air bubbles from syringe.
	Catheter too distal (PAW)	Verify PA waveform from distal lumen.
		Pull catheter back.
	RA port lies within sheath	Advance catheter.
	Thermistor against wall of PA	Reposition patient.
		Rotate catheter to turn thermistor away from wall. Reposition catheter.
	Fibrin covering thermistor	Check a-vDo$_2$; change catheter.
	Incorrect computation constant (CC)	Correct prior CO values (see formula above). Reset computation constant.
	Right-to-left shunt (VSD)	Use alternative CO measurement technique.
	Severe tricuspid regurgitation	
	Incorrect injectate temperature	Use closed injectate system with in-line temperature probe.
		Handle syringe minimally.
		Do not turn stopcock to reestablish IV infusion through proximal port between injections; reduce or discontinue IV flow through VIP port.
		Try to determine cause of interference.
	Magnetic interference producing numerous spikes in CO curve	Wipe CO computer with damp cloth.
	Long lag time between injection and upstroke of curve	Press start button after injection completed to delay computer sampling time.
	Uneven injection technique	Inject smoothly and quickly (10 ml in ≤ 4 seconds).
	RA port partially occluded with clot	Always check catheter patency by withdrawing, then flushing proximal port before CO determinations.
	Catheter partially kinked	Check for kinks, particularly at insertion site; straighten catheter; reposition patient.
	Cardiac dysrhythmias (PVC, AF, etc.)	Note ECG during CO determinations.
		Try to inject during a stable period.
		Increase the number of CO determinations.
	Marked movement of catheter tip	Obtain x-ray film to determine position of tip.
		Advance catheter tip away from pulmonic value.
	Marked variation in PA baseline temperature	Use iced temperature injectate to increase signal/noise ratio.
		Increase the number of CO determinations.
		Inject at various times during respiratory cycle.
	Curve prematurely terminated	Press start button after injection completed to delay computer sampling time.
	Right-to-left shunt	Use alternative CO measurement technique.

Irregular upslope of CO curve

Irregular downslope of CO curve

*RV, right ventricle; RA, right atrium; CO, cardiac output; VSD, ventricular septal defect; PA, pulmonary artery; PAW, pulmonary artery wedge; a-vDo$_2$, arteriovenous oxygen content difference; PVC, premature ventricular contraction; AF, atrial fibrillation.

From: Daily E, Schroeder J: Techniques in bedside hemodynamic monitoring, *5th ed. St. Louis, MO: CV Mosby, 1994, pp. 183–184. Cardiac output waveforms from: Gardner P:* Cardiac output: Theory, technique and troubleshooting. In Underhill SL, Woods S, Froelicher E, et al: Cardiac nursing, *2nd ed. Philadelphia: JB Lippincott, 1989, p. 465.*

Ventilatory Troubleshooting Guide

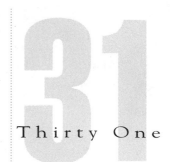

Thirty One

Problem	Causes	Management
Low exhaled tidal volume (TV)		Ventilate patient as necessary with manual resuscitation bag if exhibiting signs and symptoms of respiratory insufficiency and problem cannot be immediately corrected. Obtain appropriate assistance.
	Patient-related: Cuff leak caused by: • Insufficient air added to cuff • Higher airway pressures, which create the need for higher cuff pressures to seal the trachea • Hole in cuff • Leak in air inflation port • Displaced endotracheal tube	Evaluate for cause of leak. Inflate cuff properly to minimally occlude trachea and provide effective ventilation. • If leak is in cuff, call for assistance in reintubation. Attempt to maintain ventilation in the interim by increasing TV to compensate for gas escaping or try leaving patient on ventilator and sealing mouth and nose with hands. Inform and reassure patient. Observe for potential gastric distension caused by leakage of air into stomach. Maintain gastric suction. • If leak is in air inflation port, seal port by placing three-way stopcock or leaving syringe on port. Tape syringe hub to prevent cuff deflation. • If endotracheal tube is displaced, reposition or obtain assistance as necessary.
	Factors that increase airway resistance and/or decrease compliance (see Increased Airway Pressure) will increase inspiratory pressures and set off the high airway pressure alarm, causing the volume which is not delivered to be dumped from the ventilator. (Volume-cycled ventilators deliver the prescribed volume unless the pressure limit is exceeded.)	• Assess and correct causes of increased airway pressure (see Increased Airway Pressure). Increase airway pressure upper limit as necessary to allow for air delivery (last step after other assessments and management).
	Bronchopleural air leak, which results in passage of air from airways to pleural space.	• Refer to respiratory acidosis section for management.
	Ventilator-Related: Loose, cracked, ill-fitted connectors or humidifier.	• Check for loose, cracked, or ill-fitted humidity jar. Realign jar and tighten as necessary. Replace cracked jar.
	Loose tubing, connections.	• Check for and tighten loose tubing connections.
	Tears in tubing.	• Change tubing as necessary.
	Flow rate may become too high because of a combination of high ventilator TV, rate, or flow rate settings. High flow rates may result in an inability to deliver the total prescribed volume.	• Be aware of potential volume loss resulting from combinations of high ventilator TV, respiratory rate, or peak flow settings, which exceed capabilities of the ventilator. (The effect of higher flow rates on volume delivery should be evaluated for the particular ventilator.) Correct problem by lowering the flow rate

(continued)

Problem	Causes	Management
		(decrease peak flow or lengthen inspiratory time; lower dialed-in respiratory rate or volume settings. • Support patient with manual resuscitation bag if unable to correct problem within 10 to 15 seconds. Call for assistance to change ventilators.
No exhaled TV	**Patient-related:** Patient disconnected from ventilator. Large cuff leak; endotracheal tube displaced so that cuff is above the vocal cords (may lead to inability to seal the pharyngeal area despite addition of large volume of air to cuff).	• Check patient to ensure that adaptor is attached to tracheostomy or endotracheal tube. • Evaluate and correct cuff leaks, endotracheal tube displacement.
	Ventilator-related: Tubing disconnections, large tears in tubing, dislodged temperature sensing bag; loss of wall electrical or compressed air source.	• Evaluate for disconnected tubing, holes in tubing, loss of power or air/oxygen source.
Increased airway pressure	**Patient-related:** Higher airway pressures are required to deliver the prescribed volume because of various factors that increase airway resistance, including secretions, mucous plugs, endotracheal tube factors (becomes kinked or narrowed, biting on orally placed tube), bronchospasm or decreased lung compliance, including pneumothorax, atelectasis, pulmonary edema. The upper airway pressure alarm sounds when the peak inspiratory pressure reaches the alarm limit which is set. Endotracheal tube in right mainstem bronchus. Inspiratory pressures can become higher because of resistance of the chest wall to expansion, abdominal pressure against the diaphragm, chest-wall injury, external restrictions, abdominal contractions during coughing or breathing efforts. Coughing because of tracheal irritation caused by jarring of the endotracheal or tracheostomy tube; air leak around cuff, which causes air and secretion movement; head movement; tip of tube touching carina. Need for communication of concerns and problems; may not be sufficiently informed or comprehending explanations regarding inability to verbally communicate; alternative methods of communication are not used or are inappropriate or ineffective. Increased respiratory rate from anxiety, fear, pain, inadequate oxygenation, inadequate ventilation (hypercarbia), acidemia, or central nervous system malfunction. The higher the breathing rate, the faster the flow rates. If the ventilator peak flow rate is set too low or inspiratory time is too long, the patient will be	• Suction as necessary. • Assess for difficulty passing suction catheter through tube or observable kinking. Notify physician as necessary. • If patient bites on tube, explain purpose of tube, reason for not biting. • Anchor tube using tape or commercially designed tube holder if necessary. • Auscultate chest regularly to detect changes in breath sounds that may coincide with increased inspiratory pressures. • Notify physician of decreased breath sounds. Obtain chest x-ray film to evaluate for proper endotracheal tube placement. Mark tube depth and anchor tube securely. • Reposition patient for optimal ventilation. Increase upper pressure limit dial 10 to 15 cm H_2O higher than the pressure required for ventilation when certain positions that create higher pressures are necessary for patient management. • Evaluate for causes of coughing (minimal or no volume delivery may occur if the high airway pressure alarm sounds because, when the set pressure limit is reached, inspiration is discontinued and expiration begins). • Avoid jarring or moving tube during turning. • Evaluate for optimum cuff inflation. Add air to cuff as necessary to "just seal" the trachea from air leakage that irritates airway and causes cough. • Chest x-ray studies to evaluate for proper tube placement. • Evaluate with physician whether patient is a candidate for weaning/extubation, which will resolve the problem. • Explain reason for inability to communicate verbally and implement alternative method(s) to meet needs. Anticipate needs, ask "yes or no" questions. • Convey calm, confident, reassuring approach; explain procedures. • Evaluate for causes of increased ventilatory requirements, patient "fighting the ventilator" or "out of phase." Implement measures to correct problem(s). Provide calm, confident, reassuring approach. Explain interventions and use touch to relieve anxiety and fear. Provide analgesics as appropriate. Evaluate for

(continued)

Problem	Causes	Management
	attempting to exhale during the ventilator inspiratory phase. Forceful contraction of the thoracoabdominal musculature during the inspiratory phase causes the ventilator pressure limit to be exceeded, thus terminating air delivery prematurely.	increased work of breathing caused by inadequate oxygenation or ventilation caused by air leaks in the ventilator system. • Evaluate whether inspiratory flow rate setting is set optimally to match patient's breathing pattern. Observe chest/abdomen during inspiratory phase and evaluate whether patient appears to exhale (as evidenced by chest/abdominal contraction) during ventilator inspiratory cycle. Readjust peak flow dial higher or shorten inspiratory time and/or increase respiratory rate setting (higher setting results in increased flow rate) as necessary to match fast patient's inspiratory phase. • Observe trends in airway pressures which may signal changes in compliance. • If patient has status asthmaticus, provide sedation with morphine sulphate; pharmacologically paralyze as ordered to ensure optimal chest-wall compliance (decreases respiratory muscle activity and peak inspiratory pressures) and provide for adequate ventilation. Maintain on full ventilator support to minimize energy expenditure and maintain normal carbon dioxide levels. Provide bronchodilators, steroids, antibiotics as ordered.
	Ventilator-related: Airway upper pressure limit alarm is set too low.	• Set upper pressure limit 10 to 15 cm H_2O higher than the patient's maximum inspiratory pressure.
	Unusually high TV for the patient.	• Evaluate whether the patient is receiving too much TV (normal: 10 to 15 ml/kg normal body weight; 10 ml/kg in chronic lung disease). • Increase upper pressure limit. • Monitor for adverse effects of PEEP (see Decreased CO).
	Compliance may be decreased when PEEP is applied, probably as a result of overdistension of alveoli.	• Increase upper pressure limit. • Monitor for adverse effects of PEEP (see Decreased CO).
Respiratory alkalosis	**Patient-Related:** Factors that may increase respiratory rate or ventilation, including anxiety, restlessness, discomfort, pain; hypoxemia; central nervous system malfunction; metabolic acidosis; sensation of dyspnea caused by underlying lung pathology.	• Assist in decreasing feelings of anxiety and fear through calm, confident, reassuring approach, providing explanations and other measures to decrease stress. • Evaluate ventilator for proper functioning (receiving prescribed TV flow rate adjusted to match breathing pattern). • Check Pao_2, provide adequate oxygenation. • Evaluate and treat metabolic disturbance when warranted. • Consider different ventilation mode. • Consider that hyperventilation may not be corrected by various interventions because of central nervous system malfunction. Allow state of respiratory alkalosis.
	Mechanical hyperventilation ($Paco_2$ less than 28 mm Hg) may be used as therapy to decrease intracranial pressure.	• Mechanically hyperventilate as prescribed for purpose of decreasing intracranial pressure.
	Ventilator-related: High tidal or minute volume settings on ventilator which cause overventilation, decreased $Paco_2$, increased pH.	• Set initial TV at 10 to 15 ml/kg and set rate at 8 to 12 breaths/minute. If patient has chronic obstructive pulmonary disease, select TV of about 10 ml/kg to reduce the risk of barotrauma and hyperventilation. Check arterial blood gases in about 20 minutes.

(continued)

Problem	Causes	Management
		• Decrease TV or respiratory rate if high. (Note: Decreasing respiratory rate setting while on assist/control mode will not correct the problem if the patient is triggering the ventilator. Decreasing TV may not correct the problem in patients who can maintain their desired Paco₂ level by increasing their respiratory rate.)
	Too frequent or too many sighs.	• Eliminate or decrease sighs.
	Machine sensitivity dial is set on positive side (versus negative 2 cm H₂O) causing machine to automatically cycle without patient effort, resulting in hyperventilation (Paco₂ below normal).	• Maintain sensitivity setting so that it takes –2 cm H₂O effort before a ventilator cycle can be initiated. • If patient is on PEEP, readjust sensitivity dial so that it is –2 to –3 cm H₂O less than the set PEEP value (e.g., for PEEP 5 cm H₂O, set sensitivity dial at plus 2 or 3 cm H₂O). Note: Some ventilators automatically reset sensitivity value when PEEP is applied. • When patient is on PEEP therapy, avoid air leaks in cuff or ventilator system (air leaks may cause loss of PEEP value and machine self-cycling occurs because sensitivity is set at a positive value).
	Sensitivity needle (airway pressure needle) becomes maladjusted so that it rests at –2 cm H₂O level rather than resting at zero point, causing machine to self-cycle.	• Prior to placing patient on ventilator and prn, check ventilator sensitivity needle (airway pressure needle) to make sure it rests at zero point on airway pressure meter. Call respiratory therapist to readjust needle back to the zero point. Maintain 2 cm H₂O negativity until airway pressure needle. If ventilator does not have sensitivity dial with specific markings, regulate sensitivity setting by observing airway pressure needle. Regulate sensitivity dial so that the airway pressure needle registers 2 cm negativity with patient inspiratory effort.
Respiratory acidosis	**Patient-related:** Inadequate TV to provide adequate gas exchange. Insufficient respiratory rate. Some COPD patients have chronically elevated Paco₂ levels.	• Increase TV. • Maintain Paco₂ at the patient's normal baseline level. Do not attempt to overventilate to a normal Paco₂ level if the patient has COPD with chronic carbon dioxide retention. • Make changes gradually to patient's baseline Paco₂ and pH. (Rapid changes may cause respiratory alkalosis with risk of cardiac arrhythmias, tetany, seizures.)
	Increased carbon dioxide production from the use of total parenteral nutrition (TPN) regimens containing high glucose loads. When carbohydrate (glucose) calories in TPN exceed a patient's metabolic demands, the surplus glucose is converted to fat through biochemical process associated with increased carbon dioxide production with small increase in oxygen consumption. Increased ventilation is observed as a result of increased carbon dioxide production. In mechanically ventilated patients unable to increase their minute ventilation (e.g., patients with chronic lung disease, those with normal lungs who develop compromised lung function because of acute lung disorder), the increase in carbon dioxide production is paralleled by an increase in Paco₂. Low ventilation to perfusion ratio of alveoli because of increased airway resistance or decreased compliance problems.	• Monitor effects of nutrition therapy on respiration, including measurements of minute ventilation, respiratory rate, oxygen consumption, carbon dioxide production, arterial blood gases. If increases in ventilation or carbon dioxide, or both, are noted after TPN has begun, the amount and source of nonprotein calories should be evaluated. • Particularly observe for TPN induced acidosis in patients with chronic lung disease or marginal ventilatory reserve, who are on partial ventilator support (for example, IMV, CPAP, pressure support). • Discuss observations with physician so that changes can be made to limit glucose infusion and substitute fats for a portion of energy.
	Bronchopleural air leak results in passage of air from airways to pleural space. Increased leak may occur because of factors tending to increase peak airway pressure during inspiration, such as high peak flow rate and high airway resistance. Increased mean	• Implement measures that minimize the bronchopleural pressure gradient, maintain adequate oxygenation and ventilation (pH greater than 7.30), keep lungs expanded, and control underlying disease process. Suggested conservative management includes:

(continued)

Problem	Causes	Management
	intrathoracic pressure throughout the respiratory cycle, as occurs with a long inspiratory phase, inflation hold, expiratory retard, PEEP, and CPAP, will increase leak throughout the breath. Higher negative suction pressure will augment leak independent of factors as outlined here.	—Deliver lowest number of mechanical breaths compatible with adequate ventilation (spontaneous ventilation if possible). —Reduce exhaled TV to 10 ml/kg or less. —Adjust ventilator to minimize time spent in inspiration (short inspiratory time or high peak flow rate). —Avoid inflation hold and expiratory retard. —Avoid or minimize PEEP/CPAP. —Use lowest effective level of chest tube suction. —Explore positional differences on decreasing leak. —Sedate patient with or without paralysis if spontaneous movements accentuate leak. —Treat underlying cause for respiratory failure while maintaining nutritional and respiratory care support.
	Ventilator-related: Patient not receiving prescribed TV because of air leaks. Increased dead space on ventilator tubing. Reduction of volume delivered to the patient because of tubing system compliance and gas compression. This correction is generally in the range of 3 to 5 ml/cm H_2O of peak inspiratory pressure for adult ventilator circuits; however, may be negligible on some ventilator circuits.	• Evaluate and correct air leaks (refer to Low/No exhaled TV sections. • Remove dead space tubing. • Be aware of reduced delivered volume, which may be significant if high inflation pressures are required. • Increase TV as necessary to provide adequate ventilation.
Thick secretions	**Patient-related:** Dehydration. Infection.	• Maintain accurate intake, output, weight, CVP, LAP, PAWP recordings. Notify physician of abnormalities. • Maximize systemic hydration. • Monitor sputum for changes in color, amount, consistency. Obtain culture and sensitivity if indicated. If signs of infection, check with physician regarding antibiotics. Monitor for improvements after treatment initiated. • Suction as necessary if secretions present.
	Ventilator-related: Heating unit set too low or not functioning properly. Insufficient water in humidifier jar.	• Check sensor that monitors temperature of inspired humidified gas (should be located close to patient airway). Maintain temperature at 98°F. • Notify respiratory therapist that heating unit not functioning properly. • Add water to refill line as necessary. Do not allow water to decrease below the refill line, which decreases effective humidification. • Drain water from tubing every two hours and prn.
Tracheostomy/endotracheal tube discomfort	**Patient-related:** Insufficient attention to observing patient's airway, guiding tubing, and providing extra tubing during turning or other movement. Tube jarred with turning. Tube not secured adequately. Improvement in gas exchange because of improvement in disorder that caused increased oxygen requirement.	• Obtain necessary assistance so that one person can pay attention to guiding tubing and prevent pulling or jarring during patient activities. • Disconnect the patient from the ventilator, turn and reconnect. Do not leave off ventilator longer than 10 to 15 seconds. (Disconnection may be undesirable for patients requiring high oxygen concentrations, PEEP, or if they are paralyzed or sedated.) • Stabilize tracheostomy or endotracheal tube with one hand when reconnecting the ventilator adapter. • Anchor tube securely with ties or tape. • Position ventilator tubing on support system to minimize polling. • Recheck arterial blood gases in 15 to 20 minutes.

(continued)

Problem	Causes	Management
	Ventilator-related: Oxygen concentration setting on ventilator is too high.	• Decrease inspired oxygen concentration. • Recheck arterial blood gases in 15 to 20 minutes. • If on PEEP therapy, consider withdrawal of PEEP if Fio_2 less than 0.5. • Decrease PEEP in increments of 3 to 5 cm H_2O and evaluate arterial blood gases within 20 minutes. • Refer to Decreased CO section for other management procedures related to PEEP.
Low Pao_2/O_2 saturation	**Patient-related:** Various abnormalities causing ventilation-perfusion disturbances and shunting, such as secretions, bronchospasm, pulmonary edema, pulmonary embolism. Arterial blood gas drawn immediately after suctioning. Changes in position causing alveolar hypoventilation, ventilation-perfusion disturbances. Right mainstem bronchus intubation, pneumothorax causing decreased ventilation.	• Correct pathophysiologic state causing the abnormal oxygenation. • Hyperoxygenate before and after suctioning as necessary (refer to Arrhythmias during suctioning section). • Wait at least 15 to 20 minutes after suctioning before obtaining blood gas measurement. • Assess whether certain positions cause decreased Pao_2. Refrain from placing in positions which precipitate respiratory discomfort, unsafe drops in Pao_2, or obtain order to increase Fio_2 and/or TV for goals of maintaining adequate oxygenation, ventilation. • Evaluate for, and correct, tube malposition, pneumothorax. • Obtain chest x-ray film as necessary.
	Ventilator-related: Oxygen concentration setting on ventilator is too low. Air leak around tracheostomy or endotracheal tube cuff, or in ventilator system, or both, leading to inadequate oxygenation, ventilation, loss of PEEP therapy. Inaccurate oxygen percentage from oxygen source failure or oxygen analyzer error.	• Increase Fio_2; add inspiratory pause, PEEP as necessary to avoid unsafe high oxygen concentrations. • Evaluate for air leaks, and correct (see Low/No exhaled TV). • Notify respiratory therapist to determine accuracy of oxygen analyzer or whether oxygen concentration is being delivered. • Provide oxygen as necessary to maintain acceptable Pao_2.
Decreased cardiac output (CO) with hypotension	**Patient-related:** Significant stimulation (hypoxemia, hypercarbia, acidemia) of the autonomic system in a patient requiring ventilator support. Physiologic stress is frequently compounded by a state of anxiety and fear. These factors lead to arterial and venous constriction, as well as myocardial stimulation. Support of ventilation usually relieves work of breathing, and reverses hypercarbia, acidemia, and hypoxemia. It also produces relaxation and sleep, and may induce unconsciousness. The combination of loss of consciousness, relief of breathing work, and improved oxygenation and ventilation often leads to a profound and sudden decrease in sympathetic stimulation to the cardiovascular system, which results in arteriolar and venous relaxation and a significant increase in the vascular space. Sudden "relative hypovolemia" may occur because the patient cannot mobilize extravascular fluid rapidly. Positive ventilator pressure increases intrathoracic pressure and accentuates interference with venous return, making relative hypovolemia significant. Intravascular volume depletion; when PEEP therapy produces significant reductions in cardiac output despite intravascular volume augmentation, an element of ventricular dysfunction may be involved.	• Be aware of potential hypotension following institution of positive pressure ventilation. Monitor blood pressure, pulse, rhythm. • Stabilize cardiovascular system by correcting relative hypovolemia with appropriate intravenous fluid administration. • Elevate lower extremities 20 to 30 degrees from horizontal position if hypotension is severe. • During this period, augment spontaneous ventilation initially by manual ventilation (using technique which maintains synchrony with the patient's varying inspiratory efforts and leads to a profound and sudden decrease in sympathetic stimulation to the cardiovascular system, which results in arteriolar dilatation and allow the patient to "fight" the positive pressure, which increases intrathoracic pressure. • Make sure the manual ventilation bag is capable of providing adequate oxygenation and ventilation to meet the patient's requirements. • Place patient on ventilator when relaxed. Shorten inspiratory time or increase peak flow dial as necessary to simulate normal breathing pattern. • Monitor vital signs, hemodynamic parameters, if pulmonary artery catheter in place, including: (1) arterial-venous oxygen content difference and CO measurements (aids assessment of perfusion and oxygen

(continued)

Problem	Causes	Management
		extraction); (2) intrapulmonary shunt calculations (aids assessment of pulmonary effects of PEEP); and (3) pulmonary artery occlusion pressures (aids in the assessment of intravascular fluid administration). Notify physician of abnormalities. • Administer IV fluids to correct intravascular hypovolemia.
	Patients with airflow obstruction may trap air so that alveolar pressure remains positive at end-expiration, even when PEEP is not applied intentionally. This "autoPEEP" effect can cause increased intrathoracic pressure and severely depress CO. It is likely to develop if gas exchange is prolonged by increases in thoracic compliance or resistance, or if the time for exhalation is shortened by a high ventilatory requirement. Auto-PEEP can develop whenever the minute ventilation is great enough that the lung cannot empty to its usual relaxed volume between inflations. The magnitude of intrinsic PEEP increases with decreased duration of expiration.	• Evaluate auto-PEEP in patients with airflow obstruction (performed by occluding expiratory port at end-expiration by the ventilator or pressing end-expiration hold button on some ventilators) and observe positive pressure registered on airway-pressure manometer. No spontaneous respiratory efforts should be present nor any gas flow from a supplemental source, such as that used in some IMV systems or medication nebulization. • Treat hemodynamic effects of auto-PEEP by measures that lower mean intrathoracic pressure. 　—Adjust inspiratory time or peak flow setting to allow maximal time for exhalation between cycles (shorten inspiratory time or increase peak flow) and to avoid progressive increases in end expiratory lung volume, hyperinflation. 　—Reduce minute ventilation to minimal amount consistent with acceptable pH. 　—Try higher TV (not usually effective if minute ventilation remains unchanged) or IMV. 　—Correct fever, agitation, metabolic acidosis, to diminish ventilatory requirements. 　—Continue medical therapy for treatment of airflow obstruction. • Administer fluids to correct hypovolemia. • Administer inotropic agents as necessary. • Increase PEEP in increments of 3 to 5 cm H_2O. Monitor for signs, symptoms of decreased CO. Evaluate arterial blood gases within 20 to 30 minutes of setting change.
	Level of PEEP is unnecessarily high for therapeutic goal of adequate arterial oxygen content without significant reduction in CO at F_IO_2 below 0.5. Oxygen concentrations greater than 0.5 over prolonged periods can result in oxygen toxicity	• Use the lowest level of PEEP necessary to correct severe hypoxemia (result PaO_2 greater than 60 mm Hg under most circumstances) while allowing a reduction of the FiO_2 below 0.5. • Provide PEEP if an FiO_2 of greater than 0.5 is required for more than 24 hours to achieve a PaO_2 greater than 50 to 60 mm Hg. 　Note: "Enough" PEEP has been applied when, in the presence of adequate perfusion and hemoglobin content, a PaO_2 of at least 60 mm Hg is achieved at an FiO_2 of 0.4 or less.
	Ventilator-Related: Positive pressure ventilation and PEEP may decrease CO by impeding venous return, which decreases right and subsequently left ventricular stroke volume. Other factors proposed may include release of humoral substances during lung expansion, which depress left ventricular function and CO reduction secondary to endocardial blood supply impairment. Factors that may increase positive intrathoracic pressure and mean airway pressure include high TV, PEEP, continuous mechanical ventilation and increased respiratory rate (more positive pressure).	• May need to decrease TV to avoid high peak inspiratory pressures. • Use TV and PEEP that maintain "optimal compliance". • Avoid use of inspiratory pause or hold. • May try shortening inspiratory time or increasing peak flow to shorten the amount of time that positive pressure remains in the thorax and prevent "fighting" of positive pressure, which unduly increases intrathoracic pressure. • Use lowest PEEP level necessary to meet therapeutic goal. • Increase FiO_2 and remove PEEP as necessary until the patient is hemodynamically stabilized.
	A higher intrapleural pressure and lower CO may be produced when PEEP is used on control mode and	• May try IMV or CPAP mode if compatible with cardiovascular and clinical stability to lower intrapleural

(continued)

Problem	Causes	Management
	pressure ventilation versus PEEP with spontaneous ventilation (CPAP) or IMV.	pressures and reduce harmful alterations in cardiac function.
Anxiety and fear	**Patient-Related:** Decreased ability to communicate because of tracheostomy/endotracheal tube. Fear of unknown, unfamiliar environment and people.	• Assess most effective method(s) of communication: paper and pencil, lip reading, gestures, alphabet board, cards indicating major needs, and electric larynx. Communicate method on care plan. • Ask "yes and no" questions. • Keep call light in reach at all times. • Obtain assistance if unable to interpret communications. Use touch to ease frustrations. • Evaluate and manage psychosocial factors that may be creating anxiety and fear. • Convey calm, confident, reassuring approach. • Explain all procedures, allow patient participation in decisions to the extent possible. • Maintain familiarity in environment (family visits, significant personal belongings, radio, television, clock, consistency in personnel caring for patient).
	Effects of surgery or various other interventions, which create discomfort, pain. Decreased arterial oxygenation related to suctioning.	• Identify factors creating discomfort, pain, shortness of breath, and implement measures to modify or resolve problem. • See Low PaO$_2$ and Arrhythmias during suctioning.
	Ventilator-Related: Ventilator settings not optimally adjusted to meet patient's needs. Air leaks causing patient to receive inadequate ventilation, oxygenation; incorrect settings.	• Assess whether ventilator is optimally adjusted to meet patient's needs. Readjust flow rate setting higher or inspiratory time shorter as necessary to match faster breathing pattern. • Evaluate whether prescribed TV is being delivered and whether settings are correct. Manually ventilate as necessary. • Efficiently identify and correct problem using a calm, confident approach.
Arrhythmias during or after suctioning	**Patient-Related:** Suctioning induces arterial desaturation. Other adverse effects include bronchoconstriction, vasovagal reactions, cardiac arrhythmias, unexplained cardiovascular collapse and sudden death. There are considerable differences in the rate of fall in oxygen tension. Variables affecting the degree of hypoxemia include: (1) the ratio of suction catheter size to endotracheal tube size, (2) the duration of suctioning, (3) whether or not hyperoxygenation was performed before or after suctioning, (4) the patient's initial PaO$_2$, (5) the magnitude of pulmonary shunt, (6) suction induced alveolar collapse, (8) the ability to breathe spontaneously.	• Implement measures to minimize or prevent suction related hypoxemia and vagal reactions: —Assess need for suctioning. Suction only as necessary, not on a "routine" basis. —Use catheter no greater than half the diameter of the tube through which it is passed. —Inform patient that you will be suctioning. —Insert catheter without applying suction. —Spend less than 15 seconds total time off ventilator. Limit applied suction time to 10 seconds. —Administer hyperoxygenation (100% O$_2$) with a manual resuscitation bag or the ventilator for 3 to 5 breaths before and after each suctioning pass. —Use ventilator for hyperoxygenation when PEEP > 10 cm H$_2$O or when removal from ventilator results in distress or hypoxemia. —Monitor blood pressure, heart rate, rhythm during suctioning procedures. If arrhythmias or significant changes in heart rate occur, discontinue suctioning and ventilate patient immediately using 100% O$_2$ for several breaths. Be certain that vital signs have returned to baseline values before repeating suction process. —Modify procedure for pre- and post-hyperoxygenation to fit the individual patient's psychologic requirements.

(continued)

Problem	Causes	Management
	Large lung volumes have been reported to cause bradycardia and hypotension.	• Assess whether an increase in Fio_2 or mechanical hyperinflation with oxygen is needed to raise the Pao_2 to a sufficient level. If mechanical hyperinflation is needed, avoid large changes in pH (respiratory alkalosis) which may produce hazards related to myocardial and central nervous system excitability. • Stop hyperinflation if serious hypotension or bradycardia is observed. • Be knowledgeable about oxygen delivery performance of resuscitation bag or device used (oxygen delivery varies with different types). If the Fio_2 is increased on the ventilator, keep in mind that a variable lag time will elapse before the patient receives the increased oxygen concentration because of the "washout" time of the ventilator. • Keep patient on the ventilator during atrial pressure measurements. • Consider use of an adapter that allows the patient to remain on the ventilator during suctioning. 　NOTE: May produce smaller decreases in Pao_2 than does suctioning when the ventilator is removed. This method may be preferred if patient is unresponsive to increased oxygen concentrations because of large pulmonary shunts.
	Ventilator performance during suctioning is a critical factor in determining whether suctioning through an adapter in a closed airway can be done safely. If suctioning is performed in a closed airway system and suction flow exceeds volume of gas supplied by the ventilator, negative airway pressure can reduce lung volume and cause alveolar collapse and arterial desaturation.	• Be alert to potential complications of hypoxemia during closed airway suctioning related to suction flow exceeding gas delivery by the ventilator. Discontinue method.
	Receptors for the vagus nerve are found throughout the tracheobronchial tree, to the level of the carina. Stimulation of this nerve produces slowing of the heart rate. Mechanical ventilation increases intrathoracic pressures to Valsalva levels. The increased intrathoracic pressure that occurs during Valsalva's maneuver (coughing, vomiting, lifting, the act of defecating) causes rapid changes in preload and afterload. During strain, venous return to the heart is decreased and systolic and pulse pressures decrease. Paroxysms of coughing without taking a deep breath are Valsalva strains at high expiratory pressures.	• Monitor blood pressure and heart rate during suctioning procedure. Discontinue suctioning if significant decrease in blood pressure and heart rate occurs and ventilate patient. • Be alert to potential complications related to coughing against the obstruction of the suction catheter plus additional increased intrathoracic pressure if the closed airway system is in place. Monitor for slowing of heart rate, decreased blood pressure. • Remove the catheter from the trachea when the patient coughs. • If the closed airway suction system has been used, evaluate whether the problem is resolved by the method of removing patient from the ventilator and suctioning. Discontinue use of closed airway suction system.
Incorrect PEEP setting	**Patient-Related:** Unable to accurately read airway pressure gauge for determining PEEP setting because of patient's fast respiratory rate, irregular respiratory pattern or incomplete exhalations, or both.	• Adjust PEEP while the patient is on the ventilator unless difficulty arises in making accurate adjustments because of certain breathing patterns, which prevent accurate observation of the airway pressure needle. In this case, adjust PEEP by removing patient from ventilator, attaching test balloon to ventilator and adjusting PEEP. Obtain assistance of second person to support patient by manual resuscitation bag. • Reset sensitivity setting so that it is 2 or 3 cm H_2O less than the dialed-in PEEP value (step not necessary on some ventilators where the sensitivity automatically readjusts when PEEP is applied).

(continued)

Problem	Causes	Management
	Air leak in patient (cuff site) or ventilator system causing inability to maintain end-expiratory pressure. If air leak is corrected, the previously set PEEP value will register higher if PEEP was set while an air leak was present in the system.	• Evaluate and correct air leaks (see Low/No Exhaled Volume). • Recheck PEEP value after leak is corrected, readjust PEEP as necessary.
	Ventilator-Related: PEEP incorrectly set on machine.	• Assess whether PEEP is correctly set. Reset as necessary.
	Ventilator sensitivity setting is set so that the machine self cycles; the airway pressure needle may rest at a positive value, which results in a false appearance of PEEP.	• Set sensitivity dial so that it is 2 or 3 cm H_2O less than the dialed-in PEEP value. • Rule out the possibility of machine self-cycling by decreasing sensitivity temporarily to -2 cm H_2O (or significantly less than the PEEP setting, if on higher levels) and noting whether the respiratory rate decreases or the prescribed PEEP value registers on the airway pressure gauge. Correct air leaks.
	If air leaks develop in the ventilator system or cuff, ventilator self-cycling occurs because of loss of PEEP with a machine sensitivity setting at a positive value.	• Be suspicious of machine self-cycling if the patient does not appear to be generating muscle activity to assist or is obviously not assisting (effects of drugs) despite high respiratory rate. • Prevent air leaks, which may lead to loss of PEEP and machine self-cycling.
Pneumothorax/tension pneumothorax	Defective PEEP value or regulator.	• Change PEEP valves. Notify respiratory therapy of problem maintaining desired PEEP level.
	Patient-Related: Underlying lung pathology (COPD, emphysematous blebs, lung surgery), which makes some persons more susceptible to the effects of positive pressure.	
	Ventilator-Related: Positive pressure created by ventilator, which causes pulmonary barotrauma. High-volume or high-pressure settings, PEEP.	• Use PEEP only as necessary. • Maintain minimal PEEP levels necessary for adequate oxygenation. • Try ventilator modes with low mean airway pressure levels to decrease mean intrathoracic pressure. • Monitor for signs, symptoms of pneumothorax, tension pneumothorax. Notify physician of abnormalities. • If symptoms are mild, obtain chest x-ray film and notify physician immediately. • If tension pneumothorax occurs: —disconnect patient from ventilator and ventilate with manual resuscitation bag —increase FiO_2 to 1.0 —have someone else notify physician immediately, prepare chest tube insertion equipment for immediate use and set up chest drainage unit —have a large-bore needle ready for insertion as a life-saving maneuver for tension pneumothorax. NOTE: Needle thoracentesis is performed using a medium or large-bore needle, which is inserted into the affected hemithorax anteriorly through the second or third interspace in the midclavicular line. The needle should pass through the middle of the interspace to avoid intercostal blood vessels. • Reassure, remain with the patient. • Obtain chest x-ray film. • Monitor arterial blood gases every one to two hours until stable.
Inability to tolerate IMV mode	**Patient-Related:** Increased work of breathing from various physiologic factors that increase airway resistance, decrease lung	• Support on ventilator mode which provides patient comfort.

Problem	Causes	Management
	compliance, decrease respiratory muscle strength, endurance or alter mechanics of breathing, includes: • Secretions, infection	• Suction airway as necessary. Provide call light so that capable patient can inform of need. • Provide medications as ordered for management of respiratory infection.
	• Narrowed airway because of endotracheal tube. (Airway resistance has been reported to increase three-fold and the work of breathing almost twofold by size 7 to 9 mm endotracheal tubes. Even a 9 mm tube increased work of breathing 77.6 percent above baseline.)	• Consider endotracheal tube diameter as one of the factors which may increase airway resistance and work of breathing. • Change to different mode of ventilation or add pressure support if it provides breathing comfort. • Use t-tube method for weaning from the ventilator when physiologically stable. Suggest extubation after a short t-tube trial (20 to 30 minutes) or some patients may not need t-tube trial.
	• Bronchospasm. • Certain positions which provide less than optimal ventilation-perfusion matching. • Acute or chronic lung disorder, or both.	• Evaluate, treat bronchospasm. • Place in positions that maximize ventilation and breathing comfort (usually with head of bed elevated). • Evaluate whether the patient is physiologically stable enough to be on partial ventilator support.
	• Inadequate IMV rate or volume to maintain adequate ventilation for the patient under effects of narcotics and anesthetics. • Decreased respiratory muscle strength and endurance from effects of malnutrition.	• Provide necessary ventilator support for goals of breathing comfort, ability to rest and sleep, and maintain normal ventilation, oxygenation. May try increasing rate or volume, or both, if settings are low, otherwise switch to assist/control mode, particularly if patient is not tolerating IMV mode.
	Increased carbon dioxide production resulting from the use of TPN regimens containing carbohydrate (glucose) concentrations. Increased respiratory rate and ventilation may be observed as a result of the increased carbon dioxide production. (See Respiratory Acidosis.)	• Observe for TPN-induced hypercapnic acidosis in patients with chronic lung disease or marginal ventilatory reserve who are on partial ventilatory support (for example, IMV, CPAP, pressure support). • Discuss observations with physician so that changes can be made to limit glucose infusion and substitute fats for a portion of energy. • Provide optimum ventilator support by placing on assist/control mode. • Support patient on the ventilatory mode, which provides respiratory comfort, usually assist/control mode. • Thoroughly assess and correct any physiologic and equipment factors interfering with success. • Wean only as tolerated using t-tube method. Abide by proper procedure, which includes suctioning as necessary, optimum positioning, close monitoring and provision of a reassuring, confident and consistent approach. Provide ventilator support as necessary to avoid physiologic decompensation and deterioration of patient trust and confidence.
	Ventilator-Related: Various equipment factors can significantly increase resistance and work of breathing, which cause various signs and symptoms of respiratory distress. These include resistance in the IMV demand valve, or system, and in the ventilator breathing circuit. A significant increase in resistance results if the flow rate delivered by the IMV apparatus is lower than the patient's spontaneous inspiratory flow rate or if the demand valve requires significant airway pressure deflection to initiate air flow during spontaneous breathing. Resistance varies in the various ventilator breathing circuits. Persons with COPD are at high risk for development of inspiratory muscle fatigue	• Become knowledgeable about the particular IMV system in use, including specific capabilities, limitations, correct setup, and usual problems. • If patient develops respiratory distress after placement on IMV mode, switch to assist/control mode (or previous mode of respiratory comfort). Notify respiratory therapy for problem identification and management.

(continued)

Problem	Causes	Management
	which may precipitate acute respiratory failure. Weaning failures may be the result of improper use of the IMV method, which can unnecessarily prolong the length of time that patients spend on the ventilator. Delay of the weaning process and extubation may also occur due to gradual reduction in ventilatory rate.	
	Deleterious effects on hemodynamic status may occur when patients with poor left ventricular reserve are changed from controlled mechanical ventilation to IMV. Oxygen consumption can increase significantly at lower IMV rate.	• Monitor for deleterious effects of partial ventilator support on hemodynamic status, particularly in some patients, such as those in cardiogenic shock, whose clinical status requires a low oxygen consumption.
	Myocardial ischemia has been shown to occur more often on CPAP versus full ventilator support. Mechanical ventilator support may be beneficial to the failing heart in several ways: optimizes left ventricular end-diastolic volume (increases intrapleural pressure which decreases right heart preload; increased airway pressure may restrict left ventricular filling); in clinical states of compromised oxygen delivery (cardiogenic shock), full ventilatory support may decrease inspiratory oxygen demands and release oxygen for use by other systems; patients can be safely sedated and sympathetic outflow is decreased, which prevents hypertension and tachycardia thereby decreasing left ventricular strain.	• In the presence of cardiogenic shock, provide optimum ventilator support to decrease inspiratory oxygen demands.
	Kinked tubing, obstruction of tubing with water.	• Drape tubing to avoid kinks and optimum drainage of water into water traps. Empty water from tubing every two to four hours.
	Setting incorrectly calculated, set on machine.	• Evaluate whether IMV settings are correctly dialed on ventilator. Correct errors or notify respiratory therapy as necessary.
	Inappropriate inspiratory time or flow rate setting.	• Evaluate for appropriate inspiratory time or peak flow setting by observing speed of chest expansion on positive pressure breaths. (Rapid rise of the chest and airway pressure needle may be indicators that the inspiratory time is too short or peak flow too fast.) Notify respiratory therapy or make appropriate inspiratory time or peak flow adjustments.
	Incorrect assembly of IMV setup, malfunctioning IMV valve which creates additional resistance.	• Switch to assist/control mode or settings that provide optimum ventilation, oxygenation, and breathing comfort or ventilate patient using manual resuscitation bag if unfamiliar with machine settings. Notify respiratory therapy for correction of problem.
	Not receiving prescribed TV because of air leaks in ventilator system or cuff.	• Check whether machine is delivering prescribed positive pressure breaths by observing digital display on some ventilators or by switching to assist/control mode and evaluating volume delivery on other ventilators (see Low/No Exhaled TV).
	Some IMV systems are not synchronized with the patient's inspiratory efforts (i.e., the machine breaths are initiated at any point during the respiratory cycle). Asynchrony may create feelings of discomfort and frustration, especially with higher IMV rates. Stacking of breaths may increase intrapleural pressure, cause overdistension of alveoli and barotrauma.	• Switch to assist/control mode as necessary. If ready for weaning, use t-tube method, extubate.

Adapted from: Grossbach I: Trouble shooting ventilator and patient-related problems/parts I and II. Critical Care Nurse. *1989;6(4&5):58–70,64–78.*

Cardiac Rhythms, ECG Characteristics and Treatment Guide

(continued)

Rhythm	ECG Characteristics	ECG Sample	Treatment
Normal sinus rhythm (NSR)	• Rate: 60 to 100 beats/minute • Rhythm: Regular • P waves: Precede every QRS; consistent shape • PR interval: 0.12 to 0.20 second • QRS complex: 0.04 to 0.10 second	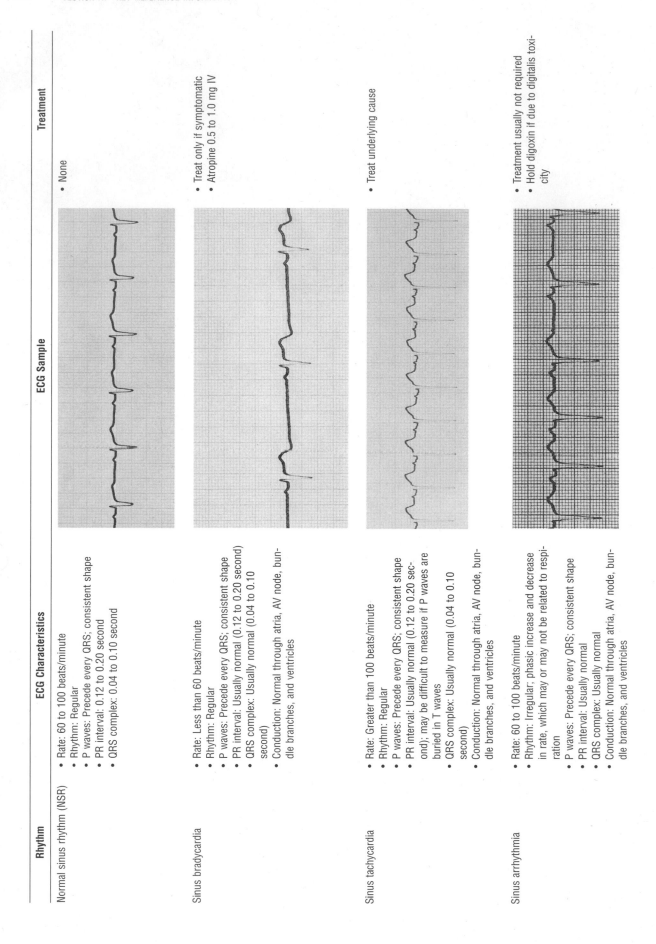	• None
Sinus bradycardia	• Rate: Less than 60 beats/minute • Rhythm: Regular • P waves: Precede every QRS; consistent shape • PR interval: Usually normal (0.12 to 0.20 second) • QRS complex: Usually normal (0.04 to 0.10 second) • Conduction: Normal through atria, AV node, bundle branches, and ventricles		• Treat only if symptomatic • Atropine 0.5 to 1.0 mg IV
Sinus tachycardia	• Rate: Greater than 100 beats/minute • Rhythm: Regular • P waves: Precede every QRS; consistent shape • PR interval: Usually normal (0.12 to 0.20 second); may be difficult to measure if P waves are buried in T waves • QRS complex: Usually normal (0.04 to 0.10 second) • Conduction: Normal through atria, AV node, bundle branches, and ventricles		• Treat underlying cause
Sinus arrhythmia	• Rate: 60 to 100 beats/minute • Rhythm: Irregular; phasic increase and decrease in rate, which may or may not be related to respiration • P waves: Precede every QRS; consistent shape • PR interval: Usually normal • QRS complex: Usually normal • Conduction: Normal through atria, AV node, bundle branches, and ventricles		• Treatment usually not required • Hold digoxin if due to digitalis toxicity

Sinus arrest

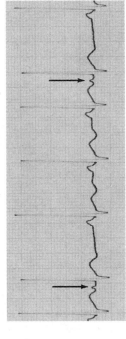

- Rate: Usually within normal range, but may be in the bradycardia range
- Rhythm: Irregular due to absence of sinus node discharge
- P waves: Present when sinus node is firing and absent during periods of sinus arrest. When present, they precede every QRS complex and are consistent in shape.
- PR interval: Usually normal when P waves are present
- QRS complex: Usually normal when sinus node is functioning and absent during periods of sinus arrest, unless escape beats occur
- Conduction: Normal through atria, AV node, bundle branches, and ventricles when sinus node is firing. When the sinus node fails to form impulses, there is no conduction through the atria.

Treatment:
- Treat underlying cause
- Discontinue drugs that may be causative
- Minimize vagal stimulation
- For frequent sinus arrest causing hemodynamic compromise, atropine 0.5 to 1.0 mg IV may increase heart rate
- Pacemaker may be necessary for refractory cases

Premature atrial contraction

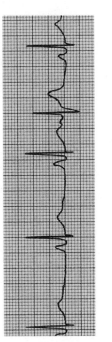

- Rate: Usually within normal range
- Rhythm: Usually regular except when PACs occur, resulting in early beats. PACs usually have a noncompensatory pause.
- P waves: Precede every QRS. The configuration of the premature P wave differs from that of the sinus P waves.
- PR interval: May be normal or long depending on the prematurity of the beat. Very early PACs may find the AV junction still partially refractory and unable to conduct at a normal rate, resulting in a prolonged PR interval.
- QRS complex: May be normal, aberrant (wide), or absent, depending on the prematurity of the beat
- Conduction: PACs travel through the atria differently from sinus impulses because they originate from a different spot. Conduction through the AV node, bundle branches, and ventricles is usually normal unless the PAC is very early.

Treatment:
- Treatment usually not necessary
- Treat underlying cause
- Drugs (e.g. quinidine, disopyramide, procainamide) can be used if necessary

Wandering atrial pacemaker

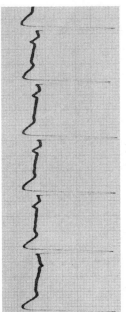

- Rate: 60 to 100 beats/minute. If the rate is faster than 100 beats/minute, it is called multifocal atrial tachycardia (MAT).
- Rhythm: May be slightly irregular
- P waves: Varying shapes (upright, flat, inverted, notched) as impulses originate in different parts of the atria or junction. At least three different P-wave shapes should be seen.
- PR interval: May vary depending on proximity of the pacemaker to the AV node

Treatment:
- Treatment usually not necessary
- Treat underlying cause
- For symptoms from slow rate can use atropine
- With rate >100, drugs to decrease atrial ectopy (e.g., quinidine) and/or slow ventricular rate (e.g., verapamil, propranolol) may be necessary

(continued)

Rhythm	ECG Characteristics	ECG Sample	Treatment
Atrial tachycardia	• QRS complex: Usually normal • Conduction: Conduction through the atria varies as they are depolarized from different spots. Conduction through the bundle branches and ventricles is usually normal. • Rate: Atrial rate is 150 to 250 beats/minute. • Rhythm: Regular unless there is variable block at the AV node • P waves: Differ in shape from sinus P waves because they are ectopic. Precede each QRS complex but may be hidden in preceding T wave. When block is present, more than one P wave will appear before each QRS complex. • PR interval: May be shorter than normal but often difficult to measure because of hidden P waves • QRS complex: Usually normal but may be wide if aberrant conduction is present • Conduction: Usually normal through the AV node and into the ventricles. In atrial tachycardia with block some atrial impulses do not conduct into the ventricles. Aberrant ventricular conduction may occur if atrial impulses are conducted into the ventricles while the ventricles are still partially refractory.	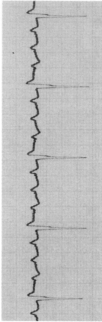	• Eliminate underlying cause and decrease ventricular rate • Sedation • Vagal stimulation • Vasopressors • Digitalis (unless it is the cause of atrial tachycardia with block) • Propranolol, verapamil, or diltiazem • Cardioversion for significant symptoms • Quinidine to prevent recurrences
Atrial flutter	• Rate: Atrial rate varies between 250 to 350 beats/minute, most commonly 300. Ventricular rate varies depending on the amount of block at the AV node, most commonly 150 beats/minute and rarely 300 beats/minute. • Rhythm: Atrial rhythm is regular. Ventricular rhythm may be regular or irregular due to varying AV block. • P waves: F waves (flutter waves) are seen, characterized by a very regular, "sawtooth" pattern. One F wave is usually hidden in the QRS complex, and when 2:1 conduction occurs, F waves may not be readily apparent. • FR interval (flutter wave to the beginning of the QRS complex): May be consistent or may vary • QRS complex: Usually normal; aberration can occur • Conduction: Usually normal through the AV node and ventricles	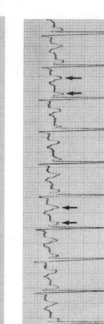	• Treatment depends on hemodynamic consequences of arrhythmia • Cardioversion for markedly reduced cardiac output • Verapamil, diltiazem, or propranolol to slow ventricular rate • Quinidine or procainamide ONLY after prior treatment to ensure adequate AV block

(continued)

(continued)

Atrial fibrillation

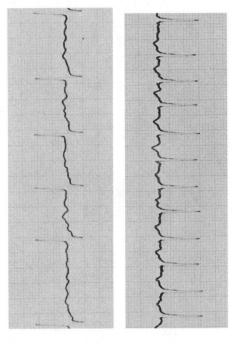

- Rate: Atrial rate is 400 to 600 beats/minute or faster. Ventricular rate varies depending on the amount of block at the AV node. In new atrial fibrillation, the ventricular response is usually quite rapid, 160 to 200 beats/minute; in treated atrial fibrillation, the ventricular rate is controlled in the normal range of 60 to 100 beats/minute.
- Rhythm: Irregular. One of the distinguishing features of atrial fibrillation is the marked irregularity of the ventricular response.
- P waves: Not present. Atrial activity is chaotic with no formed atrial impulses visible. Irregular f waves are often seen and vary in size from coarse to very fine.
- PR interval: Not measurable since there are no P waves
- QRS complex: Usually normal; aberration is common
- Conduction: Conduction within the atria is disorganized and follows a very irregular pattern. Most of the atrial impulses are blocked within the AV junction. Those impulses that are conducted through the AV junction are usually conducted normally through the ventricles. If an atrial impulse reaches the bundle branch system during its refractory period, aberrant intraventricular conduction can occur.

- Eliminate underlying cause, decrease atrial irritability, and decrease ventricular rate
- Digitalis, verapamil, diltiazem, or propranolol to decrease ventricular rate
- Quinidine, procainamide, flecainide, or amiodarone to decrease atrial irritability
- Cardioversion for hemodynamic instability

Premature junctional complexes

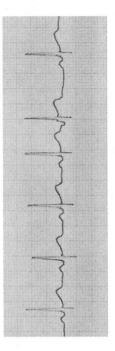

- Rate: 60 to 100 beats/minute or whatever the rate of the basic rhythm
- Rhythm: Regular except for occurrence of premature beats
- P waves: May occur before, during, or after the QRS complex of the premature beat and are usually inverted
- PR interval: Short, usually 0.10 second or less, when P waves precede the QRS
- QRS complex: Usually normal but may be aberrant if the PJC occurs very early and conducts into the ventricles during the refractory period of a bundle branch
- Conduction: Retrograde through the atria; usually normal through the ventricles

- Treatment usually not necessary
- Quinidine or procainamide sometimes used

Rhythm	ECG Sample	ECG Characteristics	Treatment
Junctional rhythm	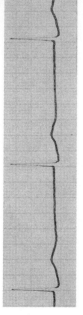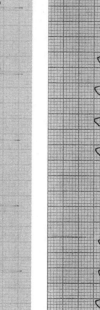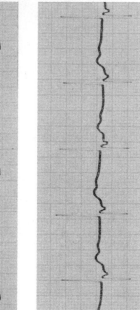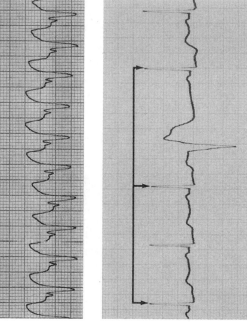	• Rate: Junctional rhythm, 40 to 60 beats/minute; accelerated junctional rhythm, 60 to 100 beats/minute; junctional tachycardia, 100 to 250 beats/minute • Rhythm: Regular • P waves: May precede or follow QRS • PR interval: Short, 0.11 second or less if P waves precede QRS • QRS complex: Usually normal • Conduction: Retrograde through the atria; normal through the ventricles	• Treatment rarely needed unless rate too slow or too fast to maintain adequate cardiac output • Atropine used to increase rate • Verapamil, propranalol, quinidine, or digitalis used to decrease rate • Cardioversion for rapid rate with severely reduced cardiac output • Withhold digitalis if digitalis toxicity suspected
Premature ventricular complexes		• Rate: 60 to 100 beats/minute or the rate of the basic rhythm • Rhythm: Irregular because of the PVCs • P waves: Not related to the PVCs. Sinus rhythm is usually not interrupted by the premature beats, so sinus P waves can often be seen occurring regularly throughout the rhythm. • PR interval: Not present before most PVCs. If a P wave happens, by coincidence, to precede a PVC, the PR interval is short. • QRS complex: Wide and bizarre; greater than 0.10 second in duration. May vary in morphology (size, shape) if they originate from more than one focus in the ventricles. • Conduction: Wide QRS complexes. Some PVCs may conduct retrograde into the atria, resulting in inverted P waves following the PVC.	• Eliminate underlying cause • Acute treatment with lidocaine, procainamide, or bretylium IV • Disopyramide, quinidine, propranolol, amiodarone, tocainide, mexiletine, or sotalol for long-term control

(continued)

(continued)

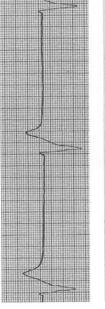
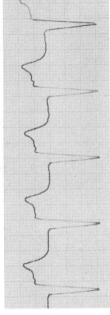

Ventricular rhythm

- Rate: Less than 50 beats/minute for ventricular rhythm and 50 to 100 beats/minute for accelerated ventricular rhythm
- Rhythm: Usually regular
- P waves: May be seen but at a slower rate than the ventricular focus, with dissociation from the QRS
- PR interval: Not measured
- QRS complex: Wide and bizarre
- Conduction: If sinus rhythm is the basic rhythm, atrial conduction is normal. Impulses originating in the ventricles conduct via muscle cell-to-cell conduction, resulting in the wide QRS complex.

- Treatment of accelerated ventricular rhythm only if symptomatic (e.g., with suppressive therapy as for VT)
- For ventricular escape rhythms, increase rate or use temporary pacemaker

Ventricular tachycardia

- Rate: Ventricular rate is faster than 100 beats/minute.
- Rhythm: Usually regular but may be slightly irregular
- P waves: P waves may be seen but will not be related to QRS complexes (dissociated from QRS complexes). If sinus rhythm is the underlying basic rhythm, regular. P waves are often buried within QRS complexes
- PR interval: Not measurable because of dissociation of P waves from QRS complexes
- QRS complex: Wide and bizarre; greater than 0.10 second in duration
- Conduction: Impulse originates in one ventricle and spreads via muscle cell-to-cell conduction through both ventricles. There may be retrograde conduction through the atria, but more often the sinus node continues to fire regularly and depolarize the atria normally.

- Treatment depends on how rhythm is tolerated
- Lidocaine, procainamide, bretylium, or magnesium sulfate for patients without severe symptoms
- Cardioversion preferred (defibrillation OK) for severely symptomatic VT
- CPR required for pulseless VT
- Prevent recurrences with drugs used for PVCs

Ventricular fibrillation

- Rate: Rapid, uncoordinated, ineffective
- Rhythm: Chaotic, irregular
- P waves: None seen
- PR interval: None
- QRS complex: No formed QRS complexes seen; rapid, irregular undulations without any specific pattern
- Conduction: Multiple ectopic foci firing simultaneously in ventricles and depolarizing them irregularly and without any organized pattern. Ventricles are not contracting.

- Immediate defibrillation
- CPR required until defibrillator available
- Lidocaine, procainamide, magnesium sulfate, or bretylium commonly used adjuncts
- Epinephrine used to convert fine VF to coarser VF
- After conversion of rhythm, use IV antiarrhythmics to prevent recurrence

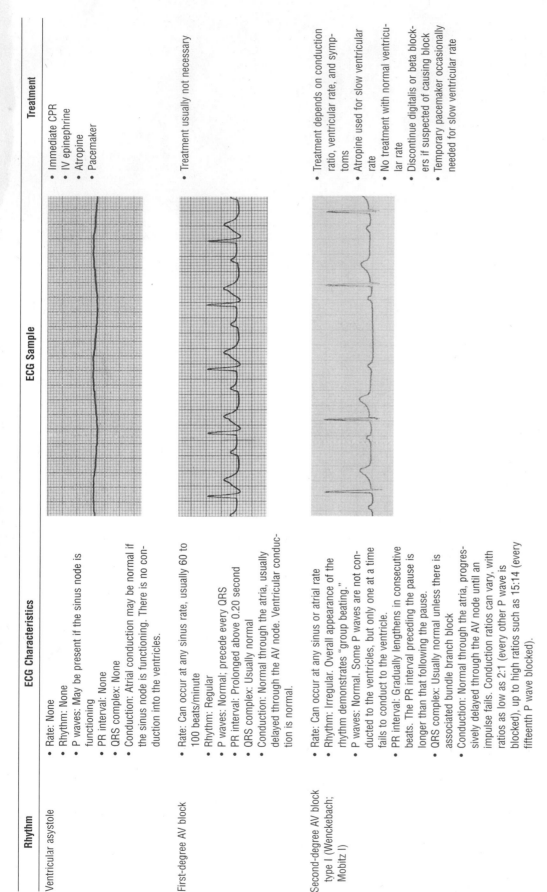

Rhythm	ECG Characteristics	ECG Sample	Treatment
Ventricular asystole	• Rate: None • Rhythm: None • P waves: May be present if the sinus node is functioning • PR interval: None • QRS complex: None • Conduction: Atrial conduction may be normal if the sinus node is functioning. There is no conduction into the ventricles.		• Immediate CPR • IV epinephrine • Atropine • Pacemaker
First-degree AV block	• Rate: Can occur at any sinus rate, usually 60 to 100 beats/minute • Rhythm: Regular • P waves: Normal; precede every QRS • PR interval: Prolonged above 0.20 second • QRS complex: Usually normal • Conduction: Normal through the atria, usually delayed through the AV node. Ventricular conduction is normal.		• Treatment usually not necessary
Second-degree AV block type I (Wenckebach; Mobitz I)	• Rate: Can occur at any sinus or atrial rate • Rhythm: Irregular. Overall appearance of the rhythm demonstrates "group beating." • P waves: Normal. Some P waves are not conducted to the ventricles, but only one at a time fails to conduct to the ventricle. • PR interval: Gradually lengthens in consecutive beats. The PR interval preceding the pause is longer than that following the pause. • QRS complex: Usually normal unless there is associated bundle branch block • Conduction: Normal through the atria, progressively delayed through the AV node until an impulse fails. Conduction ratios can vary, with ratios as low as 2:1 (every other P wave is blocked), up to high ratios such as 15:14 (every fifteenth P wave blocked).		• Treatment depends on conduction ratio, ventricular rate, and symptoms • Atropine used for slow ventricular rate • No treatment with normal ventricular rate • Discontinue digitalis or beta blockers if suspected of causing block • Temporary pacemaker occasionally needed for slow ventricular rate
Second-degree AV block type II (Mobitz II)	• Rate: Can occur at any basic rate • Rhythm: Irregular due to blocked beats • P waves: Usually regular and precede each QRS. Periodically a P wave is not followed by a QRS complex. • PR interval: Constant before conducted beats. The PR interval preceding the pause is the same as that following the pause.		• Pacemaker usually needed • CPR for slow rate and severely decreased cardiac output • Atropine

(continued)

(continued)

- QRS complex: Usually wide due to associated bundle branch block
- Conduction: Normal through the atria and through the AV node but intermittently blocked in the bundle branch system and fails to reach the ventricles. Conduction through the ventricles is abnormally slow due to associated bundle branch block. Conduction ratios can vary from 2:1 to only occasional blocked beats.

- Treatment necessary if patient symptomatic
- Atropine may increase ventricular rate
- Pacemaker may be required

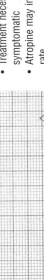

High AV block

- Rate: Atrial rate less than 135 beats/minute
- Rhythm: Regular or irregular, depending on conduction pattern
- P waves: Normal; present before every conducted QRS, but two or more consecutive P waves may not be followed by QRS complexes
- PR interval: Constant before conducted beats; may be normal or prolonged
- QRS complex: Usually normal in type I and wide in type II advanced blocks
- Conduction: Normal through the atria. Two or more consecutive atrial impulses fail to conduct to the ventricles. Ventricular conduction is normal in type I and abnormally slow in type II advanced blocks.

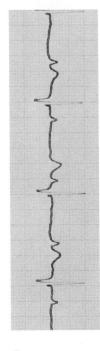

- Pacemaker
- Atropine usually not effective
- With severely decreased cardiac output, perform CPR until pacemaker available

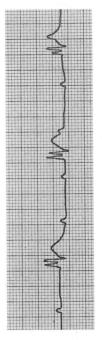

Third-degree AV block

- Rate: Atrial rate is usually normal; ventricular rate is less than 45 beats/minute.
- Rhythm: Regular
- P waves: Normal but dissociated from CRS complexes
- PR interval: No consistent PR intervals because there is no relationship between P waves and QRS complexes
- QRS complex: Normal if ventricles controlled by a junctional rhythm; wide if controlled by a ventricular rhythm
- Conduction: Normal through the atria. All impulses are blocked at the AV node or in the bundle branches, so there is no conduct on to the ventricles. Conduction through the ventricles is normal if a junctional escape rhythm occurs, and abnormally slow if a ventricular escape rhythm occurs.

Rhythm	ECG Characteristics	ECG Sample	Treatment
Ventricular paced rhythm with capture	• Rate: Depends on type of pacemaker • Rhythm: Regular • P waves: Absent, or present but dissociated from QRS complexes • PR interval: None • QRS complex: Pacemaker spike followed immediately by wide, bizarre QRS complex		• None
Ventricular paced rhythm without capture	• Conduction: Abnormal • ECG characteristics depend on nature of intrinsic rhythm • Pacemaker spike has no fixed relationship to QRS complexes		• If hemodynamically stable, elective correction/replacement of pacemaker • If hemodynamically unstable, treatment as for third-degree AV block

■ Index